MW01362724

Your Career in

Physical Medicine

Roberta C. Weiss, LVN, Ed.D.

Allied Health Curriculum Specialist
Vocational and Staff Development Educator

Your Career in Physical Medicine

SAUNDERS

An Imprint of Elsevier

SAUNDERS
An Imprint of Elsevier
The Curtis Center
Independence Square West
Philadelphia, PA 19106

Library of Congress Cataloging-in-Publication Data

Weiss, Roberta C.
Your career in physical medicine / Roberta C. Weiss. — 1st ed.
p. cm.
ISBN-13: 978-0-7216-6453-8 ISBN-10: 0-7216-6453-9
1. Medicine, Physical—Vocational guidance. I. Title.
[DNLM: 1. Physical Medicine. 2. Physical Therapy. 3. Career Choice. 4. Allied Health Personnel. 5. Sports Medicine. WB 460 W432ya 1997]
RM705.W45 1997
617'.03—dc21
DNLM/DLC 97-10170

YOUR CAREER IN PHYSICAL MEDICINE

ISBN-13: 978-0-7216-6453-8
ISBN-10: 0-7216-6453-9

Printed in the United States of America

Last digit is the print number: 9 8 7

This book is lovingly dedicated to Martha and Harry Friedman,

two very special people in my life, for all of their love and support while I worked on this project.

Preface

With all of the major technological break-throughs, the ever-changing and increasing costs in medical care, and the constant need to fill new positions in all health-related disciplines, the delivery of health care, as we once knew it, no longer exists. Instead, we are rushing to meet the demands of a society whose members, because they live longer, are in greater need to be cared for by professionals who have been trained in a number of occupations within the same educational discipline. According to the United States Department of Labor, if trends continue the way they seem to be moving, health care will continue to be one of the fastest growing industries in our economy. Employment in health-related occupations is projected to grow from 8.9 million in 1994, to 12.8 million by the end of the twentieth century. Most employers agree that persons trained in more than one occupation will have the greatest opportunity to fill these millions of jobs.

Your Career in Physical Medicine is a textbook based on the concept of training a professional in more than one occupation within the same health care discipline. It is written in simple comprehensive language, and is accompanied by photographs and basic illustrations that have been created to provide the reader with a well-rounded introduction to the principles and techniques involved in the various allied health occupations in the field of physical medicine.

This author and educator firmly believes that there are many adequate textbooks in use that provide information for the person interested either in advanced techniques in physical or rehabilitative medicine, or in one specific area of interest. However, only *Your Career in Physical Medicine* covers more than one occupation in that field.

The text consists of 31 chapters and covers concepts and hands-on skills and techniques involved in the study of basic health career opportunities, scientific principles and medical terminology, systems of health and healing, chiropractic assisting, massage therapy, physical therapy, sports medicine assisting, personal fitness training, and administrative and job-seeking skills for the physical medicine worker. To assist readers in their understanding of the subject matter, each chapter is also accompanied by performance objectives and terminology words at the beginning of the chapter, and a short summary of the material at the end of the chapter. In addition, to assist both the student and the instructor, the text is also accompanied by a *Teacher's Resource Package,* which covers such concepts as teaching methodologies and strategies, resources and references, clinical and classroom activities, and an in-depth glossary of medical terms used in the study of physical medicine.

Acknowledgments

I would like to extend my deepest gratitude and appreciation to all those who have assisted me in the preparation and development of this textbook, including: My very dear friend and colleague, Ms. Marla Keeth, LVN, Coordinator of the Health Careers Academy at Blair High School, Pasadena Unified School District/Los Angeles County Regional Occupational Programs, who acted as photographer, and who provided sustenance, in giving of her time by allowing her students to be photographed and worked with the actual patients and clients, for the preparation of this project; the highly professional health careers students enrolled in Blair High School's Health Careers Academy, for their time, expertise, and participation while being photographed and kept available for the many hours needed for the photo session for this text; Dr. Mark Anthony, D.C., Ceptembre-Joy Anthony, Massage Therapist, and Art Tedasco, for their time and expertise, and for the use of the Anthony Chiropractic Clinic; Curtis Beyer, Massage Therapist, and Betsy Raulerson, for their expertise, encouragement, and friendship, all of which were needed during the production of this textbook; the staff and clients of Professional Sports Care, for all their time and assistance in order to take photographs during actual work-out sessions; Debbie Ogilvie, for all her time and energy in bringing me and my "new" concept to the right person at Saunders; Peg Waltner, Developmental Editor, for her help and great patience while working with me during the many phases of producing this textbook; and finally, to Lisa Biello, for all of her guidance and inspiration, not only because she was willing to take a chance on something that had never been done before, but because of her genuine sense of kindness and concern for others.

Contents

Your Career in

Physical Medicine

Section

I

Introduction to Health Careers

1

Career Opportunities in Physical Medicine

Performance Objectives

Upon completion of this chapter, you will be able to:

1. Discuss career opportunities available in physical medicine.
2. Describe the training required at various levels of health care providers in the field of physical medicine.
3. Distinguish between divisions within health care facilities.
4. Discuss some of the desirable personal characteristics and technical skills required of a physical medicine worker.
5. Identify several potential duties of the physical medicine worker.
6. List potential employers of physical medicine workers.

Terms and Abbreviations

Diagnostic services services within a medical facility which deal with identifying pathological conditions or diseases.
Environmental services services within a medical facility which provide properly furnished facilities for safe use by patients and staff.
General services services within a medical facility which include admitting, feeding, and medicating patients and preserving records concerning both patients and medical personnel.
Patient care services services within a medical facility which manages the activities of daily living for patients.
Therapeutic services services within a medical facility which treats pathological conditions and diseases.

We give periods of time descriptive names in order to indicate what was important about that particular time. For example, when we speak of the Stone Age, we are referring to a time when humans had stone tools and simple survival skills. Now commentators are saying that we live in the Information Age. Computers and electronic technology make global transfer of data instantaneous. Thus, workers and employees in the health care industry must be versed in information systems for recording, storing, and retrieving data related to the health and wellness of those entrusted to their care. In addition to being skilled in the various clinical skills required of the physical medicine worker, as a health care provider you will also be expected to use various types of machines, equipment, computers, and information systems, since these are often necessary to interpret specific data and information.

History of Physical Medicine Health Care Services

Early in the twentieth century, the clinical or hands-on aspects of a medical practice were quite simple. A doctor performed all the procedures, clinical tests, and treatments on his or her own, or, in some cases, had only one assistant who helped in all aspects of the practice. More recently, clinical health care providers, in particular those associated with the administration of physical and rehabilitative procedures, have become a necessity in almost all health care facilities and in most private medical practices and clinics. As a result of the great changes made in health care technologies and the ever-increasing role of the physical medicine health care provider, the person trained in more than one of the physical and therapeutic disciplines and medical services continues to gain more and more authority, along with increased responsibility. There are now exciting possibilities for both variety and specialization in the workplace.

Careers in physical medicine are in many facets of the health care industry. Physical therapy, sports medicine and fitness training, chiropractic care, and massage therapy workers can all be found in small and large hospitals, multispecialty clinics and outpatient centers, urgent care centers, private medical offices, private and nonprofit physical therapy centers, fitness centers, clinical trials companies, and health insurance companies. These positions can also be found in skilled nursing facilities, board and care homes, and retirement hotels. Ambitious members of the physical medicine team may also choose to work for private health care registries, government agencies, and in some cases, their own business. All members of the physical medicine team are concerned with providing care and treatment to patients who need their services. This includes caring for patients suffering from disorders of the musculoskeletal and nervous systems, as well as others who may be debilitated from diseases affecting other body systems. The procedures you will provide to patients can range from something as basic as taking and recording a patient's blood pressure, temperature, pulse, and respiration to performing more advanced therapeutic treatments, such as assisting a paralyzed patient to walk again or providing therapeutic massage on an injured athlete. In addition to the skills which you will need to work with patients with weakened bones and muscles, you will also be expected to be knowledgeable and skilled in working with other members of the health care team. You will have to learn how to gain access to records about a patient's health and treatment, and at the same time, learn what you can and cannot do with those records.

Training and Education

No matter what aspect of physical medicine services you choose to work in, the fact that you have selected an occupation in the health care industry says a lot about you and your interest in helping others. Unfortunately, however, while many people wish to work in the health care industry, not all are cut out to do so. Only you can make that decision.

To be successful in your position, it's important to possess both the appropriate educational and technical skills, as well as interpersonal skills necessary to communicate effectively with others. In addition to being a compassionate person, you must also be dependable and punctual. You must be flexible and well organized. You should be able to work well under pressure, and take pride in both yourself and the job you are doing. You should not have so much pride that you are unable to accept positive criticism, and you must be able to follow rules and detailed instructions. Above all, you must like working with people, and when doing so, be tactful.

Most allied health occupations in the field of physical medicine do not require national licensing or certification in order to work in a specific position. However, all assistants and technicians working under the physical medicine umbrella must have a sense of understanding and comprehension. Therefore, as a member of this health care discipline, most employers require their workers to have a high school diploma or its equivalent. It goes without saying that to be successful in physical medicine you should also receive some advanced technical training in the field you plan to work in. This generally includes both didactic and theoretical training, as well as many hours of training in the hands-on operations of the medical equipment which you will work with. It also includes some comprehension and understanding of computer training and basic office machines, medical terminology, and a basic understanding of anatomy and physiology. Most workers receive this training as part of an overall educational program in a vocational or adult school, community college, or as part of a regional occupational program.

Physical Medicine Careers and Employment Opportunities

Health care facilities and private medical practices use many different names and titles for their physical medicine and rehabilitative workers. Doctors' offices and clinics often hire orthopedic and chiropractic assistants, physical therapy aides, and massage therapists to perform many of the therapeutic procedures required for their patients. Larger health care institutions often have job titles such as physical medicine technicians and rehabilitation technicians. No matter what your job title may be, there are certain tasks that are commonly required by all of these jobs. These include taking and recording vital signs, proper use of medical asepsis and body mechanics, understanding and being able to use the proper medical terminology and medical abbreviations as part of your charting, being able to determine the differences between the anatomical and physiological functions of patients, and having an understanding of such concepts as medical law and ethics, confidentiality, and preserving patients' rights.

During the normal workday, you will come in contact with a wide variety of people. In addition to dealing with the many kinds of patients and their individual problems and personalities, you will also interact with nursing staff, doctors and pharmacists, laboratory and radiology technicians, supervisors, housekeepers, hospital volunteers, and many other people who work as members of the hospital staff, as well as visitors seeking understanding and answers about their loved ones. You must always be prepared to communicate with surgeons, who may use very technical terms, as well as patients, some of whom may speak very little English. Such diversity in your work may at times create an environment filled with great rewards, while at other times may seem challenging and frustrating.

Employment Opportunities

Over the past several decades, employment opportunities for physical medicine workers have expanded far beyond the one-person clinical or medical assistant, who was only responsible for assisting the doctor and for such basic tasks as answering the telephone. Where a physician's office once offered the only jobs for someone interested in the field, today the options are much more extensive.

Medical care has never been more expensive or competitive. Insurance companies are not willing to pay for unnecessary procedures, so many different institutions are competing with one another to provide patient services. In today's economy, the health care institution and the private medical practice must run in a cost-efficient manner if they are to survive. Because of the escalating costs of health care and the great demand put on health care providers in today's ever-changing, highly technological health care world, there is an increased need to train people in more than one occupation within the same medical discipline.

Ten years ago, it was acceptable to hire one person to complete only one task. The employee, for example, who was hired to work as a physical therapy aide only worked as a physical therapy aide. Today, however, that same person might be expected to work in the rehabilitation therapy department as a massage therapist or orthopedic assistant, or in a fitness center as a sports medicine assistant or personal fitness trainer.

Today there are many different types of health care facilities and institutions which can be very rewarding places of employment for the physical medicine worker. These include general acute care hospitals, where patients are hospitalized for anywhere from one day to a few weeks; specialized hospitals, which have facilities that provide care for specific problems, such as spinal injury hospitals or facilities for chronic disorders; long-term care facilities, also known as convalescent hospitals, which concentrate on providing care to the elderly; and outpatient clinics, which generally house several doctors with varied specialties who combine their practice. Other types of facilities which may employ physical medicine workers include private physicians' practices, rehabilitation centers, health maintenance organizations, private fitness clubs, athletic teams, chiropractic offices, and home health care and rehabilitative care agencies.

In addition to working in a health care facility, the physical medicine worker may also seek employment within university medical schools, research centers, pharmaceutical and medical supplies companies, laboratories, insurance companies, and in some cases, even freelance self-employment.

Hospital Organization and Medical Specialties

If you choose to work in the hospital environment as a member of the physical medicine team, it is very important for you to understand how modern medical facilities function. These facilities must have a well organized chain of command that informs each employee who his or her immediate supervisor is. Such organization provides an efficient way for the facility to fulfill its mission and purpose.

An example of a hospital organization chart is shown in Table 1-1. Each service has specialized departments. These departments are determined by the type of service that is provided.

Medical Specialties

If you are working in the hospital or clinical environment, more than likely you will come into contact with many different medical specialties. A medical specialist is a physician who devotes him- or herself to a single branch of medical knowledge. You may find

Table 1-1
Organizational Chart of a Health Care Facility

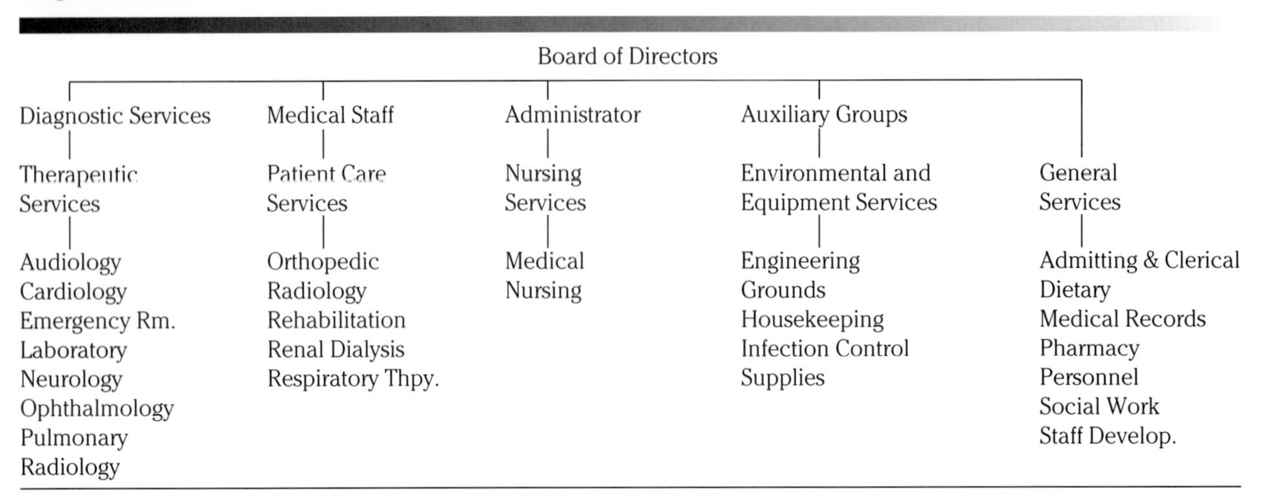

Table 1-2
Medical Specialties

Specialty	Name of Physician	Description of Specialty
Allergies	Allergist	Deals with diagnosis and treatment of body reactions resulting from sensitivity to foods, pollens, dust, medicine, or other substances
Anesthesiology	Anesthesiologist	Administers various forms of anesthesia in surgery or diagnosis to cause loss of feeling or sensation
Cardiology	Cardiologist	Deals with the diagnosis and treatment of diseases of the heart
Dermatology	Dermatologist	Deals with the diagnosis and treatment of diseases of the skin
Endocrinology	Endocrinologist	Deals with the diagnosis and treatment of diseases of the endocrine system and the hormones produced by the ductless glands
Family Practice	Family Practitioner	Diagnoses and treats diseases by medical and surgical methods for all members of the family
Gastroenterology	Gastroenterologist	Deals with the diagnosis and treatment of diseases of the digestive system
Gynecology	Gynecologist	Deals with the diagnosis and treatment of disorders of the female reproductive system
Internal Medicine	Internist	Diagnoses and treats diseases of adults
Neurology	Neurologist	Diagnoses and treats diseases of the nervous system and brain
Obstetrics	Obstetrician	Cares for women during pregnancy, childbirth, and the interval immediately following
Oncology	Oncologist	Diagnoses and treats cancer
Ophthalmology	Ophthalmologist	Diagnoses and treats disorders of the eye and prescribes glasses
Orthopedics	Orthopedist	Diagnoses and treats disorders of the muscular and skeletal systems
Otolaryngology	Otolaryngologist	Diagnoses and treats disorders of the eyes, ears, nose, and throat
Pathology	Pathologist	Studies and interprets changes in organs, tissues, cells, and changes in the body's chemistry to aid in diagnosing disease and determining the type of treatment which may be necessary
Pediatrics	Pediatrician	Deals with the prevention, diagnosis, and treatment of children's diseases
Proctology	Proctologist	Diagnoses and treats diseases of the rectum
Psychiatry	Psychiatrist	Diagnoses and treats mental disorders
Radiology	Radiologist	Uses radiant energy, including x-rays, radium, cobalt, etc., in the diagnosis of diseases
Urology	Urologist	Diagnoses and treats diseases of the kidneys, bladder, ureters, and urethra, and of the male reproductive system

yourself working in an area that deals often with one branch of medicine, such as physical therapy. Table 1-2 provides you with a list of the definitions of most of the present-day medical specialties and the names of the physicians practicing those specialties.

Summary

In this chapter, we discussed the very involved and rapidly changing field of physical medicine and the various occupations and workers involved in this very demanding yet highly rewarding branch of medicine. We determined that there are many varied career opportunities available to graduates of this field, both in private and public health care agencies and institutions, as well as for fitness centers, athletic teams, and insurance companies and preventative health care maintenance organizations. We also talked about some of the personal characteristics and technical skills which are necessary to be successful as a professional member of the physical medicine team, and defined the basic level of training for these occupations. Finally, we defined the various types of medical specialties and the name of each of the medical specialists involved in the many branches of medicine, noting that all of these are available to the physical medicine worker as a means to employment.

Review Questions

1. What is the name of the service provided for patients within a health care facility which is responsible for treating pathological conditions and diseases?
2. What is the name of the service provided for patients within a health care facility which is responsible for managing the activities of daily living for patients?
3. What is the name of the service provided for patients within a health care facility which is responsible for properly furnishing the facility for safe use by all patients and staff?
4. What is the name of the service provided for patients within a health care facility which is responsible for admitting, feeding, and medicating patients, and preserving records which concern both patients and medical personnel?
5. Give at least three examples of departments that would be found under diagnostic services:

   a. ____________

   b. ____________

   c. ____________
6. Give at least two examples of an auxiliary group working within a health care facility:

   a. ____________

   b. ____________
7. Under what service would the Pharmacy be found within a health care facility?
8. Under what service would Staff Nurses be found within a health care facility?
9. Under what service would the Physical Therapy department be found within a health care facility?

2

Health, Wellness, Fitness, and Illness

Performance Objectives

Upon completion of this chapter, you will be able to:

1. Define health, wellness, illness, and disease, and briefly explain the relationship of each to the other.
2. Briefly discuss nontraditional views of health and illness.
3. Compare the meaning of health, wellness, and fitness.
4. Identify and briefly discuss health beliefs and behaviors.
5. Identify and briefly discuss the five basic stages of illness.
6. Identify and briefly discuss the 11 sequential stages of illness.
7. Describe what is meant by sick role behavior.
8. Explain the effects illness has on family members.
9. Discuss the effects of hospitalization.
10. Identify patterns and trends which influence health and illness.
11. Explain the historical changes leading to a sedentary lifestyle.
12. Describe the importance of an organized program of exercise.

Terms and Abbreviations

Aerobic exercise exercise to improve the capacity of the heart and the lungs in order to deliver oxygen to the body during sustained activity.
Disease an alteration in the body's functions which results in a reduction of capacities or a shortening of the normal life span.
Fitness the state of being physically and mentally healthy and sound.
Health the state of complete physical, mental, and social well-being, and not merely the presence of disease or infirmity.
Health status the state or health of an individual at a given time.
Holistic health an approach to health care that considers the whole to be more than the sum of the parts.
Illness a highly personal state in which the individual feels unhealthy or ill.
Model or paradigm an abstract outline or a theoretical depiction of a complex phenomenon.
Wellness the active process through which an individual becomes aware of and makes choices that lead to a more successful existence.

Health is an ever-changing, evolving concept basic both to the study of medicine and to the delivery of administrative and hands-on care giving. For centuries, the concept of disease was the yardstick by which all health was measured, and it wasn't until as late as the nineteenth century that health care providers even began to deal with how the diseases occurred. More recently, there has been an increased emphasis on health.

There is no consensus regarding the definition of

health. There is knowledge about how one can attain a certain level of health, but health itself cannot be measured. According to the World Health Organization (WHO), *health* can be defined as a state of complete physical, mental, and social well-being, and not merely the absence of disease or infirmity. Because this definition was proposed during a time when many thousands of soldiers were returning home with their World War II injuries and traumas, many health care providers of the time thought this definition to be impractical. Today, however, some view it as a possible goal for all people, while others consider complete well-being unobtainable.

Because health is such a complex concept, much research has been completed regarding how it can be measured. Out of this research, specific *models* or *paradigms* were developed to explain health, and in some instances, its relationship to illness. The five models of health care delivery which are most widely accepted include the clinical model, the ecological model, the role performance model, the adaptive model, and the eudaimonistic model.

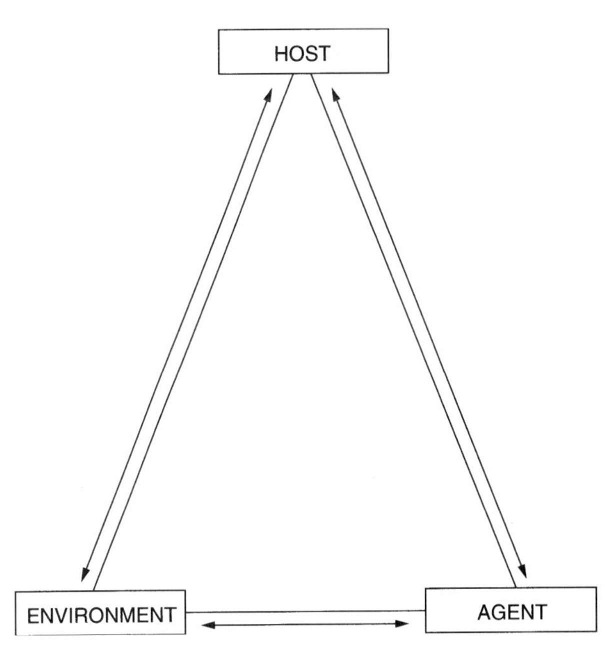

Figure 2-1
Ecological model of health care delivery. (Reprinted with permission from Weiss, R.C. *Your Career in Administrative Medical Services.* Philadelphia: W. B. Saunders, 1996, p. 10.)

Clinical Model of Health Care Delivery

The narrowest interpretation of health care delivery seems to be the clinical model. According to this model, all people are viewed as physiological systems with individual and related functions, and health is a concept used to identify the absence of signs and symptoms of disease or injury.

In the clinical model, disease is seen as the opposite of health and a relatively passive state of freedom from illness. The extreme of health, according to this model, is the absence of any signs or symptoms of disease, while the presence of such signs or symptoms is considered to indicate extreme illness. Today, the focus of many medical practices is to relieve the signs and symptoms of disease and thus eliminate the malfunction and pain of patients. When the signs and symptoms of the disease are no longer present in a person, the physician often considers that individual's health as being restored. These practitioners, therefore, base the care and treatment of their patients on the clinical model of health care delivery.

Ecological Model of Health Care Delivery

The ecological model of health care delivery is based upon the relationship of all humans to their internal and external environments. The model covers three concepts (Figure 2-1): the host, which is a person or group of people who may or may not be at risk of acquiring an illness or a disease; an agent, which can be any factor within either the internal or the external environment, that by its very presence or absence can lead to illness or disease; and the environment, either the internal or the external, which may or may not predispose the person to the development of a disease or illness.

Role Performance Model of Health Care Delivery

The role performance model of health care delivery adds the social and psychological implications and standards to the concept of health. In this concept of health care delivery, health is defined in terms of the person's ability to fulfill his or her role in society, that is, to be able to perform work. According to this model, people who can fulfill their roles are considered healthy even if they appear clinically ill. The emphasis of the delivery of health care, according to this model, therefore, should be placed upon a person's capacity rather than his or her commitment to roles and tasks.

Adaptive Model of Health Care Delivery

The focus on the adaptive model of health care delivery is based upon adaptation. According to this model, diseases are seen as the person's inability to adapt and the treatment is seen as an ability to restore the person to a state in which he or she can cope with illness or disease.

Eudaimonistic Model of Health Care Delivery

The eudaimonistic model of health care delivery incorporates the most comprehensive view of health. Health, according to this model, is seen as an actualization or realization of a person's total potential, and the highest aspiration of an individual is his or her fulfillment and complete development. Illness, according to this model, is seen as a condition or situation that prevents one from being able to self-actualize.

Developing a Personal Definition of Health

As you begin your journey into a career as a health care provider, you will soon realize that health is a highly individual perception. Meanings and descriptions of health vary considerably, and an individual's personal definition of health may not necessarily agree with that of health care professionals.

There are several factors that influence a personal definition of health. These include the developmental status of that person, social and cultural influences, previous experiences which may influence a person's perception of health, and one's self-expectations.

Wellness, Disease, Illness, and Fitness

The concept of wellness has received increasing attention in recent years. Some people believe that wellness and health are the same, while others believe that the two differ. In one respect, wellness is very similar to self-actualization as it is defined by the eudaimonistic model of health care delivery; it can only exist as a relatively passive state of freedom from illness in which the individual is at peace with his or her environment.

Wellness can be defined as an active process through which an individual becomes completely aware of choices that can lead to a more successful existence. These choices are influenced by the person's self-concept, his or her culture, and the environment. Wellness, therefore, is seen through a continuum whose extremes are total wellness and premature death (Figure 2-2).

Disease and Illness

Disease is a medical term which is used to describe any alteration in a person's body functions which results in a reduction of his or her capacities or a shortening of the normal life span. Intervention by physicians has always been the goal of eliminating or decreasing the disease process. Primitive people thought that disease was caused by outside forces or spirits. Later on, however, this belief was replaced by the single-cause theory. Increasingly, a number of factors are considered to interact in causing disease and determining a person's response to a given treatment.

Illness, while it may or may not be related to disease, differs from it in that it is defined as a highly personal state in which a person feels unhealthy or ill. Someone who feels pain or nausea tends to modify his or her behavior in some way and thus may consider him- or herself ill. An individual could have a disease—for example, a growth in the intestine—and not feel ill. According to researchers in the theory of illness and disease, for a person to feel ill, the physician must be able to determine if that person meets three distinct criteria. First, there must be a presence of symptoms, such as an elevated temperature or pain. Second, the perceptions of the illness must be describable by the person, for example, good, bad, or sick. Third, the ability to carry out daily activities, such as a job or schoolwork, must be affected.

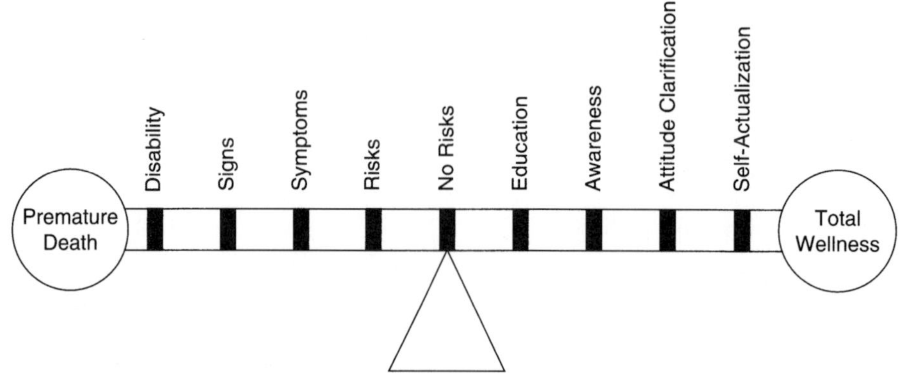

Figure 2-2
Continuum between total wellness and premature death. (Reprinted with permission from Weiss, R.C. *Your Career in Administrative Medical Services.* Philadelphia: W. B. Saunders, 1996, p. 11.)

Relationship of Health, Illness, and Disease

Health and Illness

One's state of health or illness can be considered either as points along one continuum, as related but separate entities, or as completely separate entities. A continuum of well-being, or health, is a grid or graduated scale in which peak wellness is at one end and death is at the other. Such a continuum accommodates a wide range of normal health, which reflects the fact that no one ever attains perfect health and not everyone becomes sick.

Illness and Disease

Traditionally, health care providers have dealt with diseases at a subsystem level. Subsystems are those aspects of the human body which are subsumed by the larger system of the whole body. A subsystem, for example, may be a cell, an organ, or an organ system. Only recently have medical practitioners started looking at a person as an entity or as a whole being. Health care providers, such as those employed in physical medicine, by contrast, have traditionally viewed the person as an entity, meaning that they have viewed the patient from a holistic point of view. Physical medicine providers today base their scope of practice on the multiple-causation theory of health problems or illness. For example, unemployment, pollution, lifestyle, and stressful events may all contribute to illness. In effect, these can all be considered subsystem problems, that is, problems which stem from systems in which the patient is a subsystem (Figure 2-3). Therefore, the concept of illness must include all aspects of the person as well as the biologic and genetic factors that contribute to disease. Illness, then, is influenced by a person's family, his or her social network, the environment, and culture.

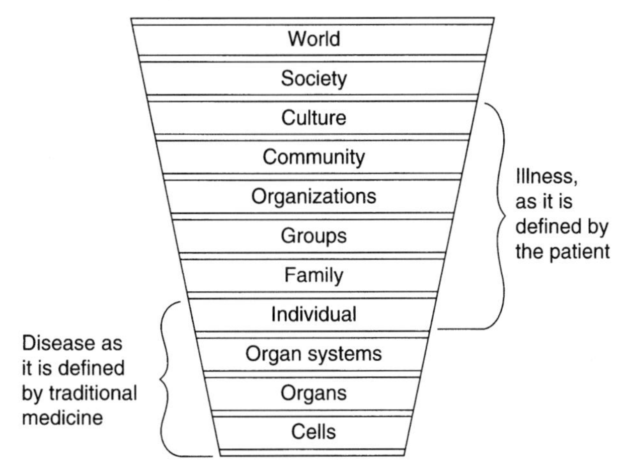

Figure 2-3
Systems hierarchy differentiating illness from disease. (Reprinted with permission from Weiss, R.C. *Your Career in Administrative Medical Services.* Philadelphia: W. B. Saunders, 1996, p. 12.)

Fitness and Wellness

Our ancestors definitely had the right idea. They kept their bodies in good, healthy condition through the physical activities required in their daily existence. In some instances, fitness was actually required for their very survival. Walking was necessary for travel, unless one was lucky enough to own a horse. Hunting was often required in order to put food on the table. And farming was needed to provide the family with fresh vegetables, fruits, and grains. Needless to say, there was little time left for leisurely pursuits, such as nonrequired exercise.

As our society progressed and technology developed, men and women were freed from many tasks requiring hard physical labor. Tasks became mental rather than physical. Today, more work is performed by the pushing of a button rather than the pulling of a hoe.

Generally, people now seem to be living longer because of better nutrition. However, although leisure time is more available to us, many of us do not get enough physical exercise in order to keep fit. *Fitness,* as it is most simply defined, is the state in which one achieves complete physical and mental health and soundness. And in order to achieve this, fitness must be developed and maintained throughout one's lifetime by a program of planned activities.

Achieving Complete Fitness

According to the American Medical Association, there are six steps which are necessary to achieve a complete state of fitness. These include

- Meeting your daily dietary needs as they are indicated by the food group pyramid.
- Regularly participating in a vigorous, sustained exercise program using all body parts.
- Securing proper medical preventive services and care in emergencies.
- Helping to prevent dental disease through proper personal and professional care.
- Choosing healthful play and contributing to society through satisfying work.
- Planning for adequate sleep and rest.

Exercise, Fitness, and Wellness

Even though you may be a busy person, running from here to there, thinking that you're getting plenty of exercise, that doesn't necessarily mean that you are actually getting enough exercise or are physically fit. However, there is a definite relationship between a person who is very busy and one who is fit. When you are in good physical condition, you generally feel good. Feeling tired, sore, or listless, means that you can't do as much. Therefore, regular exercise is important for many reasons. One of the most important is that it helps maintain a state of good health and mental and physical fitness.

Participating in a regular exercise program is part of achieving good health. Physical activity allows us to work off our frustrations. It also helps to relieve stress and tension, and release anger. It provides us with a sense of well-being. Moreover, it is an essential part of the required treatment in aiding our bodies and our minds in the recovery process. Rehabilitative exercise is generally a prescribed treatment after musculoskeletal surgery, as well as part of the therapeutic plan following accidents, injuries, and debilitating illnesses. Some forms of exercise even help us to build up our endurance by strengthening our cardiovascular system. These are called *aerobic exercises.* They help our body by increasing the capacity of our heart and lungs to deliver oxygen to the rest of our body.

Understanding the Concept of Holistic Health

The concept of *holistic health* is based upon the belief that the whole is more than the sum of its parts. When using a holistic approach to health care, you must consider the events affecting the whole person. Illness is viewed as an opportunity for growth; health is a dynamic state of being that, for each person, moves back and forth along a continuum. The extremes of the continuum in holistic health are highest health potential and death; good health, normal health, mild illness, illness or poor health, and critical illness are points along the continuum (Figure 2-4).

In the holistic model of health care delivery, wellness is seen as an ever-changing growth toward fulfilling a person's potential. It considers the person's needs, abilities, and disabilities. A critical assumption in holistic health is that the perception of health is an individual decision, encouraging self-responsibility and self-control. Therefore, health can exist in the presence of illness. For example, a man who is feeling pain in his heart may perceive himself as being near or at the point of highest health potential along the highest health potential–death continuum if he feels he is functioning to his highest potential relative to his pain.

Health Beliefs and Behaviors

The *health status* of a person is the health of that person at a given time. In its general meaning the term may refer to anxiety, depression, or acute illness and thus describes the individual as a whole. Health status can also describe such specifics as a person's vital signs, such as a pulse rate and a body temperature. The health beliefs of an individual deal with those concepts pertaining to his or her health which that individual person believes to be true. Such beliefs may or may not be founded on fact.

Health behaviors are those actions which a person takes in order to understand his or her state of health, maintain an optimal state of health, prevent illness and injury, and reach his or her maximum physical and mental potential. Behaviors such as eating wisely, exercising, paying attention to signs of illness, following treatment advice, and avoiding known health hazards (such as smoking) are all examples. The ability to relax, achieve emotional maturity, lead a productive life, and give way to self-expression also affect one's state of health.

Influences Affecting One's State of Health

There are many variables which affect or influence one's state of health. Some of these are internal factors, such as the person's genetic makeup, and others are external, such as the person's culture and physical environment.

Of the many internal and external factors influencing how one achieves his or her state of health, there are ten which have a direct effect on the person:

1. genetic makeup;
2. race and culture;

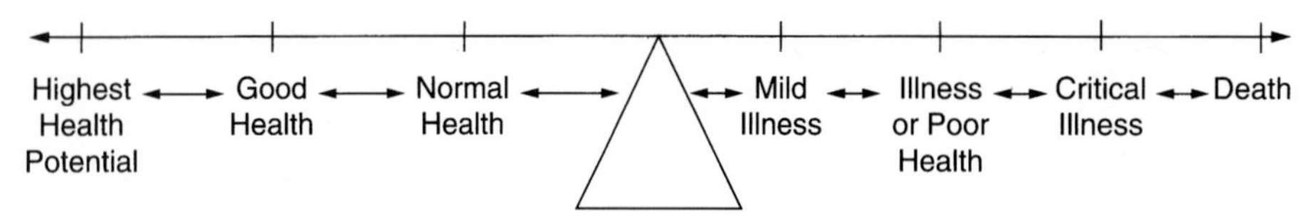

Figure 2-4
Health-illness continuum representing the holistic health model. (Reprinted with permission from Weiss, R.C. *Your Career in Administrative Medical Services.* Philadelphia: W. B. Saunders, 1996, p. 13.)

3. the sex, age, and developmental level of the person;
4. the mind-body relationship, meaning how that person allows his or her emotional responses to affect his or her body function;
5. lifestyle;
6. physical environment;
7. occupation and standard of living the person enjoys;
8. family makeup and support network;
9. self-concept; and
10. the geographic area of residence.

Factors Influencing One's Health Behavior

In addition to those factors which influence one's state of health, there are other factors that also influence one's health behavior. Culture and family influences are two examples. People can usually control their health behaviors and can choose healthy or unhealthy activities. In contrast, people have little or no choice over their genetic makeup, age, sex, physical environments, or culture.

Individual behavior is based upon one's own perceptions and modifying factors which influence one's own life.

Individual perceptions generally include

- the importance of health to the person.
- the perceived control over one's own life.
- any perceived threat of a specific illness.
- any perceived susceptibility toward a specific illness or disease.
- the perceived seriousness of a specific illness or disease.
- the perceived benefits of preventive action toward a specific illness or disease.
- the perceived value of early detection.

Individual factors that modify a person's perceptions generally include

- demographic variables, such as the person's age, sex, and race.
- interpersonal variables, such as the person's concern for significant others, family patterns of health care, and interactions with health care professionals.
- situational variables, such as the cultural acceptance of specific health-related behaviors.

Stages of Illness

Throughout the evolution of medicine and health care, scientists and researchers have described the various stages of illness. These stages, according to most researchers, are classified according to basic or physical stages, and sequential stages.

Basic Stages of Illness

There are five basic stages to illness. The first stage of illness is the transition during which most people come to believe something is wrong with them. We refer to this as the symptom experience stage.

The basic stage at which a patient signals an acceptance of his or her illness is called the acceptance of the sick role. This is the second basic stage. At this time, the patient has generally decided that his or her symptoms or concerns are sufficiently severe to suggest that they are sick.

Medical care contact is the third basic stage of illness. During this stage, patients seek the advice of a health care provider, either on their own initiative, or at the urging of significant others. When people go through this stage, they are usually seeking three types of information: validation of a real illness; explanation of the symptoms in understandable terms; and reassurance either that they will be all right or a prediction of what the outcome will be.

During the fourth basic stage of illness, known as the dependent patient role stage, the patient has already had his or her illness validated by the health care professional. The person now sees him- or herself as a patient, dependent on the professional for help. Often during this stage, the person becomes reluctant to accept a professional's recommendation.

The final basic stage of illness is the recovery or rehabilitation stage. During this time, the patient learns to give up the sick role and return to former roles and functions. For people suffering from acute illnesses, the time as an ill person is generally short, and recovery is usually rapid if it occurs. Thus, they find it relatively easy to return to their former lifestyles.

Sequential Stages of Illness

There are 11 sequential, or consecutive stages of illness. Many of these stages vary in duration, and some may occur simultaneously. They usually include the following.

1. *Symptoms experience:* during this time the patient begins to experience actual symptoms, such as pain. He or she may also become more aware that there may a problem, and begins to respond with fear or anxiety, while giving the symptoms a label and a meaning.
2. *Self-treatment:* during this time, the patient often tries to treat him- or herself, especially if it is believed that the symptoms are not serious.

3. *Communication to significant others:* during this time, the patient will begin to communicate and confide their symptoms to support persons, significant others, or health care providers.
4. *Assessment of symptoms:* during this time, the assessment of the patient's symptoms may be made by the patient, support persons, or a health care professional.
5. *Assumption of the sick role:* at this point, the person has accepted his or her illness, has been declared sick, and has accepted the role of being a sick person.
6. *Expression of concern:* during this stage, support persons and friends begin to offer the patient sympathy and express concern; some people may even recommend practitioners to their sick friend.
7. *Assessment of probable efficacy of treatment or appropriateness of treatment:* during this time, the person may begin to assess the variety of treatments available; a number of variables may affect this assessment, including previous experience and availability of information.
8. *Selection of a treatment plan:* during this time, a treatment plan may be selected with or without the advice of a health care professional; such factors as cost, time, knowledge, and effects are often involved during the selection process.
9. *Implementation of treatment:* during this stage, the patient allows the health care practitioner to implement the prescribed treatment.
10. *Evaluation of the effects of treatment:* during this stage, the patient begins to see and accept the possible outcomes of his or her treatment, including a full recovery with a change in treatment, recovery with some disability, or no recovery. At this time, the patient may also choose to exercise his or her right to completely reject or terminate all treatment.
11. *Recovery and rehabilitation:* during this final stage, the patient begins to make his or her gradual return to usual social roles.

Sick Role Behavior

Sick role behavior has to do with activities which are undertaken by those who consider themselves ill, for the purpose of getting well. Such behavior usually includes four aspects: the patient's inability to be held responsible for their own condition; allowing the patient to be excused from certain social roles and tasks; encouraging the patient to try to get well as quickly as possible; and assisting both the patient and his or her family members in seeking competent health care and treatment.

Effects of Illness on Family Members

A person's illness often affects the family or significant others. The kind of effect and its extent depend chiefly on three factors: which member of the family is ill, the seriousness and length of the illness, and what cultural and social customs that family holds.

Changes which most frequently occur in a family include role changes, task reassignments, increased stress due to anxiety about the outcome of the illness for the patient and conflict about unaccustomed responsibilities, financial problems, loneliness as a result of separation and pending loss, and change in social customs.

Each member of the family may be affected differently, depending, for example, on whether a grandparent, a parent of a nuclear family, or a child is ill. Each of these people plays a different role in the family, and each supports the family in different ways. Parents of young children, for example, have greater family responsibilities than parents of grown children.

The degree of change that family members experience is often related to their dependence on the sick person. For example, when a child is ill, there are few changes other than added responsibilities directly related to the child's illness. When the mother is ill, however, many changes are often necessary because other family members must assume her functions.

Effects of Hospitalization

Normal patterns of behavior generally change with illness; with hospitalization, however, the change can be even greater. Hospitalization usually disrupts a person's privacy, autonomy, lifestyle, roles, and economics.

When a person enters a hospital or other health care institution, such as a skilled nursing care facility, the greatest loss comes to the patient's privacy. Privacy is a comfortable feeling reflecting a deserved degree of social retreat. It is a personal, internal state that cannot and should not be imposed upon without an agreement by the person seeking the privacy. The boundaries of privacy are considered to be highly individual. People need varying degrees of privacy and establish their boundaries for it. When these boundaries are crossed, they feel invaded. Hospital personnel sometimes show little concern for their patients' privacy. Patients are asked to provide information that often they consider private; they may share a room with a stranger; and their health is frequently discussed with many health care providers.

A person's autonomy deals with those activities a person seeks which allow him or her to be completely independent and self-directed without outside control. People vary in their sense of autonomy; some are accustomed to functioning independently in most of their activities, while others are accustomed to direction from others. Hospitalized patients frequently give up much of their autonomy. Decisions about meals, hygienic practices, and sleeping habits are frequently made for them. The loss of individuality is often difficult to accept, often leading to the patient feeling dehumanized.

Hospitalization also makes a drastic change in a person's lifestyle and social role. Many hospitals determine when people wake up and when they should go to sleep. Food in a hospital is usually mass produced, and individual differences in taste are not always accommodated.

Hospitalization not only affects a person's lifestyle; it frequently affects their life roles. A woman or man may no longer be capable of earning wages; a single parent may be unable to fulfill his or her normal parental responsibilities. Such changes not only affect the patient's physical and emotional well-being, but just as important, hospitalization can often place a genuine financial burden on patients and their families. Even though many people have health insurance, it may not reimburse all costs; in addition, many patients lose wages while they are hospitalized.

As a health care provider, you can become aware of costs sustained by the patient, and by doing so, can provide care and treatment that is as economical as is safely possible. For example, you can use only the minimum supplies necessary for providing a particular treatment. You can also support activities that promote health and that return patients to their normal activities as soon as possible.

Patterns and Trends in Health and Illness

The health of most Americans throughout the United States is steadily improving. This is primarily due to early preventative efforts based on new knowledge obtained through research; improvements in sanitation, housing, nutrition, and immunization essential to disease prevention; and individual members of society taking measures to promote health and prevent disease. There are other factors, or health risks, however, that according to the U.S. Surgeon General, people set up for themselves which make them more susceptible to illness and disease. These factors include cigarette smoking, alcohol and drug abuse, injuries sustained from automobile and other types of accidents, and occupational risks suffered as a result of not following safety standards in the work place. All of these risks present challenges to the health care worker, especially members of the physical medicine team, whose goal is to promote and provide the patient with care and treatment relative to his or her musculoskeletal system, as well as to the body as a whole.

Measuring Trends in Health Care Delivery

Evidence of current health status and changes in the last few decades are measured in various ways. Measurements are made of longevity or life expectancy; the way people feel about their health; mortality rates and causes; morbidity rates and causes; the type of health behaviors people practice; and the amount and kind of health services used.

Longevity of Life Expectancy

In 1960, life expectancy at birth was about 70 years of age. By 1983, it nearly reached 75 years. Differences, however, exist between races and between males and females. In 1982, for example, the life expectancy for a Caucasian male was 71.5 years of age. For a Caucasian female, it was 78.8 years of age. For an African-American male, it was 64.9 years, while it was 73.5 years for an African-American female.

How People Feel About Their Health

The way a person feels about his or her health is one way in which a person's health status can be ascertained. Over the past several years, people of all ages have generally held the same perception of their health status. In 1981, for example, when most people were asked how they felt about their state of health as compared to other people of the same age, approximately 87.3 percent said they felt good or excellent. What is most interesting is that about 70 percent of people who stated they felt good or excellent were elderly persons.

Summary

In this chapter, we discussed the concepts of health and wellness, fitness and exercise, and illness and disease, as well as the relationship that each of these have to one another. We also talked briefly about nontraditional views of health and illness, as well as health beliefs and behaviors, the basic and sequential stages of illness, what is meant by sick role behavior, and the effects illness has on both the patient and family members. Finally, we discussed the effects of hospitalization and the role it plays in caring for an ill person, and identified various patterns and trends which influence both health and illness.

Review Questions

1. Briefly define *disease.*
2. Briefly define *health.*
3. Briefly define *wellness.*
4. Briefly define *illness.*
5. What model of health care delivery is based upon the relationship of all humans to their internal and external environments?
   a. eudaimonistic
   b. adaptive
   c. ecological
6. What model of health care delivery incorporates the most comprehensive view of health?
   a. eudaimonistic
   b. adaptive
   c. ecological
7. What model of health care delivery sees disease as a failure in the person's ability to adapt?
   a. eudaimonistic
   b. adaptive
   c. ecological
8. Health ______________ are defined as those actions which a person takes in order to understand his or her state of health and prevent illness or injury.

3

Medical Law and Ethics

Performance Objectives

Upon completion of this chapter, you will be able to:

1. Delineate the difference between medical law and medical ethics.
2. Discuss the Code of Ethics that members of the physical medicine team are morally bound to follow.
3. Identify at least four examples of ethical behavior for the physical medicine professional.
4. Discuss the Patient's Bill of Rights.
5. Discuss the need to license medical personnel.
6. Explain the Rule of Personal Liability.
7. Briefly discuss the Good Samaritan law.
8. Demonstrate an understanding of specific patient consent forms.
9. Discuss the legal implications of a patient's medical record.

Terms and Abbreviations

Defamation any attack on a person's reputation; called "libel" when the written word is used and "slander" when the spoken word is used.

Duty of care a lawful obligation which protects the patient by requiring the health care worker to provide safe care to the patient.

Ethics moral standards and principles.

Good Samaritan law a law, differing in various states, that protects a health care worker from a malpractice suit when coming to the aid of a person in an emergency situation.

Informed consent the act of informing the patient of the risks and alternatives to a medical procedure and the patient acknowledging the assumed risks by signing a consent form.

Malpractice literally, "bad practice" by a professional; any care below an expected standard which results in injury.

Medical practice acts statutes dealing with licensing of medical personnel.

Negligence occurs when any member of the health care delivery system fails to do something for a patient that another person of the same training and position would do under the same or ordinary circumstances.

Patient's Bill of Rights a document produced and adopted by the American Hospital Association which states what a patient has the right to expect during his or her medical treatment.

Reasonable care acts or services performed by a health care professional who is then protected by law if it is proven that he or she acted reasonably compared to fellow workers.

Rule of Personal Liability dictates that all health care workers be held responsible for their own conduct.

The laws and ethical codes of conduct for the medical profession must be understood by all members of the physical medicine team. These laws and ethics codes protect all members of the medical profession, as well as the patient.

Medical ethics have been important in the study

of medicine as far back as 400 B.C., when Hippocrates wrote the Hippocratic Oath, a document which first developed the standards of medical conduct and ethics. Today, many individual health care professional associations have adopted their own codes of ethics in order to govern their health care workers. Members of the physical therapy team, the sports medicine team, and the chiropractic team all have ethical codes that provide guidelines for their professional behavior.

The practice of medicine today exists within a framework of laws. Such laws governing medical practices may vary from state to state, so it is important to know your state's laws governing the physical medicine worker, as well as federal and local statutes.

Understanding Medical Ethics and Medical Law

Medical *ethics* are concerned with whether the physical medicine worker's actions are right or wrong, whereas medical law focuses more on whether one acted legally or illegally. Ethical behavior deals with behavior that is specific and represents the ideal conduct for a certain group. Each group of health care professionals who require a license to function in their position have drafted and adopted specific codes of ethics. These ethics are based upon moral principles and practices. If accused of unethical behavior by a medical worker's professional association, you can be issued a warning or in some cases even be expelled from the association.

Medical law is concerned with the legal conduct of the members of the medical profession. There are federal, state, and local laws which must be followed, and violation of such laws may subject the offender to civil or criminal prosecution. Professional licenses can be taken away, fines can be levied, and prison sentences can be imposed. Often, the line between what is unethical and what is illegal can be unclear. If you, as a member of the health care delivery system, decided, for example, you were going to be rude to a patient, that is unethical behavior. But if you decided to inform the patient's neighbor of his or her disease, that is illegal behavior. In addition, you can also be sued by a patient for *defamation,* which is considered an attack on a person's reputation. This is called "libel" when the defamation is written, and "slander" when spoken.

Another example of the difference between unethical and illegal behavior concerns the viewing of a friend's chart in a part of the hospital where you do not work. If you read it out of curiosity, that is unethical. If you talk about it, that is illegal. If an action is illegal, it is always unethical. However, it can be unethical without being illegal. Remember, ethics represent the highest standards of behavior.

Ethical Behavior

As a member of the physical medicine team, you are responsible for displaying ethical behavior at all times. This means maintaining the highest level of ethical conduct. To accomplish this, you should always:

- Respect the rights of all patients to have opinions, lifestyles, and beliefs that are different from your own.
- Remember that everything seen, heard, or read about a patient is considered confidential and does not leave the job site.
- Be conscientious in doing your work, doing the best you can at all times.
- Be ready to be of service to patients and co-workers at any time of the workday.
- Let the patient know that it is a privilege for you to assist him or her.
- Follow closely the specific rules of ethical conduct prescribed by your employer.

The Patient and the Health Care Worker

The Patient's Bill of Rights

Awareness of the patient's rights is the responsibility of all members of the health care team. Because this is such a vital and important aspect of providing care and treatment to the patient, the American Hospital Association (AHA) felt it was necessary to establish a document which identified what the patient could expect from those individuals who cared for the patient. As a result, the *Patient's Bill of Rights* was adopted by the organization. The intent of such a document is to make both members of the health care system and patients aware of what the patient has a right to expect. According to the AHA, the patient has a right to:

- Considerate and respectful care.
- Obtain from their physician complete, current information concerning their diagnosis, treatment, and prognosis in terms that they can be reasonably expected to understand.
- Informed consent, which should include knowledge of the proposed procedure, along with its risks and probable duration of incapacitation; in addition, the patient has a right to information regarding medically significant alternatives.
- Refuse treatment to the extent permitted by law, and to be informed of the medical consequences of such action.
- Have case discussion, consultation, examination, and treatment conducted discretely, and have those not directly involved in the patient's care be granted permission by the patient for their presence.

- Expect that all communication and records pertaining to his or her care be treated in a confidential manner.
- Expect the hospital to make a reasonable response to request for services, and the hospital must provide evaluation, service, and referrals as they may be indicated by the urgency of the case.
- Obtain information as to any relationship of the hospital to other health care and educational institutions, insofar as his or her care is concerned, and the relationship among individuals, by name, who are treating the patient.
- Be advised if the hospital proposes to engage in or perform human experimentation affecting his or her care or treatment, and the right to refuse to participate in such research projects.
- Expect reasonable continuity of care.
- Examine and receive an explanation of the bill regardless of the source of payment.
- Know what hospital rules and regulations apply to his or her conduct as a patient.

The Athlete's Bill of Rights

In addition to having an understanding of patient's rights, those of you who choose to work in the field of sports medicine may encounter some situations or circumstances for which you must also be concerned about the rights of the athlete. It is for this reason that the American Medical Association created its Committee on the Medical Aspects of Sports. According to the committee, all players who are engaged in athletic sports and competition are responsible for playing fair, giving his or her best, keeping fit and in training, and conducting him- or herself with credit to the sport and the school or organization which he or she is representing. In turn, says the committee, the athlete has the right to expect the highest degree of protection against injury through the implementation of good technical instruction, proper regulation and conditions of play, and adequate health supervision.

The committee further states that according to these rights, all athletes have the right to expect:

- Good coaching through careful conditioning and technical instruction.
- Good officiating through comprehension of all rules and regulations governing athletic competition.
- Use of good equipment and playing facilities.
- Good health supervision, including a thorough preseason history and medical examination, and the presence of a physician at all contests who is also available during all practice sessions, and who has medical control of all health aspects of athletics.

Licensing of Health Care Workers

The medical profession and many of the individual health care professions are legally regulated throughout the United States by the issuing of licenses and certificates. All 50 states require the licensing of hospitals. The statutes dealing with the individual licensing and certification of the individual health care professionals are commonly referred to as *medical practice acts.*

Licenses can be revoked or suspended when a medical professional has been found guilty of violating various statutes involved in the licensing process. Grounds for losing a medical license include serious crimes such as murder, rape, and arson. Crimes of moral turpitude, such as tax crimes, minor sexual offenses, and false statements while applying for a license can also be grounds for loss of the license. Other crimes which may cause the worker to have his or her license suspended or revoked include incapacity due to insanity, or excessive use of alcohol or drug addiction.

Protection Under the Law

In the health care environment, both the patient and the health care worker must be assured protection under the law. For the patient, this means being assured of safe care. For the health care professional, it means being protected from irresponsible law suits.

The patient is protected by a process known as *duty of care.* This entitles the patient to safe care by making it mandatory that he or she be treated by meeting the common or average standards of practice expected in the community under similar circumstances. The duty of care also provides that the patient be treated with *reasonable care,* that is, protection of the health care professional by law if it can be proven that he or she acted reasonably as compared to fellow workers of the same or similar training in a situation of the same nature. If it is proven that the health care worker failed to meet such a standard and harm comes to the patient as a result, negligence may be proven.

Negligence is the failure to give reasonable care or the giving of unreasonable care. The patient is harmed because the health professional did something wrong or failed to do something that he or she should have done under the circumstances.

The Good Samaritan Law and Medical Malpractice

The *Good Samaritan law* is a law which, in its entirety, addresses the problem of medical malpractice suits for a physician or any trained health care professional who comes upon an accident scene and attempts to render aid to the victim. The law, which has been enacted in all 50 states, encourages members of health care professions to offer treatment without fearing the possibility of a malpractice suit. Laws throughout the country do differ, so it is wise to check the law in your own state in order to determine what professional liability may exist during an emergency situation.

The term *malpractice,* unfortunately, is a term that is familiar to all of us, because of the large number of lawsuits filed and settled throughout the country. For the medical worker, it seems that the higher the educational level and requirements of the worker, the greater is the likelihood that they may be responsible for their actions.

When used in the medical professions, malpractice refers to any misconduct or lack of skill that results in the patient's injury. A patient who thinks that his or her physician has been negligent in diagnosing and treating an illness or accident may file a medical malpractice claim. Most claims are generally made against physicians, however, any employee working in the health care environment can be named in a malpractice lawsuit. Most insurance companies who issue medical malpractice policies on physicians take into account that the policy will also cover the physician's employees as well, but medical office or hospital employees may also wish to purchase their own insurance policy, which is usually quite inexpensive.

Physicians are liable for the actions of their employees while the employees are on duty; for example, a laboratory assistant who accepts a lab specimen from two patients and then mislabels the specimens, consequently causing one patient to be told that his specimen is normal and the other being administered antibiotics. Subsequently, the patient who has been told that everything was all right develops an infection which could have been prevented if the antibiotics had been administered. In this case, the doctor could be sued for the negligence of the employee mislabeling the specimens.

In health care, under the *Rule of Personal Liability,* all individuals are held responsible for their own personal conduct. In a medical malpractice suit, such as the example previously described, both the physician and the laboratory assistant could be held jointly liable for medical malpractice.

You can also be held jointly responsible if you work for a doctor who is involved in an illegal act and you are aware of the crime, but fail to report it. Physicians must also report crimes that they learn about when practicing medicine, such as a shooting, child or elder abuse, or rape. As a member of the physical medicine team, you can also be held jointly responsible with the physician if you fail to report such crimes. In some cases, protecting patient confidentiality and the patient's right to complete privacy of their records does not apply. Births, deaths, communicable diseases, and crimes are all examples of times when the physician is bound by law to report what has occurred. If you fail to report these types of cases, you may also be held liable.

In some instances, the law is very specific regarding confidentiality and reporting of information. In cases dealing with patients suffering from AIDS, for example, there are laws and regulations which take into account the confidential nature of the patient's illness. However, these regulations seem to be constantly changing. Therefore, it is important that you keep current about the law and regulations regarding confidentiality and patient's records in treating this disease in the state in which you are working.

Obtaining Patient Consent

When a doctor makes a diagnosis and recommends a specific mode of treatment, the patient has the responsibility whether or not to accept such diagnosis and treatment. The physician has the responsibility of informing the patient in words that he or she can understand as to the risks and alternatives of any suggested procedure. The patient has the responsibility of deciding whether or not to accept all the explained risks. Once it is ascertained that the physician has properly explained the procedure and the patient fully understands it and the risks, a consent form must be signed by the patient, indicating that he or she fully accepts the risk of the procedure. The process is called *informed consent.* As part of your responsibility, you may be asked to prepare the consent form (Figure 3-1) for any type of procedure, whether it is to be performed in the office or in the hospital. Consents are also required before an experimental procedure or prior to any other unusual procedure taking place. Consent forms are also used prior to the administration of any experimental medications.

In cases where the patient may have difficulty with understanding or speaking the English language, the consent form must be translated or prepared in the patient's native language. A patient who has not been properly informed through the informed consent process can sue the physician for medical malpractice.

Specific guidelines have been established in regard to the details and the signing of the consent form. These include the following:

- Always make sure that the patient fully understands the consent form and realizes what he or she has signed; patients who are mentally handicapped should be given an explanation that can

Patient or someone acting for the patient agrees to the following terms of hospital admission.

1) **MEDICAL TREATMENT:** Patient will be treated by his/her attending doctor or specialists. Patient authorizes Hospital to perform services ordered by the doctors. Special consent forms may be needed. Many doctors and assistants (such as those providing x-rays, lab tests, and anesthesiology) may not be Hospital employees and are responsible for their own treatment activities.
2) **GENERAL DUTY NURSING:** Hospital provides only general nursing care. If the patient needs special or private nursing, it must be arranged by the patient or by the doctor treating the patient.
3) **MONEY AND VALUABLES:** The Hospital has a safe in which to keep money or valuables. It will not be responsible for any loss or damage to items not deposited in the safe. The Hospital will not be responsible for loss or damage to items such as glasses, dentures, hearing aids and contact lenses.
4) **TEACHING PROGRAMS:** The Hospital participates in programs for training of health care personnel. Some services may be provided to the patient by persons in training under the supervision and instruction of doctors or hospital employees. These persons may also observe care given to the patient by doctors and hospital employees. Photos or video tapes may be made of surgical procedures.
5) **RELEASE OF INFORMATION:** The Hospital may disclose all or any part of the patient's medical and/or financial records (INCLUDING INFORMATION REGARDING ALCOHOL OR DRUG ABUSE), to the following:

   a. **Third Party Payors:** Any person or corporation, or their designee, which is or may be liable under a contract to the hospital, the patient, a family member, or employer of the patient, for payment of all or part of the hospital's charges, including but not limited to, insurance companies, utilization review organizations, workman's compensation payors, hospital or medical service companies, welfare funds, governmental agencies or the patient's employer;

   b. **Medical Audit:** The Hospital conducts a program of medical audit and the patient's medical information may be reviewed and released by employees, members of the medical staff or other authorized persons to appropriate agencies as part of this program.

   c. **Medical Research:** Information may be released for use in medical studies and medical research.

   d. **Other Health Care Providers:** Information may be released to other health care providers in order to provide continued patient care.

   I understand that the authorization granted in items 5. a, b, c and d may be revoked by me at any time, except to the extent to which action has been taken in reliance upon it. The authorization will stay in effect as long as the need for information in items 5. a, b, c and d exist.

I have read and understand this Admissions Agreement, have received a copy and I am the patient, the parent of a minor child or the court appointed guardian for the patient and am authorized to act on the patient's behalf to sign this Agreement.

Harriet Culver — WITNESS Bertha C. Young — PATIENT / PARENT OF MINOR CHILD / COURT APPOINTED GUARDIAN (PLEASE CIRCLE THE CORRECT TITLE)

October 6, 19XX 1:00 p.m. — DATE

MEDICAL POWER OF ATTORNEY A.R.S. §14-5501: I appoint ______________________ as my agent to act in all matters relating to my health care, including full power to give or refuse consent to all medical, surgical and hospital care. This power of attorney shall be effective upon my disability or incapacity or when there is uncertainty whether I am dead or alive and shall have the same effect as if I were alive, competent, and able to act for myself.

______________ WITNESS ______________ PATIENT

FINANCIAL AGREEMENT

I agree that in return for the services provided to the patient, I will pay the account of the patient, and/or prior to discharge make financial arrangements satisfactory to the hospital for payment. If the account is sent to an attorney for collection, I agree to pay reasonable attorney's fees and collection expenses. The amount of the attorney's fee shall be established by the Court and not by a Jury in any court action. A delinquent account may be charged interest at the legal rate.

If any signer is entitled to hospital benefits of any type whatsoever under any policy of insurance insuring patient, or any other party liable to patient, the benefits are hereby assigned to hospital for application on patient's bill. However, IT IS UNDERSTOOD THAT THE UNDERSIGNED AND PATIENT ARE PRIMARILY RESPONSIBLE FOR PAYMENT OF PATIENT'S BILL.

IN GRANTING ADMISISON OR RENDERING TREATMENT, THE HOSPITAL IS RELYING ON MY AGREEMENT TO PAY THE ACCOUNT, EMERGENCY CARE WILL BE PROVIDED WITHOUT REGARD TO THE ABILITY TO PAY.

Bertha C. Young — PATIENT ______________ OTHER PARTY AGREEING TO PAY

Harriet Culver — WITNESS ______________ RELATIONSHIP TO PATIENT

October 6 19XX — DATE

09-1542 1-84

Figure 3-1
Consent form. (Reprinted with permission from LaFleur, M.W. and Starr, W.K. *Health Unit Coordinating.* Philadelphia: W. B. Saunders, 1986, p. 483.)

be understood completely, with as few confusing terms as possible.

- The patient must never be forced to sign the consent form, and must not be allowed to sign it under the influence of alcohol or drugs.
- All signatures must be witnessed, dated, and signed in ink, with full legal names used.
- Any adult over 18 years of age may sign his or her own consent unless the patient is incompetent and has a guardian, or there is an emergency, in which case two physicians must sign the consent form.
- Married minors may sign their own consent for treatment.
- Unmarried minors must have a consent signed by one parent or legal guardian, however, consent of both parents is usually suggested; a stepparent may not sign a consent form.

- An emancipated minor, who is under the age of 18 and who has been declared by a court of law to be legally responsible for his- or herself, may sign his or her own consent form.
- Because any break in the skin may be considered an operation, a consent form must be signed in order to avoid liability for battery.
- Telephone consents are valid in an emergency situation, provided that the telephoned consent is witnessed by two people, and is immediately followed by a written confirmation.
- A consent is valid for a reasonable time after signing, as long as there is no change in the anticipated procedure.

Patient Medical Records and the Law

The patient's medical record is considered a legal document and as such is the property of the physician if the patient is an outpatient, and the property of the hospital if the patient has been hospitalized. It is extremely important that these records be as accurate, complete, up to date, and as neat as possible, in order to protect members of the medical staff from any future litigation, as well as evidence of truth if there is a lawsuit or court case regarding the patient's care or treatment. While all patient records are considered confidential, any or all parts of it may be subpoenaed and used during a court action. Therefore, most hospitals and private medical practices make it a standard practice to obtain a signed release of information form from the patient when they are first seen or admitted to the hospital.

If you are required to write in the patient's medical records, always remember to use only permanent ink, and never erase an entry. If an error has been made, simply cross the error out, using only one line, initial it, and rewrite the correct entry above or next to the original entry. No documentation written in pencil or with erasures is acceptable, and any record with either of these can be rejected automatically as legal evidence.

Summary

In this chapter, we discussed some of the very important concepts dealing with medical law and ethics, including the differences between each and what constitutes medical negligence and medical malpractice. We also talked about ethical behavior on the part of the physical medicine worker, as well as the role of both the patient's bill of rights and the athlete's bill of rights, and what the patient and athlete have the right to expect from their health care professionals. In addition, we talked about the need to license medical personnel, and the purpose of the rule of personal liability and the Good Samaritan law. Finally, we talked about patient consent forms and defined the legal implications of the patient's medical record.

Review Questions

1. A patient's ______________ is a document which states what a patient has the right to expect during his or her medical treatment.
2. Briefly define the Good Samaritan law.
3. ______________ pertains to any attack on a person's reputation.
   a. ethics
   b. negligence
   c. defamation
4. ______________ pertains to any member of the health care delivery system failing to perform or to do something for a patient that another person of the same training and position would do under the same or ordinary circumstances.
   a. negligence
   b. defamation
   c. malpractice
5. ______________ pertains to any care which is provided to a patient which is below an expected standard and which can result in injury.
   a. negligence
   b. defamation
   c. malpractice
6. Briefly define what is meant by *duty of care.*
7. When the written word is used to defame someone, it is called ______________; when the spoken word is used to defame someone, it is called ______________.
8. Briefly explain the concept of *medical ethics.*
9. Give at least two examples of ethical behavior:
   a. ______________
   b. ______________

4

Health and Safety in the Physical Medicine Environment

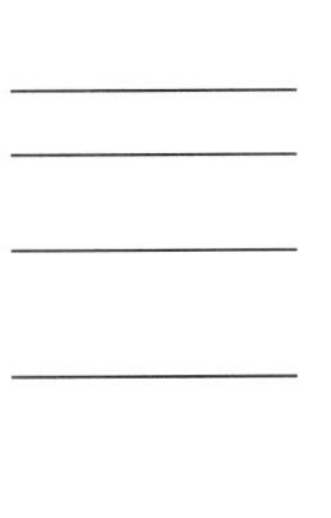

Performance Objectives

Upon completion of this chapter, you will be able to:

1. Identify factors associated with making people more susceptible to infection than others.
2. Explain the difference between medical and surgical asepsis.
3. Describe and be able to demonstrate how to perform correct handwashing techniques.
4. Explain the relationship between good body alignment and practicing good body mechanics.
5. Identify specific types of activities that will ensure a safe environment for both patients and members of the physical medicine health care team.
6. Identify potential emergency situations and how to respond to them.
7. Discuss the skills necessary to provide privacy for patients seen in the hospital and in other physical medicine environments.
8. Discuss methods for maintaining treatment rooms within the physical medicine environment.

Terms and Abbreviations

Alignment having parts in their proper relationship to one another.
Asepsis the absence of disease-producing organisms.
Bacteria one-celled microorganisms that can cause fermentation, decay, and, in some cases, disease.
Bacteriology the study of bacteria.
Balance keeping an object in a steady position, or stable.
Base of support the area on which an object rests; when the body is upright, the feet form the base of support of the body.
Body mechanics the efficient use of the body during activity.
Center of gravity the point at which the mass of the body is centered.
Infection process that occurs when pathogens attack a person and produce signs and symptoms of an illness.
Line of gravity the imaginary vertical line that passes through the center of gravity.
Medical asepsis medical techniques used to reduce the number and prevent the spread of pathogens.
Nosocomial infection an infection acquired by the patient while being cared for in the hospital.
Pathogen any disease-producing organism.
Posture the position of the body parts in relation to one another.
Susceptible having a very low resistance to disease.

For as many years as there have been people living on earth, they have suffered from infectious diseases. For a very long time, however, it was thought that an infection might be part of the actual healing process. No one knew how or why infections were transmitted. Physicians would move from one patient to another without ever washing their hands or changing their dirty lab coats. And who ever heard of wearing sterile gloves or isolation gowns? It wasn't until as recent as the middle of the nineteenth century that the germ theory of disease was even suggested.

Asepsis and Infection Control

Asepsis is defined as the absence of microorganisms that are capable of causing disease. As it is now practiced, asepsis is based upon the many discoveries of scientists from around the world. One of the greatest of these was Louis Pasteur. Born in France, Pasteur made tremendous strides in the prevention and treatment of disease. It is for all his work that he is considered the founder of *bacteriology,* the study of *bacteria,* microorganisms that may cause disease. In fact, today there are millions of people around the globe who owe their lives to this man. It was his work that ultimately proved that germs could be spread through the air, but the spread of such germs could in fact be controlled. In addition, he also proved that these germs could be killed. Because of his knowledge and his work in bacteriology, Pasteur was also one of the very first to practice surgery with the use of antiseptics to prevent infection.

Susceptibility and Infection

Some people tend to be more susceptible to infection than others. One factor has to do with the age of the person. The very young and the very old seem to develop infections easily. This is because a small child does not have the mature immune system that is needed to fight off infections. Nor does the elderly person, simply because of his or her age.

People with disabilities or who have body systems weakened because of their disabilities also seem to be more susceptible than others to infection. One example of this is the patient who suffers from a spinal cord injury becoming more susceptible to urinary bladder infections because of their inability to empty the bladder effectively. Another example is the patient who has been diagnosed with multiple sclerosis also being more susceptible to pneumonia because of impaired lung capacity and muscle paralysis.

People who are well nourished are less susceptible to infection than those who are malnourished. Nutrition plays an important role in the prevention of infection and in recovery from illness. Without proper nourishment, our bodies would not be able to function properly. A good diet, therefore, can provide the substances the body needs to repair itself.

Ingestion of medications can also increase one's incidence of infections. Drugs used in the treatment of leukemia, for example, will decrease the number of white blood cells manufactured by the body. These cells are part of the body's immune system and are necessary to fight infection.

Patients who have been diagnosed with acquired immune deficiency syndrome (AIDS) also have a weakened immune system. These patients are very *susceptible* to many kinds of infections, that is, they have a very low resistance to disease.

The Infection Cycle

Microorganisms move from place to place in a cycle (Figure 4-1). If the cycle is broken, the microorganisms cannot grow, spread, or cause disease. A person with an *infection* acts as a reservoir for the microorganisms, allowing them to grow and multiply. The infection may be spread by the hands, bed clothes or linens, and equipment. Microorganisms can even be transmitted by a simple cough or a sneeze. The person exposed to and receiving the organism is called the host. The infectious agent may enter the host via an opening in the skin or any opening of the body (mouth, nose, eyes, ears, etc.). If the host is unable to fight off the infecting organism, that person will begin to show signs or symptoms of a disease or an infection.

Germs and microorganisms are everywhere. They are in the air, in the soil, in the food and water we consume, and even on other people. The skin is called our first line of defense, and if this is broken, germs and organisms may enter the body.

In order for an infection to occur, the environment for the microorganisms to grow and multiply must be just right. This means that food and moisture are needed. Oxygen is also needed, except in those cases where the microorganisms are anaerobic, that is, not requiring oxygen for growth. There are a few bacteria which fall into this category. One common example of an anaerobic bacteria is the one that causes tetanus. It generally grows well in a puncture wound because it is anaerobic. Bacteria needing oxygen for growth are called aerobic bacteria. Normal

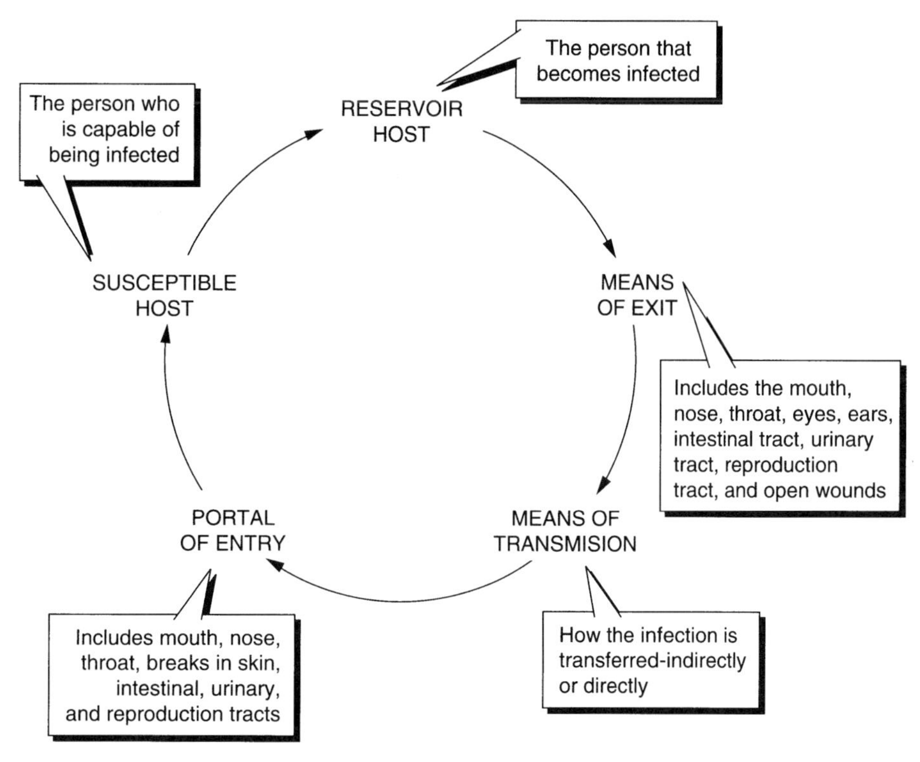

Figure 4-1
The infection cycle. (Reprinted with permission from Weiss, R.C. *Your Career in Administrative Medical Services.* Philadelphia: W. B. Saunders, 1996, p. 25.)

body temperature is best for most bacteria to grow and multiply. High temperature kills most microorganisms, while low temperatures retard and tend to slow the growth rate. Finally, many bacteria need darkness to grow and multiply. When exposed to light, they die. Food, moisture, oxygen, warm temperature, and darkness all encourage the growth of bacteria. In order to break the infection cycle, you must modify at least one or more of these factors.

Practicing Medical and Surgical Asepsis

The most common means by which organisms are transmitted are the hands, since they carry germs to the mouth, eyes, nose, and to other people. The best way to inhibit this transmission is through the practice of medical and surgical asepsis.

Medical asepsis is the practice of reducing the numbers and preventing the spread of microorganisms. It can be accomplished in a number of ways, such as covering your nose and mouth when you sneeze or cough, washing your hands before you handle food and after you have used the restroom, washing your hands before and after you have treated a patient, wearing a clean uniform or lab coat each day to work, practicing good body hygiene, and keeping dirty items such as linen and equipment separate from clean items in your department.

Surgical asepsis is the practice of eliminating all microorganisms, both *pathogenic* (or "disease-producing") and nonpathogenic. Examples of surgical asepsis include using sterile equipment for giving injections, performing venipuncture, starting IVs, and surgery, and using sterile dressings and bandages to cover open wounds.

One of the most important tasks you will be faced with in health care is to provide the very best possible surroundings for you and the patients entrusted to your care. A clean, dry, light, and airy environment will help prevent the growth of pathogens and *nosocomial infections,* which are infections acquired by the patient while in the hospital.

One of the easiest and best ways of preventing the spread of bacteria is through using correct handwashing techniques. Figure 4-2 shows the correct procedure for handwashing. It is a skill used not only for your protection but also for those around you—patients, co-workers, and visitors. You will wash your hands before and after doing treatments and at any other time your hands become dirty.

When washing your hands, always remember to use plenty of flowing water, a good germicidal soap, and friction. It is the friction, or strong rubbing movement of both hands against each other, that loosens the bacteria from the skin. The water is directed so that it flows from the wrist down toward the fingers.

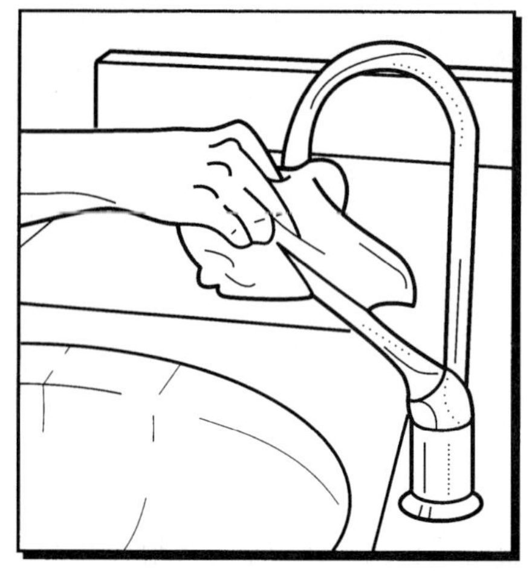

Step 1: Never touch sink with your uniform.

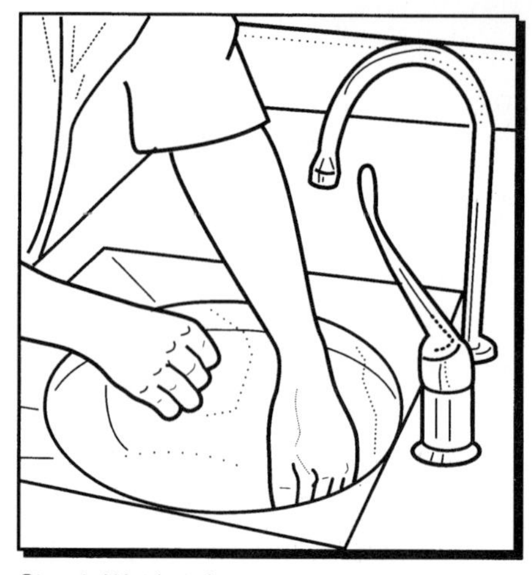

Step 2: Wet hands.

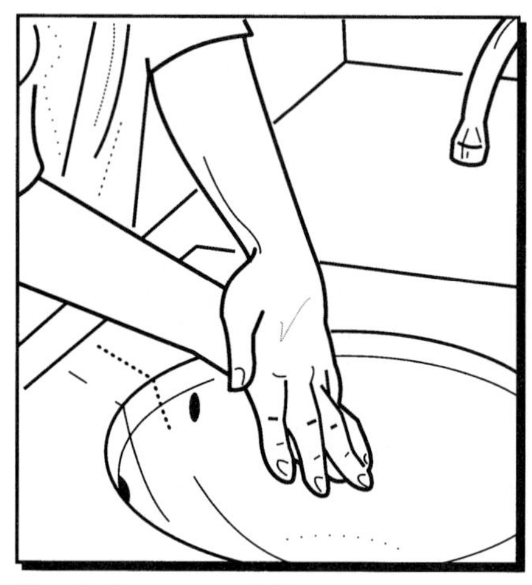

Step 3: Use strong rubbing movements.

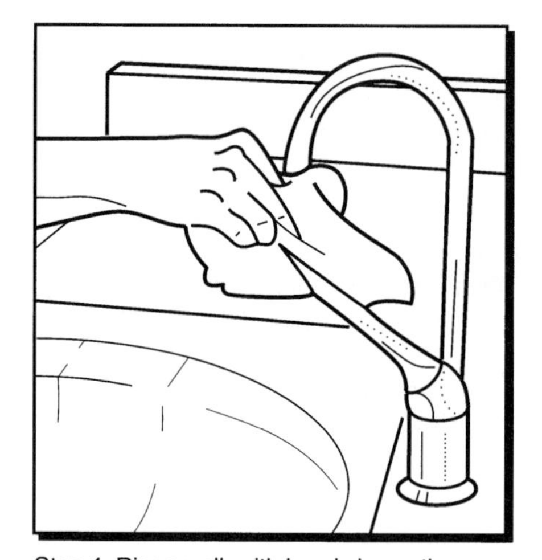

Step 4: Rinse well, with hands lower than wrist.

Figure 4-2
Steps in handwashing to prevent spread of bacteria. (Reprinted with permission from Weiss, R.C. *Your Career in Administrative Medical Services.* Philadelphia: W. B. Saunders, 1996, p. 26.)

This carries the suds and dirt down the drain. Never lean against the sink or allow your uniform or lab coat to touch it. After drying your hands with a paper towel, before you discard it in the trash, you must always remember to use the towel to turn off the faucet. After you have finished washing your hands, you may also apply some lotion to them to prevent any chapping and to keep the skin soft.

Medical Asepsis in the Physical Medicine Environment

In most large medical facilities, the physical medicine and rehabilitative medical services department and the physical therapy department are generally self-contained or within very close proximity to one another. This makes it easier to keep these areas clean and thus prevent the growth and spread of bacteria and microorganisms. Tables and equipment have adequate space between each item so that they may be kept spotlessly clean.

All articles that are used in these departments must be cleaned after each use. This prevents the spread of pathogens between patients. It also protects your co-workers from the possibility of contracting an infection from a patient. In the past, many hospitals placed articles in the direct sunlight to destroy pathogens. Since this is not very practical today, equipment may be soaked in an antiseptic solution or wiped off with a disinfectant.

Antiseptics are used to inhibit and stop the growth of pathogens, yet they are mild enough to be used on the skin. A disinfectant is used to stop the growth of the pathogenic organisms, but it is harmful if used directly on the skin. Sterilization is a process used to kill all microorganisms. Items which have been sterilized are usually marked or wrapped in special containers to maintain their cleanliness until they are to be used.

It is the responsibility of all members of the physical medicine, rehabilitation, and physical therapy departments to be on guard continuously against the spread of infections. If you start to perform a procedure on a patient and suddenly remember that you failed to wash your hands since working with your last patient, you must immediately stop the procedure and wash your hands. A clinician who observes that medical aseptic techniques are not being followed and does nothing to correct it is not safe to practice as a member of the health care profession. Nothing should ever be assumed when practicing asepsis.

Following Universal Precautions

In today's medical and health care facilities, all departments practicing within the physical medicine environment must practice universal precautions to prevent the spread of communicable diseases and infections. All patients and staff are considered possible carriers of potentially harmful pathogens. Blood and body fluids carry many pathogens. Body fluids that may be infected include blood, sputum, urine, stool, and drainage from open wounds. In order to decrease the risk of accidental exposure to body fluids, the department in which you work will have strict infection control procedures that must be followed by all members of the staff. This is especially true when working with patients who have open wounds. These precautions are for all patients, and they stress prevention of exposure and possible infection. As a member of the physical medicine health care delivery team, you should make yourself aware of the infection control procedures followed by your department and the facility.

Providing for a Healthy and Safe Environment

Health care workers are active people. In the performance of your work, you will use a variety of movements. You may be required to reach, pull, lift, stoop, sit, stand, carry objects, push wheelchairs and stretchers, and stand at the treatment area or a patient's bedside. Your body must be in good physical condition. This means being constantly aware of how to most effectively and efficiently use your muscles. Doing so will prevent injury to yourself as well as your patients.

Practicing Good Body Mechanics

Body mechanics is the efficient use of the body during an activity. Good posture is insurance for health and happiness. *Posture* refers to the position of your body and the relationship of its individual parts to one another. Once you know your faulty posture habits and have a corrected posture image, you can begin to control *alignment.* Your movements will be safer and more efficient. You will feel tall, poised, and graceful. You should always remember to practice good posture in your walking, sitting, and working. It will decrease the fatigue you may be experiencing during the day. Figure 4-3 shows the correct alignment of body parts.

The most common complaint of all health care workers, particularly those working in physical medi-

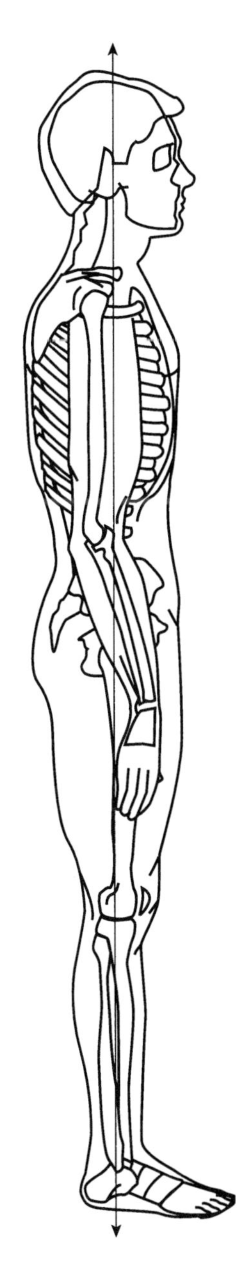

Figure 4-3
Correct postural body alignment. (Reprinted with permission from Weiss, R.C. *Your Career in Administrative Medical Services.* Philadelphia: W. B. Saunders, 1996, p. 27.)

cine and rehabilitation medical services, is low back pain. Often this involves lifting a load while twisting around at the waist. It may result in severe muscle strain, or in some cases even disc herniation or rupture. It is costly in loss of salary and medical expenses. The important point is that it is preventable.

When the parts of the skeletal system are aligned, balance can be maintained (Figure 4-4). *Balance* is the maintaining of an object in a steady position so that it does not tip or fall. To maintain balance, the body must have a wide *base of support.* In a standing position, the feet are the base of support. The *center of gravity* is located at the center of the pelvis just below the umbilicus. To maintain balance, the center of gravity must fall within the base of support (between the feet). When the center of gravity falls out-

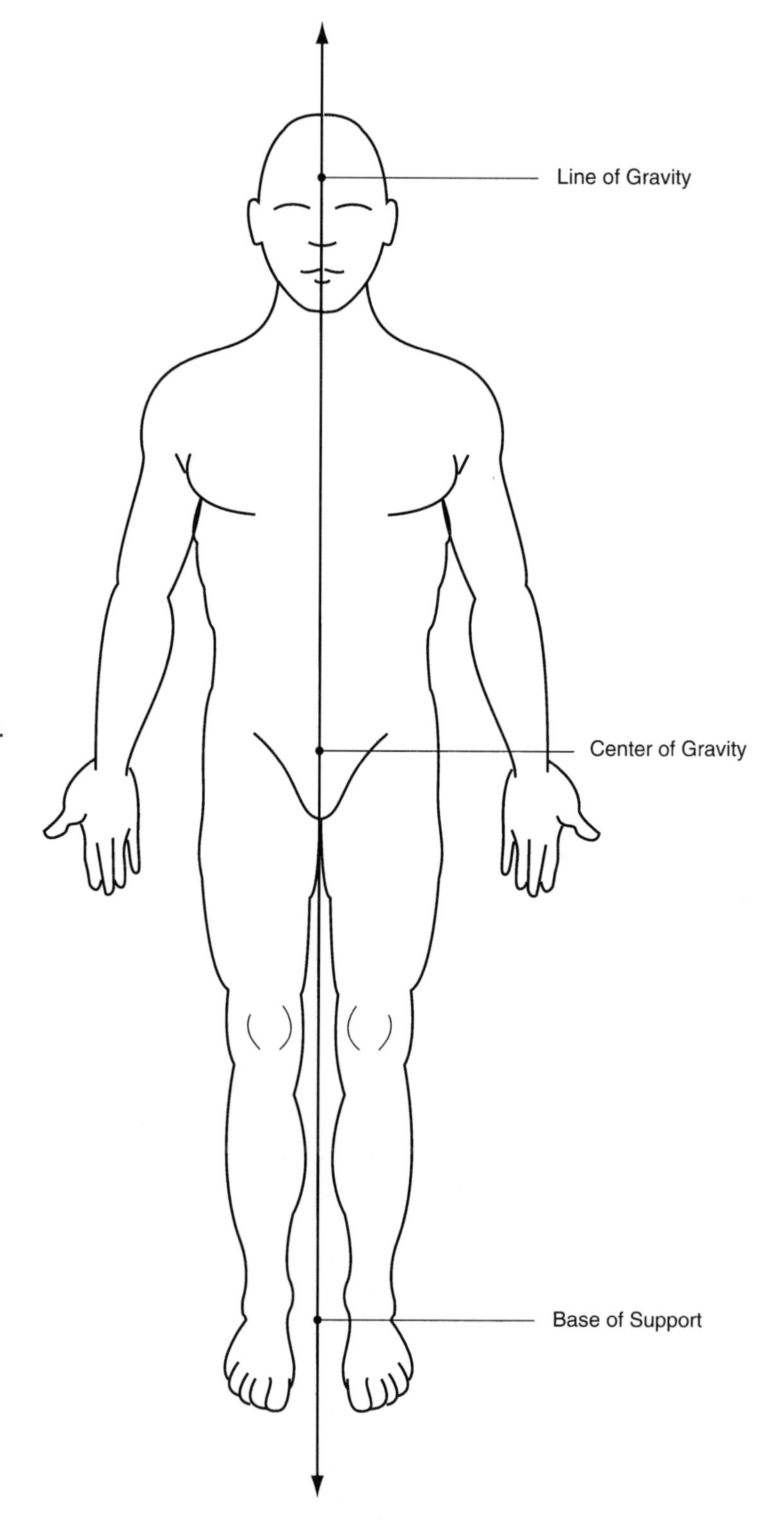

Figure 4-4
Maintaining balance through body alignment. (Reprinted with permission from Weiss, R.C. *Your Career in Administrative Medical Services.* Philadelphia: W. B. Saunders, 1996, p. 28.)

side of the base of support, you will lose stability or balance. The *line of gravity* is an imaginary vertical line that passes through the center of gravity.

In order to use your muscles most efficiently and prevent the possibility of muscle strain or other injury, there are certain guidelines you can follow when lifting objects or helping patients. These include:

- Always remembering to size up the load and never lifting more than you feel comfortable lifting. When in doubt, get help!
- Always remembering to stand with your feet shoulder width apart or with one foot slightly in front of the other.
- If you have to squat, always remember to bend at your knees, never at your waist. The latter will only add more stress to your back.
- Always remembering to bring the load close to your body, using a firm grip with both hands.
- Always remembering, when lifting an object, to tighten your abdominal muscles, and then lift the load using your leg muscles.

It's important to remember that even lifting very light loads can result in injury if you do not use proper body mechanics. Using good posture and body mechanics in your everyday work will decrease the amount of energy expended and provide more ease and grace in your movements. The knowledge of proper body mechanics and alignment will help you prevent injury to yourself and to others (Figure 4-5 on p. 30).

Providing a Safe Environment

The makeup of the physical medicine or physical therapy departments are important to the well-being of the patient. The goal is to have a therapeutic or healing environment. Therefore, it is the responsibility of all members of the physical medicine team to provide continuously for safety, privacy, and order.

You must be constantly alert to provide safe care in every treatment and procedure done for each and every patient. A safe environment will help prevent injuries and potential lawsuits. Falls, which are among the leading causes of lawsuits in the hospital environment, can be prevented by taking a few thought-out precautions, including:

- Keeping the floor clean and dry and putting things away as soon as you are through using them.
- Cleaning up all spills immediately after they occur.
- Checking with the nursing station before you perform a procedure on a patient whose level of consciousness or orientation you are unsure of.
- Giving extra attention to patients with vision or hearing impairments.

Any time you are required to use an electrically operated piece of equipment, you must make sure it is in proper working condition. Make sure there are no frayed wires or faulty plugs. Report equipment problems to your supervisor, and move faulty equipment out of patient care areas so that it will not be used accidently.

Another aspect to creating a safe environment is providing for your patient's privacy. Privacy is the legal right of every patient, and anytime you are required to perform a procedure, you must also provide for the patient's privacy. Always remember to knock before entering a patient's room or a treatment area. If you are performing a procedure that requires the patient to disrobe, always make sure that you only expose the part of the body needed for the procedure. And if you must perform the procedure in the patient's hospital room, make sure you remember to have the privacy curtain pulled around the patient. Remember, as health care workers, we are accustomed to situations that would be embarrassing to the average person. Therefore, always be aware of providing for the privacy of each of your patients.

Finally, another very important aspect of a safe environment is knowing your hospital or facility floor plan regarding exits, locations of fire extinguishers, and how to use them. Make a point of finding out how to report a fire. Many clinics and hospitals have special code words which alert the entire building of fires and emergencies. You should know these codes and be aware of your responsibilities if an emergency does occur in your facility.

Common Emergencies

A safe environment also means being aware of potential crisis or emergency situations and then responding appropriately. Patients want to feel that you will know what to do if an emergency does occur. Naturally, any emergency should be reported to your supervisor immediately.

A common emergency is fainting, which is the temporary loss of consciousness. This occurs quite often and is not considered a serious malady. It is generally associated with illness or emotional stress. The patient shows pallor, sweating, and a slow, weak pulse that later becomes rapid. To treat the patient, first check the pulse, respiration, and blood pressure, and make sure the airway is open, elevate the patient's feet, and provide supportive care.

Another type of common emergency which you may encounter is a convulsive seizure. This is a disorder of the central nervous system which is character-

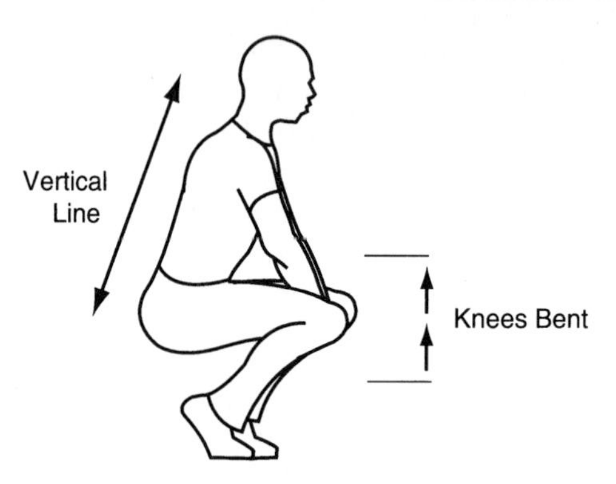

A. Lifting Heavy Objects

Figure 4-5
Using correct body alignment to prevent injuries. (Reprinted with permission from Weiss, R.C. *Your Career in Administrative Medical Services.* Philadelphia: W. B. Saunders, 1996, p. 30.)

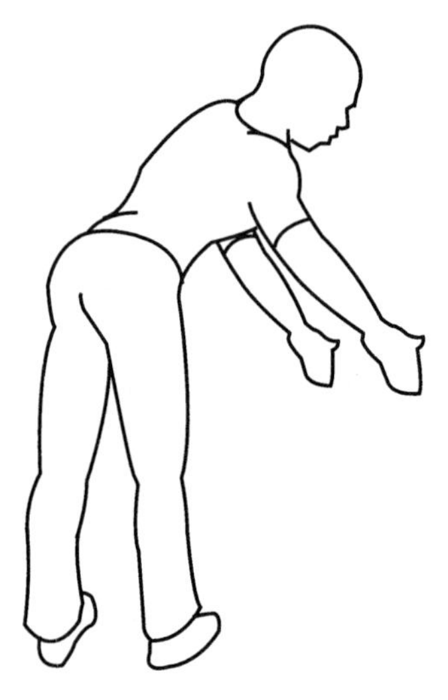

B. Twisting Incorrectly

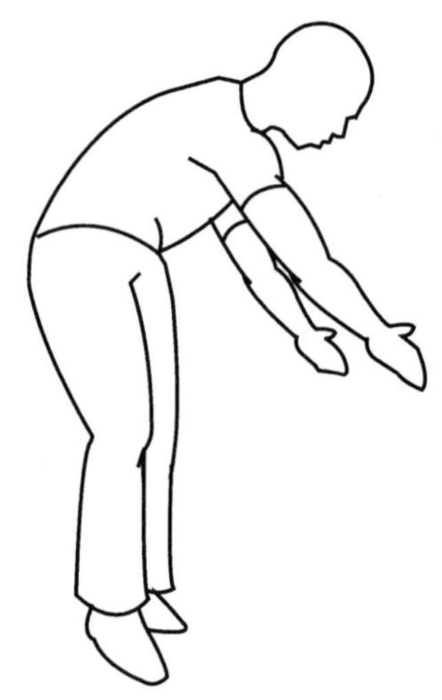

Twisting Correctly

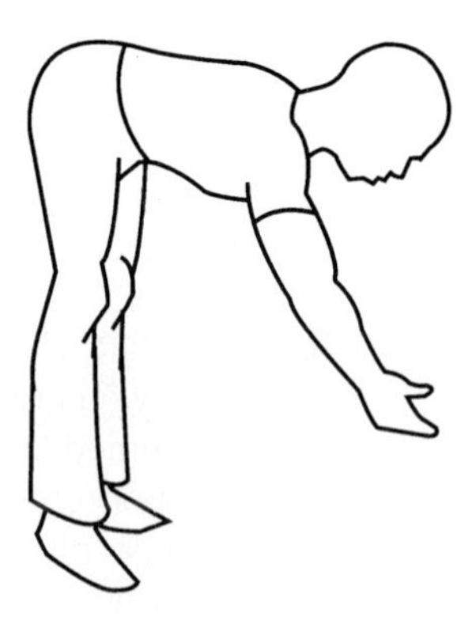

C. Bending Incorrectly

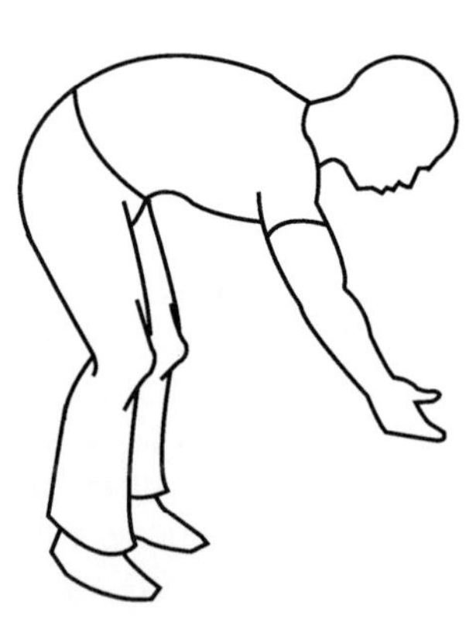

Bending Correctly

ized by recurrent attacks. It generally involves changes in the patient's level of consciousness, motor activity, or sensory phenomena. The onset is usually sudden and lasts only a brief time. The individual convulses, falls to the floor, and, in some cases, exhibits violent, involuntary muscle contractions.

The aim of treatment during a seizure is to prevent the person from injuring him- or herself. Move furniture out of the way, loosen the clothing around the person's neck, and place a pillow or soft roll under the person's head. After the seizure is over, the patient will be sleepy and lethargic. Rest should be encouraged.

A fall, which may lead to contusions, sprains, or dislocations, is another common emergency, and as we have already noted, is one of the leading causes of lawsuits in the hospital environment. A contusion or bruise is an injury to muscle and soft tissue as a result of a blunt force. Discoloration occurs when small capillaries break and leak into the tissue. The area is usually quite painful and generally causes swelling.

To treat a sprain, gently apply cold compresses or ice packs to the area. This will cause vasoconstriction, which slows the internal bleeding and thus decreases the pain. The injured part should be elevated and wrapped in an elastic bandage for compression and support.

An emergency which could have a deadly result is cardiac arrest. In this very critical situation there is a sudden stoppage of the heart. The patient loses consciousness, stops breathing, and has no pulse and no heart sounds. Time is the most important factor in resuscitation. You must quickly assess the situation and call for help. A delay of more than four to six minutes could result in irreversible brain damage. As a member of the community, as well as the health care delivery team, you must be familiar with standard cardiopulmonary resuscitation (CPR) techniques, and if necessary, begin rescue breathing or CPR immediately.

Maintaining the Treatment Area

By keeping your department neat, you will be doing a big part toward helping to keep things running smoothly. You will also find that your own work, as well as everyone else's, is much easier once there is a system for keeping everything in order. As soon as possible, you should learn exactly where different articles, equipment, and supplies are kept and always return them to the same place. This keeps the shelves, cabinets, and treatment rooms in a state of readiness. Shelves should be labeled so that everyone will know at a glance where a particular item is located. Tabletops should be kept clear and clean so that there is always work space. Wastebaskets should be emptied regularly, and the rest of the department should be kept clean and in perfect working order.

Equipment should be checked often and cleaned with the recommended disinfectant after being used. Moveable equipment should be placed where it will not tilt or roll. Water should be drained from the autoclave or sterilizer after each use. And it is a good idea to frequently check with your supervisor for any ideas or suggestions regarding changes in the normal cleanup routine of the department.

An inventory is also important in any department. A good reference file, listing the names, addresses, and telephone numbers of the companies from which supplies and equipment can be ordered should be kept. Prices and order numbers of supplies and equipment are usually listed with information supplied from the company. Supplies on hand should be checked often so that new supplies may be ordered before they are needed, but do not order more supplies than will be used in a reasonable length of time. Storage space should be available for anything that is ordered. If you are required to keep the inventory for your department, always make sure that you have your list approved by the department supervisor before you make out a requisition or take an order.

Any equipment needing repairs should be reported to your supervisor as soon as possible. Never try to repair the equipment or take advice from another employee who is not qualified to repair the equipment because more damage and greater costs may result. Most equipment requires certification as being safe before it can be used for patient care or client use.

Medical supplies are very expensive. Therefore, you should only use what is necessary and return reusable supplies to their proper places. In some institutions, supplies are ordered for each individual receiving treatment. This is especially true when ordering medications, dressings, and bandages. Wise use of medical supplies in your department will decrease the cost of the patient's medical care, which will ultimately decrease the costs for the medical facility, thus putting additional monies back into your pocket in the form of increases in salary.

Summary

In this chapter, we discussed the important aspects of health and safety in the health care environment. We talked about medical and surgical asepsis and infection control procedures, noting the importance of each in the protection of the patient, the client, and the health care worker. We also discussed awareness of posture and maintenance of good body alignment and use of proper body mechanics. We explained the role safety played in the health care environment and discussed some of the more common emergencies which could be avoided through the proper maintenance of a safe clinical environment. Finally, we discussed how to properly maintain the physical medicine environment and its individual treatment areas and departments, noting that it is the responsibility of all members of the health care delivery team to maintain the department and its individual surroundings in a state of readiness and order.

Review Questions

1. Briefly define the concept of *medical asepsis.*

2. What does the term *alignment* mean?

3. A one-celled microorganism which is capable of causing fermentation, decay, and in some cases disease, is called ______________.

4. What type of infection is acquired by the patient while being cared for in the hospital?
   a. bacteriological
   b. nosocomial
   c. viral

5. ______________ pertains to keeping an object in a steady position or stable.
   a. alignment
   b. center of gravity
   c. balance

6. The point at which an object rests, when the body is upright, is called:
   a. base of support
   b. center of gravity
   c. line of gravity

7. An ______________ is a process which occurs when pathogens attack a person and then produce signs and symptoms of an illness.

8. Briefly explain the *infection cycle.*

9. What is the easiest and best way a health care provider can prevent the spread of bacteria?

10. What is the name of the process used to kill all microorganisms?
    a. disinfection
    b. sterilization
    c. sanitization

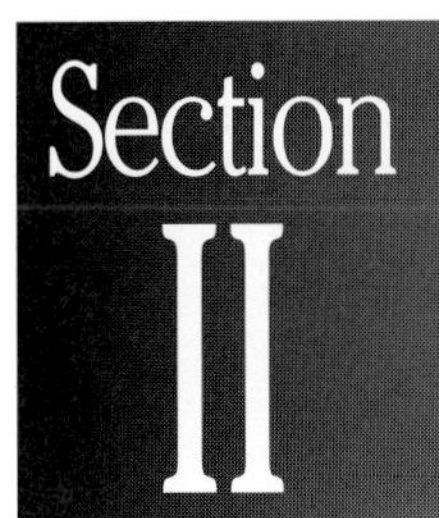

Scientific Principles in Physical Medicine

5

Basic Structure and Function of the Human Body

Performance Objectives

Upon completion of this chapter, you will be able to:

1. Identify the various systems of the human body and briefly explain the individual structures, components, and functions of each.
2. Identify common disorders of each of the systems of the body.

Terms and Abbreviations

Arthritis disease of the musculoskeletal system in which there is an inflammation of bones at the joints with accompanying pain and swelling of the joints.

Fracture a common bone injury in which there is a break in a bone; may be a simple fracture, a compound fracture in which there is a break in the skin, or a greenstick fracture in which the fracture is incomplete and which is most often seen in children.

Ligaments structures which hold bones together.

Musculoskeletal system all the bones, joints, and muscles in the body.

Prostatism any condition which results in the obstruction of the prostate gland along with retention of urine in the bladder.

Tendons structures which attach muscles to bones.

The human body is a miraculous piece of work which consists of many individual structures, organs, and systems, all of which work both independently and as part of a team whose overall goal is the ongoing preservation of life. While you may not be involved in the actual hands-on care and treatment of patients, other than those suffering from a disorder or injury of the musculoskeletal system, as a member of the physical medicine health care team it is still important for you to have a basic understanding of the rest of the individual systems that make up the human body so that you can better comprehend why patients seek medical care in the first place. A basic knowledge of these very important concepts will almost guarantee you the ability to perform your job in a much more efficient and effective manner.

Systems of the Human Body

The human body is comprised of nine systems. These include the musculoskeletal system, the digestive system, the circulatory system, the respiratory system, the nervous system, the integumentary system, the urinary system, the endocrine system, and the reproductive system.

The Musculoskeletal System

The *musculoskeletal system,* which is made up of all the bones, joints, and muscles of our body, provides us with the ability to stand erect while at the same time protects us from falling and injuring our-

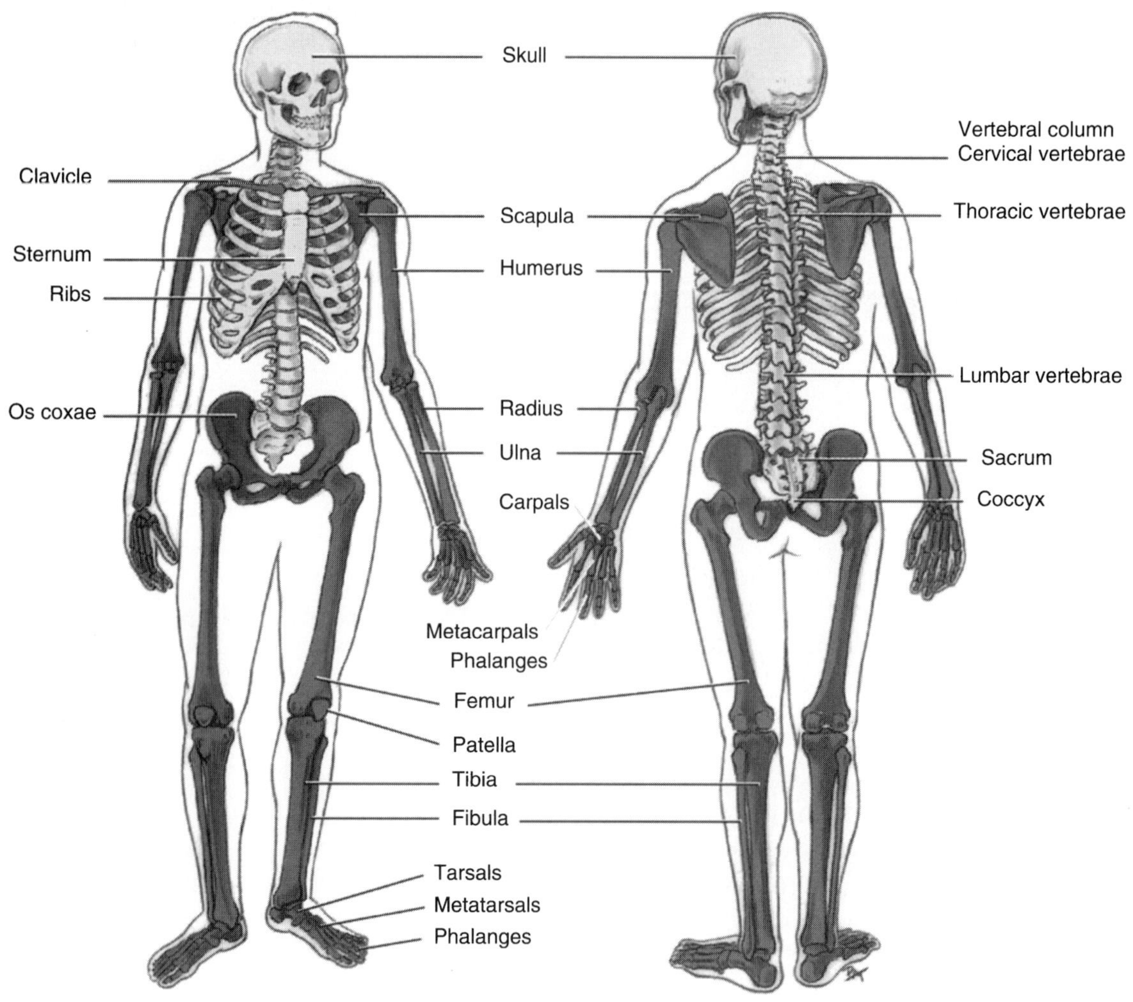

Figure 5-1a
The skeletal system. (Reprinted with permission from Applegate, E.J. *The Anatomy and Physiology Learning System.* Philadelphia: W. B. Saunders, 1995, p. 101.)

selves (Figures 5-1a, 5-1b, and 5-1c [on p. 38]). The three types of muscles which are found in this system include skeletal, or voluntary muscles, which are connected to bone and make it possible for voluntary movement, such as walking or picking up an object from the floor; smooth, or involuntary muscles, which cannot be controlled by our will, but rather, by the autonomic nervous system, which includes such muscles as those found in the digestive and respiratory systems; and cardiac muscle, which makes up the heart wall.

All the bones of the body together make up the skeleton. The skeleton has three general functions: movement, because skeletal muscles are attached to bones; support of the body; and protection of our vital organs, such as the heart or our liver.

The point at which two bones come together is called a joint. There are many different kinds of joints, each with a different function. Some joints allow us to bend our elbow, fingers, or knees. These are called hinge joints. Another type of joint is called an immovable joint, such as the junctions of the bones of the adult skull. These joints help protect our brain.

Tendons and ligaments are actually parts of the musculoskeletal system. *Tendons* attach muscles to bones, while *ligaments* hold the bones together at the joints.

Common Disorders of the Musculoskeletal System

The most common injury or disorder of the musculoskeletal system is a *fracture,* which is any break in a bone. While there are several different types of fractures, the most commonly seen include *simple fractures,* which occur without resulting in a break in the skin, *compound fractures,* which involve breakage of soft tissue with the broken bone protruding through the skin, and *greenstick fractures,* which are incomplete breaks in the bone fibers, and which most often occur in children.

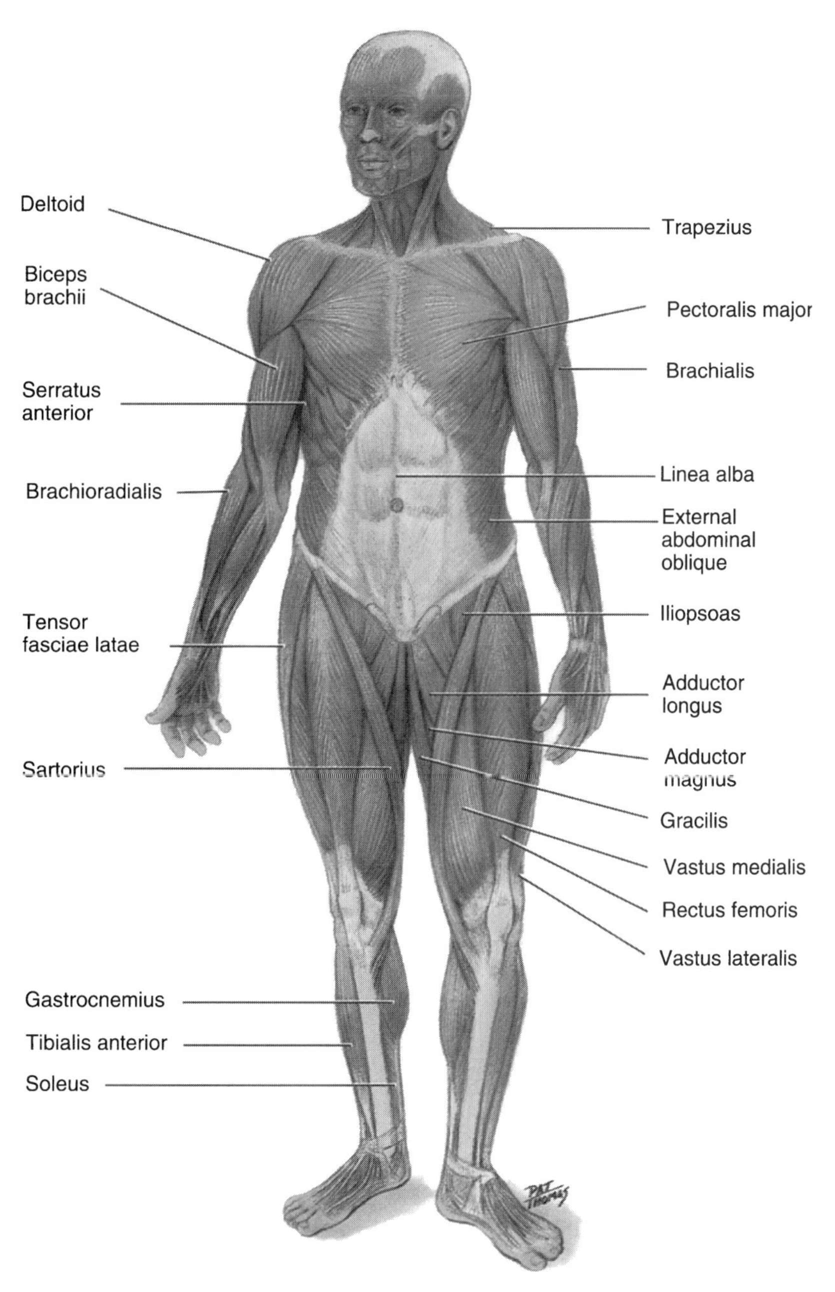

Figure 5-1b
The muscular system (anterior view). (Reprinted with permission from Applegate, E.J. *The Anatomy and Physiology Learning System.* Philadelphia: W. B. Saunders, 1995, pp. 145–146.)

In addition to fractures, the most common disorders and injuries to the musculoskeletal system include dislocations, sprains, and strains. A dislocation, which is almost always accompanied by torn or stretched ligaments, is a bone injury in which a bone is moved from its normal position in a joint. A sprain is an injury that occurs when a joint moves too far, thus resulting in overstretching or tearing of the ligaments. Back sprains or sprained ankles are common types of injuries. Muscle strains result from simply overworking the muscles. They are usually accompanied by a great deal of soreness and pain.

A disease considered quite common to the musculoskeletal system is *arthritis.* It is a disorder involving an inflammation of the bones at the joints, which is often accompanied by pain and swelling of the joints. Arthritis is most often seen in older patients.

The Digestive System

The digestive system includes the mouth, throat, esophagus, stomach, small and large intestines, and closely associated glands and organs (Figure 5-2 on p. 39). Its function is to digest food, or to change it from an insoluble to a soluble form. This is accomplished through a process of action between the chemicals and the digestive juices.

The first part of the digestive tract is the mouth. Here the food is torn apart and then ground up by the teeth. Digestion begins in the mouth as saliva mixes

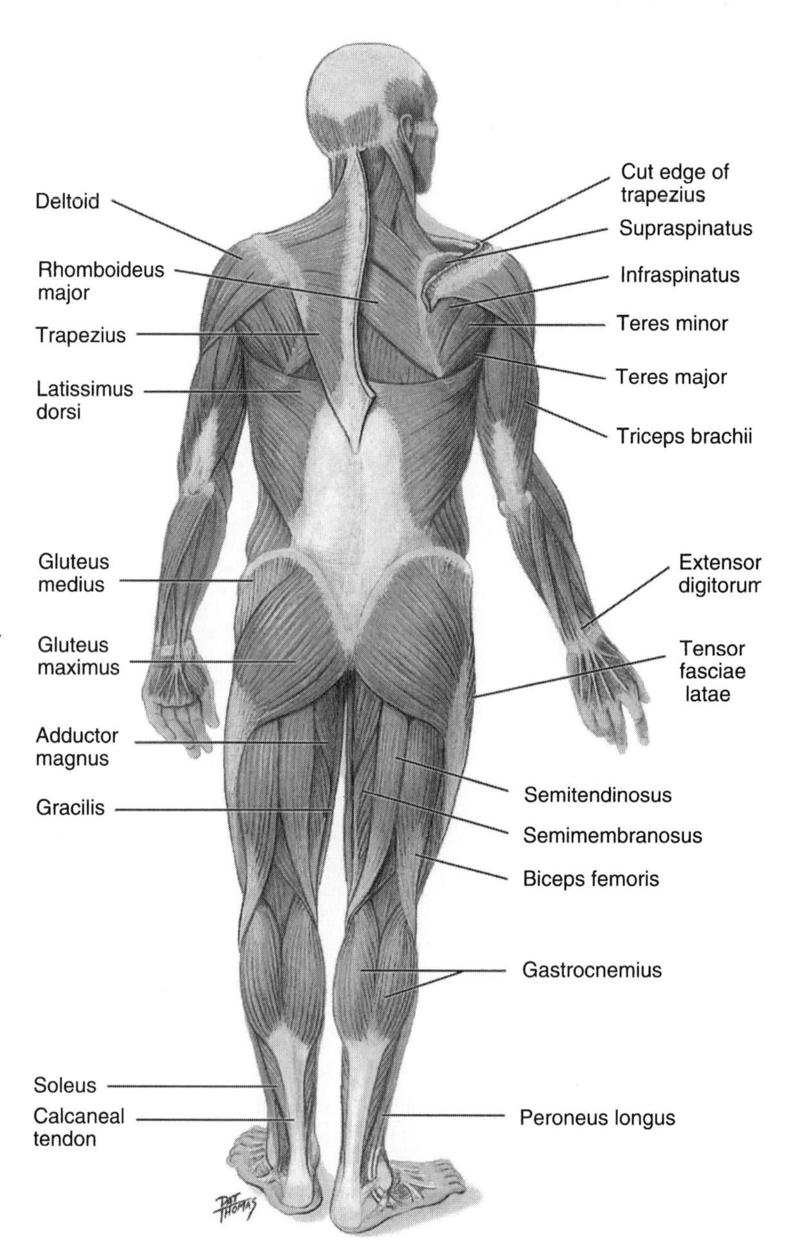

Figure 5-1c
The muscular system (posterior view). (Reprinted with per-mission from Applegate, E.J. *The Anatomy and Physiology Learning System.* Philadel-phia: W. B. Saunders, 1995, pp. 145–146.)

with and then acts on the food. The food then passes through the throat or pharynx as it is swallowed and eventually goes through the esophagus to the stomach. Food remains in the stomach from four to six hours. During this time, it is churned by the action of smooth muscles in the stomach and is mixed with digestive juices secreted by stomach glands.

Food passes from the stomach into the small intestine, which is about 20 feet in length and is arranged in coils and loops held in place by a thin sheet of tissue called the mesentery. The small intestine is divided into three parts. The first part is called the duodenum, which is eight to ten inches long. The second part is called the jejunum, which is six to nine feet long. The final part of the small intestine is called the ileum. Most digestion occurs in the duodenum. Bile from the liver and juice from the pancreas empty into the duodenum. These juices, along with the secretion of glands in the small intestine, carry on most of the digestion of the food. The digested food is then absorbed from the lining of the small intestine and enters the bloodstream.

After food has been carried through the small intestine, the undigested food residue eventually moves into the large intestine. The large intestine consists of the cecum, the appendix, the ascending, transverse, and descending colons, the rectum, and the anus. The last part is the external opening of the digestive system. Food is not digested in the large intestine, but water and minerals are absorbed there. The food is moved through the entire digestive tract by wavelike contractions of the intestines called peristalsis.

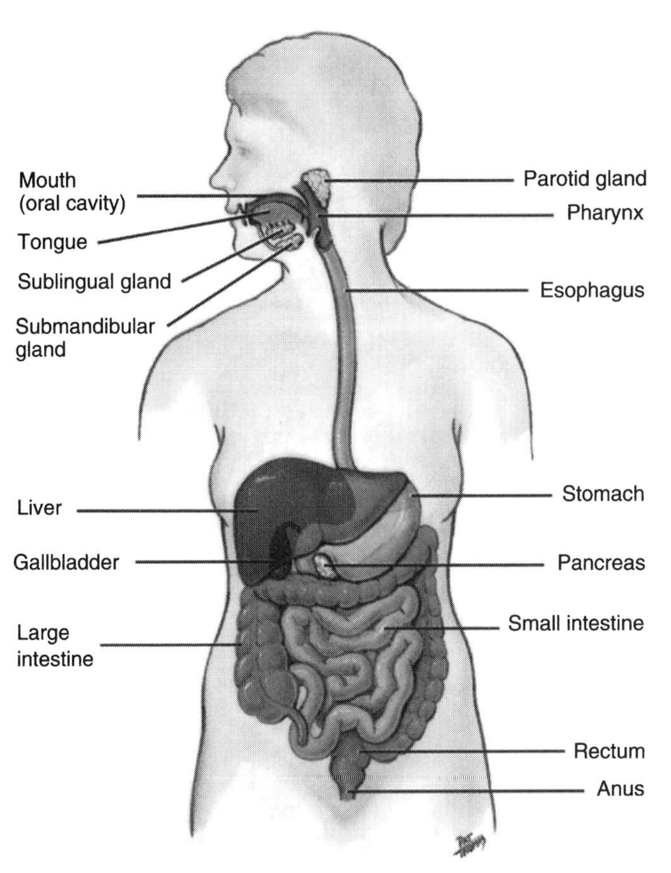

Figure 5-2
The digestive system. (Reprinted with permission from Applegate, E.J. *The Anatomy and Physiology Learning System.* Philadelphia: W. B. Saunders, 1995, p. 328.)

Disorders and diseases of the digestive system are very common. Many of these include inflammatory conditions. Those most often seen include appendicitis, which is an inflammation of the appendix; cirrhosis, which is a chronic liver disease, often caused by excessive alcohol intake; constipation, an abnormal delay in, or infrequent bowel movements; diarrhea, abnormally frequent, watery bowel movements; gastritis, an inflammatory condition of the stomach lining; and heartburn, which is a burning sensation experienced in the stomach. Other conditions seen frequently include hepatitis, which is an inflammation of the liver, nausea, and ulcers, which occur in an area of the stomach or small intestine where the tissues are gradually disintegrating.

The Circulatory System

The circulatory system is made up of the heart, blood vessels, and blood (Figure 5-3 on p. 40). Its main function is to send the blood throughout all parts of our body, carrying with it digested food and oxygen, and then return it to the heart carrying waste products of metabolism.

The heart is a hollow, cone-shaped organ which is about the size of your fist when it is closed. It has four separate chambers, and is located in the center of the chest cavity with the tip pointing slightly to the left. It is well protected by the ribs and sternum. The function of the heart is to pump blood to every part of the body.

Blood vessels of the circulatory system include the arteries, which carry blood away from the heart; veins, which return the blood to the heart; and capillaries, which are small vessels that connect arteries to veins. The blood vessels you are most likely to find discussed at your facility are the aorta, which is the largest artery of the body, located along the spinal column, and the coronary arteries and veins that supply the heart.

The blood which is carried throughout our body is a very complex fluid. It is made up of red blood cells, called erythrocytes, white blood cells, called leukocytes, and platelets. The red blood cells carry oxygen to every cell in the body. The white blood cells destroy pathogenic bacteria and thereby help the body to combat diseases caused by bacterial infection. Platelets are involved in the clotting mechanism of blood.

The lymphatic system is also part of the circulatory system. Lymph is a clear, colorless fluid which is formed in tissue spaces throughout the body. It collects in tiny lymph capillaries and is eventually carried to even larger lymph vessels until finally it empties into the blood. The lymph vessels pass through the lymph nodes, which then filter out any foreign

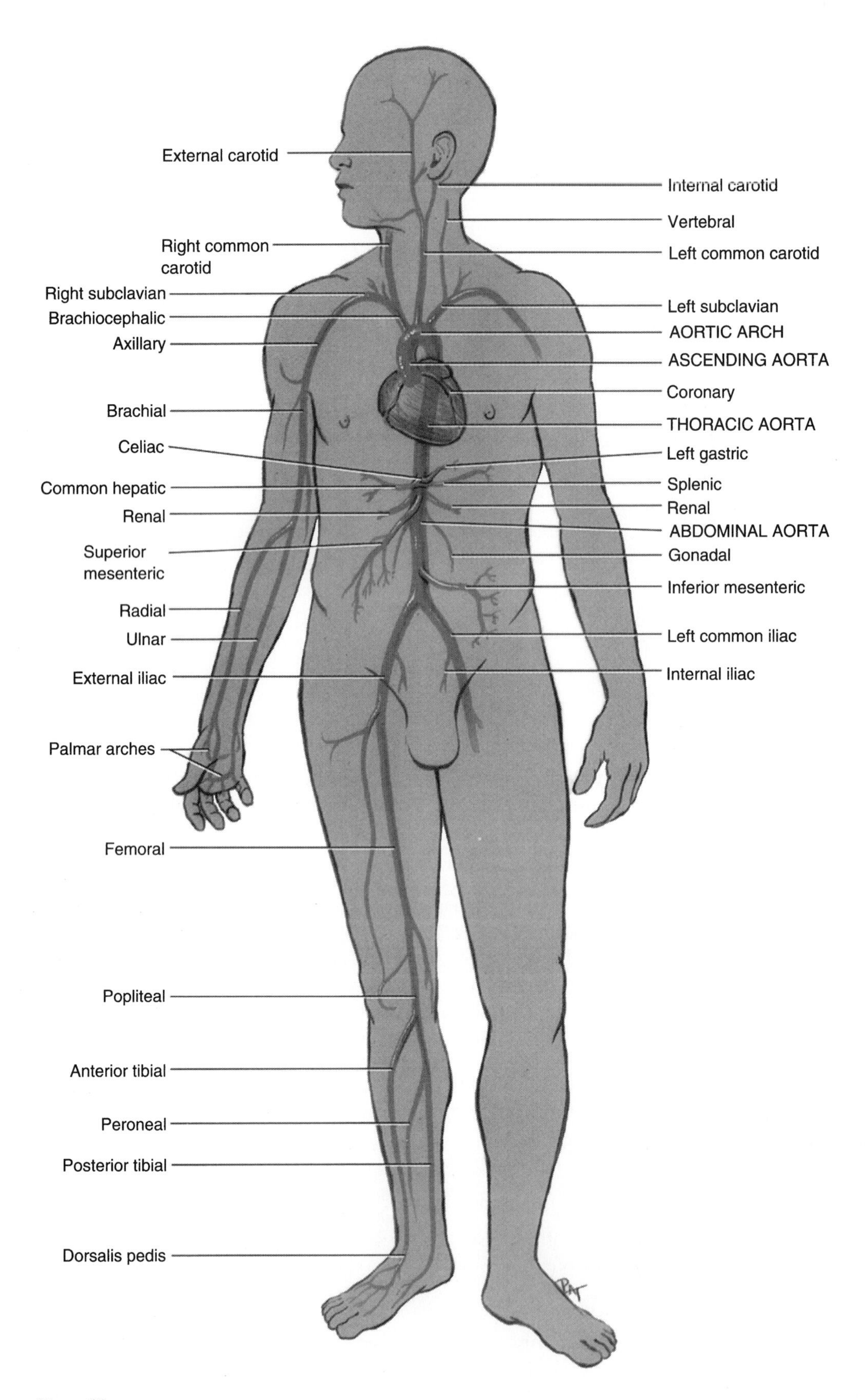

Figure 5-3
The circulatory system. (Reprinted with permission from Applegate, E.J. *The Anatomy and Physiology Learning System.* Philadelphia: W. B. Saunders, 1995, p. 272.)

particles. Sometimes lymph nodes become infected because they filter out bacteria which may then invade the nodes themselves.

When discussing the circulatory system, we must also mention pulse and blood pressure. Pulse is the rhythmic throbbing which can be felt in an artery as a result of the heart beating. The pulse rate, rhythm, and strength are all indicators of health or the presence of disease. Blood pressure is the pressure that blood exerts on the inside walls of blood vessels. The systolic blood pressure is the pressure measured during the time in which the heart muscle is contracting. Diastolic blood pressure is the pressure measured during the time the heart muscle is relaxing. Blood pressure is reported as two figures, systolic pressure over diastolic pressure, such as 120/80.

Many patients coming into the medical office or being admitted into the health care facility will have diseases and disorders of the circulatory system. The most common of these include the following:

- *anemia:* a condition in which the blood is deficient in the number of red blood cells or in hemoglobin.
- *arteriosclerosis:* a condition in which there is a thickening, hardening, and loss of elasticity of the blood vessels.
- *congestive heart failure:* a condition which occurs when there is a failure of the heart to maintain an adequate output of blood in order to meet the demands of the body.
- *coronary occlusion:* an obstruction of a coronary artery.
- *myocardial infarction:* also referred to as a heart attack, in which damage to the heart muscle has occurred as a result of diminished blood supply to the heart muscle from a coronary occlusion.
- *hemorrhage:* extensive loss of blood.
- *Hodgkin's disease:* a disease of unknown cause, which affects the lymph nodes.
- *hypertension:* an abnormally high blood pressure.
- *heart murmur:* an abnormal heart sound.
- *phlebitis:* an inflammation of a vein.
- *varicose veins:* dilation of veins, often occurring in the legs.

The Respiratory System

The function of the respiratory system is to bring air containing oxygen into the body and at the same time eliminate carbon dioxide and water. Each body cell must have a constant supply of oxygen and must also get rid of carbon dioxide.

Figure 5-4 illustrates the structures of the respiratory system, which include the nasal cavities; the sinuses; the pharynx, which is the throat; the larynx, or voice box, which contains the vocal chords that make speech possible; the trachea, a short tube extending from the larynx to the bronchi; the bronchi, which lead to the lungs; the lungs are a pair of lobed organs found

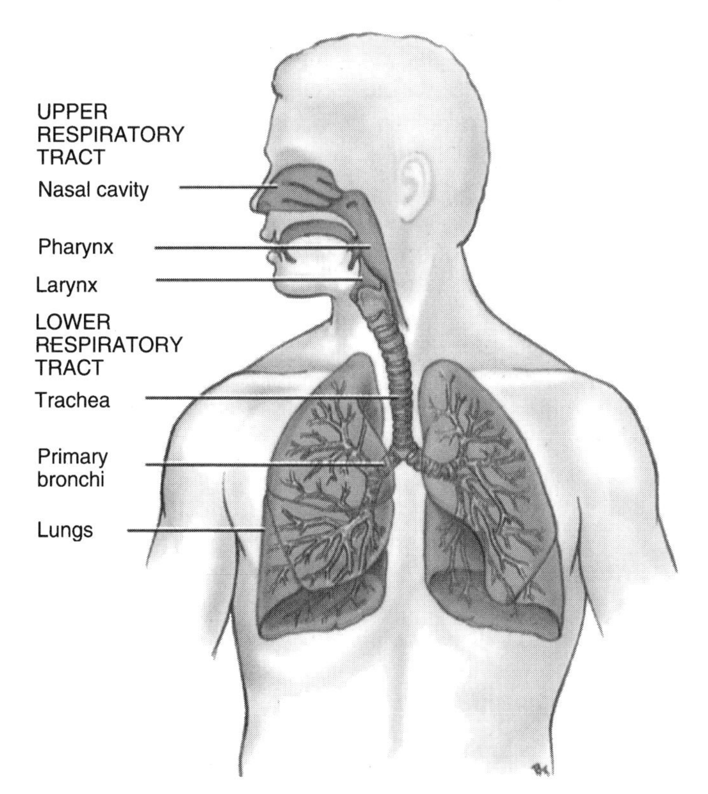

Figure 5-4
The respiratory system. (Reprinted with permission from Applegate, E.J. *The Anatomy and Physiology Learning System.* Philadelphia: W. B. Saunders, 1995, p. 306.)

in the thorax or chest cavity; and the diaphragm, a sheet of muscle that separates the abdominal and chest cavities. The contraction of the diaphragm forces air into the lungs. The pleura is the membrane that covers the lungs and lines the chest cavity.

Air is brought into the lungs as the diaphragm contracts. It then passes through the nasal cavity, the pharynx, larynx, trachea, bronchi, and finally into the lungs. The actual exchange of oxygen with carbon dioxide takes place through the thin cell walls of the alveoli by the process of diffusion. Oxygen from the alveoli enters the blood and is carried to every cell. Carbon dioxide then returns to the alveoli and is eventually exhaled.

The most common disorders of the respiratory system include

- *asthma:* an allergic reaction in which the bronchioles swell, making breathing difficult.
- *bronchitis:* an inflammatory condition of the bronchi.
- *common cold:* the most widespread of all communicable diseases, characterized by swollen and inflamed mucous membranes and discharge from the nose and throat.
- *emphysema:* a condition which causes a swelling of the alveoli due to chronic bronchial obstruction, and which is common in heavy smokers.
- *influenza:* a disease characterized by inflammation of the upper respiratory tract, with generalized aches and pains, and which is highly contagious.
- *pleurisy:* an inflammation of the pleura.
- *pneumonia:* an inflammation of the alveoli of the lung which may be caused by bacteria or viruses.
- *tuberculosis:* either an acute or chronic condition caused by the tubercle bacillus usually affecting the respiratory system.

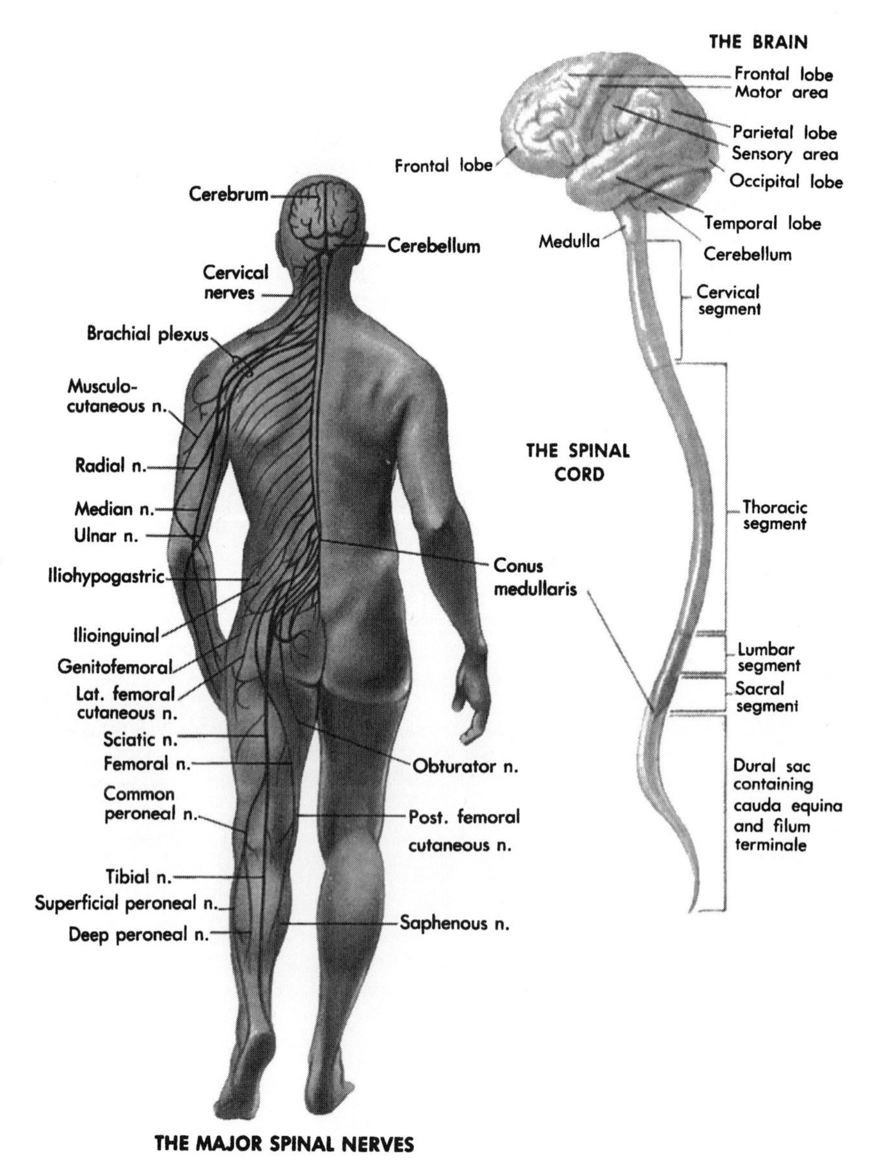

Figure 5-5
The nervous system: (a) Brain and spinal nerves; (b) autonomic nerves. (Reprinted with permission from Bonewit, K. *Clinical Procedures for Medical Assistants,* 3rd ed. Philadelphia: W. B. Saunders, 1995 plates 13 and 14.)

The Nervous System

The nervous system is our body's main communications system. It consists of three parts: the central nervous system, which is made up of the brain and the spinal cord; the peripheral nervous system, consisting of the nerves extending to the outlying parts of the body; and the autonomic nervous system, which controls all of our involuntary functions, such as the digestive system or the respiratory system (Figures 5-5a and 5-5b). The nervous system also includes the sensory organs, structures which make up our eyes and ears, our sense of taste, smell, touch, temperature, pain, pressure, and balance.

Common disorders of the nervous system generally include cerebrovascular accidents, often referred to as stroke, in which there is a destruction of brain tissue as a result of hemorrhage from blood vessels of the brain; epilepsy, which is a chronic disorder with abnormality of brain functions, sometimes referred to

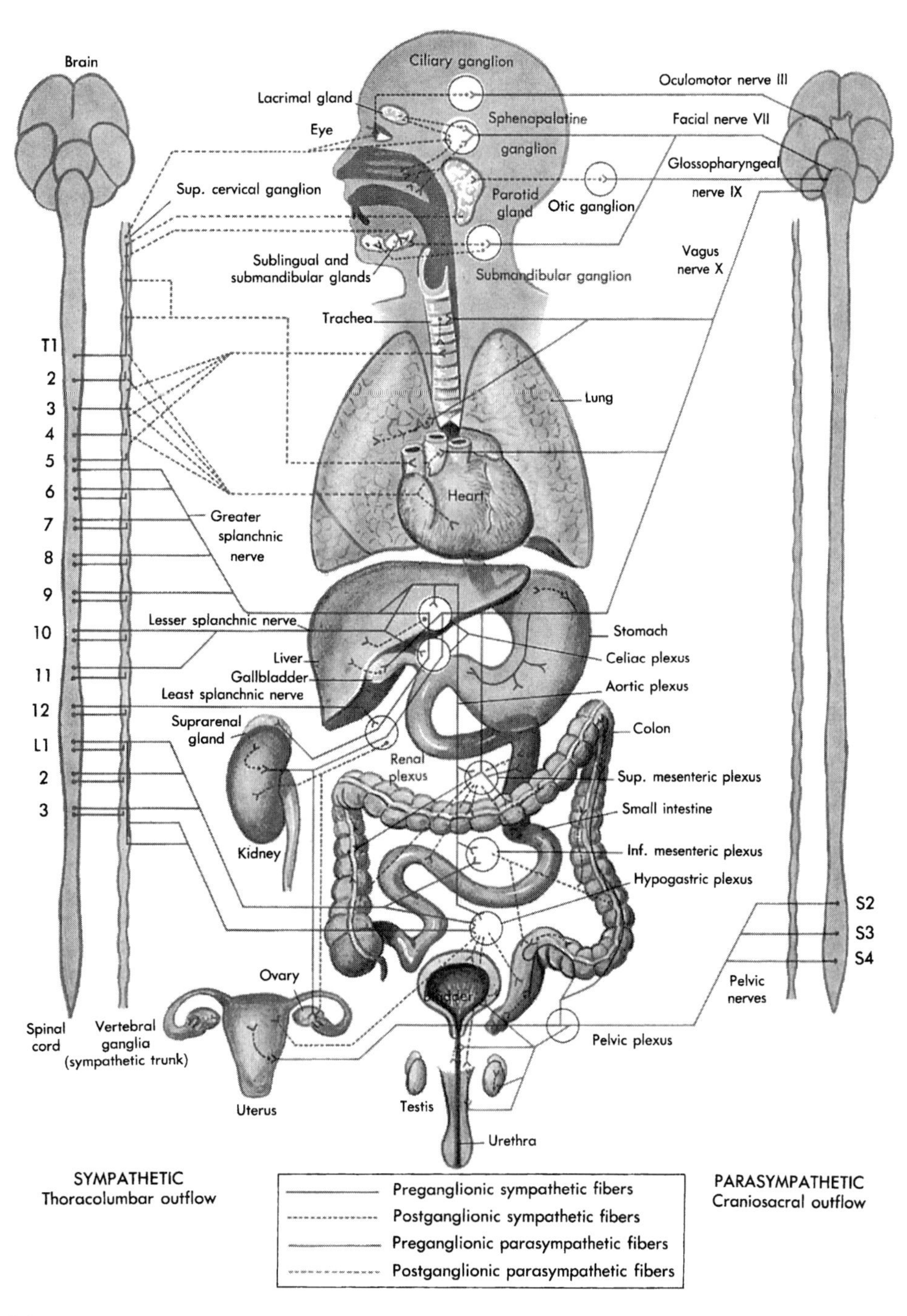

(b)

Figure 5-5
(Continued)

as convulsive seizures; meningitis, an inflammatory condition involving the membrane covering the brain and the spinal cord; paralysis, which is a temporary or permanent loss of functions, often accompanied by loss of sensation or voluntary motion; poliomyelitis, a less commonly seen acute viral disease which may destroy nerve cells and cause paralysis; shingles, a condition caused by a formation of blisters along the course of a nerve, most often affecting the intercostal nerves; and vertigo, often referred to as dizziness.

The Integumentary System

The skin, which is the largest organ of the body, is made up of a thin layer that covers the entire body (Figure 5-6). Sometimes called the integument or integumentary system, its function includes excreting excess waste materials, protection of deeper tissues, regulation of body heat, and providing us with information about the environment, such as temperature, pain, or pressure through its receptors. The integumentary system also has accessory organs. These organs include the hair, nails, sweat glands, and the oil glands.

Common disorders of the integumentary system include wounds, or lesions, and skin diseases, such as athlete's foot, acne, and fever blisters.

The Urinary System

The primary function of the urinary system is the excretion of the body's waste products. Figure 5-7 shows the parts of the urinary system. The kidneys are a pair of bean-shaped organs located on the back of the abdominal wall. Their function is to filter waste materials from the blood. The ureters are tubes that extend from the kidneys to the urinary bladder. The urinary bladder is the sac in which urine is collected. The urethra is the tube from the urinary bladder that extends to the exterior, or outside of the body.

The blood flows to the kidneys where waste products such as urea, uric acid, and various salts are filtered out. The waste product, urine, flows from the kidney through the ureters to the urinary bladder. The filtered and cleansed blood is then returned to the circulatory system. The urine is excreted from the bladder through the urethra.

Common disorders of the urinary system include cystitis, which is an inflammatory or infectious condition of the urinary bladder; nephritis, or Bright's disease, in which there is severe inflammation of the kidneys; uremia, a condition in which wastes normally excreted by the kidneys are retained in the blood; and urinary calculi, which are kidney stones.

The Endocrine System

The endocrine system is made up of several glands that produce hormones (Figure 5-8). Hormones are chemical substances that regulate the function of other organs.

The pituitary gland is located at the underside of the brain. It secretes several different hormones, each

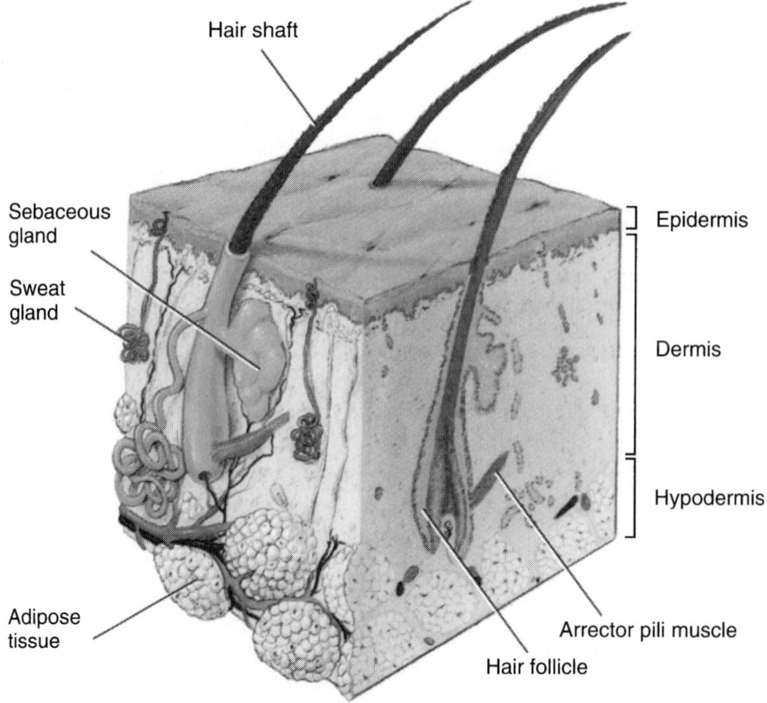

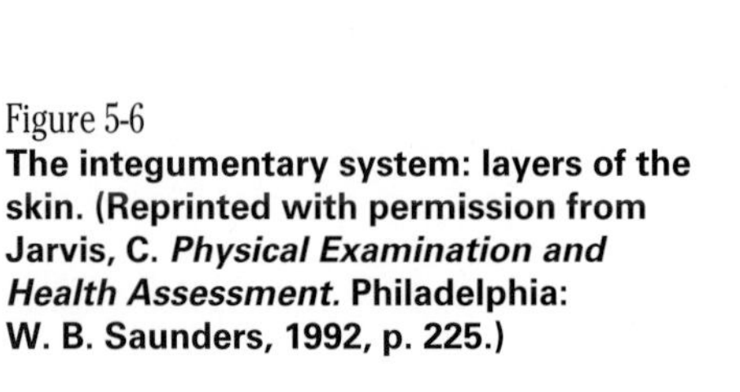
Figure 5-6
The integumentary system: layers of the skin. (Reprinted with permission from Jarvis, C. *Physical Examination and Health Assessment.* Philadelphia: W. B. Saunders, 1992, p. 225.)

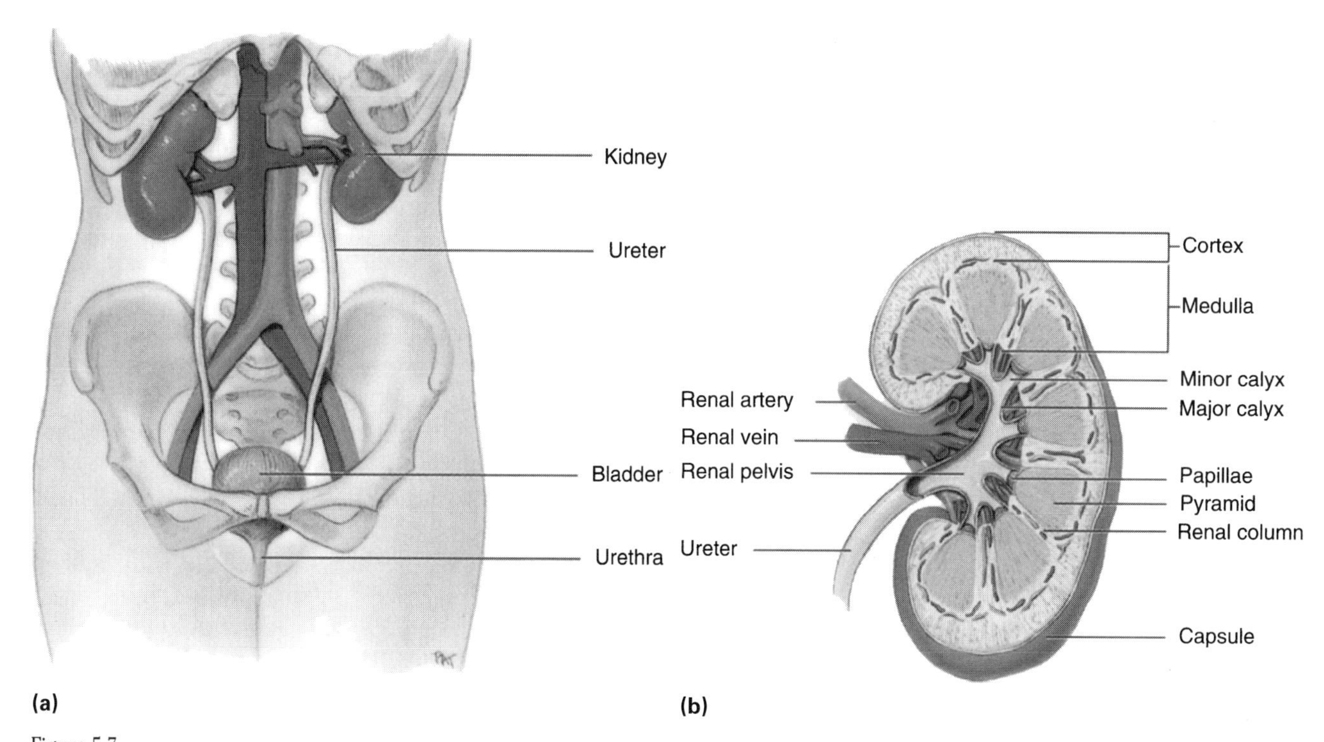

Figure 5-7
(a) The urinary system; (b) the kidney. (Reprinted with permission from Applegate, E.J. *The Anatomy and Physiology Learning System.* Philadelphia: W. B. Saunders, 1995, p. 372.)

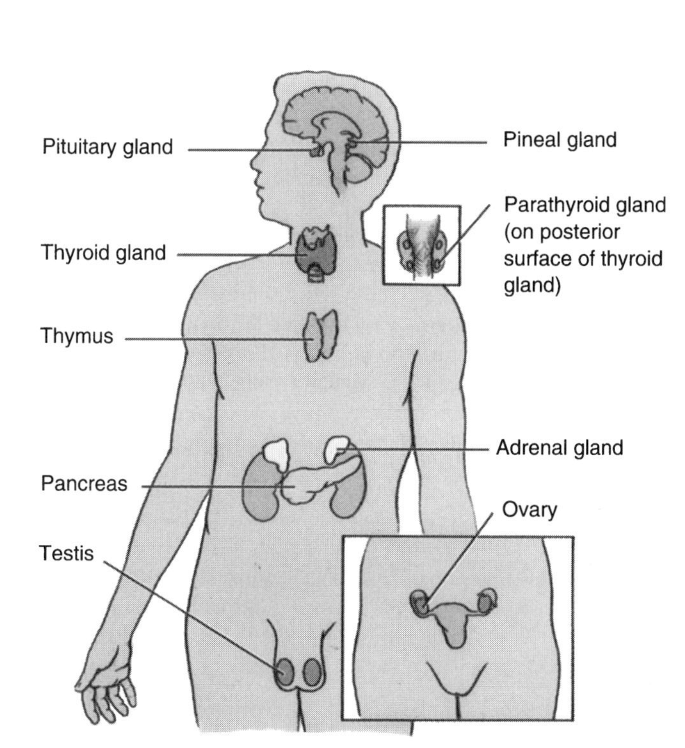

Figure 5-8
The endocrine system. (Reprinted with permission from Applegate, E.J. *The Anatomy and Physiology Learning System.* Philadelphia: W. B. Saunders, 1995, p. 208.)

having a different function. Some of the functions are the control of the activity of other glands, the control of body growth, and the contraction of involuntary muscles. Because the pituitary is involved in so many body functions, it is often referred to as the "master gland." Acromegaly is a disease of adults that results from hyperactivity of the anterior pituitary. The bones of the face, hands, and feet widen. Dwarfism, a condition in which patients are abnormally small, and gigantism, in which patients are abnormally large, may result from a deficiency or an excess of a hormone that controls body growth.

The thyroid gland is located just below the larynx in the neck. Its main function is to help control our growth and metabolism. The secretion of the thyroid gland is called thyroxine. An enlargement of the thyroid gland is called a goiter. Goiters may result from a lack of iodine in the diet, which is necessary for the proper functioning of the thyroid. If there is an overexertion of thyroxine, an exophthalmic goiter can result. In the patient suffering from this disease, we often see the characteristic bulging eyes, a strained appearance of the face, intense nervousness, and a very rapid metabolic rate.

The other glands found in the endocrine system include the two pairs of parathyroid glands which are embedded in the thyroid and which control the use of the calcium and phosphorus by the body; the two adrenal glands, located just above each kidney, and which are responsible for controlling the release of energy in order for us to meet emergency situations, and for use of water and salt by the body; and the islands of Langerhans, which are small groups of cells located in the pancreas that secrete insulin. Insulin controls the rate of glucose metabolism and regulates blood glucose concentration. While the islands of Langerhans are located in the pancreas, they do not produce digestive juices and have no digestive function.

The sex glands are also part of the endocrine system. In the male they are called the testes, and in the female they are the ovaries. The testes produce hormones that regulate the production of sperm cells and the development of male secondary sex characteristics. The hormones produced by the ovaries regulate the development and activity of the female reproductive system. They are also responsible for the development of the female secondary sex characteristics and for body changes that occur during pregnancy.

Two glands which are little understood by most scientists are the thymus gland and the pineal gland. The thymus gland is located in the chest just behind the sternum. It produces hormones that stimulate the production of lymph tissue and lymphocytes. It also functions in immune reactions. However, its function is not well understood. We know that it is present at birth, but begins to atrophy after about the age of 16. The pineal gland, which is located in the cranial cavity at about the middle of the brain, is also little understood.

The disease most often associated with the endocrine system is called diabetes mellitus, which results from a lack of insulin being produced in the islands of Langerhans. Without enough insulin, the body is unable to use glucose. Patients with diabetes must control the disease by regulating their glucose intake. They do this by taking additional insulin at regular intervals.

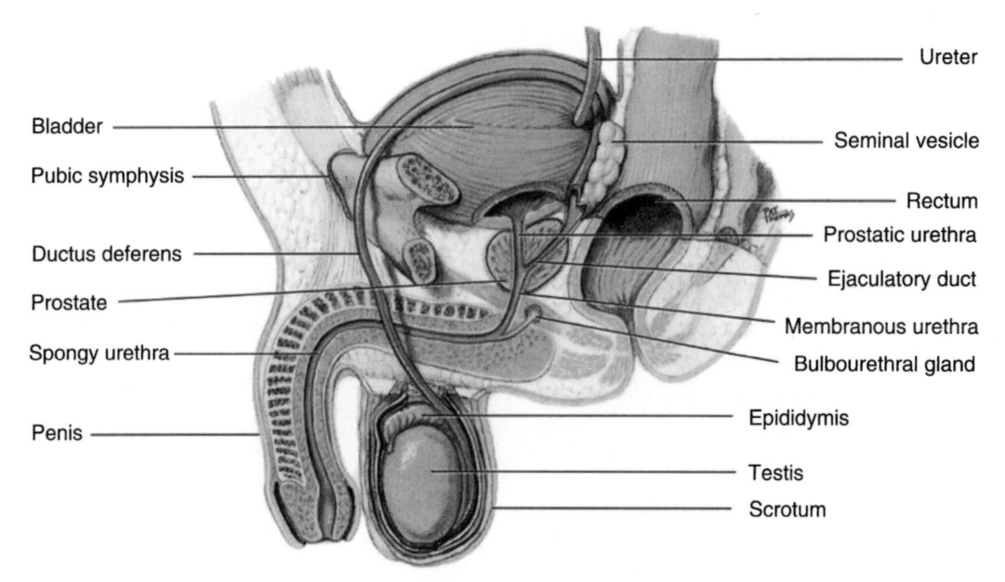

Figure 5-9
The male reproductive system. (Reprinted with permission from Applegate, E.J. *The Anatomy and Physiology Learning System.* Philadelphia: W. B. Saunders, 1995, p. 392.)

The Reproductive System

The reproductive system includes both the internal and the external reproductive organs. Its purpose is to generate reproductive cells, called ovum in the female, and sperm in the male.

The male reproductive system includes the scrotum, testes, penis, and prostate gland (Figure 5-9). The scrotum is a sac or pouch suspended between the thighs, which contains a pair of testes. The testes produce sperm cells and male sex hormones. The penis is the male organ of reproduction and urination, located in front of the scrotum. The prostate gland surrounds the neck of the bladder and the urethra and produces a fluid that helps sperm cells keep their motility.

The female reproductive system includes the ovaries, fallopian tubes, uterus, vagina, and the vulva (Figure 5-10). The ovaries produce egg cells, called ova or ovum, and female sex hormones. They are located in the upper part of the pelvic cavity. The fallopian tubes are ducts which lead from an area near the ovary to the uterus, and which carry the egg cells from the body cavity to the uterus. The uterus is the

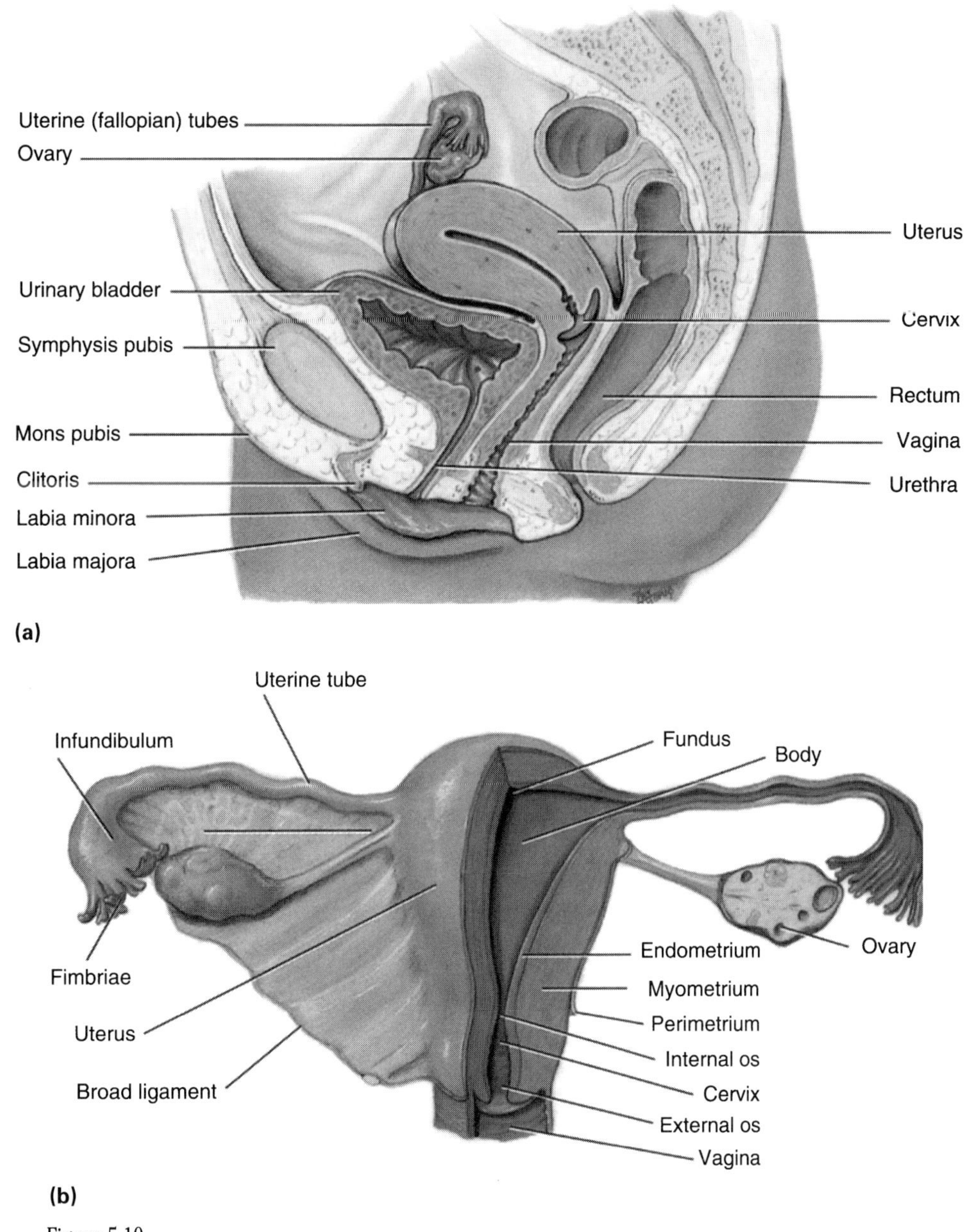

Figure 5-10
(a) The female reproductive system; (b) the uterus and uterine tubes. (Reprinted with permission from Applegate, E.J. *The Anatomy and Physiology Learning System.* Philadelphia: W. B. Saunders, 1995, pp. 400, 403.)

organ that contains and nourishes the embryo during pregnancy. The vagina, which is often referred to as the birth canal, is the muscular tube connecting the uterus with the exterior of the body. The vulva is the external part of the female reproductive system.

The union of the female's ovum with the male's sperm is called fertilization. This union usually occurs in the fallopian tubes, with the fertilized egg continuing its passage down through the tube until it reaches the uterus. Six to eight days after fertilization takes place, the ovum becomes implanted in the uterine wall. The duration of pregnancy is about 40 weeks or 280 days. At the end of the pregnancy, hormones stimulate contractions of the uterine wall, and birth occurs.

If an ovum is not fertilized by the sperm, a phenomenon known as menstruation occurs. It is the discharge of bloody fluid from the uterus at about 28-day intervals. Ova are produced at about the middle of this 28-day period. The uterine wall prepares for the implantation of a fertilized egg; however, when fertilization does not occur, the lining of the uterine wall sloughs off and is discharged. This loss of uterine lining leaves some areas bleeding. Thus, blood is discharged from the uterus. The entire menstrual cycle is controlled by hormones.

There are many disorders of the reproductive system. However, the most commonly seen include dysmenorrhea, which is painful menstruation; leukorrhea, which is a vaginal discharge; orchitis, an inflammatory condition of the testes, which is often due to trauma, mumps, or other infections; salpingitis, which is an inflammatory condition of the fallopian tubes; and sterility, a less often seen condition, in which either the male or the female may be unable to reproduce.

Summary

In this chapter, we talked briefly about the basic structure and function of the human body. We discussed the fact that there are nine systems of the human body, and each of these systems has individual structures which function both independently and as part of a group in order to provide us with the necessary processes and functions required to live. We also talked about some of the more commonly seen disorders and medical conditions associated with each of these systems.

Review Questions

1. A common bone injury in which there is a break in a bone is called a:

   a. dislocation

   b. fracture

   c. sprain

2. A disease of the musculoskeletal system in which there is an inflammation of bones at the joints with accompanying pain and swelling of the joints is called:

   a. dysentery

   b. athlerosclerosis

   c. arthritis

3. What is the name of the structures that are responsible for holding bones together?

4. What structures make up the digestive system?

5. Blood vessels that carry blood away from the heart are called_______________. Blood vessels that carry blood toward the heart are called_______________.

6. Briefly explain the function of the respiratory system.

7. What is the medical term used to describe a heart attack?

8. Briefly explain the function of the urinary system.

9. Briefly explain the function of the nervous system.

6

Applied Anatomy and Physiology of the Musculoskeletal System

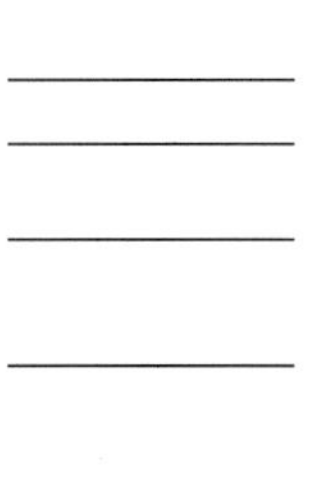

Performance Objectives

Upon completion of this chapter, you will be able to:

1. Briefly define the functions of the skeletal system.
2. Describe different types of bone tissue.
3. Discuss the functions of a long bone.
4. Identify the materials required for building bone.
5. Briefly describe the different types of bones.
6. Identify bones in both the axial and appendicular skeleton.
7. Discuss the role cartilage plays in the skeletal system.
8. Describe different types of joints and explain their movements.
9. Explain common disorders of bones, joints, and muscles.
10. Briefly define the functions of the muscular system.
11. Identify and briefly explain different types of muscles.
12. Explain how muscles contract.
13. Explain what is meant by the "origin" and the "insertion" of a muscle.

Terms and Abbreviations

Amphiarthrosis refers to a joint that is slightly moveable.
Articular cartilage a covering of the epiphyses that provides protection and helps ensure smooth joint movement.
Articulation the point at which two bones come together to form a joint.
Bursa a sac or cavity found between bones in joints or between tendons and bones.
Cancellous bone tissue a type of bone tissue which is characterized by several open spaces among bone processes, and which has a sponge-like appearance.
Cartilage specialized connective tissue made up of cells which have been embedded in a collagenous matrix, and which makes up part of the skeleton.
Compact bone tissue a type of bone tissue that is hard, dense, and has no open spaces.
Diaphysis the long, main portion or shaft of a bone.
Diarthrosis a joint that is freely moveable, such as a rotary joint.
Endomysium tissue that covers individual cells in a muscle.
Endosteum the lining of the medullary canal of bones.
Epimysium tissue that covers the outside surface of muscle, and which is made up of fibrous connective tissue.
Epiphysis the end of a long bone, which is covered with articular cartilage at the joints.
Haversian canals channels or canals which run longitudinally throughout compact bone.
Insertion the place of attachment of a muscle to a bone which it moves.
Medullary cavity the hollow shaft of a long bone.
Origin the more fixed end or attachment of a muscle.
Osteoblast bone cells that form bone.
Osteoclast bone cells that destroy bone tissue.
Osteocyte bone cell.
Perimysium the fibrous connective sheath that surrounds individual bundles of muscle fibers.

Periosteum the white, fibrous, protective covering on the outer surface of bone.
Synarthrosis an immovable joint.
Volkmann's canals channels that run horizontally through compact bone, extending from the periosteum to the Haversian canals.

The human body is often compared to a smooth-running machine with many intricate parts to it, all of which must work together to promote good health, growth, and life itself. As we have already discussed in Chapter 5, the body is a combination of organs and systems supported and protected by a framework of bones called the skeleton. The muscles working upon the skeleton provide us with all the basic movements which are needed as we work and play through each day of our lives.

The Skeletal System

The human skeleton (Figure 6-1) is the framework of our body. It is made up of 206 bones. These bones give form and shape to the various parts of our body. They also protect delicate organs, such as our brain and our spinal cord. Bones also act as levers; muscles are attached to the bones to make movement. Bones also act as a storehouse for minerals by manufacturing some of the body's blood cells.

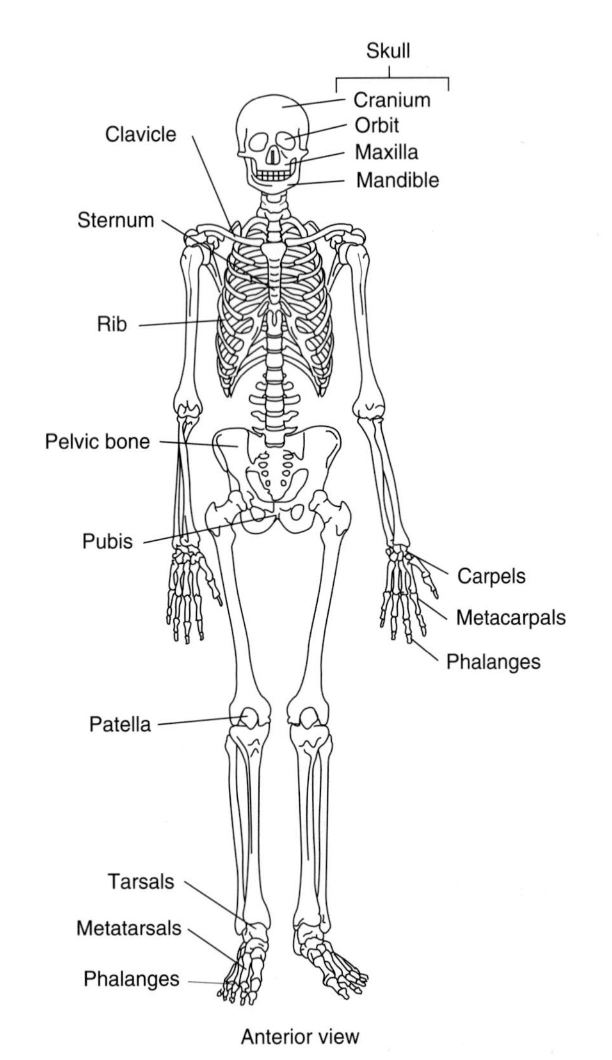

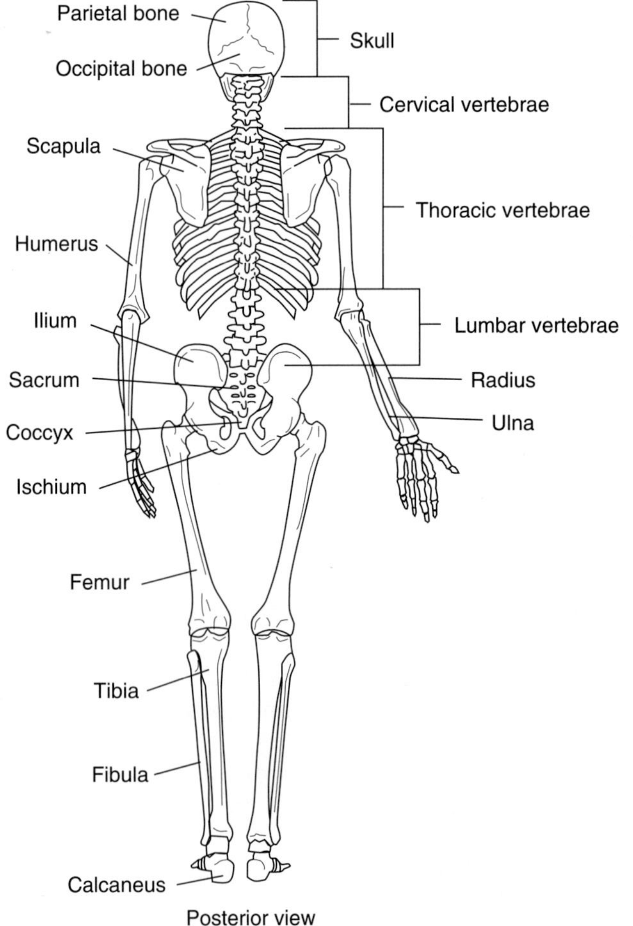

Figure 6-1
The human skeleton.

Functions of the Skeletal System

The human skeleton has five basic functions. These are providing support to the body; providing sites for muscles to attach, thus making movement or locomotion possible; protection of body parts; producing blood cells; and storing fat and mineral salts, especially of calcium and phosphorus.

Structures of the Skeletal System

Bone is a type of connective tissue made up of many collagen fibers impregnated with compounds of calcium and phosphorus. These minerals give bone its characteristic hardness and actually account for about two-thirds of its weight.

There are two types of bone tissue. The first, called *cancellous bone tissue,* has many open spaces, giving a spongy appearance. Blood vessels from the outer bone cover, called the *periosteum,* infiltrate the spaces in cancellous bone tissue, providing food and oxygen, and remove waste products of metabolism. Cancellous bone also contains red marrow which produces blood cells.

The second type of bone tissue is called *compact bone tissue.* It is much more dense than cancellous bone tissue, and on microscopic examination it appears as many circles. These circles are actually bony plates arranged concentrically around tiny channels or canals, called *Haversian canals.* These channels run longitudinally throughout the compact bone. There are also horizontal channels through compact bone, called *Volkmann's canals.* These microscopic channels extend from the periosteum to the Haversian canals and to the inner *cavity* of bones. Like the Haversian canals, they also contain minute blood vessels and nerves. Both the Haversian canals and the Volkmann's canals provide us with a means of transporting food, oxygen, and metabolic wastes, and also communicate a nerve supply throughout bone tissue.

Bone is considered living tissue, made up of cells called *osteocytes.* There are two types of osteocytes. The first are called *osteoblasts.* These tiny structures, which actually form collagen fibers using calcium and phosphorus, are most frequently found in the periosteum and endosteum. The second type, called *osteoclasts,* are bone cells that destroy bone tissue.

Our bodies require many regulatory substances in order to build bone tissue. These include compounds of calcium and phosphorus, which are essential for bone production; vitamins A, C, and D, which are necessary for the proper absorption of mineral compounds; and the hormone parahormone, produced by the parathyroid glands, and which is required for the proper regulation of calcium and phosphorus levels in the blood. Deficiencies in any of these minerals, vitamins, and hormones can result in serious disorders of the skeletal system.

Structure of a Long Bone

Before we can actually discuss the different types of bones found in the human body, it is important that you first have a basic understanding of the gross structure of all bones. To better comprehend what each of these structures looks like, let's look at a diagram of a long bone (Figure 6-2).

The long, main portion or shaft of the bone is called the *diaphysis.* It appears hollow and cylindrical in shape and is made up primarily of compact bone. The cylindrical shape of the bone gives it the ability to accommodate maximum strength and support with minimum weight.

The ends of the long bones are called *epiphyses.* Their rounded shapes provide maximum space for muscle attachment, and their cancellous bone makeup and spongy-like appearance make the epiphyses more able to withstand shocks and jolts without harm.

The periosteum is a white, fibrous protective covering on the outer surface of the bone, well supplied with blood vessels, nerves, and lymph vessels. It is essential for bone growth and maintenance.

The hollow shaft of a long bone is called the *medullary cavity.* This cavity, which contains yellow

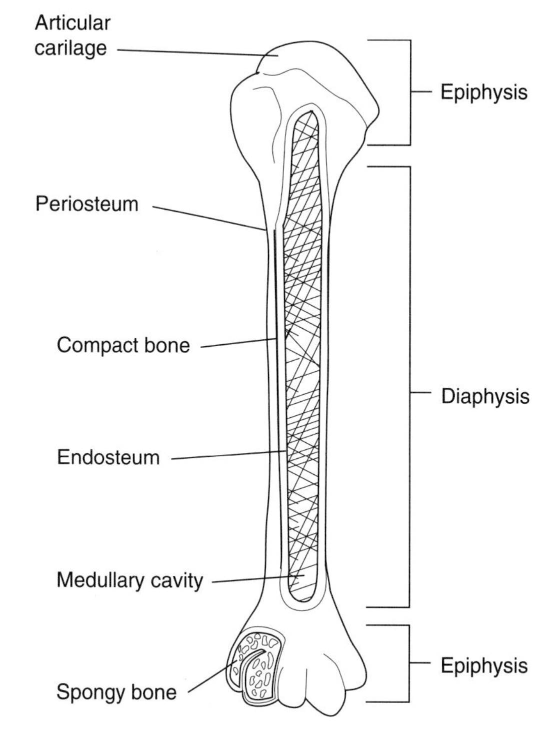

Figure 6-2
Long bone.

bone marrow, is lined with the *endosteum,* which is primarily composed of osteoblasts with a few osteoclasts.

Articular cartilage covers the epiphyses in areas where the ends of separate bones meet to form a joint. This cartilage provides protection for the bone ends and helps to ensure smooth movement of the joints.

Types of Bones

As we have already stated, the human body is made up of over 200 bones, each of which has been modified for its specific function. They can be divided into five broad groups according to their size and shape. These groups include long bones, short bones, flat bones, irregular bones, and sesamoid bones.

Long bones are found in the upper and lower arm, the upper and lower leg, and the fingers and toes. They are mainly composed of compact bone, although cancellous bone may be found in the epiphyses.

Short bones, which include the bones of the wrist and ankle, are made up of cancellous bone covered with compact bone. These bones are most responsible for providing strength.

Flat bones, which include the ribs, the scapulae, and some of the bones of the skull, consist of an inner portion of cancellous bone with an outer layer of compact bone. Because of the broad, flat shape of these bones, they provide protection for vulnerable body parts and large areas of muscle attachment.

Irregular bones have unusual and specialized shapes. Their overall function is articulation, and their irregular shape makes it possible for them to fit smoothly in order to form joints. Some examples of irregular bones include the vertebrae of the spinal column, the bones of the inner ear, and some of the facial bones. Irregular bones are made up of inner cancellous bone covered with an outer layer of compact bone.

Sesamoid bones, which are small, rounded bones found next to joints, are covered with cartilage or ligaments. Their primary function is to help eliminate friction in joints and thus increase the efficiency of motion in hinge joints. The patella, or kneecap, is an example of a sesamoid bone.

The Axial and Appendicular Skeletons

The human skeleton is usually divided into the axial and appendicular skeletons. The axial skeleton (Table 6-1) refers to bones arranged around the long axis of the body. These include the bones of the skull, the vertebral column, the ribs, the sternum, the three small bones of the ear, and the hyoid bones.

The Axial Skeleton

Bones of the Skull

The bones of the skull include those of the cranium, which enclose and protect the brain, and the facial bones, which include the bones of the nose, cheeks, and the jaws. There are 8 cranial bones and 14 facial bones. The cranial bones include the frontal, occipital, parietal, temporal, sphenoid, and ethmoid bones (Figures 6-3a and 6-3b on p. 54). These bones form immoveable or *synarthrotic* joints, and their surfaces are united by a thin, fibrous membrane which gives greater protection from possible injury. In an infant, space between the cranial bones provides room for growth of the skull. These spaces are called fontanels, and are protected from injury by the fibrous membrane. Bone formation continues as the child grows and the fontanels close.

The Facial Bones

The facial bones (Figure 6-4 on p. 55) include the palatines, which form the hard palate of the mouth and the lateral nasal wall, the nasal bones, the upper jaw or maxillae, the lower jaw or mandible, and the cheekbones, or zygomatic (malar) bones. The lacrimal bones, which are found at the inner side of the eye cavity, have a tiny groove that accommodates a portion of the tear or lacrimal duct. The vomer bone forms the lower and back portions of the nasal septum. And the nasal conchae or turbinate bones, extend from the lateral wall of the nasal cavity.

The Bones of the Middle Ear and the Hyoid Bone

The tiny bones of the middle ear, which are vital to hearing, are included in the axial skeleton although they are not actually a part of either the axial or appendicular skeleton. They include the maleus (hammer), the incus (anvil), and the stapes (stirrup).

The hyoid bone is a small U-shaped bone located between the larynx and the mandible. It is quite unique in that it does not attach to any other bone, but rather is suspended from the styloid process of the temporal bone of the skull. It is very important because it provides an attachment for some of the muscles of the tongue.

Table 6-1
The Axial Skeleton

Bones of the Skull			Number of Bones	
Cranium	frontal		1	
	occipital		1	
	parietal		2	
	temporal		2	
	sphenoid		1	
	ethmoid		1	(8)
Facial bones	turbinate		2	
Upper jaw	maxilla		2	
	nasal		2	
Cheek	zygomatic (malar)		2	
Lower jaw	mandible		1	
	lacrimal		2	
	palatine		2	
	vomer		1	(14)
Spinal column	vertebrae			
	cervical	1–7	7	
	thoracic	8–19	12	
	lumbar	20–24	5	
	sacral	25–29*	5	
	coccygeal	30–33**	1	(26; 30 in child)
Chest (thorax)	ribs (12 pair)		24	
	sternum (including xiphoid process)		1	(25)
Inner ear bones	malleus		2	
	incus		2	
	stapes		2	(6)
Horseshoe-shaped bone	hyoid		1	(1)

*These fuse in adults to form the sacrum.
**These fuse in adults to form the coccyx.

The Spinal Column and Vertebrae

The vertebrae make up the spinal column (Figure 6-5 on p. 56). They protect the delicate nerves and structures that run through the column, and also help to make posture possible. In adults, there are 26 vertebrae, and in children there are 33. This difference is because in adulthood several vertebrae fuse together. The vertebrae are numbered for convenience in identifying them. The first seven are called cervical vertebrae, and are numbered C1 through C7. The next 12 are called the thoracic vertebrae, and are numbered T1 through T12. These provide dorsal attachment for the ribs. The next five are called the lumbar vertebrae, and are numbered L1 through L5, followed by five sacral vertebrae. The last vertebrae are called the coccygeal vertebrae. In children, there are four to five separate coccygeal vertebrae, which ultimately fuse together in adults to form the coccyx.

The Ribs

There are 12 pairs of ribs which protect the delicate structures of the heart and lungs. These ribs attach to the vertebrae from the back, and to the sternum in the front. The first seven pairs attach directly to the sternum, and the last five pairs attach dorsally but are held in place ventrally by strong cartilage that binds them to the sternum. The last pairs do not actually attach directly to the sternum, and thus are referred to as "floating ribs." This gives the rib cage greater flexibility.

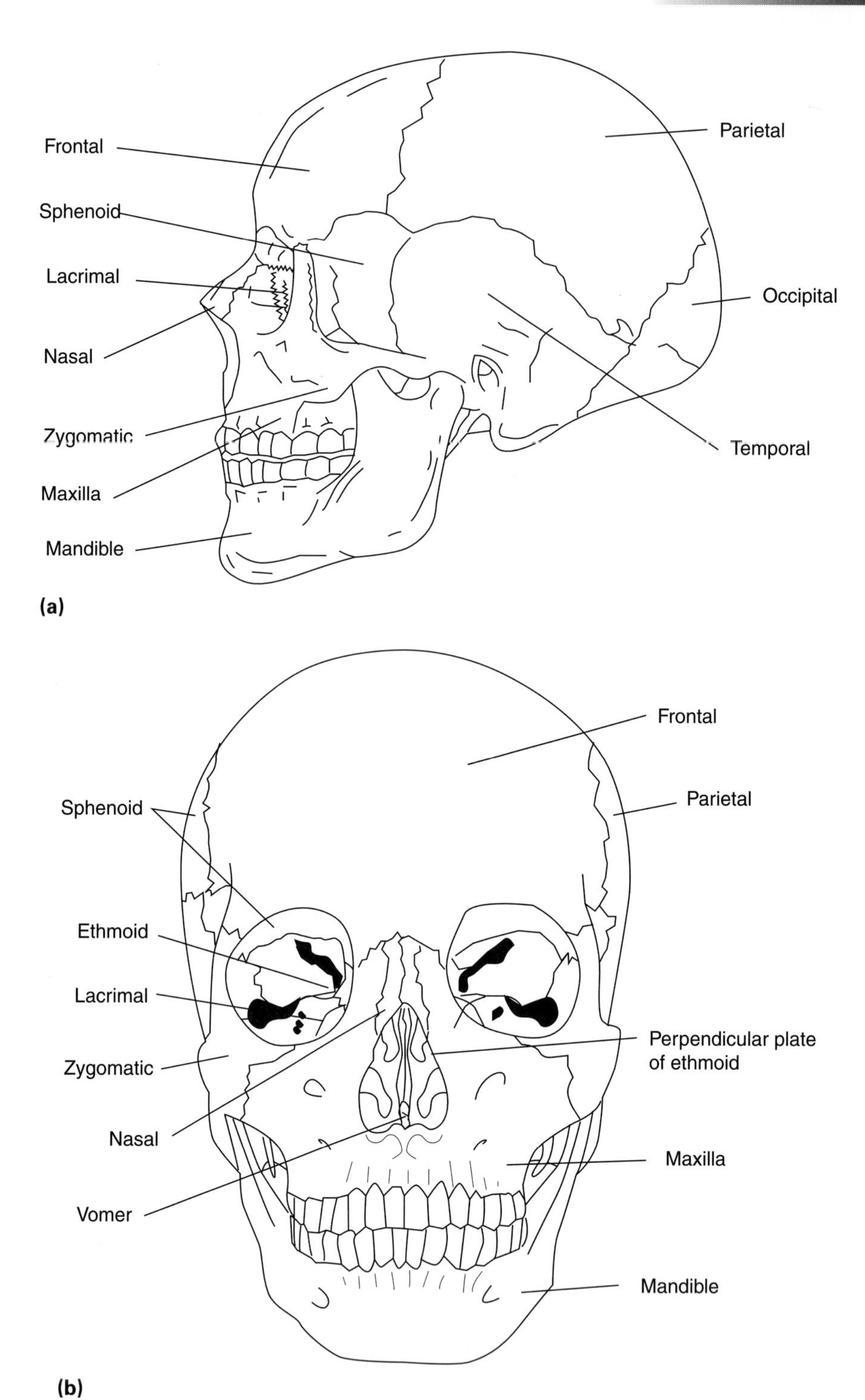

Figure 6-3
Bones of the skull: (a) Lateral view of the skull; (b) front view of the skull.

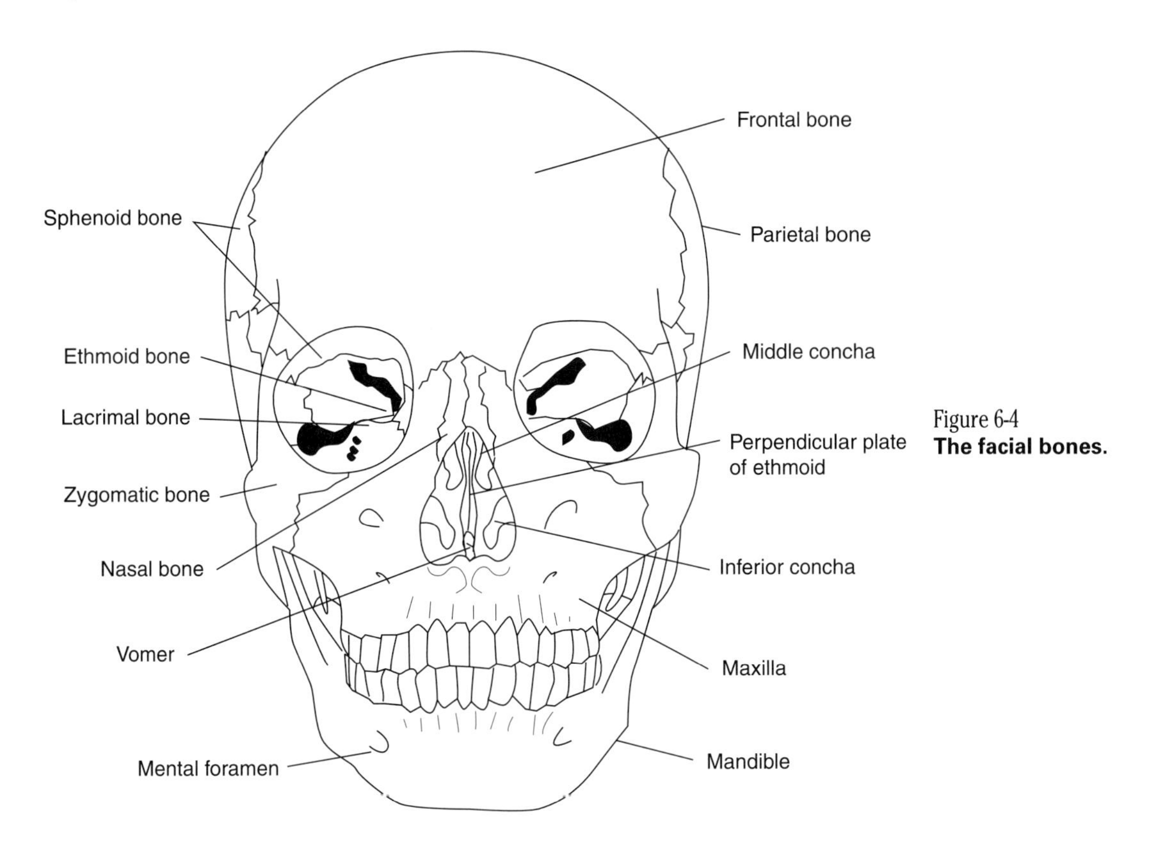

Figure 6-4
The facial bones.

The Appendicular Skeleton

The appendicular skeleton (Table 6-2 on p. 57) includes all of the bones of the upper and lower extremities. This includes the bones of the shoulder girdle, the bones of the pelvic girdle, or hip, and the bones which make up the feet and toes.

The shoulder girdle consists of the clavicle and scapula, the humerus of the upper arm, the radius and ulna of the lower arm, the carpals of the wrist, the metacarpals of the hand, and the phalanges or fingers of the hand.

The bones which make up the pelvic girdle, or hip, include the ilium, the ischium, and the pubis, which all fuse together in adulthood to form the innominate or hipbone. The bones of the leg include the femur or thigh bone, the patella or kneecap, the tibia, and the fibula. And the bones of the ankle, feet, and toes, include the tarsals, the metatarsals, and the phalanges.

Joints and Movement

Joints or *articulations* are points at which two bones come together (Figure 6-6a on p. 57). And movement of any heavy bones, such as those of the upper or lower extremities, would be next to impossible if it were not for joints.

There are several kinds of joints found in the human body, all of which are classified according to their specific function or movement. Some are referred to as immoveable, because of their ability to provide stability and protection. Two examples of immovable joints include the sacrum and the skull. Other joints, such as those which make up the vertebrae of the spinal column and those which attach the ribs to the sternum, or breastbone, are called amphiarthrosis or partially moveable. The amount of movement from these types of joints are very small.

There are several moveable joints which provide us with the ability to move our fingers, elbows, and knees. These are referred to as hinged joints, since they function in the same way as the hinge of a door. Pivot joints provide us with the capability to rotate certain structures. The ability of the head to rotate on the vertebral column is one example of a pivot joint. Other joints are *diarthrosis,* allowing us complete freedom of movement in all directions. These are called ball-and-socket joints. The shoulder joint is one example of a ball-and-socket joint. And some joints have only one bony surface, thus allowing the bone to glide over another bony surface. These are called gliding joints. The wrist is an example of a gliding joint.

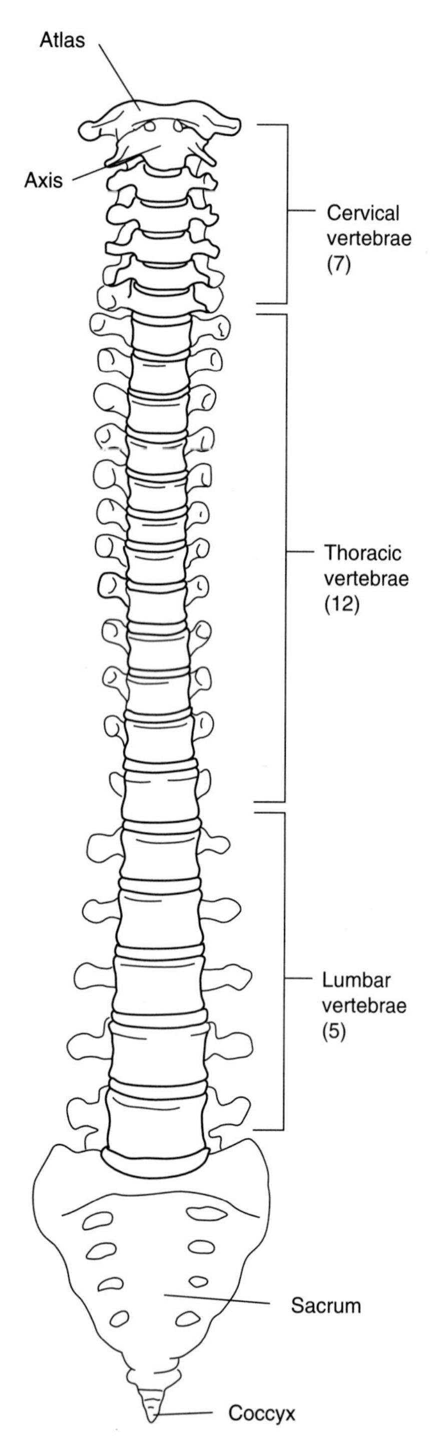

Figure 6-5
The spinal column and vertebrae.

The type of movement at a specific joint is determined by the structure of the individual joint. And as we have already stated, it would be impossible for us to maneuver or move any part of our body without the use of our joints.

As Figure 6-6b (on p. 58) shows, there are several different types of movement that individual joints can accomplish. Flexion, for example, gives the joint the ability to decrease the size of an angle, while extension is just the opposite, in that it allows the joint to straighten. A good example of flexion and extension is the movement of the elbow. While flexion brings the forearm close to the humerus and thus decreases the size of the angle, extension allows the arm to straighten.

Abduction is a motion that provides a bone with the ability to move away from the body, while adduction makes it possible to move the bone toward the body. If you move your foot away from the side of your body, that's an example of abduction; returning the foot to the side is adduction. Rotation is the movement which allows a bone to move on its own axis, such as your skull having the ability to move on the axis of the spinal column. Turning your head from side to side is an example of rotation. Finally, circumduction, which is the action of one end of a bone moving in a circle while the other end remains stationary, involves all of the movements of flexion and extension, abduction and adduction, and rotation. A good example of circumduction is moving your outstretched arms in a complete circle.

Diseases and Disorders of Bones and Joints

There are many diseases and disorders of the skeletal system and the joints. These range from degenerative disorders of the joints to fractures of the bone itself. Some of the most common of these include arthritis, osteoporosis, rickets, curvatures of the spine, and gout.

When we discuss arthritis, we are actually referring to many different conditions of the skeletal system which may cause pain and deformity in the joints. In some forms of arthritis, the skin and connective tissues may also be affected.

There are several types of arthritis. Rheumatoid arthritis is one of the more serious types because it not only affects the bones and joints but may also affect other body systems, such as the lungs, muscles, skin, blood vessels, and the heart. The cause of rheumatoid arthritis is still unknown, but it has symptoms very similar to that of an infection. The structures located within the joint become greatly inflamed, eventually causing total destruction and deformity of the joint itself. Eventually, pain limits movement, and contractures begin to develop.

Another form of arthritis is called osteoarthritis, or degenerative joint disease. This is a condition which will affect all of us to some degree as we grow older. In osteoarthritis, the joints which are affected just wear out. While the cause of osteoarthritis is still unknown, it seems to occur more often in older

Text continues on p. 60

Table 6-2
The Appendicular Skeleton

Common Name	Technical Name	Number of Bones	
Upper Extremities			
Shoulder girdle	clavicle		
	scapula	2	
Upper arm	humerus	2	
Lower arm	radius	2	
	ulna	2	
Wrist	carpals	16	
Hand	metacarpals	20	
Fingers	phalanges	28	(64)
Lower Extremities			
Hip girdle	ilium (these fuse in the adult to form the innominate or hipbone)		
(pelvic girdle)	ischium		
	pubis	2	
Thigh	femur	2	
Lower leg	tibia	2	
	fibula	2	
Kneecap	patella	2	
Ankle	tarsals	14	
Foot	metatarsals	10	
Toes	phalanges	28	(62)

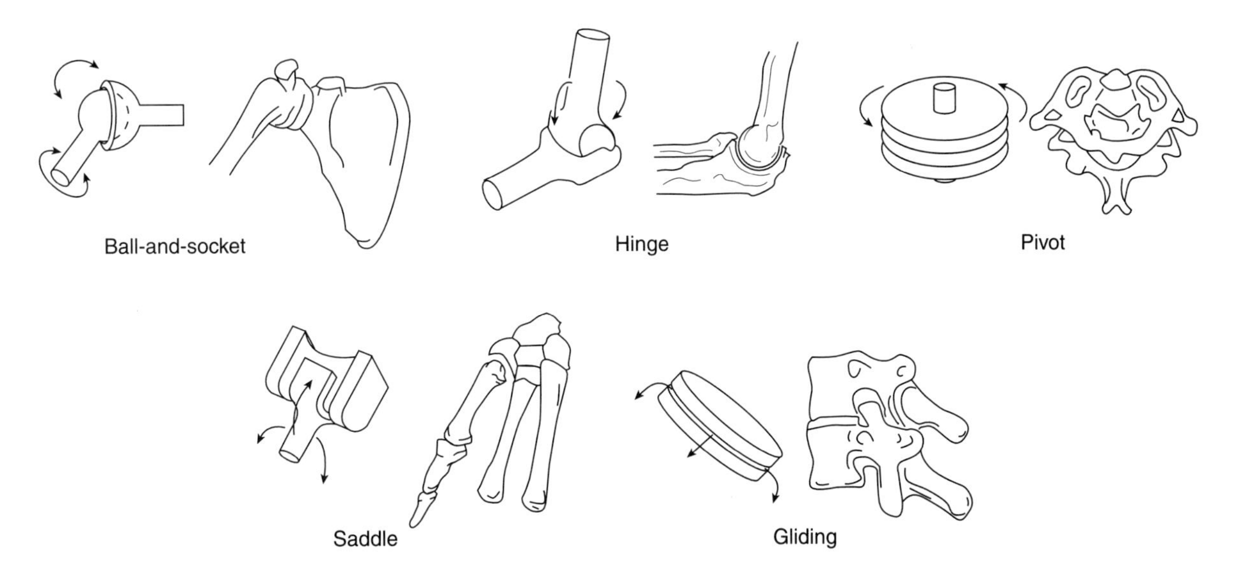

Figure 6-6a
Types of joint movement.

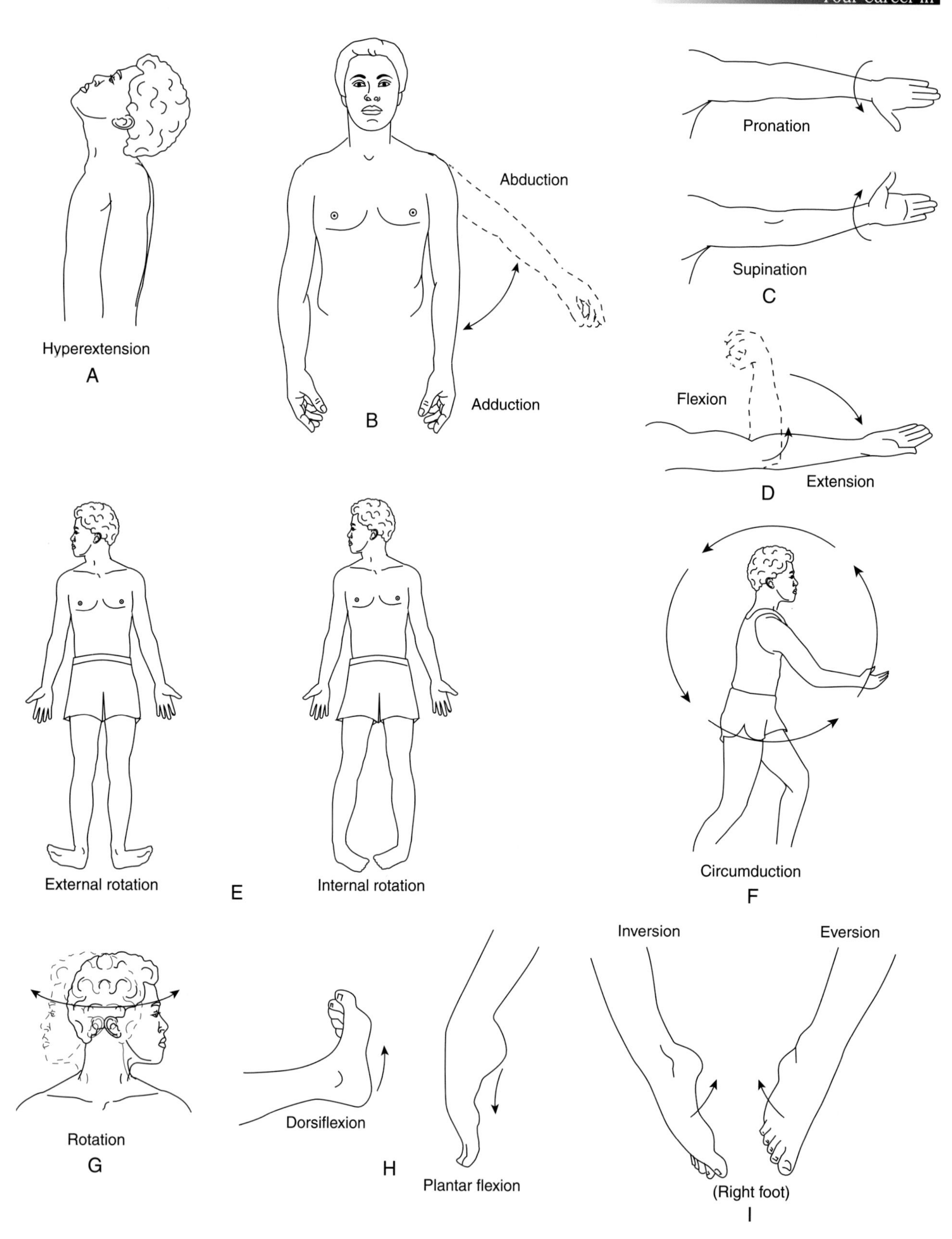

Figure 6-6b
Types of joint movement.

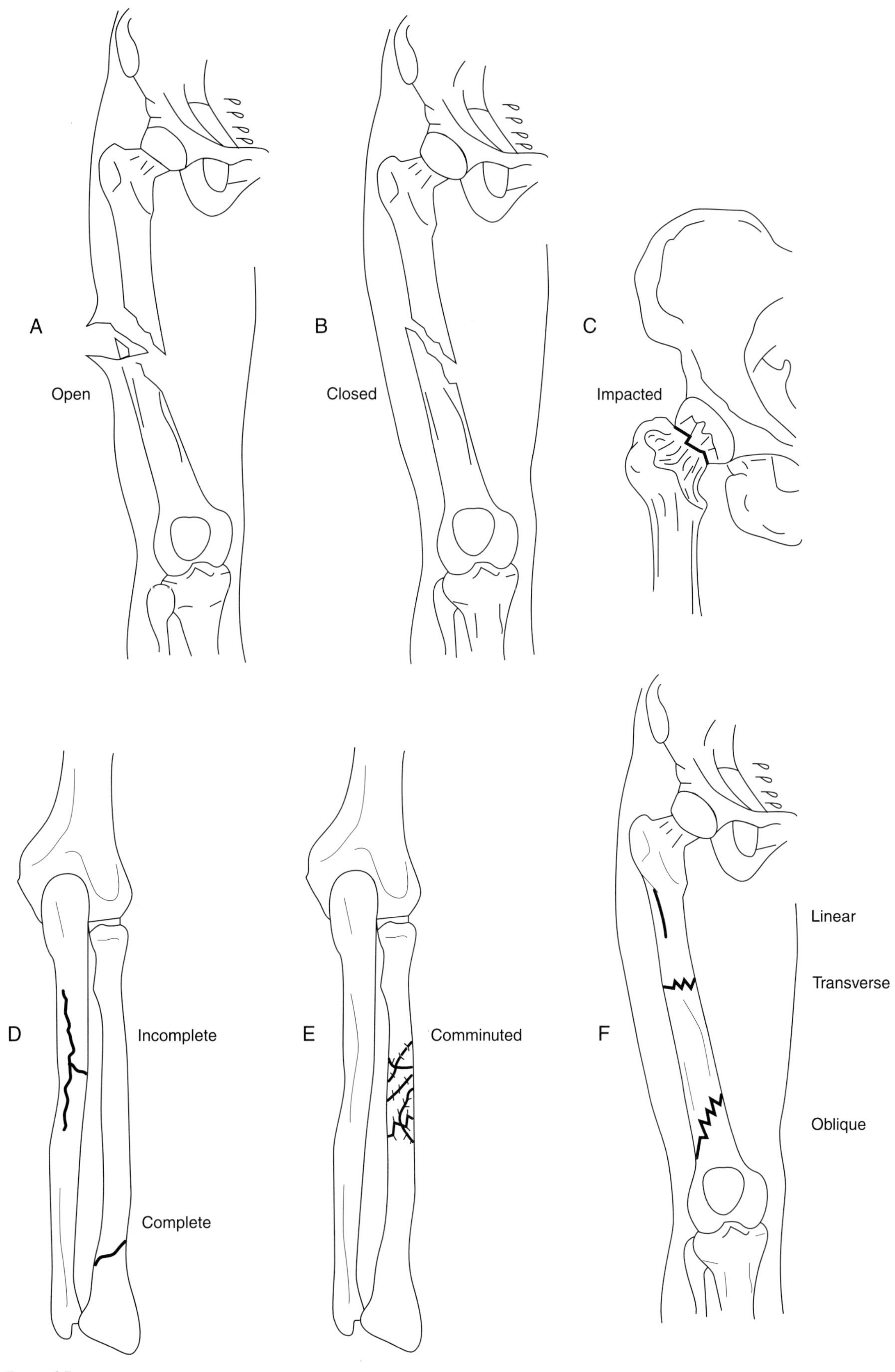

Figure 6-7
Types of fractures.

patients who have suffered some type of joint trauma or in patients who are obese.

Infectious arthritis is caused by a bacterial infection. While other bacteria have been known to cause this form of arthritis, the most common offender appears to be gonococcus. In this condition, the patient's knee, wrist, and ankle are the joints most commonly affected, and the arthritis almost always occurs at the same time the patient has a genital gonorrheal infection.

A form of arthritis that affects over one million people each year is gout. When present, gout generally affects only one joint, usually the big toe, and is characterized by crystal deposits in and around the affected point.

A disorder of the skeletal system which is seen most commonly in elderly women or in patients who have been confined to bed for long periods of time is osteoporosis. In this condition, there is a loss of mineral from the bone itself, thus causing the bones to become brittle and fracture more easily.

Two diseases which affect both the bone and the joints are rickets and bursitis. Rickets often affects infants and children who do not have enough vitamin D in their diets, thus causing the bones not to harden properly, resulting in deformation and bending of the bones. Bursitis is an inflammatory condition of the *bursa* or fluid-filled sacs in and around joints and tissues where friction would occur.

In addition to suffering from degenerative and inflammatory diseases of the skeletal system and joints, some patients may also experience some type of curvature of the spinal column. The most common of these include kyphosis, which is an exaggeration of the natural posterior curve, thus causing the patient to walk with a hunchbacked appearance; scoliosis, which is a side to side curvature of the spine; and lordosis, which is an exaggerated in-

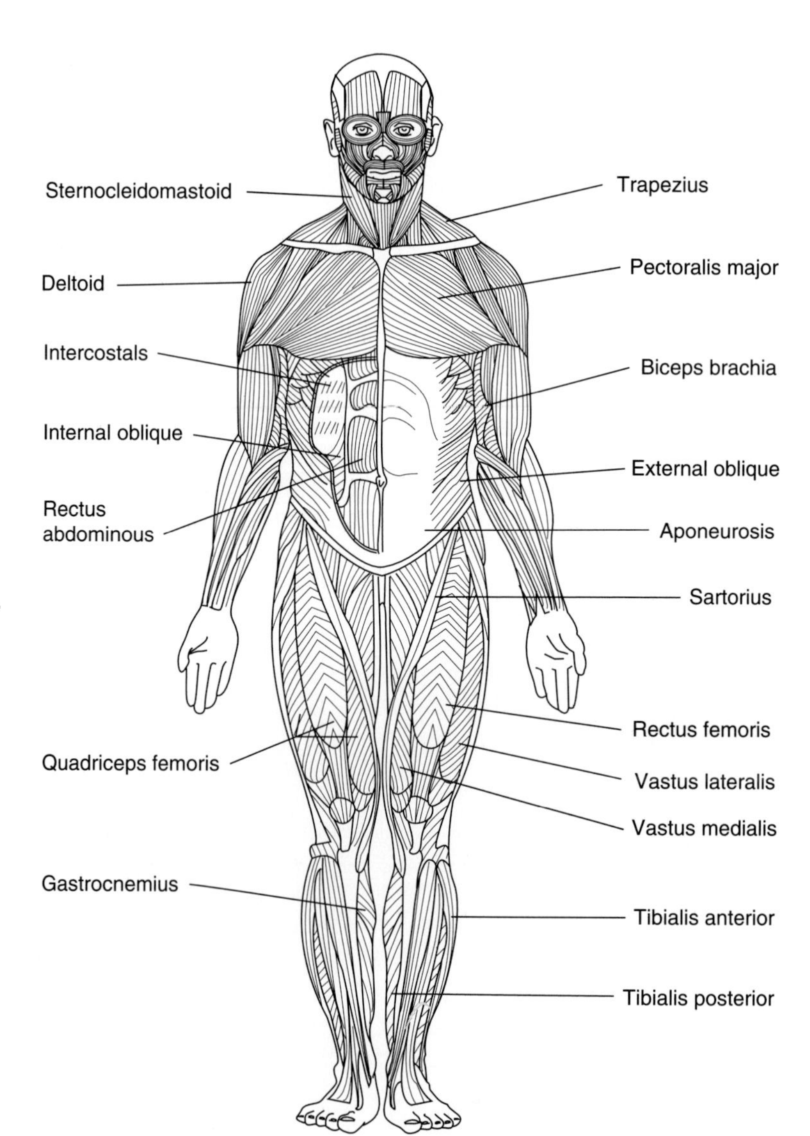

Figure 6-8a
The muscular system (anterior view).

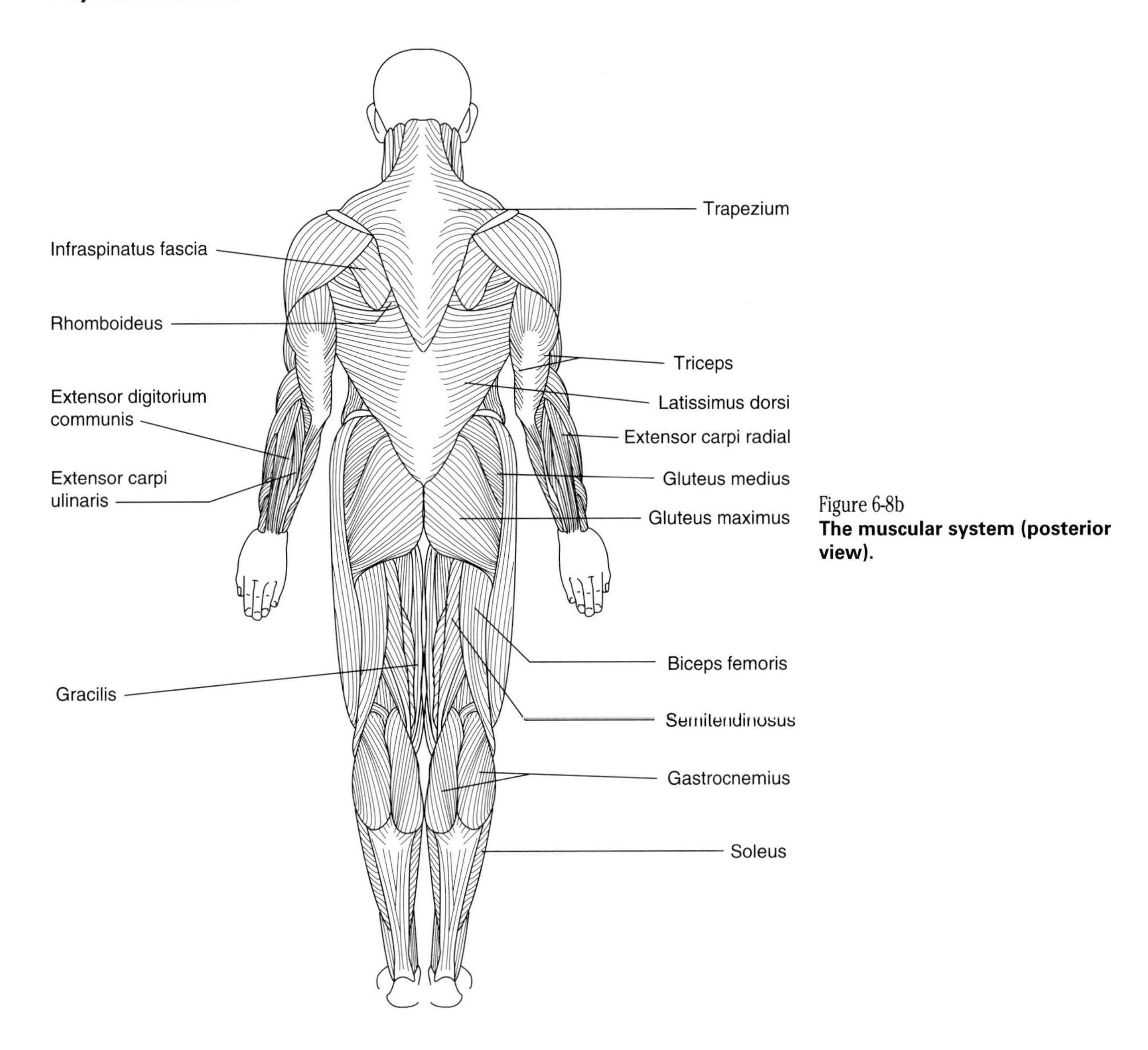

Figure 6-8b
The muscular system (posterior view).

ward curvature of the lumbar region of the spinal column.

Fractures of the Skeletal System

No discussion of the disorders and injuries of the skeletal system would be complete without mentioning fractures. A fracture is a break in a bone. It may be either closed (simple), or open (compound), as shown in Figure 6-7 (on p. 59). An open fracture involves a break in the skin, as well as the bone, causing the bone ends to protrude through the skin. A closed fracture can be classified as greenstick, complete, comminuted, or spiral. Greenstick fractures occur most often in children because their bones are much more flexible and tend to bend (like a green stick) rather than break. The greenstick fracture is incomplete. A complete fracture occurs when the two ends of the bone separate at the site of the break. A comminuted fracture is the result of a complete fracture of the bone into more than two pieces. When this type of fracture occurs, surgery is generally indicated to reset the bone fragments. Spinal fractures, which are not often seen, generally result from twisting injuries, such as those suffered in skiing accidents.

Sprains and Dislocations

A sprain is an injury to the ligaments or connective tissue that supports a joint. A dislocation, on the other hand, is the actual separation of the bones which make up the joint. Many times, because of the severity of the trauma causing a joint to dislocate, a muscle strain or sprain may also occur with the dislocation. This type of dislocation is often characterized by an abnormal position and deformity of the affected joint.

The Muscular System

The muscular system (Figures 6-8a and 6-8b on pp. 60 and 61) has three basic functions. The first, and perhaps the single most important function, is to provide our body with its ability to move. One only has to suffer the inability to move, or have limited motion to realize just how important our muscles are to us. Another function of muscles is to maintain body positions or posture. This is how we are able to stand, sit, kneel, stoop, or assume any other posture. A third important function of the muscles are their ability to help maintain our body's temperature. Because of the size, or mass of muscles, they are able to produce large amounts of body heat that can later be transported throughout our body by means of circulating blood. (See Table 6-3 for the common muscles.)

There are three types of muscle tissue (Figure 6-9). These include striated muscles, smooth muscles, and cardiac muscles. Striated or skeletal muscles, along with the bones of the skeletal system, make it possible for us to move all the parts of our body. This includes not only our arms and legs, but also, our internal organs, such as our diaphragm when we breathe, or the beating of our heart. Striated muscles, which are also called voluntary, and which attach themselves to bone, make up about 40 to 50 percent of our entire body weight.

Smooth muscles give our body its ability to control certain activities below our level of consciousness. For this reason, they are often referred to as involuntary muscles. Because internal organs or viscera are also controlled by smooth muscles, they may also be called visceral muscles.

The muscle which can only be found in the heart is called cardiac muscle. It is both an involuntary muscle and a striated muscle because of its physical characteristics and its ability to combine with other types of muscles.

Table 6-3
Common Muscles

Name	Origin	Insertion	Action
deltoid	spine of scapula, clavicle, acromial process	lateral surface of humerus	abducts arm
trapezius	occipital bone, 7th cervical, and all thoracic vertebrae	acromial process of clavicle and spine of scapula	draws scapula toward spinal column; rotates scapula to lift shoulder
latissimus dorsi	vertebrae, iliac crest	humerus	extends upper arm
triceps brachii	scapula	ulna	abducts upper arm
gluteus maximus	ilium, sacrum, coccyx, sacrotuberous ligament	femur	extends thigh; rotates outward
gastrocnemius	femur	tarsal	extends foot; flexes lower leg
sternocleidomastoid	sternum, clavicle	temporal bone	flexes head; rotates head toward opposite side
pectoralis major	clavicle, sternum, costal cartilage of ribs	humerus	flexes upper arm; adducts upper arm anteriorly; flexes supinated forearm
biceps brachii	scapula	radius	supinates forearm and hand
external oblique	lower eight ribs	iliac crest and pubis	compresses abdomen
flexor carpi radialis	humerus	second metacarpal	flexes hand; flexes forearm
vastus medialis	femur	tibia	extends leg
vastus lateralis	femur	tibia (patellar tendon)	extends leg
tibialis anterior	tibia	tarsal, metatarsal	flexes foot; inverts foot
serratus anterior	ribs	scapula	pulls shoulder forward; abducts and rotates upward
intercostals	rib, lower border	rib, upper border	elevates ribs
sheath of rectus abdominus	ossa coxae	ribs, xiphoid process	compresses abdomen; flexes trunk
sartorius	anterior, superior iliac spines	tibia	adducts and flexes leg; permits crossing of legs

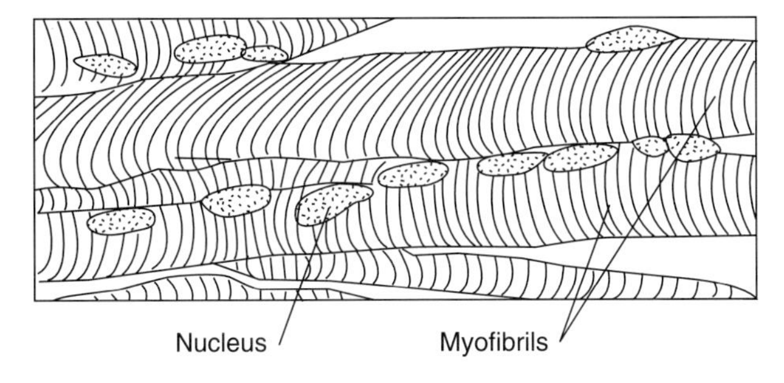

A. Striated (voluntary) muscle cells

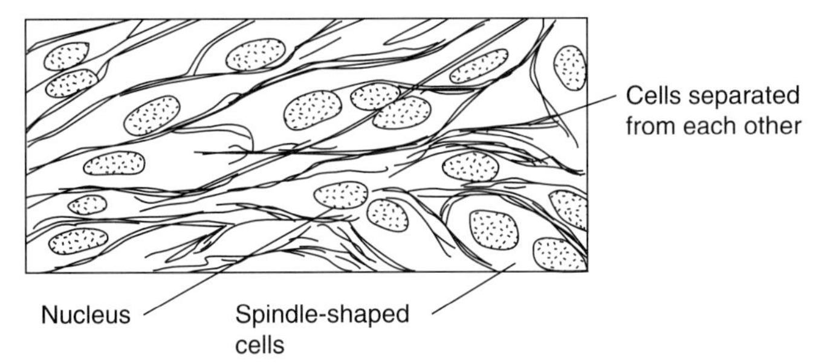

B. Smooth (involuntary) muscle cells

Figure 6-9
Types of muscle.

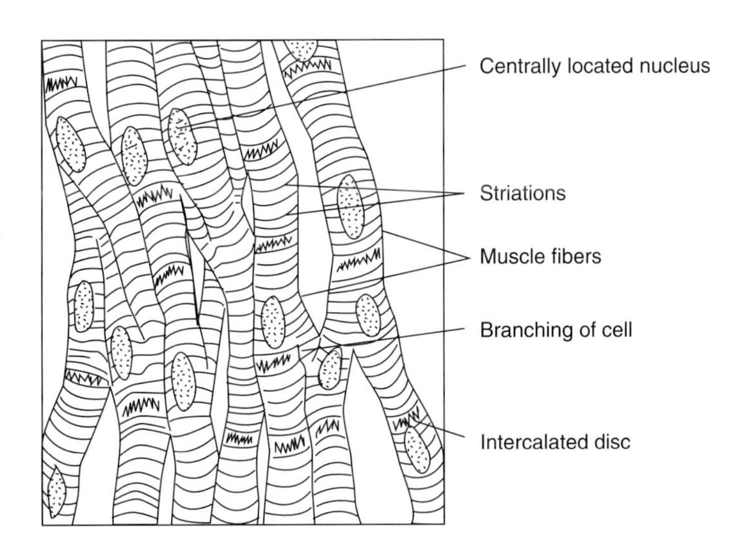

C. Cardiac muscle cells

Skeletal Muscle Structure

All muscles are made up of three parts (Figure 6-10 on p. 64). The outside surface, which is covered by a fibrous connective sheath, and which folds inward to cover individual bundles of muscle fibers is called the *epimysium.* Once the epimysium surrounds each individual bundle, it becomes known as the *perimysium.* It then extends in order to cover individual muscle cells, where it becomes known as the *endomysium.* These three parts are structured in such a way as to be continuous with the fibrous tissue that eventually forms a tendon. Tendons are continuous with the periosteum of bone, where they firmly attach muscles to the bones and ultimately move when muscles contract.

Skeletal muscle cells are unique in that they have many nuclei. They are made up of many long, slender threads called myofibrils, which are strands lying next to one another and extending lengthwise

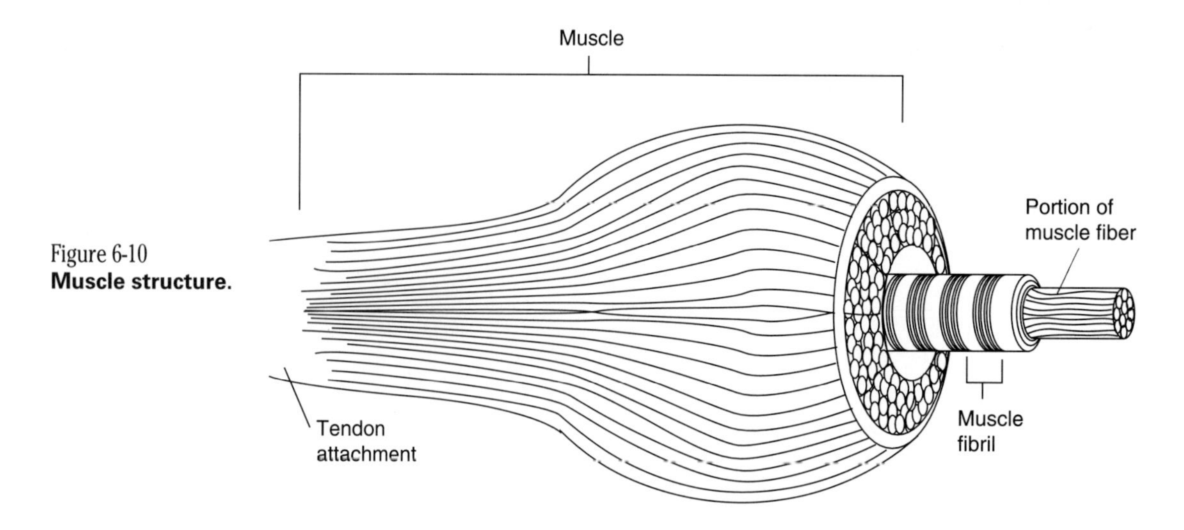

Figure 6-10
Muscle structure.

throughout the cell. These myofibrils are in turn made up of smaller strands called myofilaments, which consist of bands of protein.

Energy and Muscle Contraction

While much occurs at the cellular level of the muscles in order to make it possible for them to move, the most profound changes have to do with creating energy so that they are able to contract. Energy is required for all muscle contraction. This energy is supplied to the cells by aerobic respiration in which glucose combines with oxygen with the release of energy. If the oxygen supply is inadequate for cellular needs, as in strenuous or prolonged exercise, pyruvic acid provides energy without using free oxygen. This is commonly referred to as anaerobic respiration. When the pyruvic acid breaks down to release the energy, lactic acid, which accumulates in the tissues and causes a feeling of fatigue, is given off. What results is a process known as oxygen debt, a condition occurring because of the body's inability to supply enough oxygen for adequate aerobic respiration. When oxygen debt does occur, there may be muscle cramping or spasms following prolonged exercise.

Muscle Action

As we have already stated, movement is a major function of our muscular system. However, the only movement muscles are capable of is contraction followed by relaxation. Skeletal movement is accomplished by the pulling action on bones to which the muscles are attached.

All individual muscle cells contract when they are stimulated. And this stimulation is determined or affected according to specific factors. These include oxygen and food supply, the number of fibers stimulated, and the extent to which activity is required.

For a muscle to be able to move, it must have two or more attachments. These attachments are generally to bones. The more fixed end or attachment of the muscle to bone is called its *origin.* The place of attachment of a muscle to a bone which it moves is called its *insertion.* Therefore, when you bend your elbow, you can observe the origin of the biceps brachii at the scapula, which does not move, and the insertion at the radius, which does move.

Most of the muscles which make up our body are modified for their specific type of action. Terms used to describe these functions include the following.

- *flexor:* muscle that bends at a joint.
- *extensor:* muscle that extends a part or increases the angle of a joint.
- *abductor:* muscle that moves a part away from the midline of the body.
- *adductor:* muscle that moves a part toward the midline of the body.
- *rotator:* muscle that revolves a part on its axis.
- *sphincter:* circular muscle that closes an opening.

Disorders of the Muscular System

Like the bones which make up our body, muscles are also subject to many diseases and disorders. Two common degenerative disorders seen in the muscular system include muscular dystrophy, a degeneration of the muscle cells that eventually causes the muscles to waste away and atrophy; and myasthenia gravis, a very poorly understood disease causing great muscle weakness and fatigue. In myasthenia gravis, the nerve impulses fail to initiate normal muscle contractions, eventually causing the patient to have the appearance of drooping eyelids and an inattentive appearance.

In addition to degenerative disorders, a muscle can become permanently shortened because of a formation of fibrous tissue replacing the muscle cells. If this occurs, a contracture develops. Myalgia, or muscle pain, is often seen in muscle cramps and muscle spasms. Muscle cramps are painful, spasmodic, muscle contractions of longer duration. A muscle spasm is a sudden, involuntary muscle contraction of a much shorter duration. If myositis occurs, there is a severe inflammation of the muscle tissue.

Summary

In this chapter, we discussed the applied anatomy and physiology of the musculo-skeletal system, and the role these very important systems play in our everyday lives. We briefly discussed the function of both the bones and the muscles, and identified the various motions and movements of each of the individual structures that make up these two systems. We also discussed some of the most frequently seen disorders of the bones and muscles.

Review Questions

1. A ______________ refers to a joint that is slightly moveable.
2. Briefly explain the difference between cancellous bone tissue and compact bone tissue.
3. An osteoblast refers to:
   a. bone cells that form bone
   b. bone cells that destroy bone tissue
   c. a bone cell
4. What is the name of the long, main portion or shaft of a bone?
5. A sac or cavity found between bones in joints or between tendons and bones is called:
   a. bursa
   b. cartilage
   c. endosteum
6. ______________ refers to the place of attachment of a muscle to a bone which it moves, while ______________ pertains to the more fixed end or attachment of a bone.
7. What is the name of the fibrous connective sheath that surrounds individual bundles of muscle fibers?
8. True or False: An immovable joint is called a synarthrosis.
9. What is the name given to small rounded bones found next to joints, which help eliminate friction and increase efficiency in hinge joints?
   a. zygomatic
   b. ethmoid
   c. sesamoid
10. What is the name of the white fibrous protective covering on the outer surface of bone?

7

Applied Kinesiology and Physical Medicine

Performance Objectives

Upon completion of this chapter, you will be able to:

1. Identify areas of study in kinesiology, and briefly explain how principles of kinesiology are used to improve performance.
2. Identify and briefly describe anatomical and fundamental body positions.
3. Explain how muscles are grouped according to their role in movement.
4. Identify and explain various types of exercises.
5. Identify equipment used for evaluating exercise.
6. Discuss how to plan an exercise program.

Terms and Abbreviations

Adhesions formations of new fibrous tissue which have resulted from an inflammation or surgery.
Biomechanics the substudy or subdivision of mechanics concerned with the motion of all living organisms.
Calisthenics rhythmic bodily exercises.
Circuit training a selected exercise activity which has been organized into a sequence or circuit for performance.
Contracture an abnormal shortening of a muscle tissue.
EMG abbreviation for electromyogram, which is a tracing of a muscular contraction.
Goniometer a device used to determine range of motion in order to measure angles.
Kinesiology the study of human movement using the principles of both anatomy and mechanics.
Kinetic a term used to define motion.
Mechanics the study of the motion of a body and the effect of force on it.
Overload increasing the demand on the body past that point to which it has adapted.
Posture the position of the body and the relationship of its parts to one another.
Range-of-motion exercises exercises used to move each joint through full normal movement.
ROM abbreviation for range of motion.
Repetition the process of repeating an exercise or an activity.

When we want to define human movement as it relates to our body's anatomy and the individual principles of mechanics used as we move its various parts, we are actually talking about a very detailed science known as *kinesiology*. All human movement depends on two sets of factors. The first, body structure and function, deals with characteristics of muscles, skeletal structure, and the types and actions of joints and nerve functions which initiate and control activities. The second set of factors, which lie more within the branch of physical sciences dealing with physics, mechanics, and geometry, focuses more on the principles governing gravity, fluid resistance, friction, and the reaction of external forces in the environment, such as the ground, other people, or sports equipment. All of these factors play a great role in our body's ability to function physiologically as each and every part individually moves. Because of the principles involved in the study of kinesiology, preparation in this field is a very important part of the education of people like yourselves who are interested in working in physical medicine.

Understanding Biomechanics

When studying kinesiology, in addition to gaining a basic understanding of anatomy, the branch of science you should also become familiar with is *mechanics*. This includes the study of the motion of our body as it relates to the effects of force on it. The subdivision of mechanics concerned with the study of motion of all living organisms is called *biomechanics*. And applied biomechanics is considered part of the study of physical rehabilitation. It is also an area covered in other interdisciplinary studies, such as engineering, physical education, and aerospace sciences.

When we study biomechanics, particularly as it relates to physical medicine or rehabilitation, we must also take into account how the body moves, its positioning, alignment and balance, and its relationship to the action of muscles.

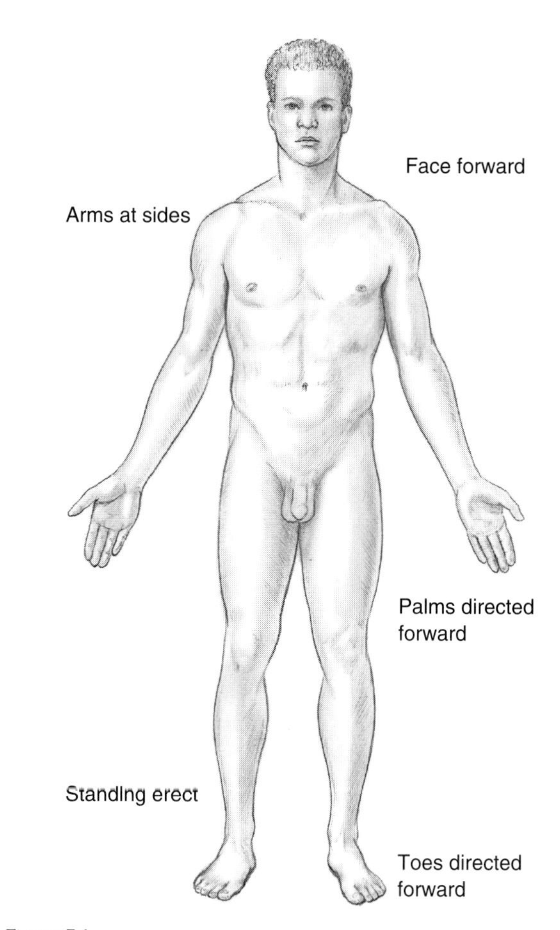

Figure 7-1
Anatomical position. (Reprinted with permission from Applegate, E.J. *The Anatomy and Physiology Learning System.* Philadelphia: W. B. Saunders, 1995, p. 14.)

Body Positions

All of the terms we use to describe how our body is positioned are based upon a standard position known as the anatomical position (Figure 7-1). When a person is standing in this position, he or she is standing erect with the head and trunk aligned, arms straight by the sides, with the palms facing forward, and the legs straight with the feet together. In kinesiology, this position is generally used as a reference point for describing all movements of the forearm, hand, and fingers.

A fundamental standing position is used as a point of reference to describe all the movements of the individual body parts except for the forearms, hands, and fingers. This position differs from the anatomical position in that the palms are turned toward the person's thighs.

Posture, Body Alignment, and Balance

The term *posture* is used to describe the position of our body as it relates to its individual parts, and those parts to one another. To gain proper alignment of your body, stand tall with all the parts of your skeleton perfectly aligned. When the parts of the skeletal system are properly aligned, balance can be maintained.

Balance refers to how we maintain an object in a steady position so that it does not tip or fall. To maintain balance, we must have a wide base of support. This means that when we are in a standing position, our feet become the base of support. The center of gravity is the geometric center of an object and is located on a person close to the center of his or her pelvis just below the umbilicus. The exact location varies with a person's age, sex, and body build. The line of gravity is an imaginary line that passes through the center of gravity and the base of support. In order to maintain balance, the center of gravity must fall within the base of support between the feet. When the center of gravity falls outside the base of support, the person will lose his or her stability or balance. The larger the base of support, the greater the stability.

Balance is important in movement when performing sports activities or any form of exercise. The ability of a person to maintain balance during such movement is called dynamic balance. It may be inverted, as in the case of gymnastics, diving, and dancing, and it is always affected by the pull of gravity, the base of support, the line of gravity, and the mass of the person.

Muscle Action and Kinesiology

The study of the muscles is very important to understanding kinesiology. Our body has about 500 individual muscles, and as we have already discussed in Chapter 6, these muscles are classified according to their function. Smooth (involuntary) muscles are grouped according to their action. These include movers, which perform specific movements, such as those that contribute most to movement (called prime movers) and those that help the prime movers (called assistant movers); antagonists, which are muscles that oppose prime movers; stabilizers, which help to stabilize a prime mover; and synergists, which increase the efficiency of prime movers by inhibiting movements in other associated joints.

Exercise and Muscle Action

There are many types of exercise to help increase muscle action. These include exercises which develop and maintain flexibility, strength, and endurance, and exercises which help to produce cardiopulmonary fitness.

Exercises used to develop and maintain flexibility can be active or passive. Active exercise in turn is either static or *kinetic*. Isometric exercise is a static activity because the muscles are contracted without moving a limb or joint. Pushing against a door frame is an example of an isometric exercise. Kinetic exercises require the muscles to contract and move one or more muscles and joints. These may be performed against resistance, as in the case of weight training, or without resistance, as in gymnastics or *calisthenics*.

Passive exercises are often grouped as either forced or nonforced. A nonforced movement is completed within the limits of a person's range of motion. That is, no pain is involved. These activities are generally used in a medical setting for rehabilitation of a physically disabled person, and often in the treatment of *contractures* and *adhesions*. Forced passive exercise goes beyond voluntary range of motion.

Exercises which are vigorous and which must be sustained in order to produce cardiopulmonary fitness are called aerobic exercises. In these exercises, the entire body must be moved. In order for an exercise to be aerobic, the heartbeat must be raised and sustained for at least 12 minutes. Some examples of aerobic exercises include brisk walking, continuous dancing, swimming, bicycling, and jogging.

A type of exercise program which organizes selected activities into a sequence or circuit, is called a *circuit training* program. A circuit is laid out so that a person does one activity, or exercise, for a specific period of time or for a set number of repetitions and then jogs or runs to another station to perform another type or exercise. At the station, the activities are designed to build strength, flexibility, or muscular endurance.

A type of training which involves alternating heavy exercise with periods of rest or light exercise is called interval training. Its purpose is to allow the body to recover energy which has been stored in muscle during the resting interval. In interval training, the time periods of exercise are about the same length but can be set at any interval appropriate to the intensity of the exercise. The number of repetitions, intensity, and distance covered generally depends on the sport and athlete involved. This type of exercise program is most commonly used by swimmers and track and field athletes.

Using Kinesiology as an Evaluation Tool

A person working in physical medicine and using kinesiology as an evaluation tool must be able to conduct a qualitative analysis in order to determine whether a performer is using his or her motor skills correctly and at their greatest efficiency. You must also be able to describe the skill and break it down into individual components, and at the same time determine whether anatomical and mechanical principles are being used correctly. If changes are needed, you must also be able to create, devise, and modify a plan necessary to improve performance effectively.

The initial evaluation is often recorded on a standardized form which lists the areas of evaluation. Many types of equipment are also available to aid in the assessment. These range from a simple double-armed goniometer to sophisticated computerized equipment and movie or video cameras.

Evaluating Range-of-Motion

Because of many factors, range-of-motion, or ROM, patterns vary with the individual. For this reason, norms are often quite difficult to establish. There are four basic methods for studying ROM. Three are performed directly on the person using the double-armed goniometer, flexometer, or elgon (Figure 7-2). The fourth method uses film. When this method is used, filming must be accurate in order to show a difference in the joint angles between two pictures. The camera must be at a right angle to the plane of action and the joint center must be marked to show in some way. The ROM is the difference between the joint angles shown in the first picture as the action begins and the second picture as it concludes.

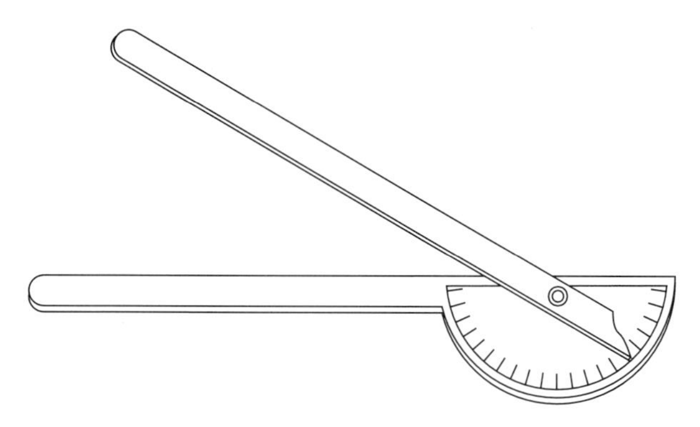

Figure 7-2
The goniometer.

A goniometer is a device used to measure angles, and therefore assesses a joint's range-of-motion. A double-armed goniometer has a stationary arm and a moveable arm which are held together by a pin. To measure the range-of-motion, the holding pin is placed over the joint center with the stationary arm aligned with the body segment. The other arm is moved with the body segment or aligned at the completion of the movement. The indicator shows the number of degrees through which the segment moved.

Evaluating Motor Skills

The easiest way to evaluate the action of a muscle is by observing and palpating it as it contracts. If the muscle lacks strength, it is sometimes difficult to feel its contraction. Therefore, this technique is often limited to the superficial muscles.

Muscle contraction, stimulated electrically, is a means of studying the action of individual muscles. It cannot analyze a series of actions, however. A machine called a muscle stimulator is required for this type of testing.

Through *electromyography (EMG),* the electrical potential generated by muscular movement is picked up by electrodes, amplified, and ultimately recorded on a graphic chart. Muscle activity can then be studied. Computers can be tied into the system to quantify the data. Physicians often use EMGs to analyze and determine defects in movement and conduction of neural impulses moving the muscles. Figure 7-3 shows a myogram of movement in two muscles; the biceps femoris and the tibialis anterior.

The use of videotape, movie film or motion pictures, and computer technology are often used to evaluate a person's motor skills. Videotape is generally used to film a specific performance. Like movie film, it can be shown in slow motion or stopped to study a specific motor skill. Videotape also lends itself well to teaching, since the flow and sequence of movement can easily be observed and then repeated for additional reinforcement.

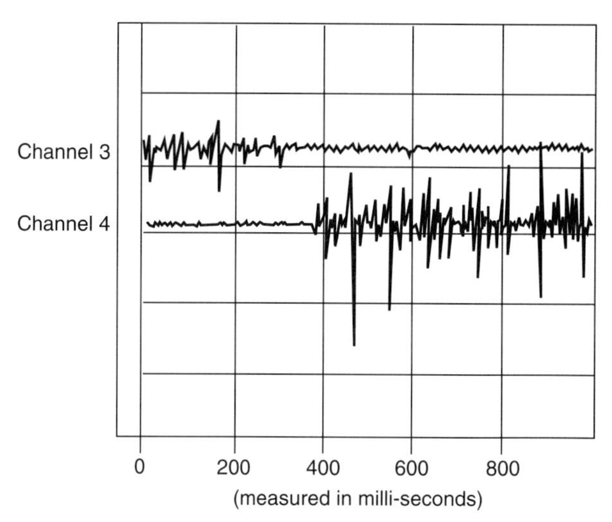

Figure 7-3
Myogram showing movement of muscles.

Computer technology used in conjunction with specific software programs is frequently used when the practitioner needs to both collect and analyze specific data which has been collected by other methods of evaluating movement and motor skills. Another purpose for using the computer is to provide a simulation. Mathematical models are developed through complex equations in order to simulate sequential patterns in movement. The models can then be used to determine the effect of altering outside forces upon a specific performance.

Planning the Exercise Program

Once you have completed the evaluation process, you are ready to begin the next step: planning the actual exercise program. However, before you can even begin to plan the program, there are certain specific considerations, or factors, which you must take into account. These include (a) determining the type of exercise or activity you want to develop, such as cardiovascular fitness, muscular strength, endurance, or flexibility; (b) the actual intensity of the chosen exercise; (c) the duration or length of time involved in each activity; and (d) the frequency of performance or how often the exercise is to be performed.

When determining the intensity of a planned exercise, the best time to accomplish it is while the person is engaged in an aerobic exercise. All intensity is judged by the rate at which the heart beats. To determine the heart rate, stop strenuous exercise but continue some movement. Then, using your fingers, locate the pulse in the neck or wrist. Count for ten full seconds. Multiply this number by six in order to establish the actual beats per minute.

Another important point to remember whenever you are planning an exercise program is that an individual should only exercise in his or her target rate zone during the aerobic portion of the program. What this means is that people who are beginning a program, or who lead a rather sedentary lifestyle, should generally stay in the 60 to 70 percent zone of their heart function. On the other hand, adults who lead a more active lifestyle should aim for at least 70 to 80 percent.

Determining Oxygen Consumption

If you are employed in a large sports medicine facility or fitness center that conducts research in kinesiology, chances are you will hear the term VO_2 Max. This term refers to the maximum volume of oxygen consumption. The volume, which generally varies with a person's size, age, and fitness, is used as an index of oxygen consumption by the body and therefore is able to indicate the degree of endurance or physical fitness.

Anyone who practices a good exercise program knows that his or her body tends to increase its metabolism during periods of activity. Following exercise, there is an oxygen debt, which leaves us with that out-of-breath feeling. Once this oxygen debt has been repaid, we immediately recover. With planned training, our body will increase its ability to take in oxygen and thus consume it much more efficiently while we are exercising.

Improving Performance

Once an exercise program has been properly planned, the study of kinesiology has also provided us with specific principles that can be applied to improve our overall performance of the activities. One principle is known as *progression*. This involves beginning the activity very slowly, and then gradually increasing the amount or frequency of the exercise being performed. This means, for example, if you are a jogger, increasing the distance you jog or decreasing the time required to run one mile. Progression should always be gradual and properly planned.

Another principle for improving your performance is *repetition*, or how many times you complete a specific exercise. Repetitions can be grouped into sets, with a rest to mark the end of a set. A push-up, for example, might be repeated five times to form one set. These repetitions could be increased to a set of eight before a rest. The number of sets can also be increased.

A third principle used to help increase our overall performance is called *overload*. Overload has to do with our body's ability to adapt to meet the increased demands placed on it. For example, if you can easily walk on a treadmill for 20 minutes, increase the time to 30 minutes.

Summary

In this chapter, we discussed the study of applied kinesiology and its relationship to physical medicine and physical performance. We explained how muscles are grouped together according to their role in movement, and identified various types of exercises. We also talked about different types of equipment used for evaluating exercise. Finally, we discussed how to properly plan an exercise program, and the principles involved in improving one's performance of such a program.

Review Questions

1. What is the name of the science that deals with the study of human movement using the principles of both anatomy and mechanics?
2. What does the abbreviation ROM mean?
3. What is the name of the substudy of mechanics that is concerned with the motion of all living organisms?
4. Briefly explain what an electromyogram is.
5. A ______________ refers to an abnormal shortening of a muscle tissue.
6. A selected exercise activity which has been organized into a sequence or circuit for performance is called a:
   a. calisthenic
   b. biomechanical
   c. circuit training
7. A group of gymnastic exercises is frequently referred to as:
   a. calisthenics
   b. biomechanics
   c. repetitions
8. ______________ is the position of the body and the relationship of its parts to one another.
9. The process of repeating an exercise or an activity is called:
   a. kinetics
   b. repetitions
   c. mechanics

8

Medical Terminology and the Medical Record

Performance Objectives

Upon completion of this chapter, you will be able to:

1. Identify specific prefixes, suffixes, and root words used in medical terms.
2. List common medical abbreviations used in the health care environment.
3. Identify body structure terms related to position, direction, anatomical planes, posture, and types of movement.
4. Explain the importance and uses of the medical record.
5. Distinguish between subjective, objective, assessment, and plan information on a patient's medical record.

Terms and Abbreviations

Prefix always placed at the beginning of a word and pertains to a word element, that when combined with a root, changes or adds to the root word's meaning.

Root pertains to the body or main part of the word, referring to the primary meaning of the word as a whole.

Suffix always placed at the end of a root and pertains to a word element used to change or add to the meaning of the word.

The discussion of medical terminology will help you to understand the many terms commonly used in medicine and in your individual department. The prefixes and suffixes of many medical terms give definite information about the meanings of the terms. If you know these prefixes and suffixes, it will be a lot easier to understand many medical words. A *prefix* is a word fragment placed in front of the basic or root word (Table 8-1). A *suffix* is a word fragment added at the end of the basic or root word (Table 8-2). The *root* word is the main body of the word, that is, the part that usually gives the meaning to the word (Table 8-3).

There are no specific rules governing the pronunciation of medical terms. A medical dictionary will give you some suggestions as to the pronunciation of words, however, in many hospitals and medical facilities, these pronunciations will vary among professionals and individual departments.

Using Medical Abbreviations

Many abbreviations for words and phrases are used in the treatment of patients to save time and space. As a member of the physical medicine team, you must learn these abbreviations so that you can follow directions and communicate with other health care workers (Table 8-4). Since the physical medicine profession has adopted many abbreviations that are commonly used by health care professionals in writing

Text continued on page 75

Table 8-1
Common Prefixes and Their Meanings

Prefix	Meaning	Word Example	Meaning of Example
a-, an-	without	apnea	without breath
ab-	away from	abnormal	away from the rule
		abduct	away from the midline of the body
ad-	toward	adduct	toward the midline of the body
albus-	white	albinuria	white or colorless urine
ambi-	both	ambidextrous	uses both hands with equal ease
anti-	against	antisepsis	preventing growth of bacteria
bi-	two; both	bilateral	pertaining to two sides of the body
circum-	around	circumrenal	around the kidneys
cyano-	blue	cyanosis	bluish skin color due to lack of oxygen
endo-	in; within	endocardium	inside layer of the heart
epi-	upon; over	epidermis	outside layer of the skin
erythro-	red	erythrocyte	red blood cell
ex-, exo-	out; away	extension	movement widening angle between two adjoining parts
glyco-	sweet; sugar	glycosuria	sugar in the urine
hyper-	above; excessive	hypertension	abnormally high blood pressure
hypo-	below	hypotension	abnormally low blood pressure
inter-	between	intervertebral disc	cartilage found between most vertebral bones
leuko-	white	leukocyte	white blood cell
lith-	stone	lithotomy	removal of a stone
nephro-	kidney	nephrology	study of the kidney

Table 8-2
Common Suffixes and Their Meanings

Suffix	Meaning	Word Example	Meaning of Example
-algia	pain	neuralgia	pain along course of a nerve
-ectomy	cutting out	thyroidectomy	surgical removal of the thyroid
-iasis	condition of	lithiasis	formation of a stone
-itis	inflammation	endocarditis	inflammation of the endocardium
-ology	study of	cardiology	study of the heart
-pathy	disease	osteopathy	disease of the bone
-phobia	fear	hydrophobia	fear of water
-plasty	repair	rhinoplasty	surgical correction of the nose

Table 8-3
Common Root Words and Their Meanings

Root	Meaning	Word Example	Meaning of Example
cardia	heart	carditis	inflammation of the heart
costa	rib	costalgia	pain in a rib
gastro	stomach	gastroenteritis	inflammation of the stomach
neuro	nerve	neuralgia	pain along a nerve
oto	ear	otitis	inflammation of the ear
pedi	foot	pedicure	care of the feet
phlebo	vein	phlebitis	inflammation of a vein
pneumo	lung	pneumonectomy	surgical removal of a lung

Table 8-4
Common Medical Abbreviations and Their Meanings

Commonly Used Abbreviations	Meaning
aa	of each
ad lib	as desired
AIDS	acquired immune deficiency syndrome
amt.	amount
ASHD	arteriosclerotic heart disease
ax	axillary
BM	bowel movement
BP	blood pressure
BRP	bathroom privilege
c̄	with
C	Celsius (Centigrade)
Cal	calorie
cc	cubic centimeter
CHF	congestive heart failure
cm	centimeter
CO	coronary occlusion
CNS	central nervous system
CPR	cardiopulmonary resuscitation
CVA	cerebrovascular accident (stroke)
DC	discontinue; discharge
DOA	dead on arrival
Dx	diagnosis
EKG	electrocardiogram
elix	elixir
F	Fahrenheit
Fx	fracture
gm (GM)	gram
gtt	drops
hema	blood
hemi	half

(Continued)

Table 8-4 *(Continued)*
Common Medical Abbreviations and Their Meanings

H&P	history and physical
Ht.	height
Kg	kilogram
L	liter
m	minim
MI	myocardial infarction (heart attack)
ml	milliliter
NG	nasogastric
NPO	nothing by mouth (nil per os)
O.D.	right eye
O.S.	left eye
O.U.	both eyes
O2	oxygen
OOB	out of bed
oz	ounce
p̄	after
P	pulse
PID	pelvic inflammatory disease
PM	afternoon
Post-op	after surgery
Pre-op	before surgery
Pt.	patient
PO	by mouth (per os)
P.R.N.	whenever necessary, or as needed
QNS	quantity not sufficient
QS	quantity sufficient
R	respiration
Rx	prescription (recipe)
s̄	without
Semi	half
Sig	write (let it be labeled)
SOB	shortness of breath
S.O.S.	if necessary
SSE	soapsuds enema
s̄s̄	half
STD	sexually transmitted disease
Stat	immediately
T	temperature
T.O.	telephone order
TPR	temperature, pulse, respiration
tr	tincture
ung.	ointment
ur	urine
URI	upper respiratory infection
V.O.	verbal order
wt.	weight
>	greater than
<	less than
♀	female; woman
♂	male; man

Table 8-4 (*Continued*)
Common Medical Abbreviations and Their Meanings

Abbreviations Related to Time	Meaning
a.c.	before meals
A.M.	morning
b.i.d.	twice a day
h	hour
h.n.	tonight
h.s.	bedtime; hour of sleep
noct.	night
p.c.	after meals
q.d.	every day
q.h.	every hour
q.2h	every 2 hours
q.i.d.	four times a day
q.o.d.	every other day
t.i.d.	three times a day
t.i.n.	three times a night
Department Abbreviations	**Meaning**
CCU	Coronary Care Unit
CS; CSR	Central Supply; Central Supply Room
EENT	Eye, Ear, Nose, and Throat
ER	Emergency Room
GI	Gastrointestinal Department
GYN	Gynecology Department
ICU	Intensive Care Unit
LAB	Laboratory
MICU	Medical Intensive Care Unit
NICU	Neonatal Intensive Care Unit
OB	Obstetrics
OR	Operating Room
PEDI	Pediatrics
P.T.	Physical Therapy
R.T.	Respiratory Therapy
X-Ray	Radiology

their notes in the patient's medical record, it is very important that you study and learn these common abbreviations so that you will be able to easily recognize their meanings.

Body Structure and Medical Terminology

The human body may be compared to a smooth-running machine. It has many parts which must work together in order to promote good health, growth, and life itself. The body is a combination of organs and systems which are supported and protected by a framework of bones known as the skeleton. The muscles working upon the skeleton provide for the movements as we work and play through each day. All of this is then protected by an external covering known as the skin, which is considered the largest of all our body organs. You will need to know the various parts of the body and how to describe them in medical terms.

The human body is divided into five specific cavities or compartments: thoracic, abdominal, pelvic, cranial, and spinal (Figure 8-1). Within the thoracic cavity are the lungs, heart, aorta, and the thymus gland. The abdominal cavity contains the stomach, liver, gallbladder, small intestine, colon, or large intestine, spleen, and the pancreas. The reproductive organs and the urinary bladder are all located within the pelvic cavity. The brain lies within the cranial cavity, while the spine is located within the spinal cavity. Various structural units make up the body. Cells, tissues, and organs are organized into individual systems. These systems include the skeletal, muscular, nervous, circulatory, digestive, respiratory, urinary, reproductive, and endocrine.

Anatomical Position

Many terms are used to describe the body and to identify the position, direction, and location of the parts of the body. In addition, these terms are also used to describe various medical characteristics of the body, such as the location of incisions or injuries on the body. In order for the health care professional to be able to read the patient's medical record and thus have a mental picture of the patient's condition, all descriptive terms are based on an accepted standard position. This standard is known as the anatomical position (see Figure 7-1 on page 67). In this position, the person is standing erect, facing forward, with the head and trunk aligned, the arms straight by the sides with palms facing forward, and the legs straight with the feet together.

Defining Position and Direction

Once you know the definition of the anatomical position, you can begin to use specific terms to describe position, direction, and location. While Figure 8-2 shows the relationship of some of these terms to one another, the following is a list of all of the terms which are used to describe the body's position and direction.

- *anterior:* toward the front or in front of; ventral.
- *posterior:* toward the back or in back of; dorsal.
- *medial:* nearest the midline.
- *lateral:* away from the midline or toward the side.
- *internal:* inward or inside.
- *external:* outward or outside.
- *proximal:* nearest the point of reference.
- *distal:* farthest away from the point of reference.
- *superior:* above.

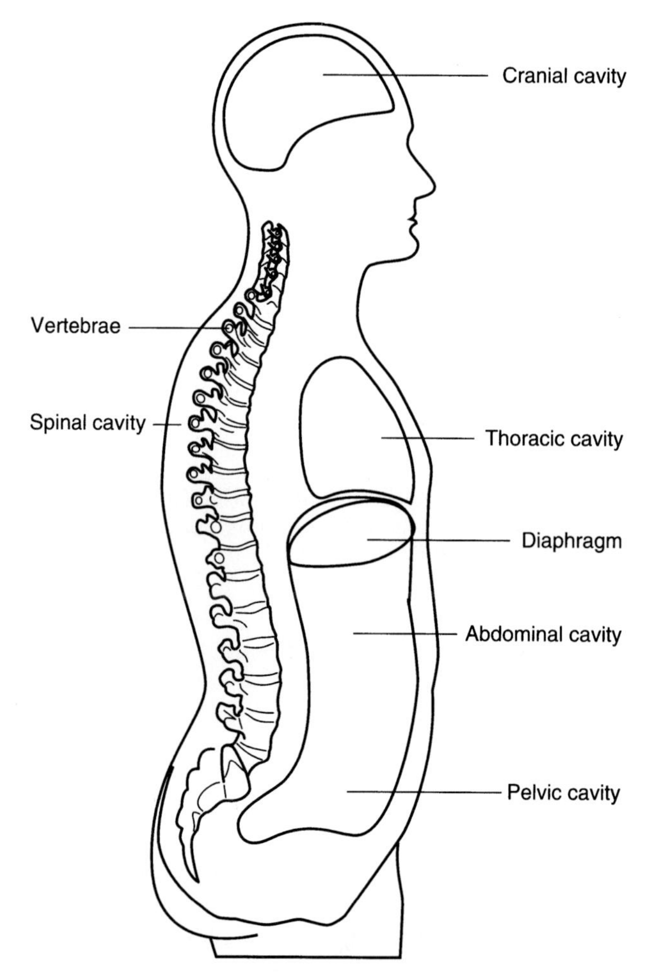

Figure 8-1
Body cavities. (Reprinted with permission from Weiss, R.C. *Your Career in Administrative Medical Services.* Philadelphia: W. B. Saunders, 1996, p. 36.)

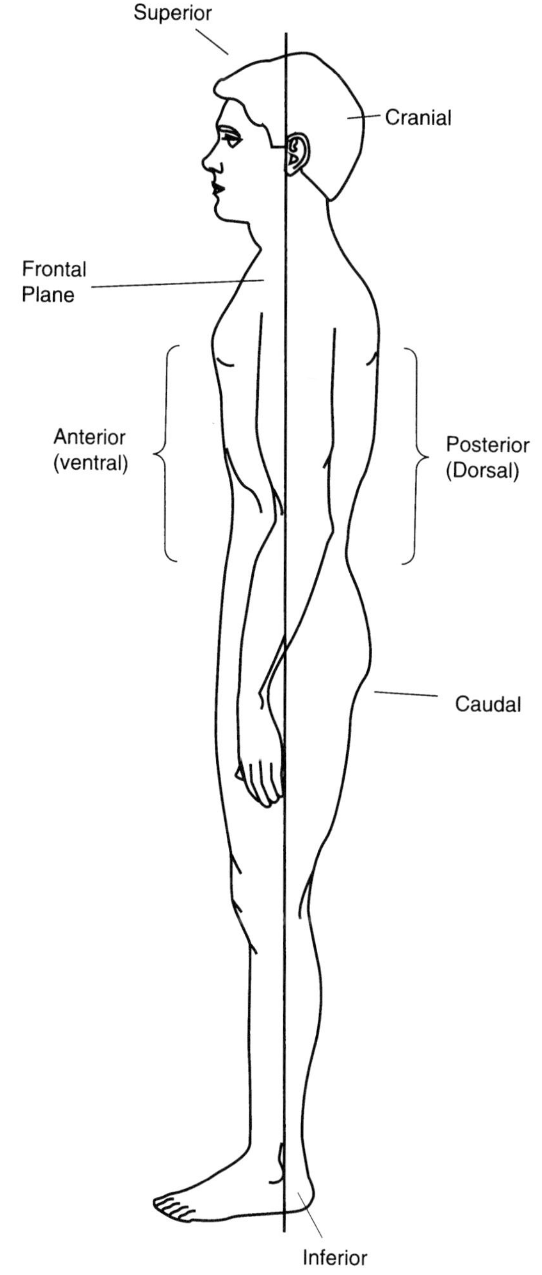

Figure 8-2
Body positions and directions. (Reprinted with permission from Weiss, R.C. *Your Career in Administrative Medical Services.* Philadelphia: W. B. Saunders, 1996, p. 36.)

- *inferior:* below.
- *cranial:* toward the head.
- *caudal:* toward the tail.

Defining Anatomical Planes

There are specific terms used to describe and identify structures, areas of the body, and certain types of movement of the extremities (Figure 8-3 on p. 78). These include

- *sagittal:* an imaginary plane that runs parallel to the long axis of the body, dividing it into right and left sections.
- *frontal:* an imaginary plane that runs through the side of the body, dividing it into anterior (front) and posterior (back) sections.
- *transverse:* an imaginary plane dividing the body into superior (upper) and inferior (lower) sections.

Defining Anatomical Postures

There are specific terms used to describe anatomical postures. These include

- *erect:* standing position.
- *supine:* lying down.
- *prone:* lying flat on the stomach, with the face down.
- *side-lying:* lying with the body positioned on either the left or right side.

Defining Types of Movement

There are specific terms used to describe various types of body movement. These include

- *flexion:* bending at a joint.
- *extension:* straightening at a joint; unbending.
- *abduction:* moving away from the center of the body.
- *adduction:* moving toward the center of the body.
- *rotation:* rolling a part on its own axis, such as the turning of the head.
- *pronation:* moving the palm from the anatomical position into a position with the palm facing posteriorly, or backward.
- *supination:* moving the palm into the anatomical position facing anteriorly, or forward.
- *eversion:* turning the foot outward.
- *inversion:* turning the foot inward.

It's very important to remember that not all joints can perform all motions. The immovable joints are, of course, incapable of performing any of them. Of the freely moving joints, only the ball-and-socket joints, such as the hip and the shoulder, can perform all motions. The hinge joints, such as those found at the knee and the elbow, are only able to flex and extend.

Understanding the Patient's Medical Record

Memory, even at its very best, is often fleeting and inaccurate; medical records, on the other hand, contain accurate and detailed facts. These facts serve as

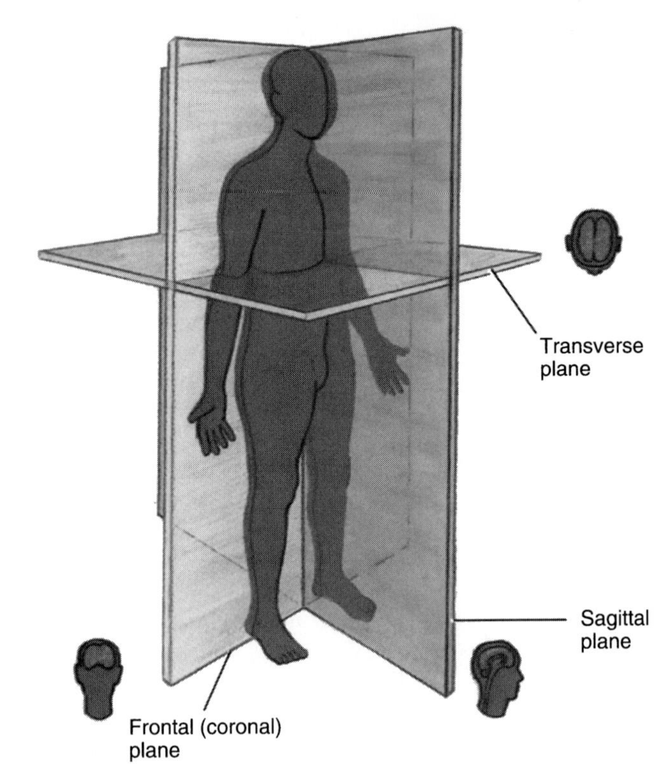

Figure 8-3
Anatomical planes. (Reprinted with permission from Applegate, E.J. *The Anatomy and Physiology Learning System.* Philadelphia: W. B. Saunders, 1995, p. 14.)

a basis for the study, evaluation, and review of the patient's medical care.

Patients' medical records have been found among the earliest Egyptian and Hindu writings. Until modern times, however, no effort was ever made to keep patients' histories in any type of systemic order. These records are of the greatest importance to the physician while the patient is under his or her care. They are also extremely valuable if the patient returns for treatment after several years. For the patient, the record has a historical value, as it is the document which forms his or her case history.

A patient's history also has great statistical value. For instance, it may be of use to the physician in evaluating a specific type of treatment, or to find out the incidence of a particular disease. The record may also be used as the basis for a lecture, an article, or a textbook. Further, patients' histories have legal importance. They may be summoned as a legal document and used in a court of law either to uphold the rights of the doctor if he or she is involved in litigation, or they may be used to confirm the claim of the patient if the doctor is called as a witness.

The medical record is used by health care practitioners to exchange information or as a means of communication. The physician, nurses, and other personnel contribute information to the record. A doctor may change a patient's care if the nurse has observed a change in the patient's condition. Likewise, after reading the notes written by the physical therapy aide, a nurse may plan specific nursing care that will allow the patient the greatest degree of comfort toward the prevention of any future musculoskeletal symptoms.

There are many different types of printed forms available for keeping medical records. Some hospitals print their own forms. Preprinted forms are useful because they save time. They also assist the recorder in remembering questions he or she want to ask. They are a way to consistently and accurately record the details of the patient's care and treatment.

The physician is always the person who initiates the treatment by checking the appropriate referral blanks or writing directions or orders for treatment in a narrative form. The request for a lab test or an electrocardiogram, for example, is then sent to the cardiovascular department or the laboratory, as soon as possible, so that the procedure or lab test can be scheduled and carried out. Usually, the hospitalized patient and the chart are brought to the department from the nursing unit. Information relating to how the testing or procedural goals are being accomplished and the patient's response to the procedure are then recorded in the medical record after the test or procedure has been completed.

Charting Notes in the Medical Record

Most large health care facilities and individual medical practices document the patient's care and treatment in the medical record by utilizing a four-point system known as SOAP notes. The SOAP abbreviation refers to the four methods in which the patient's care is identified, assessed, and ultimately, carried out.

The *S* stands for subjective symptoms which the patient may be presenting, and includes any information the patient says, family remarks made regarding the patient, and any other information stated by other health care providers. The *O* refers to any objective information, tests, or treatments which may have been provided for the patient, as well as any observations or measurements made by a member of the health care team. The assessment, or how well the patient is responding to a given treatment, is abbreviated by the *A*. It includes any professional opinions or goals of a specific type of therapy or treatment made by the health care provider. And the *P*, which pertains to the plan, is what needs to be done or what will be done for the patient, based on the objective and subjective findings and the assessment.

Not all hospitals or individual departments will use the SOAP note format. Your department may choose to set up its own method of keeping records. Some departments use 5-by-8-inch file cards and record only the visits of the patients. Others may use an 8-by-11-inch file folder which encloses individual progress notes. In any case, the SOAP format is a good way of organizing your written data, no matter what type of forms the department uses.

Writing in the Medical Record

Since the patient's medical record is considered a legal document, it should always be written in ink. The information should be factual and have meaning. Notes must be accurate, without any spelling or grammatical errors. And any errors must be properly corrected by drawing one line through the error, with the person making it writing his or her initials to verify that an error has been made and corrected. You must never scratch out mistakes and or use correction fluids. Remember, too, that all information within the medical record is confidential. This means that the record should not be used for any other reason but as a means of exchanging information between members of the professional medical staff.

Summary

In this chapter, you were introduced to medical terminology and the medical record. In doing so, we determined that a basic knowledge of medical terms will make you more knowledgeable about your patient's condition and thus allow you to read medical reports and records with greater understanding. As you continue to gain experience in the field of physical medicine, you will recognize the importance of using proper terms and abbreviations to save time and space when documenting patients' responses to medical treatments.

Review Questions

1. A ______________ is always placed at the beginning of a word.
   a. prefix
   b. suffix
   c. root
2. A ______________ is always placed at the end of a word.
   a. prefix
   b. suffix
   c. root
3. A ______________ pertains to the body or main part of a word.
   a. prefix
   b. suffix
   c. root
4. What does the term anterior mean?
5. What does the term lateral mean?
6. Define the following prefixes:
   a. anti ______________
   b. erythro ______________
   c. leuko ______________
7. Define the following suffixes:
   a. ectomy ______________
   b. itis ______________
   c. ology ______________
8. Define the following abbreviations:
   a. P.T. ______________
   b. CHF ______________
   c. H&P ______________
9. Define the following abbreviations:
   a. NPO ______________
   b. t.i.d. ______________
   c. a.c. ______________

9

Measuring Vital Signs

Performance Objectives

Upon completion of this chapter, you will be able to:

1. Briefly explain the purpose and function of vital signs.
2. Identify each of the vital signs, and briefly discuss the role each plays in the proper functioning of the body.
3. Describe variations of the body's vital signs.
4. Describe and be able to demonstrate how to properly obtain, measure, and record a patient's vital signs.

Terms and Abbreviations

Blood pressure the amount of force exerted by the heart against the walls of the arteries as it contracts and relaxes.
Pulse the beat of the heart as it is felt through the walls of the arteries.
Respiration the act of breathing in oxygen and breathing out carbon dioxide.
Sphygmomanometer instrument used to measure the blood pressure.
Stethoscope instrument used to listen to the beats of the heart as they are heard through the walls of the arteries.
Temperature the degree of body heat that is a direct result of the balance maintained between heat produced and heat lost by the body.
Vital signs important signs or measurements of the body's state of health; includes the temperature, pulse, respiration, and blood pressure.

Whether you are working in the physical therapy or rehabilitation department, or for a private orthopedic surgeon, chiropractor, or national athletic team, as a member of the physical medicine health care delivery team there is a very strong possibility that you, at some time, will be responsible for obtaining, measuring, and recording the patient's *vital signs.* After all, one of the very best tools the doctor has to evaluate the patient's cardiovascular condition is by noting any changes or variations in his or her blood pressure, temperature, pulse, or respiration.

The vital signs are considered one of the best and most measurable ways to determine one's state of health, and variation in the norm of any one or all of the vital signs can provide the physician with his or her first indication that there may be something wrong with the patient's cardiovascular system, which is the very basis for helping the patient, the client, or the athlete to meet both the physical and emotional needs of his or her musculoskeletal endurance.

Blood Pressure

Blood pressure, according to most physicians, is considered the most significant of all the vital signs. It is the amount of force exerted by the heart against the walls of the arteries, while the heart is contracting and relaxing. It consists of two readings; the systolic pressure, which is created as the force of blood is pushed against the arterial walls while the ventricles of the heart are in a state of contraction, and the diastolic pressure, which occurs when the ventricles are in a state of relaxation. When recording the blood pressure, it is identified in millimeters of mercury (mmHg). The upper number is recorded as the systolic pressure, and the lower number is recorded as the diastolic pressure.

Variations and Abnormal Blood Pressure

Like the other vital signs, blood pressure may vary according to the patient's age, sex, and whether or not he or she exercises, smokes, or drinks. Other factors, such as obesity, the taking of certain medications, and the patient's emotional state of health also have bearing on one's blood pressure. In some cases, blood pressure may increase when the patient is standing, or when it is being measured in the right arm as opposed to the left.

Normal blood pressure generally ranges between 110 to 140 systolic and 70 to 90 diastolic. The average, or what is considered the "normal" blood pressure reading for most healthy adults, is 120/80 mmHg. Because of the loss of elasticity and the buildup of fatty deposits within the walls of the arteries, blood pressure tends to increase with age, while children, on the other hand, generally tend to have a lower blood pressure reading.

Any time there is a drastic change in the patient's blood pressure there is cause to worry. If, for example, the blood pressure drops below 110/70 mmHg, the doctor may be concerned with a condition known as hypotension, or abnormally low blood pressure. This is generally difficult to diagnose because there are few symptoms associated with it. An abnormal increase of the blood pressure over 140/90 mmHg, or hypertension, on the other hand, may also give rise to worry. Hypertension is usually easier to diagnose because it is almost always accompanied by headaches, irritability, blurred vision, nosebleed, nausea and vomiting, and dizziness.

Measuring and Recording the Blood Pressure

Two instruments are used to measure the blood pressure. They are the *stethoscope* and the *sphygmomanometer* (Figure 9-1). The stethoscope consists of two earpieces, tubing, and a diaphragm, or bell, and is used to listen to the heart beating as it is heard through the walls of the artery. The sphygmomanometer utilizes an apparatus known as a manometer, which is the actual tool of measurement for obtaining the blood pressure. With the assistance of a

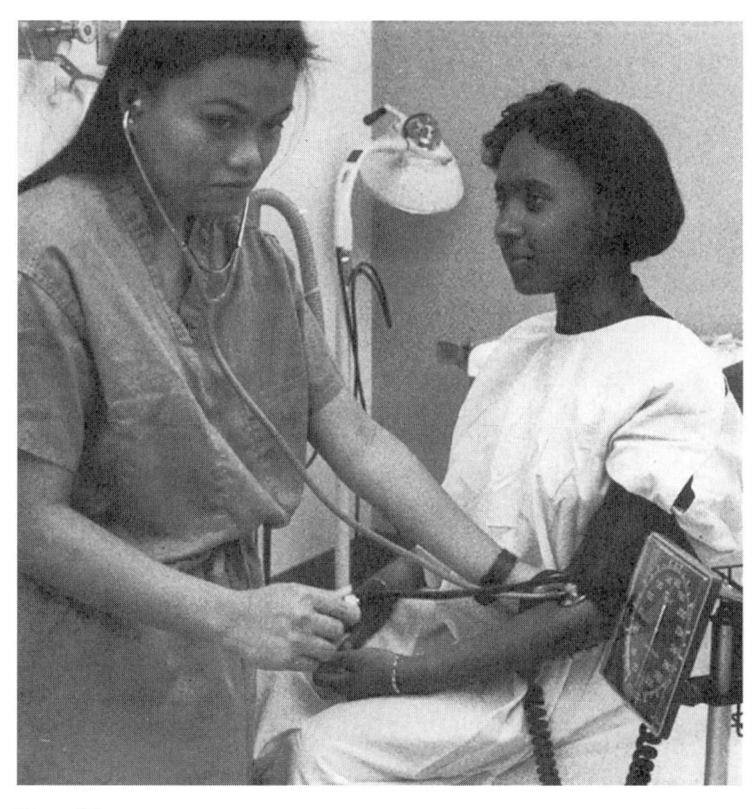

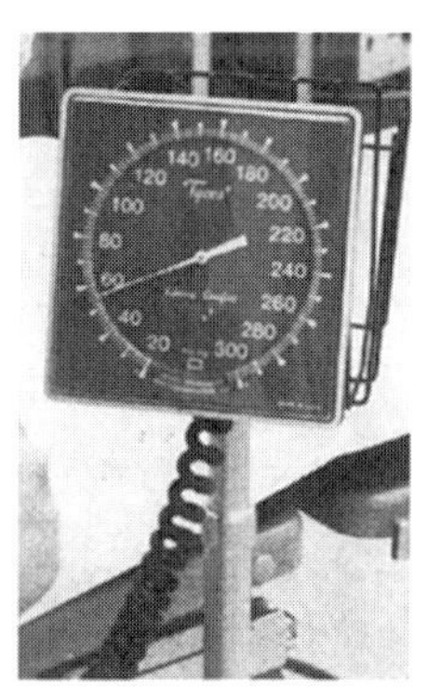

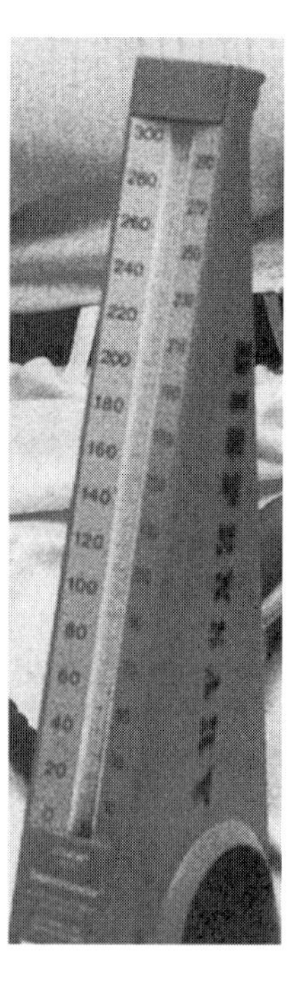

Figure 9-1
Stethoscope and sphygmomanometer. (Reprinted with permission from Weiss, R.C. *Your Career in Cardiovascular Technology.* Philadelphia: W. B. Saunders, 1996, p. 64.)

cuff, an inflation bulb, and a pressure control valve, the sphygmomanometer is wrapped around the patient's arm over the brachial artery and secured in place. The stethoscope is used to listen to the beats of the heart at the brachial artery while the sphygmomanometer is pumped up.

Procedure for Obtaining the Blood Pressure

To properly obtain the blood pressure, you should:

1. Gather the necessary equipment. This includes the sphygmomanometer, the stethoscope, and cotton balls or alcohol wipe pads to clean the earpieces.
2. Wash your hands and clean the earpieces of the stethoscope.
3. Position the patient in a sitting position with his or her arm supported. If the patient is wearing long sleeves, expose the arm by rolling up the sleeve approximately five inches above the elbow or removing the arm from the sleeve if necessary.
4. Gently place the deflated cuff evenly, yet snugly, around the patient's arm with the lower edge about one to two inches above the antecubital space, or the inside of the elbow.
5. Center the cuff over the brachial artery before securing it with clasps or velcro.
6. Locate the brachial pulse in the antecubital space by palpating it with your fingertips. Never use your thumb, since it has a pulse of its own and may therefore be deceiving when you are feeling for the brachial pulse.
7. Place the earpieces of the stethoscope in your ears and place the diaphragm or bell over the brachial artery, making sure neither one is touching the cuff.
8. With the other hand, close the air valve on the bulb by gently turning the thumbscrew in a clockwise direction; pump the air into the cuff until the level of the mercury is 10 to 20 mmHg above the palpated systolic pressure or about 180 mmHg.
9. Turn the thumbscrew counterclockwise to release the air at a slow rate so the pressure falls at a rate of about two to three mmHg per second.
10. Listen carefully for the first tapping sound; this represents the systolic pressure. Note this number on the scale of the sphygmomanometer.
11. Continue to deflate the cuff while listening to the sounds. Read the scale again when the second sound becomes dull or muffled; this second sound represents the diastolic pressure.
12. Keep deflating the cuff until you no longer hear any sounds.
13. After you no longer hear any sounds, open the valve completely and rapidly deflate the cuff. Remove the cuff from the patient's arm.
14. Record the results on the patient's chart, noting any unusual occurrences which you may have heard or seen, and identify from which arm the blood pressure was obtained.
15. Wash your hands.

Temperature, Pulse, and Respiration

Measuring the Temperature

Obtaining an accurate measurement of the patient's temperature, pulse, and respiration is just as important as obtaining the blood pressure. As with blood pressure, many factors also affect the patient's temperature, pulse, and respiration. These may include the time of day in which the measurements are taken, the sex and age of the patient, the emotional status and the degree of involvement in physical activities, and even the weather.

A patient's *temperature* is almost always obtained at the same time as the pulse and respiration. There are three methods which are acceptable for measuring the body's temperature. The most common of these is the oral method, in which a thermometer is placed under the patient's tongue and left in place for three to five minutes before it is read.

The most accurate method for obtaining the temperature is the rectal method. It involves placing the thermometer into the patient's rectum and leaving it in place for approximately five minutes. The least accurate mode of obtaining an accurate temperature is the axillary method. This is accomplished by placing the thermometer under the axilla, or armpit, and leaving it in place for approximately 10 minutes. For children, the method of choice is usually the rectal method and for children or adults who have difficulty holding an oral thermometer in place, the axillary method is considered most desirable. Whatever method is used, you must always remember to use the right thermometer (Figure 9-2).

Normal readings for body temperature usually vary one degree either way for oral, axillary, and rectal readings. The average normal reading for a healthy adult using the oral method is 98.6 degrees F. Using the axillary method, the aver-age normal reading is approximately 97.6 degrees F, and the normal reading using the rectal method is approximately 99.6 degrees F.

Procedure for Obtaining an Oral Temperature

To properly obtain an oral temperature, you should:

1. Gather the necessary equipment. This will include either an oral glass thermometer, a sheath-covered thermometer, a plastic

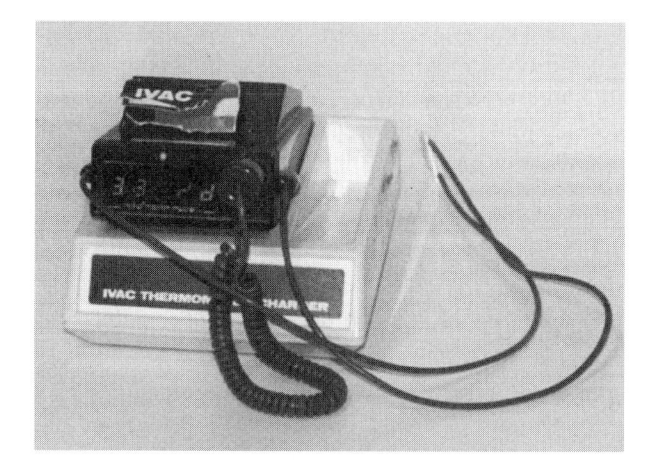

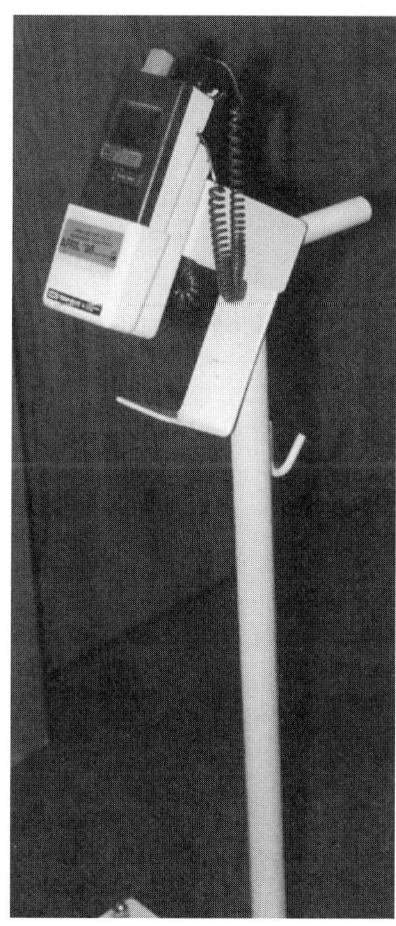

Figure 9-2
Example of two types of thermometers currently in use. (Reprinted with permission from Weiss, R.C. *Your Career in Cardiovascular Technology.* Philadelphia: W. B. Saunders, 1996, p. 66.)

thermometer, or an electronic thermometer, some tissues, a watch with a second hand, and a piece of paper and pencil to write down the reading.
2. Wash your hands.
3. If you are using a glass thermometer, remove it from its holder and wipe it with a clean tissue. Check to be sure that the thermometer is intact.
4. Read the mercury column. If it does not read below 96 degrees F, shake it down. Make sure you are standing away from any objects. Grasp the stem of the thermometer and gently shake it with a downward motion.
5. Insert the bulb end under the patient's tongue, toward the side of the mouth. Instruct the patient to hold the thermometer in place for three minutes.
6. Remove the thermometer, holding it by the stem. Wipe it from the stem end toward the bulb, and discard the tissue.
7. Hold the thermometer at eye level and locate the column of mercury. Read to the closest line and record this number on your piece of paper.
8. Wash the thermometer in cold water and soap before returning it to its proper place.
9. Wash your hands.

Procedure for Obtaining a Rectal Temperature

To properly obtain a rectal temperature, you should:

1. Gather the necessary equipment. This will include a glass rectal thermometer or the electronic thermometer with a plastic probe, a lubricant, such as K-Y Jelly, and some tissues.
2. Wash your hands.
3. Put on gloves and if you are using a glass thermometer, remove the thermometer from its holder and wipe it with a clean tissue. Make sure the thermometer is intact.
4. Read the mercury column to make sure it registers at 96 degrees F. If necessary, shake it down in the same manner as described in using an oral thermometer.
5. Place a small amount of lubricant on a tissue and apply the lubricant to the bulb end of the thermometer. Separate the buttocks with one hand and insert the thermometer about one and one-half inches into the rectum. Hold the thermometer in place for approximately five minutes.
6. Remove the thermometer, holding it by the stem, and wipe it clean from the stem end toward the bulb end and discard the tissue. Wipe the lubricant from the patient with a clean tissue.
7. Hold the thermometer at eye level and locate the column of mercury. Read to the closest line and then record your findings on a piece of paper.
8. Wash the thermometer in cold water and soap before returning it to its proper place.
9. Wash your hands.

Procedure for Obtaining an Axillary Temperature

To properly obtain an axillary temperature, you should:

1. Gather the necessary equipment. This will be the same equipment as for taking an oral temperature.
2. Wash your hands.
3. If you are using a mercury thermometer and it does not read below 96 degrees F, shake it down.
4. Wipe the area dry and place the thermometer in the patient's axilla. Instruct the patient to keep the thermometer close to the body. Leave the thermometer in place for approximately 10 minutes.
5. Remove the thermometer and wipe it clean. Read to the closet line and record this number on a piece of paper.
6. Clean and replace the thermometer in the same manner as you did with the oral thermometer.
7. Wash your hands.

Measuring the Pulse

The purpose of obtaining the measurement of a patient's *pulse* rate is to determine the strength, rate, and rhythm of the heartbeat as it is felt through the walls of the arteries. Such a pulsation, found in the arteries, is produced by the movement of blood being forced through them by the contractions of the heart.

The pulse is measured with regard to its individual rate, rhythm, and volume. The rate is a reflection of the number of pulsations, or beats, counted for a given period of time; usually a minute. The pulse rhythm refers to the intervals of time between each pulse. These intervals of time are generally described as regular, irregular, or skipping. Volume is a term used to describe the strength of the pulsations, that is, whether it is full, strong, bounding, weak, or thready. A normal pulse is most often described as being regular and strong.

A person's pulse, just like his or her blood pressure and temperature, can also be influenced by many different factors, such as age, sex, body size, metabolism, exercise, and even one's emotional state. For a normal, healthy adult, the average pulse ranges from 60 to 80 beats per minute, with 72 considered the norm. Children tend to have a much faster metabolism than do adults. The average range for a normal healthy child from age one to seven usually runs between 80 to 120 beats per minute, while kids over the age of seven generally range from 80 to 90 beats per minute. Newborns and infants have the greatest number of pulsations, with the average ranging between 130 to 160 beats.

A pulse can only be measured at a site in which it can be felt through the walls of the arteries. While there are many locations on the body where the pulse can be obtained, the location of choice is usually at the radial artery, that is, the inside of the wrist. Other locations include the brachial artery, which is located over the inner aspect at the bend of the elbow; the temporal artery, which is found at the side of the forehead at the temple; the popliteal artery, at the back of the knee; the dorsalis pedis artery, at the upper surface of the foot between the ankle and the toes; and the carotid artery, located on both the right and left sides of the anterior neck, which is most often the artery of

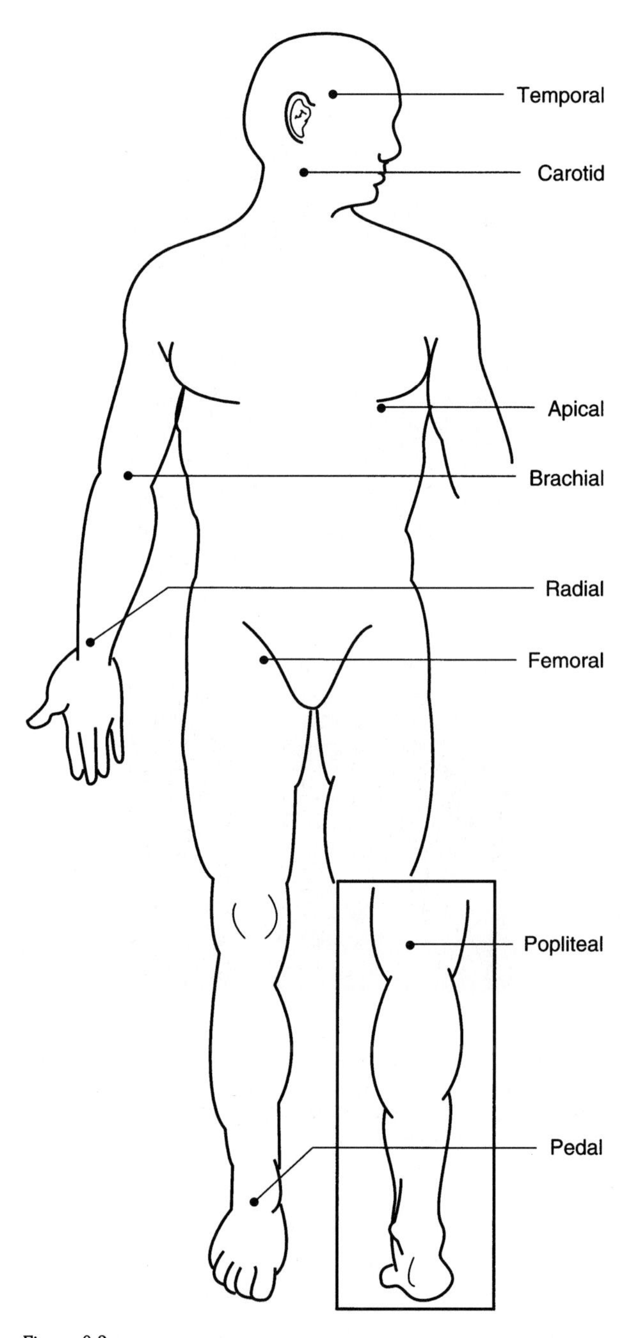

Figure 9-3
Locations of pulse sites. (Reprinted with permission from Weiss, R.C. *Your Career in Cardiovascular Technology.* Philadelphia: W. B. Saunders, 1996, p. 68.)

choice for palpitation during cardiopulmonary resuscitation. In some instances, the pulse may also be taken at the apical site, which is located between the fifth and sixth ribs and approximately two to three inches to the left of the breastbone (Figure 9-3).

Procedure for Obtaining a Radial and Apical Pulse

To properly obtain a radial pulse, you should:

1. Gather the necessary equipment. This will include a watch with a second hand and a piece of paper and pencil to record the pulse.
2. Wash your hands.
3. Identify the patient by name and identification bracelet and explain the procedure.
4. Position the patient in a sitting or lying position with the arm being used supported.
5. Hold the patient's wrist by placing your first three fingers on his or her wristbone over the radial artery. Gently apply light pressure so you can feel the pulsations. Be sure not to use your thumb to palpate the pulse, since it has its own pulse.
6. While holding the patient's wrist, count the pulse for one full minute. Note the rate, rhythm, and volume of the pulse.
7. After you have counted the pulse for a full minute, record the number, noting the rhythm and volume. Indicate at what site the pulse was obtained.
8. Wash your hands.

If you are required to obtain the patient's apical pulse, you will need to use a stethoscope, since this type of pulse can only be measured by listening to the heartbeat, and then determining the number of beats and the rhythm and volume at which these beats are produced. Once you have determined that the pulse will be obtained at the apical site, you should:

1. Gather the necessary equipment. This will include a stethoscope, alcohol and cotton balls or an alcohol wipe, a watch with a second hand, and a piece of paper and a pencil to record your findings.
2. Wash your hands.
3. Identify the patient by name and with his or her identification band, and explain the procedure.
4. Position the patient in a sitting or lying position.
5. Clean the earpieces of the stethoscope with the alcohol.
6. Warm the diaphragm of the stethoscope with your hands and then place the earpieces into your ears. Place the diaphragm over the apex of the heart, which is located in the fifth intercostal space two to three inches to the left of the breastbone.
7. Listen for the heartbeat and count the number of beats for one full minute, noting the number, rhythm, and volume of each beat.
8. After you have listened to the beats for a full minute, record the apical pulse, indicating the site used with the letter "A" enclosed in a circle.
9. Clean the earpieces of the stethoscope and return it to its proper place.
10. Wash your hands.

Measuring the Respirations

When we define the term *respiration,* we are actually referring to the process of breathing in oxygen and breathing out carbon dioxide. Such a process takes place in the respiratory control center which is located in the medulla oblongata, found in the lower portion of the brain stem. All healthy respirations occur automatically; however, the very act of breathing in and out is considered to be under voluntary control. That is why a person may attempt to hold his or her breath for a period of time, but eventually must stop to allow a breath to be taken.

The act of breathing in and out actually involves two individual processes. These are referred to as external respiration and internal respiration. External respiration takes place during the exchange of respiratory gases between the alveoli of the lungs. Internal respiration occurs during the exchange of respiratory gases between the body cells and the blood.

Like the pulse, when the respirations are measured, they are usually counted for one full minute, with special attention paid to the rate, depth, and rhythm of each respiration. The rate refers to the number of respirations per minute. It is generally described as being normal, rapid, or slow. The depth of the respirations depends upon the amount of air being inhaled and exhaled and is recorded as being shallow or deep. The rhythm is defined as the intervals of each respiration and may be described as being regular or irregular in rate and depth.

Like the other vital signs, the number of times in which a person takes in a breath of oxygen and breathes out carbon dioxide is influenced by many different factors, such as his or her age, emotional state, increase in muscular activity, such as through exercise, whether or not the person may be taking specific medications, and the presence of any diseases of the lungs or any other organs of the cardiovascular system. In some cases, certain changes in the climate and atmosphere may also affect the rate and depth of the respirations.

Procedure for Obtaining a Respiratory Rate

Obtaining a patient's respiratory rate is almost always done at the same time the blood pressure, temperature, and pulse are taken. This often occurs when the temperature is being obtained by the oral method. By inserting the oral thermometer into the patient's mouth, you are free to watch the patient's chest expand and lower as each breath is taken, usually without the patient trying to control the number of breaths being inhaled and exhaled. To obtain the respiratory rate, you should:

1. Gather the necessary equipment. This will include a watch with a second hand and a piece of paper and pencil to record the respirations.
2. Wash your hands.
3. Identify the patient by name and the identification band and explain the procedure.
4. Position the patient in a sitting or lying position.
5. Place three fingers on the patient's wrist as if you were going to take his or her pulse. As you are holding the patient's wrist, count each breathing cycle, that is, each time the patient inhales and exhales as one full breath by watching the rise and fall of the patient's chest or upper abdomen.
6. Count the number of respirations for one full minute. Then record the rate, depth, and rhythm of the respirations.
7. Wash your hands.

Summary

In this chapter, we discussed the purpose and function of the vital signs. We noted that these important signs, that is, the blood pressure, temperature, pulse, and respiration, are the best indicators for the physician to use in determining the patient's overall state of health. We also talked about specific variations of these vital signs, as well as what the normal ranges are for each individual sign. Finally, we explained the procedure for obtaining each of these signs, concluding that they are almost always obtained at the same time, when the patient is least able to influence their outcome.

Review Questions

1. The amount of force exerted by the heart against the walls of the arteries as it contracts and relaxes is called:
   a. pulse
   b. respiration
   c. blood pressure
2. The beat of the heart as it is felt through the walls of the arteries is called:
   a. pulse
   b. respiration
   c. blood pressure
3. Briefly explain the concept of *vital signs.*
4. An instrument which is used to listen to the beats of the heart as they are heard through the walls of the arteries is called a:
   a. sphygmomanometer
   b. stethoscope
   c. audioscope
5. What is the name of the instrument used to measure the blood pressure?
6. Give at least three examples of factors influencing a person's blood pressure:
   a. ____________
   b. ____________
   c. ____________
7. Why is it important never to use your thumb to feel for a patient's pulse?
8. Identify at least three locations in which a pulse rate can be taken:
   a. ____________
   b. ____________
   c. ____________
9. What method of taking a patient's temperature is most often used with small children?
   a. rectal
   b. axillary
   c. oral
10. What method of taking a patient's temperature is considered the most accurate?
    a. rectal
    b. axillary
    c. oral

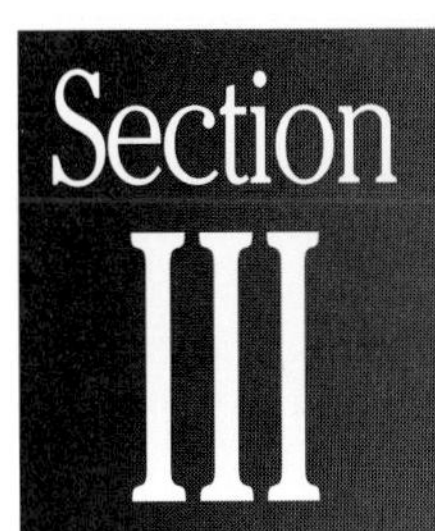

Physical Medicine and the Healing Process

10

Introduction to the Healing Process

Performance Objectives

Upon completion of this chapter, you will be able to:

1. Briefly discuss the mystery and magic of the human body, as it relates to the healing process, and in particular, its relationship to the study of physical medicine.
2. Identify and briefly discuss the six systems of healing used in the practice of physical medicine.
3. Briefly describe the differences and correlation between natural, or "nature-assisted" cures and "physician-assisted" cures, as each is related to the healing process.

Terms and Abbreviations

Chi (or **Qi**) term used in China to define the universal life energy.
Ki term used in Japan to define the universal life force.
Pneuma term used in Greece to define the universal life force.
Prana term used in India to define the universal life force.
Yin; Yang terms used in China which refer to opposite poles attracted to each other in order to produce movement and energy.

The human body is a realm of both wonder and amazement, as well as fear and reverence. Inside each of us is a greater sense of magic and astonishment than anything that could ever be contrived or created by our own imagination. All of the work that takes place in our body can barely be comprehended, much less matched by human invention. Just think of it; our heart beats 100,000 times a day; that's 2.5 billion times in the average lifetime. Our eyes perceive 10 million gradations of light. Our nose can tell the differences among thousands of odors and fragrances. Our brain takes in billions of bits of information, organizes them, and then provides us with an incredibly staggering array of responses. Who can consider the turbulence of human emotions, the insight and comprehension of one single mind, or the purity and innocence of a child's love without standing back in awe that so much magic can be contained in so measurable a package?

No artist or sculptor has yet to fully capture the mystery reflected in our eyes, the grace and strength in our hands, or the allure in our legs. Hence, the human body is the domain, or environment, in which both art and usefulness become one. Yet, it is not only with wonder that one approaches the human form, but with uneasiness and apprehension, too. You need only to listen to your own heart beat, or consider all those electrical impulses flashing across your brain, to awaken to the terrible delicacy and frailty of life.

Bridging the Gap Between Modern Medicine and Ancient Beliefs

The human body is many worlds in one. Therefore, if you ask a psychologist, a person who studies anatomy, a priest, or an artist for their views on the body, you will more than likely get four different answers, all of which would be correct. Travel to other cultures and ask the same question of Middle Eastern, Chinese, and native American healers, and each will give you a vastly differing description of the human body. Each of their accounts will also be correct. In fact, no single view of the body offers a definitive understanding.

We are living during an era in which people crave information about their bodies. We yearn for greater self-sufficiency when it comes to our health and health care. Many people would like to have the ability to heal themselves of illness or prevent disease, using methods that have fewer toxic side effects than many modern drugs. So we are turning increasingly to the tools of the ancient past, and combining them with the techniques and understanding of modern science. In no other branch of modern health care does this seem to be more evident than in the study of physical medicine. For it is the study of physical medicine that has been able to reach across and transcend the cultural lines of healing, in order to bridge the gap between the Eastern mysteries of healing one's body through faith and beliefs, with the Western philosophy of using modern technology and medical science.

Today, we continue to struggle to reconcile the two fundamental philosophies between believing and having faith in our body's ability to heal itself, and using modern medical techniques to cure the body of its ills and diseases. We want to understand our individual organs and how each functions. But we also want to see how each relates to the whole body, mind, and spirit. We search for knowledge to better understand ourselves, our bodies, and thereby live more fully healthy and satisfying lives.

The Human Body: Friend or Foe

One of the greatest shortcomings of our modern approach to health care is the belief that we are all victims of either our body's planned obsolescence or of germs—tiny agents that are invisible to the naked eye, pernicious, and arbitrarily infectious. For example, we "catch" a cold, or we "come down" with the flu, as if the illness descends mysteriously from above. How many times have you heard someone say, "She was never sick a day in her life and then suddenly she got sick." In other words, our friend was going along fine, minding her own business, when out of the blue her body broke down. She was an innocent victim of some mysterious illness.

Our methods of treatment reveal even more deeply this ingrained set of attitudes. Most treatments are designed to suppress symptoms or kill the organisms invading the body. How often do we stop to think that perhaps those symptoms are really our body's way of telling us that something in our behavior is causing an underlying disease, or that the common cold may have a beneficial effect on our health? How many of us believe that our body has the power to heal itself?

To better understand your body's language and to learn from your illnesses, you must first learn to see your body as a friend with its own operating system, its own healing powers, and its own laws for maintaining health. Too often we think of the body as an enemy, failing us when we least expected it, or when we needed it most.

Making Sense of the Body's Magic

According to history, magic has always been humanity's earliest explanation for how the body worked. Long before systematized approaches to health and the human body were organized more than 6,000 years ago, humanity's ancestors used potions, amulets, rings, and charms to rid the body of harmful demons and spirits that brought illness and suffering.

Humanity's understanding of the body began to emerge from the mists of superstition about 5,000 years ago, when the body began to be studied extensively in China, India, Greece, and Egypt. Despite their differences in language and metaphors, all of these early cultures approached the body from the same basic view. These traditional peoples saw life as an integrated whole, a unity. The body was approached as a unified system in which the physical, mental, and spiritual aspects of life were one. Moreover, each life was united with the life of the universe itself. It is one life which all things share.

In China, this ultimate unity was seen as the creator of two archetypal forces, called *yin* and *yang*. These two forces manifest in everything in the material universe and make the relative world possible. Like poles of a magnet, yin and yang attract each other and thus produce movement and energy. In China, that universal life energy is called *chi*, or *qi*.

The idea of a universal life force was common among virtually all traditional peoples. In India, it is called *prana*, in Japan, *ki*, and in ancient Greece, *pneuma*.

In some ancient societies, the healers performed crude surgeries, did autopsies, and investigated the structure and function of organs and tissues. But their investigations were often guided by simple questions such as, "What causes this to function?" or "What gives an organ life?" Their answers were that in addition to the corporeal body, there is a more fundamental entity which is this underlying energy that is life itself. This life energy infuses the entire human being, causing the body to have vitality, movement, and function. The life force also gives the body the power to heal wounds, to overcome disease and injury, and to succeed in the face of difficulty and challenge.

Death is seen as the moment the life force leaves the flesh. Without the life force, none of the bodily functions continue. The flesh is revealed as merely a matrix of earthy substances that immediately decay and return to the earth.

These ideas about life point to a major difference between early traditional societies and modern ones dominated by the tools and techniques of scientific medicine, and especially between East and West. In traditional systems, such as the Chinese and Greek, the body is seen as having the ability to cure itself of illness. The physician serves only to assist the body's own healing powers. Conversely, modern medicine uses drugs and surgery to overcome disease. Antibiotics, for example, kill a pathogen, while surgery removes organs and their related problems altogether. Rather than encourage the body's healing powers, the modern medical doctor uses medicine to deal directly with the illness or injury.

In the Chinese system, the life force flows through the body in specific channels, or meridians. These channels of energy unite the entire body into an organized whole, much like integrated circuitry unites an electric unit. But the channels of energy also make certain organs and senses particularly intimate and mutually dependent upon each other.

In the West, the body is seen as a biochemical machine in which the parts are separate and distinct. It is understood in ever-smaller units, that is, as tissues, organs, cells, molecules, and atoms. For this reason, Western science is often referred to as reductionist, meaning that it is searching for the single underlying unit that makes up the body or, in the case of disease, a single pathogen or physical impairment that gives rise to symptoms. A Western physician, therefore, would see a joint problem as confined largely to the joint and its related parts. And treatment for such a problem might consist of manipulation, physical therapy, medications, or surgery to correct the malfunctioning joint.

The understanding of a life force has larger applications—it even applies to a basketball player's attempt at a free throw. An athlete's performance, or any action for that matter, is not merely an act of biochemistry, but an attunement with this all-pervasive life force which is the underlying power of the universe. The player who is in tune with the universe in this way cannot help but be perfect in the moment. But in order to achieve that perfect unity between the body and the life force, the mind must be empty. The mind fragments and interprets experience. It tells you which parts of an experience are important and which are unimportant. But the perfect free throw lies in a state in which you are empty of "mind," empty of labels or concepts, and free to apply your skill unfettered to the task at hand. In other words, you don't think about the act. You just do it, and thereby come into harmony with the underlying life force that is creating the moment itself. By being attuned to the underlying power or truth, the basketball player and the ball he or she is attempting to throw into the hoop become one.

Systems of Healing

Peoples of traditional civilizations around the world have long included among their medical practices such therapies as diet and herbs, compresses and poultices, massage techniques and acupuncture, and purgatives and sweats. They have been particularly well developed in four major medical systems, including Chinese, Ayur-Veda of India, Greek medicine, and homeopathy.

But beyond the power and force of specific herbs or techniques lies a much more fundamental understanding of health and the healing process. Health is typically defined in traditional medical systems as a state of balance and wholeness. These systems are based on the belief that humans are unified with, and even the product of, the vast forces which maintain the universe. Illness is caused when one or more of these forces within a person is out of balance. And medicine is the means by which such a balance can once more be restored.

For the Chinese, health is achieved by creating harmony between the opposing powers of yin and yang. When the organs maintain a balanced condition, when they do not become too contracted or too expanded, the life force or qi flows smoothly throughout the body. Each organ receives optimal life force; it is capable of warding off illness and efficiently eliminating waste. However, when one or more organs becomes excessively contracted or expanded, qi flow becomes blocked. Once the life force is diminished, the organ becomes sluggish, inefficient, and stagnant. In effect, it becomes a perfect host for disease and illness.

Balance is the means to health and long life, say the Chinese, Greeks, and Indians. By eliminating extremes in behavior, life can be enjoyed fully, without excessive burdens. And protection of the life force through moderation has been, and continues to be, the key to good health and long life. Even Hippocrates, the Greek physician known today as the father of medicine, had a similar view. He taught that health is achieved by balancing four humors, or fluids, within the body. As long as these fluids remained in harmony among one another, an individual experienced good health. When they became imbalanced, one suffered illness.

In both the Greek and the Chinese systems, imbalances were often corrected by the body by merely discharging or eliminating the stagnation or excesses stored within. Hippocrates referred to this discharge as catharsis, which means the purging or cleansing of the system, especially the bowels. The common cold could, for example, serve to eliminate toxins and excesses that are the basis for disease.

Natural Cures Versus Physician-Assisted Cures

To a conventional physician, the runny nose, sneezing, cough, and watery eyes of a typical common cold are seen as merely irritating symptoms that should be eliminated as quickly as possible. Medication is designed to do just that. But from the point of view of most traditional medicines, the common cold, with its sneezing, runny nose, and frequent urination, is a highly efficient way of eliminating accumulated toxins and waste.

Hippocrates said that although health is the natural state of humans, disease is also a natural process that follows an organic pattern. During illness, there are key points at which the doctor can intercede and assist the patient in restoring his or her health. Hippocrates called these points of crises or opportune moments at which time balance and the forces of health can once more be restored. Hippocrates also implied that disease seems to serve some kind of evolutionary or growth process.

Like the Chinese, Hippocrates developed an extensive array of foods, herbs, and physical therapies which could be used to restore balance to the body. These often included proper food and drink, calmness of mind and body, and suitable exercise. Today, scientists continue to demonstrate the effectiveness of such methods.

How did traditional people discover their methods or cures? The easy answer is trial and error, however, you may not get such a response if you were to ask a Chinese healer or a native American medicine man how they arrived at their information.

According to *The Yellow Emperor's Classic of Internal Medicine,* which is the oldest and perhaps the most respected medical book in the world, methods and cures were ascertained from ancient times in which communication with Heaven occurred, thus creating the very foundation of life. Such a foundation existed between yin and yang and between heaven and earth. Therefore, the healers and medicine men preserved the natural spirit and were in complete harmony with the very breath of Heaven and were thereby in direct communication with Heaven.

Another school of thought as to how traditional people discovered their cures had to do with the role plants and animals played. According to the Cherokee Indians, for example, animals invented disease to reduce the human population. But the plant kingdom discovered the animals' plot and called a council meeting during which time the plants decided to provide healing remedies to humanity when stricken by illness. All plants were to have some healing properties, no matter how common or seemingly useless they might appear to be.

To traditional peoples, the world was alive with powers, life forces, and spirits. Mountains, rivers, trees, and boulders all possessed their own personalities and even souls. Their oneness of nature was not an abstract concept, but rather a deep and personal relationship in which people talked to the four winds, the sun, the stars, and the moon. These were minor deities, the emissaries of the Great Spirit.

The healer mediated between the human world and the world of the transcendent powers. Healers, therefore, served as both physician and religious leader. Shamans the world over called upon the powers of healing implicit in the universe to rid the sick of evil or noxious spirits. There were no conceptual boundaries between mind and body and soul. Whatever was in the spirit became manifest in the body, and vice versa. The perception of life was not linear but circular. Thus, treatment included the physical and the spiritual—foods, herbs, and physical therapy, along with ritual, jewels and crystals, and prayer.

In today's society, scientists, and in particular those who work with people involved in physical and sports medicine, and with patients who suffer from disorders and injuries which require physical therapies and holistic modalities of treatment, know that such methods work. The powers of the mind have just begun to be explored, but studies are showing that the invisible realm of thoughts, emotions, and belief systems dramatically influence health in both positive and negative ways. Studies have also shown that belief in one's own recovery can be as powerful as any medication or surgical intervention.

Modern medicine, as it continues to grow, is taking on a whole new set of views and belief systems that seems to look very much like our ancient traditions; one that is supported and transformed by our contemporary sciences and current schools of thought. The sciences of medicine and physics are also building bridges. When the physicist looks deeply into the world of the atom and its even tinier realms, he or she is discovering a unity that the ancients would have agreed with and understood.

Though they differ in language and metaphor, most traditional medical systems are based on the principles of health as being a complete state of balance or wholeness, governed by a universal life force, with illness caused as a direct result of imbalances from within the body that block the life force from flowing optimally and freely through it, and that symptoms of disease are seen as the body's effort at self-healing.

Summary

In this chapter, we briefly discussed the mystery of the human body as it relates to the healing process. We also identified and talked about the six systems of healing used in the practice of physical medicine. Finally, we described the differences and correlation between natural or "nature-assisted" cures and "physician-assisted" cures, and their relationship to the healing process.

Review Questions

1. What is the term used in China to define the universal life energy?
2. What is the term used in Japan to define the universal life force?
3. The two terms ______________ and ______________ refer to opposite poles which attract one another in order to produce movement and energy.
4. How many years ago did humanity's understanding of the human body begin?
5. In India, the universal life force is referred to as ______________.
6. In the Chinese system of medicine, the life force flows through our body through specific channels called ______________.
7. List the four major medical systems.
8. Briefly explain how the Chinese and Greeks maintain a sense of balance.
9. What is the name of the oldest, and often considered the most respected, medical book in the world?
10. What did Hippocrates call the time in which balance and the forces of health come together to be restored?

11

Systems of Healing

Performance Objectives

Upon completion of this chapter, you will be able to:

1. Identify the six basic systems of healing available to the physical medicine practitioner and health care worker.
2. Briefly explain the relationship of each system of healing to one another.

Terms and Abbreviations

Ayurvedic medicine a study of medicine, first used by the Hindus, which sees health as the basis of one's relationship with cosmic consciousness.

Catharsis the purging or cleansing of the system, especially the bowels.

Chinese medicine a form of medicine based on the view that humanity is part of a larger reaction, a greater body, that is the universe itself.

Greek medicine a study of medicine which sees all living things moving toward specific and knowable goals, with each living thing playing a part in a more grand cycle, which is essentially healthy and constructive.

Hippocrates known to modern medicine as the "father of medicine."

Homeopathy a system of healing based on the theory that a substance that produces a certain set of symptoms in a healthy person has the power to cure a sick person manifesting those same symptoms.

Meridian used in Chinese medicine, and defined as deep rivers of energy running through the body.

Modern medicine pertains to the dominant form of health care in the industrialized world today, and which is poised between an increase in the reliance upon technology and a growing awareness of the importance of disease prevention and the central role of self-care and more holistic practices.

Naturopathy system of healing which uses nontoxic healing methods derived from the best traditional healing systems from around the world, and which often includes the use of herbs.

The Yellow Emperor's Classic of Internal Medicine referred to as the oldest medical book in the world, and used as the basis of Chinese medicine.

In today's world, scientists and physicians, unlike their ancient predecessors, have the advantage of being able to cure or treat their patients by using any number of methods or systems of healing. In no other branch of medicine is this overlapping of various systems of healing as relevant as in physical medicine. In addition to implementing conventional modalities and treatments based on scientific data, these practitioners and healers also have at their fingertips the benefit of using any one of the many ancient or traditional forms, or systems, of medicine. These include those modalities found in the study of Chinese medicine, ayurvedic medicine, Greek medicine, and homeopathy.

Chinese Medicine

No other medical system deserves the description of being called traditional more than Chinese medicine. Modern Western medicine, which we often refer to as traditional, is only two centuries old. Chinese medicine, on the other hand, is at least 3,000 years old, and is still being used to treat tens of millions of people in China and other places around the world. From the view of a traditional Chinese healer, modern medicine is considered the experimental system because people have relatively little experience with it, and certainly the alternative because it is far from the precepts upon which the Chinese system is built.

Chinese medicine is based upon the concept that humanity is part of a much larger creation, a greater body, that is the universe itself. Each of us, according to Chinese medicine, is subject to the same laws that govern the stars, the planets, the trees, and the earth. In this way, Chinese medicine is essentially macroscopic, meaning that its understanding of health begins with an understanding of nature and the laws that govern it. To follow the laws of nature is to be blessed with good health, long life, and good fortune, say the Chinese. Ultimately, this path leads one to a revelation about one's own life and the life of the universe itself.

To investigate the workings of the body is, for the Chinese, to explore the nature and origin of the universe. All the forces that created and shaped the universe are present in the human being, and consequently rule our health and destiny. Health care is, according to the Chinese, therefore, a spiritual pursuit in which the healer serves as both physician and priest or religious leader.

All Chinese medicine is based on *The Yellow Emperor's Classic of Internal Medicine*, which was written approximately 2,500 years ago, and which forms the basis of Chinese medicine and the foundation for most of Asian medicine, including the systems adopted by Japan, Korea, the Philippines, and other Asian countries, except for India, which may have been influenced by the Chinese, but developed its own system, called Ayur-Veda. In fact, virtually all of the oriental health systems flourishing in the West today, including acupuncture, shiatsu, acupressure massage, macrobiotics, Do-In, and sotai, are based upon Chinese medicine.

As we previously discussed in Chapter 10, the first law of Chinese medicine is the law of yin and yang. According to the Chinese, all life and the entire material universe originated from a single unified source, called Tao, an integrated and undifferentiated whole that is present in everything. Tao created two opposing forces—yin and yang, which are primal opposites that combine to create everything in the relative world. To more fully understand the law of yin and yang, look at Table 11-1, which lists their respective characteristics.

Yin and yang are relative terms, and individual men and women can be more or less yin or yang. Some women are far more yang than some men. Each gender has an inherent or archetypal nature, according to the Chinese. Men are constitutionally more yang, women are constitutionally more yin.

Yin and yang are each incomplete without the other. By combining, they create all phenomena. Thus, everything is composed of a unique mix of both. Take the moon, for example. The moon is yin in comparison with the sun. However, the moon possesses both yin and yang characteristics, because it has both a dark side (yin) and a light side (yang).

People, too, have both yin and yang aspects. Certain characteristics within the same person can reflect both yin and yang. A passive person (yin) can be stubborn (yang), for example, or a chaotic person (yin) can also be domineering (yang).

As Table 11-1 shows, Chinese medicine divides the body into yin and yang parts. Certain organs are considered yin, while others are considered more yang. The attraction of yin and yang creates movement and energy, an energy known in China as qi, or the life force. Qi energy is all around us and infusing us, and thus permeates the entire universe, which is an infinite resource available to all.

The Body's Energy Channels

Qi flows through the body in precise and orderly patterns called *meridians*. They can be understood as deep rivers of energy running through the body. There are 14 meridians, 12 of which are associated with the organs of the body, while two have the responsibility of unifying various systems.

Each meridian runs vertically, bringing qi to specific parts of the body, and no part is left unnourished of qi, unless a meridian becomes blocked or stagnant. This causes an imbalance in the flow of life force. Such imbalances can be compared to placing a big rock in a river: behind the rock, the water becomes excessive and powerful; in the lee of the rock, the water is diminished.

Without adequate life force, tissues and organs become stagnant. They can no longer eliminate waste from cells. As the waste products accumulate, the blood-cleansing organs become stressed, and eventually their capacity to clean the blood is exceeded, causing an accumulation of toxins, such as fat, cholesterol, ammonia, uric acid, triglycerides, and carbon dioxide. The accumulation of toxins in turn creates an environment for disease to manifest itself.

In Chinese medicine, all health care is designed to balance qi and treatment is meant to bring harmony between deficiency and excess between yin and yang.

Virtually all behavior can affect the flow of qi in the body. Too much rest or complacency can make one loose and weak (yin), which can be balanced and healed by greater amounts of work and activity (yang). People who work excessively and experience

Table 11-1
Characteristics of Yin and Yang

	Yin	Yang
Cosmic bodies	earth moon	heavenly realms sun
Temperament	passive mentally active following asleep	aggressive physically active leading awake
Time of day	night	day
Season	fall and winter	spring and summer
Magnetic pole	negative	positive
Temperature	cold	hot
Density	contracted to solid	expanded and hollow
Speed	slow	fast
Relative moisture	moist to saturated	dry
Body location	feet lower extremities	head upper extremities
Organs	dense, internal organs: kidneys, lungs, heart, liver, bones	hollow, surface organs: intestines, spleen, gall bladder, skin
Height	low	high
Distance	near	far
Sides	left	right
Light	darkness	light
Sexual characteristics	female	male
Constitution	female	male

too much stress, on the other hand, need relaxation in order to restore equilibrium and health to life.

The Chinese also categorized practically every activity, food, and herb according to the yin and yang spectrum. Because these are relative values, a single object or activity can be more yang than some things, more yin than others. Exercise, for example, is considered more yang than writing, but both would be considered yang activities compared to watching television, eating, or sleeping, each of which is progressively more yin.

Acupuncture and Pulse Points

The preeminent form of therapy in Chinese medicine is acupuncture. Acupuncture is the one part of Chinese medicine that nearly all Westerners have heard of or seen, though few understand its purpose.

Since qi energy is an infinite resource permeating the entire environment, it can be directed into the body in order to restore health. An acupuncturist uses needles as antennae to direct qi to organs or functions of the body. However, the needles also can be used to drain qi where it is excessive; to warm parts of the body that are cool or stagnant; to decrease or increase moisture; and to reduce excessive heat. The acupuncturist does this by selecting specific points along specific meridian lines and then applying various needling techniques to bring about the desired results. There are as many as 2000 points, but traditional acupuncturists generally use between 150 and 200 points.

Diagnosis of health and illness is done by using several techniques, including physiognomy, or relating facial and body features to internal organs; examining the tongue, iris, and sclera of the eye; and palpating the pulse.

Pulse diagnosis was raised to a high art in China. The pulse is sensed by placing three fingers with varying amounts of pressure on the radial artery at the wrist. With pulse diagnosis, the Chinese physician is said to be able to read six organs on each wrist, or a total of 12 organs and meridians.

The Five Element Theory

Beyond the law of yin and yang, the most all-encompassing tool in traditional medicine is the five element theory. In Chinese medicine, it is considered to be the central tool, or instrument, for all diagnosing and treatment. It is used to link the seasons of the year, aspects of nature, and the body's organs, as well as specific foods, herbs, and treatments that will cure disease. It is also used for agricultural planning, healing, psychology, maintaining harmony in relationships, and even divination. This incredible tool single-handedly demonstrates the Chinese talent for seeing the unity within apparent diversity.

For our purposes, let's look at the five elements from the perspective of understanding the body and healing. According to the theory, all change occurs in five distinct stages. Each of these stages, which include summer, late summer, fall, winter, and spring, can be associated with a particular time of the year; a particular element in nature; and a pair of organs within the body. Summer is associated with fire and the heart and small intestine. These organs and season are, therefore, referred to as the fire element. Late summer, proceeding from July to mid-September, is a time between the intensity of summer and the decline of fall. It is regarded as a stable time of the year, and hence, is associated with the earth. The earth element is also associated with the stomach and spleen. Fall is associated with metal and the lungs and large intestine, and is therefore regarded as the metal element. Winter is associated with the kidneys and bladder and the winter months, from December 21 to March 21. It is known as the water element. Spring is associated with the liver and gall bladder and the tree or wood. Thus, it is referred to as the wood element.

If you plot these five stages on a circle, as shown in Figure 11-1, you can see that each stage leads to the next. Each stage of element nourishes those related organs within the element, and then passes qi onto the next stage. For example, the fire element provides qi to the heart and small intestine and then passes qi into the earth element, the stomach, spleen, and pancreas. For this reason, fire is called the mother of the earth element, because it provides life force to the earth organs. This is called the nourishing or creative cycle.

Chinese medicine is an extremely complex and sophisticated healing system. In addition to its two fundamental principles—the law of yin and yang and the five elements—it is an array of other diagnostic and medicinal tools that are themselves refinements

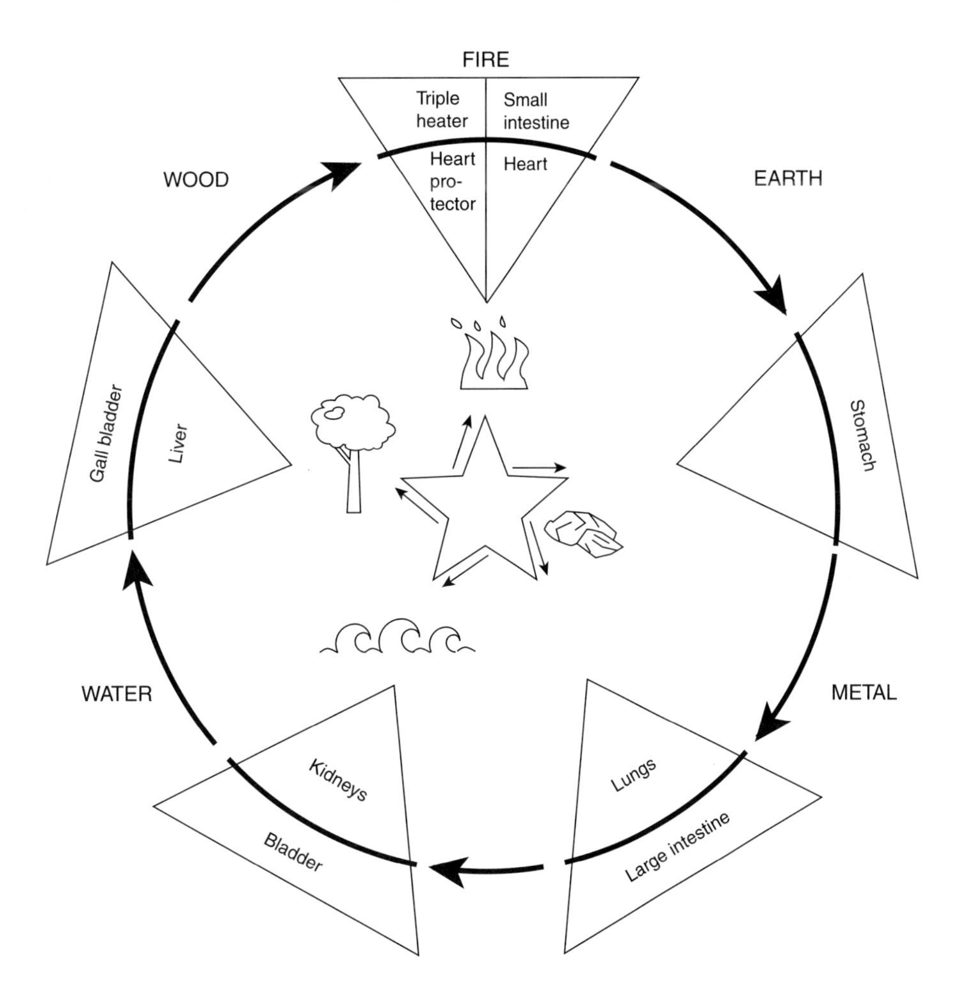

Figure 11-1
The five elements.

of this foundation. Illnesses which arise out of an imbalance within the body ultimately arise from a person's way of life, that is, his or her relationship with the universe itself. Thus, in Chinese medicine, the healer helps to restore the balance by combining the appropriate herbs, diet, and medicinal practices, along with changes in the patient's personal way of living.

Ayurvedic Medicine

Legend says that the system known as Ayur-Veda, or the knowledge of long life, was given to one of the Hindu rishis, or seers, by the God Indra. When that may have happened, no one really knows, but scholars do know that *ayurvedic medicine* goes back at least to the fifth century B.C. and is based on the Vedas, the oldest known philosophical and spiritual writings known to man.

Like the Chinese and Greek systems, Ayur-Veda sees health within a universal context. Human life, according to the Hindus, is an extension of the life of the creator, or what the Vedas refer to as cosmic consciousness. Health, therefore, is based upon one's own relationship with cosmic consciousness. The healer serves to reestablish harmony between the individual and the life of the universe by balancing universal forces within each person. These forces are both complementary and unique, competing with one another, yet at the same time maintaining their own identities and natures.

As with most traditional health systems, ayurvedic medicine is also based upon a creation myth. From a single, unified and cosmic consciousness, two forces emerged, one male and the other female, respectively called Shiva and Shakti. These two forces combined to create multiple levels of being that include cosmic intelligence, ego, and physical forms, including humankind.

Cosmic consciousness is also manifested as a life force, which the Hindus call prana. This force is considered the animating power of all life force. It not only provides vitality and endurance to each living being, but is also the basis of healing. The life force appears in physical form as the five elements, which are bound together by three forces called the Three Doshas.

Ayur-Veda teaches that the body is composed of the five great elements: earth, water, fire, air, and ether. These elements are not seen in the purely material sense, but rather, are metaphorical categories that describe functions and aspects of the human body. For example, the breakdown and absorption of food during digestion can be seen as a fire function. The earth element stands for all the mineral substances that make up the body, including those that combine in order to create bone, cartilage, and contribute to muscle formation, such as calcium. Earth is also associated with the body's solid waste. Water, of course, would represent all the liquid substances found in the body, such as blood, mucus, lymph, hormones, semen, fat, urine, and other fluids. It is also associated with the kidneys and genitals. Air is the substance that animates the body and gives it the ability to move, and thus is linked to the nervous system. Ether, the most subtle and abstract of the five elements, is the principle of form and idea from which the body draws its archetypal design. Therefore, it is most responsible for holding the body together. Since the elements are seen as interdependent functions, they are often present in the same activity. For example, while earth is responsible for bones, the activity of walking, which involves both bone and muscle, includes both earth and fire; fire, because this element is responsible for the expenditure of energy.

The Three Doshas

Having achieved form and substance, the body maintains harmony and health by balancing the three forces within it. These forces are known as the three doshas, or vata, pitta, and kapha. Vata and kapha are seen as opposites while pitta is the mediating force between the two extremes. The three doshas act on the five elements. They are the moving forces behind the substances and function represented by the five elements. When the three doshas are balanced, the body functions harmoniously. When there is an imbalance among the doshas, illness results.

Vata, which is associated with the air element, represents the force of kinetic energy within the body. It ceaselessly stimulates motion, including the function of the nervous system, muscles, heart, blood flow, and thoughts. It is the vata activity in the brain that stimulates thought; the vata activity in the heart that stimulates beating; in the muscles that creates movement; in the nervous system that sparks electrical impulses and communication.

Kapha, most closely linked with both the elements of earth and water, is the source of potential energy. It is responsible for stability, groundedness, physical strength, and holding. Kapha also causes tissue to be moist and lubricated, and therefore is associated with lymph and mucus.

Pitta is most closely associated with fire. It causes the burning of energy and the creation of heat within the body. It governs digestion, assimilation, and the metabolic processes of cells. It is linked with all the fiery aspects of life, such as hunger, curiosity, and thirst. Pitta also mediates between kinetic energy (vata) and potential energy (kapha). Just as a fire burns and endures by transforming potential energy into kinetic, so pitta utilizes the two opposite forces in order to bring about movement and endurance to bodily function.

As we have seen, each of the three doshas may be present in the same organ, depending on whether it is currently active or at rest. However, individual organs are more closely aligned with specific doshas. The three doshas and their corresponding organs are shown in Table 11-2.

Constitutional Body Types

The doshas manifest themselves in unique combinations in each one of us, and thus give rise to our individual body types that may lean toward one dosha or another. Some people have a body type that was more influenced by vata prenatally, while another will have more pitta characteristics. Each dosha creates tendencies within each of us, but because no one is perfectly balanced, one or two of the doshas will have dominated during the shaping of the constitution and the personality.

These imbalances will provide unique strengths and weaknesses, and thus create tendencies toward specific kinds of disorders and illnesses. For example, people who have the kapha body type are generally stocky and often heavyset, but frequently are surprisingly agile and athletic. If they overeat or avoid exercise, they can easily become overweight. Kapha people have a tendency toward illnesses afflicting the kapha-related organs, especially the lungs, lymph, and stomach. Because of their weight and the kapha tendency to reduce movement and circulation, they also can suffer from heart disease. The pitta body type is often athletic, muscular, extremely active, and ruddy-skinned. Those who have this kind of body are generally intense people, hardworking, and smart. They have excellent digestion, lots of energy, and usually do most things quickly. They also have fiery natures, are inspirational to others, and often have a tendency toward being the leader. Pitta body types are prone to illnesses affecting the pitta organs, especially the liver and gall bladder, blood, small intestine, and spleen. Therefore, they can easily suffer from ulcers, and should be aware of their potential toward cancer and strokes.

Greek Medicine

Hippocrates was a towering figure and in the minds of some, even a revolutionary of his day. Born in Greece in 460 B.C., he is credited with founding the first school of *Greek medicine,* dedicated to the scientific understanding of health and the human body. He refused to consider health and illness as a gift or punishment visited upon humanity by the Gods. Rather, he regarded each as the consequences of natural and orderly processes which could be understood and, in the case of illness, treated. Ironically, the man who today is called the "father of medicine" has had little influence over modern medical thinking. He is more apt to be cited as an inspiration by practitioners of alternative medicine, many of whom regard his fundamental precepts as still valid.

According to Hippocrates, all living things move toward specific and knowable goals. Each living thing plays a part in a more grand cycle, which he believed to be essentially healthy and constructive. When illness manifests itself, the body's natural tendencies are to heal itself and restore the individual to its larger social purpose.

Hippocrates believed that health is the natural state of humanity. Illness is also natural, and therefore must be governed by natural laws that are understandable. As such, illness follows a specific pattern.

Table 11-2
The Three Doshas

Vata	Pitta	Kapha
Bones, including bone marrow	Blood	Brain, especially in its capacity to store information
Brain, especially motor activity	Brain, in the synthesis of stored information, memory, and learning	Joints
Colon, when active	Eyes, when awake	Lymph
Heart	Hormones, in active phase as when stimulating an activity	Mouth
Lungs, specifically in the act of breathing	Liver	Stomach
Nervous system	Small intestine, especially during digestion and assimilation	Chest cavities
	Spleen	

The physician's job is to intervene in that process at precise moments to assist the body in healing. The healing process thus consists of a triad which includes the physician, the patient, and the conditions surrounding the patient. All three must participate in the recovery process.

Like the early pioneers of Eastern medical systems, Hippocrates understood health and illness as relative states of balance. Elements exist within the body that must be balanced for health to exist. Illness, therefore, is a state of imbalance.

Though scientific in his approach, Hippocrates had no hesitation in calling medicine an art. As a matter of fact, he believed that the art of healing was the noblest of all the arts, and as such, the physician should be responsible for studying each patient individually and should then adapt to the conditions of his or her illness. Specifically, he maintained that the physician must intercede at only the right moment in the process of healing. And once the moment has been reached, the physician must act quickly. He called these moments kairos, which is the root word for "crisis." It was during such healing crises that the body reached a moment of truth in which restoration of health or death hung in the balance. At this moment, according to Hippocrates, pepsis, or the forces of healing, could be assisted and illness overcome.

Hippocrates also maintained that the whole process of healing could have beneficial effects. Illness could serve to create a new order among the four humors, as well as eliminate poisons and wash away impurities within the system. The Greek word used was katharsis or now *catharsis,* meaning to purify, especially the digestion. Once this process of purification was complete, one could achieve a new state of being, or what Hippocrates called "a blended maturity."

Like his Asian counterparts, Hippocrates also encouraged his students and followers to be humble and to recognize the true source of healing. He taught them that the art of healing involved a combination of knowledge given to them by the gods into the fiber of the physician's mind.

Ancient Hippocratic medicine is no longer practiced as such, but its influence has formed the very basis of a medical tradition which has continued to many traditional healers practicing today. Among modern healers, Hippocratic principles are most clearly seen in the system known as naturopathy.

Homeopathy

Late in the eighteenth century, a German physician by the name of Samuel Hahnemann became discouraged by the prevailing practice of medicine, which in his day used such techniques as bloodletting and blistering to treat illness. Physicians of the time were also using a number of substances, such as mercury, which today are determined to be highly toxic to the body. Hahnemann found that these methods were not only ineffective, but more importantly, often made the patient more ill and often caused death.

Hahnemann, who considered himself a deeply spiritual man, believed that physicians were meant to assist the body's natural healing mechanisms, rather than administer chemicals that would override them. As such, his lifelong dream was to discover if God had not indeed given some law whereby the diseases of mankind would be cured.

Over a period of time, Hahnemann became disenchanted and eventually decided to drop the practice of medicine and earn his living by translating medical texts. Eventually he came upon a man by the name of William Cullen, a Scottish physician, who maintained that cinchona bark cured fever by virtue of its astringent and bitter qualities. Being the inquisitive and incredulous man he was, Hahnemann decided to test Cullen's hypothesis on himself by taking a dose of the cinchona, which contains quinine, a well-known medicine for fever and malaria. Instead of producing astringency, the cinchona caused fever and the symptoms of malaria in the healthy Hahnemann. He repeated the same experiment using other medicines with similar results.

Based on his many experiments, Hahnemann soon discovered that a substance that produces a specific set of symptoms in a healthy person also had the power to cure a sick person suffering from those same symptoms. He thus articulated the first of several principles of what would eventually be known as the new medicine of *homeopathy.* He called the principle the law of similars, which in essence states that like cures like. The name homeopathy joined the Greek words homoio, which means like, with the word pathos, for pathology or sickness.

The law of similars revealed to Hahnemann how the body reacts to disease. He maintained that the presence of an illness stimulates the body's defense system to eliminate the illness. That defensive reaction produces symptoms, which are part of the body's effort at eliminating the underlying disease. According to Hahnemann, the symptoms were not the illness, but rather, part of the curative process.

Hahnemann further maintained that the effective medicines actually produce a condition similar to the illness itself, which arouses the body's defense system against the underlying disease. In effect, the medicine makes it easy for the body to recognize the underlying disease and thus mobilize its defenses against the illness. The outward presence of this effect are symptoms.

Strictly speaking, the law of similars was not by itself a new principle either. It was known among ayurvedic physicians two thousand years earlier and was central to the medical approaches of Hippocrates. Still, it was in direct opposition to the prevailing medical approach of the West, which Hahnemann termed allopathy. Allopathic healers basically prescribed drugs to create the opposite effect of a symptom in the body. Allopaths treat swelling, for example, by administering drugs that will directly reduce swelling. Symptoms are suppressed, which Hahnemann contended causes the disease to go deeper into the body, and thus leads to a more serious condition, ultimately which is much harder to cure.

Hahnemann wanted to reduce the severity of the symptoms caused by medicine, and thus decided to reduce the size of the dosage. Eventually, he found that the smaller dose was even more effective against the underlying illness. Further experiments led Hahnemann to his next principle, which he called the law of potentiations or the law of infinitesimals. This states that the smaller the dose of medicine, the greater its potency or its effect on the body's vital force. Thus, a microdose of the medication actually strengthens the vital force against the illness. Hahnemann developed a method to dilute medicines down to infinitesimal doses by diluting the quantities and then shaking them, which today homeopaths refer to as succussion. This process is done successively until, for some dosages, only molecular amounts of the original medicine remain.

Criticism and Controversy

Homeopathy has drawn its most hostile criticism on the basis of its law of infinitesimals. This is primarily due to the fact that most orthodox physicians have maintained that there is not enough of the medicine left after diluting it to have any effect on an illness.

Hahnemann continued to believe that dilution and succession actually reduced the material substances to their spiritual essence, which, in his mind, accounted for the medicine's enhanced power. Like the native American, Greek, oriental, and ayurvedic physicians who came before him, Hahnemann maintained that the underlying reality of the physical world is essentially spiritual. But unlike many modern spiritual teachers, who view such matters as abstract, Hahnemann insisted that this underlying spiritual power was physically present in the form of energy. Later, other homeopathic physicians offered similar, if more scientific, suggestions. Thus, homeopathy embraces yet another fundamental principle of ancient or traditional medicine: the presence of an underlying spiritual energy that is the governing foundation of the material world. Like its predecessors, homeopathy is at least in part spiritual medicine.

Homeopathy has been used safely since 1810, when Hahnemann first published his findings. Since then, millions of people have relied exclusively on homeopathy for the treatment of virtually all types of illnesses. However, the success of this treatment has not come without its debates and arguments. Probably the most controversial episode involving the scientific testing of homeopathy took place in 1989, when a group of researchers led by French physician Jacques Benveniste reported findings that confirmed the effectiveness and power of homeopathic medicines. After the study was published in a well-known British science journal, it was attacked worldwide, with many scientists claiming that such findings were a delusion. Undaunted by these claims, in 1991, Benveniste reported another series of experiments that once again validated the homeopathic thesis. His work was published in the journal of the French Academy of Sciences. Sadly, many physicians and scientists today clearly believe that homeopathy remains a serious threat to modern science and medicine.

Naturopathy

Naturopathy traces its origins in the United States to a German-born healer by the name of Benedict Lust, who, in 1902, launched a newspaper called *The Naturopath and Herald of Health.* He had procured the name naturopathy from its originator, John H. Scheel, who ran a hospital in the state of New York. According to Lust, *naturopathy* has to do with the use of nontoxic healing methods derived from the best traditional healing systems from around the world. In that sense, naturopathy did not originate with Lust, or with any single person, but has its roots in Greek, oriental, and European medical traditions. With these systems, it shares a belief in an underlying life force, but not an explicit allegiance to a specific unifying principle such as yin and yang or the five elements.

Today, naturopaths employ a diversity of natural therapies, including acupuncture, homeopathy, botanical remedies, chiropractic, therapeutic massage, diet and nutrition, fasting, colonics, hydrotherapy, and compresses. Furthermore, naturopathic physicians who have attended an accredited four-year program are trained in most of the same scientific disciplines taught in conventional medical schools. Consequently, a naturopath also will occasionally employ medical tests, such as blood and urine analysis, for diagnosis. Moreover, most naturopaths acknowledge that modern medicine, including drugs and surgery, have a place in crisis intervention, though they remain committed to using nontoxic and noninvasive methods.

Like the Chinese and Greek systems, naturopaths regard illness as the body's effort at self-cleansing. Sneezing, coughing, fever, sweating, diarrhea, frequent urination, and rest are all methods, according to naturopaths, used by the body to eliminate the underlying conditions that promote illness. Pain is seen as a message from the body that something is wrong. Such conditions as inflammation are the body's method of localizing problems to allow the rest of the system to function unimpeded. Naturopaths say that the body will place toxins at specific places in an effort either to eliminate the poisons, or to keep them from getting to organs that are vital to life.

Using Herbs to Heal

Naturopaths regard the underlying life force as the source of the body's ability to heal itself; thus, medicine becomes a force to assist this life force. Among the most frequently used remedies in natural medicine, and the oldest, are herbs. The medicinal effects of herbs are categorized by their effect on the body. Some of the most common properties of herbs include the following.

- *alternative:* used to heal and purify the blood without creating side effects.
- *anodyne:* used to relieve pain.
- *astringent:* used to cause contraction and thus stop discharge.
- *antiseptic:* used to stop decay and putrefaction.
- *demulcent:* used to relieve inflammation.
- *emmenagogue:* used to promote menstruation.
- *febrifuge*: used to reduce or eliminate a fever.
- *nervine:* used to smooth the nervous system and treat disorders of the nervous system.
- *sedative:* used to promote relaxation and sleep.
- *tonic:* used to invigorate and strengthen the whole body.

Conventional Modern Medicine

Modern medicine, which is the dominant form of health care in the world today, is actually balanced between two trends: an increased reliance upon technology and highly sophisticated scientific procedures for both diagnosis and treatment of illness, and a growing awareness of the importance of disease prevention and the central role of self-care and more holistic practices. Will these two seemingly opposite trends ever merge to create a new form of medicine, one that ultimately combines the modern with the ancient, the technological with the philosophical? Before we can answer this question, we must first take a closer look at the historical background of modern medicine.

Modern medicine, which is a relatively recent development, is also known as conventional or orthodox medicine. It is also referred to as allopathy, coming from the Greek word allo, meaning "other," and pathos for "suffering disease." While modern medicine claims Hippocrates as the "father of medicine," such a claim can only be rooted in one aspect of Hippocrates' method: he was the first physician to bring scientific and analytical reasoning to health care. In the process, he set medicine apart from religion and myth. Hippocrates' method of questioning and observing the patient closely in order to recognize the underlying illness and its cause still remains among one of the most important methods of diagnosing. On the other hand, few of his ideas on the stages of disease, or his healing methods, such as diet, herbs, and a wide variety of natural remedies, are respected or used by orthodox medical doctors today.

Despite its claim on the Greek physician, modern medicine did not really emerge until the early sixteenth century when a Flemish physician by the name of Andreas Vesalius did some of the earliest experiments in anatomy. After Vesalius, an English physician by the name of William Harvey first described the circulation of blood and the functioning of the heart. In the later seventeenth century, Dutch naturalist Antonj van Leeuwenhoek created the first high-powered microscope, capable of magnifying objects 300 times, which provided an essential instrument for inquiring into the inner workings of the human body. Also during this century, French philosopher René Descartes' work crystallized the concept of mechanism and dualism, effectively creating the model of the body as a machine, separate and distinct from mind. Not long after that, Isaac Newton provided the mathematical and scientific understanding to these concepts, which ultimately became the dominant world view of the West for the next 300 years.

Many of these advances formed the very foundation for the pivotal medical discoveries which were to come throughout the nineteenth century. The most significant of these was made by French scientist Louis Pasteur, who, during the 1860s, proved that microscopic organisms, such as viruses and bacteria, could cause disease. German bacteriologist Robert Koch advanced the theory even further, stating that in order to establish the causative organism of a specific disease, there must be four conditions present. This later became known as Koch's rule.

In 1895, German scientist Wilhelm Roentgen discovered X-rays, which ultimately led the way to the development of a practical X-ray machine. By passing

X-rays, highly charged waves of energy, through the body and then onto a scientific photographic plate, scientists found that they could create an accurate image of parts of the body's interior.

The Science and Technology of Modern Medicine

Being able to use X-rays and microscopes awakened scientists to the power of new technologies that could provide them with important information. Scientific medicine was increasingly looking at the body at the cellular level for the answers to questions regarding humanity's health. This coincided with the dominant need of its day, namely, to find solutions for the leading causes of death, which at that time were pneumonia and influenza. Interestingly, by contrast, heart disease and cancer, which today are considered to be the leading causes of death, were of little or no concern during the eighteenth and nineteenth centuries.

Pasteur's work still stands as among the greatest achievements in medicine. His germ theory as the origin of disease gained overriding acceptance in the West in the early twentieth century. Since almost all illness was thought to originate from microscopic organisms, scientists began to search for the means by which these tiny creatures could be killed. The tools that seemed to offer the most promise for doing this were synthetic drugs.

It is sometimes argued that modern pharmacology is merely a more sophisticated version of the ancient practice of herbology, but in fact, the two disciplines bear only superficial resemblance to each other. Traditional herbology holds that everything about a medicinal plant is active: its shape is created by specific natural or energetic forces; its taste often indicates its influence on a body part; the time of year and method by which it is harvested affect its effect; and, finally, the plant has a spiritual origin and mythological significance. Plants have not only material substance, but what might be termed energetic or spiritual properties.

In contrast, modern pharmacology is based on the development of concentrated, purified chemical substances that are used to target one aspect of the disease process. In 1805, for example, scientists isolated and extracted morphine from opium and gave medicine its first pure painkiller. This began the practice of extracting what chemists thought were the active ingredients in plants. In 1935, the antibacterial agents called sulfonamides were formed. These were followed by the development of penicillin, streptomycin, and tetracycline in the 1940s.

Since the 1940s, thousands of new drugs have been developed. Original antibiotics, for example, proved to be miraculous agents against infectious diseases. This caused medical scientists to bask in the glory of their successes. Ultimately, they believed that a chemical cause and pharmaceutical cure for every illness would soon be found.

Along with the development of the modern pharmaceutical industry came an onslaught of new discoveries and new machines. They quickly formed the cornerstone of medical diagnosis. Among these were the recognition in 1901 of three distinct blood groups, and the increasing understanding of blood constituents and analysis. Then, in 1906, came the creation of the electrocardiograph, a machine that could be used to record the electrical impulses of the heart. By 1932, the electron microscope was developed, a machine capable of magnifying images to a power of five million. At the same time, lower-dose X-ray machines were discovered, making X-rays safer; more sensitive photographic technology provided clearer pictures; and radioactive dye was combined with X-ray technology to provide more accurate images of human organs.

Still later, scientists developed such highly technological procedures as computerized axial tomography (CAT) scanning and magnetic imaging (MRI), so that three-dimensional pictures of the interior parts of the body could be produced. Blood and urine analysis became highly sophisticated, with doctors relying heavily upon such tests for diagnosis.

During the time in which the growth in pharmacology and technology was taking place, surgery passed through a similar evolution. Dating back more than 6,000 years, at least to the ancient Egyptians and Peruvians, the principles of modern surgery originated with such innovators as Ambroise Paré, a Frenchman who in 1542 bound a wound by securing strips of cloth to the skin and then joined the strips with stitches.

World War II also played a role in shaping the course of modern medicine, when wound treatment provided surgeons with an understanding of how the body's immune system could be suppressed so that it could accept skin grafts, foreign implants, and transplanted organs. With this new knowledge, the first coronary bypass was performed in 1951 by a Canadian physician, Arthur Vineberg, in Montreal, and the first heart transplant in 1967 by South African surgeon Dr. Christiaan Barnard.

The New Medicine

Today, Western medicine stands as a monolith on the world stage. Few other spheres of human endeavor have developed so rapidly and in such a singular fashion. In the United States, it employs millions of people and accounts for a huge share of the country's gross national product. In terms of sheer influence over the daily life of most people, the health care industry is perhaps unrivaled.

Ironically, modern medicine is now in the throes of a revolution, in part because the disease patterns of the Western world have changed. Today, the leading causes of death in the U.S. are no longer infectious diseases, but rather, degenerative ones, such as illnesses of the heart and arteries, cancer, and diabetes. Studies have determined that these illnesses are caused primarily by lifestyle factors, such as dietary habits, stress, and patterns of thinking, feeling, and behaving. In other words, the leading killer diseases no longer fit into the germ theory paradigm. Modern medicine's failure to cure these illnesses, which do not really fit its worldview, and its enormous drain on many Western societies' economies, have revealed the system to be highly inflexible to the prevailing needs of modern life. The medical industry remains strongly wedded to crisis intervention, and its overreliance on extremely expensive tests, procedures, and technologies today threatens to bankrupt entire nations. At the same time, many common drugs and surgical procedures continue to undergo insufficient testing, or cause terrible side effects, raising doubts about the efficacy of some of medicine's methods and the accuracy of its claims.

Though most of orthodox medicine adheres stubbornly to its technological and pharmaceutical methods, a new and powerful trend is underfoot, which emphasizes the prevention of illness and the use of simpler, noninvasive methods of healing. Better diet, more active lifestyles, and healthier interpersonal relationships are the core constituents of this route to health. These trends lead us right back to where we began; the role and relationship of physical medicine, a practice which encompasses all systems of healing, from massage therapy, to homeotherapy; from chiropractic, to the laying on of hands; from the use of herbal compounds, to the stretching of muscles. In other words, to the healing process.

Summary

In this chapter, we discussed the six systems of healing which have been used throughout Eastern and Western civilization. We identified these systems as Chinese medicine, ayurvedic medicine, Greek medicine, homeopathy, naturopathy, and conventional modern medicine, and concluded that all of these systems are used in the study and in the practice by today's physical medicine practitioner.

Review Questions

1. What is the name of the study of medicine first used by the Hindus, that sees health as the basis of one's relationship with cosmic consciousness?
2. Who is known as the "father of medicine"?
3. What is the name of the system of healing which supports the theory that a substance that produces a certain set of symptoms in a healthy person has the power to cure a sick person manifesting those same symptoms?
4. What is the name of the system of healing that uses nontoxic healing methods derived from other healing systems from around the world, and which often includes the use of herbs?
5. What does the term *catharsis* mean?
6. List at least three health systems currently in use that are based upon Chinese medicine.
7. Briefly explain the difference between *yin* and *yang*.
8. What is the preeminent and most important form of therapy in Chinese medicine?
9. Briefly explain the *five element theory*.

Chiropractic Assisting: Basic Concepts and Applications

12

Introduction to Chiropractic

Performance Objectives

Upon completion of this chapter, you will be able to:

1. Briefly explain the meaning and philosophy of chiropractic and its relationship to the study of medicine.
2. Discuss the education, training, and role of the doctor of chiropractic and the chiropractic assistant.

Terms and Abbreviations

CA abbreviation for chiropractic assistant.
Certificated chiropractic assistant a chiropractic assistant who has received additional training and education in chiropractic philosophy, terminology, and various physical diagnostic procedures, and who has been certified by the Chiropractic Board of Examiners.
Chiropractic the branch of the healing arts which is based on the premise that good health greatly depends upon a normally functioning nervous system.
Chiropractic assistant a professional aid to the doctor of chiropractic, under whose direct guidance and supervision, he or she performs various administrative and clinical duties, and who assists in the preparation, control, and care of patients.
DC abbreviation for doctor of chiropractic.
Doctor of chiropractic refers to a physician who gives particular attention to the relationship of the structural and neurological aspects of the body in health and disease.

Chiropractic is a branch of the healing arts, and as a science, is based on the premise that good health depends, in part, upon a normally functioning nervous system. When body structures, such as cells and organs, are functioning normally, a state of health or normal physiology is said to exist. However, when the body's physiology is abnormal, a disease state begins.

The science of chiropractic teaches us that within the body there are well-established survival mechanisms designed to maintain a state of good health, and such innate intelligence is working in our body all the time, even when we're not aware of it. Think about what you had for breakfast this morning. Did you have to tell your body to digest it? Did you tell your heart how many times to beat, or your lungs when to breathe? You see, the greatest miracle of our body is that it has the ability to function and keep us well, that is, as long as we make sure that there is no interference. Since chiropractic does not use drugs or surgery to maintain the body's state of health, it is often referred to as a natural method of health care.

The Chiropractic Approach to Health Care

Doctors of chiropractic are physicians who consider the human body to be an integrated being, and as such, give special attention to spinal mechanics and neurologic, osseous, muscular, and vascular relationships. Therefore, their viewpoint and approach to health care and disease prevention and maintenance may differ considerably from that of the medical doctor.

In chiropractic, for example, disease is seen as an abnormal function, and abnormal function is function which is out of time and phase with one's environment. In other words, to the chiropractor, disease is viewed as a condition which occurs when the environment is disturbed. And this disturbance leads to a disruption of the nervous system, thus preventing the patient from achieving a normal adaptive response.

Maintaining Health Through Chiropractic

The chiropractic approach to well-being typifies our society's new and changing attitude toward health. It is based on the concept of health maintenance rather than treating one's disease. The basic recognition prevailing in chiropractic is the understanding that being well differs from relieving one's symptoms. Most concerned, thinking people have recognized that being symptom-free does not necessarily mean you are well.

Chiropractic also provides us with an understanding that health is not a commodity that can be purchased in a tablet or bottle, but rather, can only be obtained and maintained by allowing the natural recuperative powers of the body to function properly and unimpaired. Therefore, the effectiveness of chiropractic health care can only be measured by the benefits realized during one's entire lifetime.

Philosophy of Modern Chiropractic

Modern chiropractic reflects the rediscovery of therapeutic manipulation, which was first founded in the United States by Dr. D.D. Palmer in 1895. It is a type of medical practice which uses the same time-honored methods such as consultation, case history, physical examination, laboratory analysis, and X-ray examination. However, it differs from general medical practice in that it emphasizes structural examination on the spine.

Scope of Practice

Spinal analysis and adjustment have always been emphasized within the practice of chiropractic, but they by no means reflect the sole scope of practice used by the majority of chiropractic practitioners. In fact, several forms of therapy now gaining popularity within all the healing arts can thank chiropractic pioneers for their development in this country. Many physical therapy modalities, for example, were perfected by chiropractors and their use taught in chiropractic colleges long before the profession of physical therapy was created. History records that the use of physiologic therapeutic devices within the healing arts was initiated and developed in this country by nonallopathic professions, with pioneer chiropractors offering major leadership in both application and development.

Another important aspect to chiropractic is therapeutic nutrition. Unfortunately, however, even during the enlightenment of today, it is allowed only a few hours of instruction in medical schools.

And while oriental acupuncture and acupressure have received much publicity within the popular press and interest within the majority profession since the late 1960s, peripheral stimulation used in chiropractic to elicit certain physiologic reactions has been known and commonly applied within the practice of chiropractic since the turn of the century. It has always been an attribute of chiropractic to seek and develop conservative health care measures.

The Chiropractic Team

The person in charge of the chiropractic team, is the *doctor of chiropractic (DC).* While this person may also be referred to as a chiropractor or chiropractic physician, the doctor of chiropractic is a physician who gives particular attention to the relationship of the structural and neurologic aspects of the body in health and disease. In order to care for the human body in health and disease, and as a member of the health care delivery team, the chiropractic physician must be well educated in diagnosis and case management.

Working directly under the supervision and direction of the chiropractic physician is the *chiropractic assistant (CA).* This person acts as a professional aid to the chiropractor, and as such, is generally responsible for performing various technical duties, office and administrative functions, and often assists in the preparation, control, and care of patients.

Upon licensing by a credible agency, such as the Chiropractic Board of Examiners, a chiropractic assistant may choose to become a *certified chiropractic assistant.* Such certification can only be awarded to an assistant who has received the appropriate education and training in chiropractic philosophy, terminology, various physical diagnosis procedures, anatomy and physiology, clinical laboratory procedures, ethics and jurisprudence, radiological technology, adjunctive therapy, and basic office procedures. Certification is a type of licensure which allows an assistant to perform certain diagnostic, therapeutic, and rehabilitative services that are beyond the legal scope of uncertified chiropractic assistants. While there is a growing trend to have assistants obtain specific certification and continuing education in the application of roentgenographic equipment, physiologic therapeutics, and other clinical procedures, these requirements vary from state to state.

Role of the Chiropractic Assistant

Because of the increase in the number of chiropractic physicians, the need to seek skilled assistants has also grown. The field offers many personal rewards, such as above-average salaries and abundancy in job opportunities for growth and advancement.

While physicians in private practice have employed assistants for many years, the paraprofessional profession in chiropractic was slow to grow until about 15 years ago. It is now rapidly accelerating. Most DCs employ at least two CAs, and many have five or more. The primary reasons for this accelerated need for more CAs are advancing technology requiring skilled assistance, the administrative complexities involved in helping patients with insurance claims, the increase in office automation and computerization, and the rising costs in hospitalization which encourage more services to be performed in-office as opposed to in the hospital.

Qualifications of the Chiropractic Assistant

In your role as a chiropractic assistant, the doctor will delegate many duties to you. However, the final responsibility for any decision is always that of the doctor. It is therefore necessary that the DC be looked to for leadership and policy. It is the role of the chiropractic assistant to administer this policy.

The chiropractic assistant is generally involved in two basic, but often neglected, phases of work: human relations and economics. All experience and ability should be directed toward these aspects of the practice. Many attributes of an efficient assistant are taught in the classroom; they are basic personality traits, such as courtesy, intelligence, cooperativeness, tactfulness, and resourcefulness.

Tact and understanding are basic qualifications, as are discretion and good judgment. It is important to know when to talk and when to listen. Your personality should be cheerful and respectful, radiating interest in your patients' concerns. However, relating your personal life troubles has no place in communications with patients.

Trustworthiness, loyalty, and honesty are other basic qualifications. The doctor must be able to have full trust and confidence in your actions. Greater responsibilities can not be given to you unless minor responsibilities are held with respect.

A chiropractic assistant must be loyal to his or her doctor, the practice, and the profession. Indiscreet criticisms always have a way of coming home to roost. An honest, straightforward manner is necessary. The doctor should never have a reason to question your truthfulness as he or she may have cause to act quickly on your word without further investigation.

Accuracy, having a good business sense, and efficiency are also basic qualifications. Skill in recording the doctor's instructions, taking instrument readings, and being aware of a patient's verbal and nonverbal communications are necessary qualifications for every chiropractic assistant. Accuracy in administrative routines and diagnostic and therapeutic procedures is essential in health care.

Finally, using common sense and good judgment are two fundamental qualifications of the CA. The doctor should feel that office procedures will be carried out effectively in minimum time and according to high standards without a great deal of direct supervision.

Duties and Responsibilities of the Chiropractic Assistant

In a well-managed office, the chiropractic assistant serves as another brain and another pair of hands. He or she does those duties that do not require the special knowledge, skill, or training of the doctor. In a sense, the assistant acts as a partner, performing details and office functions that the DC does not have the time to do.

Each chiropractic practice reflects the individual personality or personalities of the doctor or doctors involved. Since we all vary in our genetic and conditioned personality structure, it is unlikely that the duties of an assistant in one practice will be identical with those in another, even if several other major practice characteristics are similar. Duties of any given assistant thus will be determined as much by the personality and goals of the doctor in charge as they will be by the type and size of the practice itself.

Most chiropractic assistants serve either in an administrative or clinical capacity. However, in some offices, the assistant may be responsible for completing tasks in both areas. In the administrative role, the assistant functions in a nontechnical nature, carrying out such tasks as answering the telephone, performing billing and collections procedures, and acting as an administrative assistant to the chiropractor. In the function of a clinical assistant, the CA is often required to perform many varied and technical procedures, such as assisting in physical diagnostic procedures, X-ray film processing, in-office laboratory tests, auxiliary therapeutic applications, massage and muscle therapy, rehabilitative procedures, and posture training. All of these duties are performed under close supervision of the chiropractic-employer.

As you can see in Table 12-1, the role of the chiropractic assistant is both broad and varied. You may be called upon to carry out numerous administrative and secretarial functions, serve as a business manager, prepare examination and therapeutic setups, and help the chiropractor during various parts of the examination and treatment procedure.

It's also important that you understand that your work as a chiropractic assistant is often determined by the office's needs, as well as the assistant's ability. Another factor is that of legal requirements. In some states, you may be permitted to perform X-ray exposures, apply physical therapy applications, and execute therapeutic massage on your patients. In other states, however, your position and the procedures you perform may require licensing or certification. In either case, however, the chiropractic assistant always functions under the direct supervision of his or her chiropractor-employer.

Working in the Professional Chiropractic Office

Whenever you work around people, especially those who are sick or are not feeling at their greatest capacity, one of your most important goals should be to act in the most professional way possible. That means never showing a lack of interest toward your patients, always making sure you provide for his or her privacy, and avoiding unnecessary interruptions whenever the chiropractor is working with the patient. It also means maintaining a professional ethical standard throughout your work.

Ethics and the Chiropractic Assistant

As in any health care environment, there are certain ethical standards which the chiropractic assistant is expected to maintain. These include the main-

Table 12-1
Chiropractic Assistant Responsibilities

Administrative Responsibilities

- Opens office and contacts chiropractor's answering service for messages.
- Answers telephone, schedules appointments, sends appointment reminder cards to or telephones patients.
- Explains general office procedures to patients and answers questions about procedures.
- Obtains basic new-patient information and makes up their chart and pulls charts of scheduled patients.
- Assists patients in completing office forms, receives payments, and makes receipts.
- Files, types correspondence, transcribes chiropractor's dictation, processes mail, prepares calendar.
- Performs general office management, including billing, insurance processing, and banking procedures.
- Prepares and mails statements to patients, maintains office business supplies, supervises petty cash.
- Other administrative responsibilities as required by chiropractor-employer.

Clinical Responsibilities

- Takes and records vital signs, height, and weight, and records routine reevaluation data.
- Conducts general posture analysis with instrumentation and teaches good health habits.
- Assists DC in certain therapeutic applications and conducts certain auxiliary therapeutic applications.
- Records clinical findings for DC during examinations and orients patient to equipment used during therapy.
- Conducts therapeutic massage and passive exercises and teaches prescribed home therapy and rehabilitative techniques.
- Explains necessity of patient cooperation for optimal recovery.
- Prepares patient X-ray identification markers and conducts assigned X-ray patient positioning, exposure, processing, and film-filing functions, as required by chiropractor.
- Maintains inventory control of clinical supplies and checks arriving shipments of clinical supplies.
- Other technical responsibilities as required by chiropractor-employer.

tenance of privileged patient information and protection of the doctor-patient relationship, never making derogatory remarks about another doctor or employee, and always being courteous to patients, other staff members, and your employer.

Another important aspect to adhering to professionalism in your office has to do with the human relations element. Remember, good human relations is always good business, and should therefore be just as important and of primary concern to the chiropractic assistant as it is to the chiropractor. When the chiropractor is busy with other patients or duties, it is often the chiropractic assistant who first meets the patient entering the office. First impressions are lasting impressions. Thus, as far as the patient is concerned, your attitude is often the one which most reflects the attitude of the office.

The first responsibility of the office is the responsibility of the assistant in greeting the patient, welcoming the patient, and putting him or her at ease. Most of the patients you will encounter in the office are generally apprehensive, nervous, and often extremely sensitive. By creating an atmosphere which is both friendly and professional, the patient will feel more at ease and therefore more receptive to both the chiropractor and the treatment the patient may need.

Professionalism on the Job

All members of the health care team play an important role in developing a professional office atmosphere. Health care is a serious business, and as such, professionalism must always be conveyed to patients in a subtle manner through office routine, office appearance, and personnel appearance and attitudes.

Experienced assistants should help orient new assistants to the office's team approach to patient care. Using the terms "we" when talking with patients, or "our" when referring to the office should become automatic if you are truly to become a member of the office team. Also, try to limit your discussions with patients to office matters, and do this in a friendly manner. This does not mean you cannot be a good listener. Conversations with fellow staff members should also be limited to office-related matters during office hours. Habitual chatting reduces the time and opportunities for self-development in your career.

The office telephone is the primary link between the practice and the community. Therefore, personal telephone calls during office hours should be brief and limited to the needs of the situation.

Convey a Professional Image

The chiropractic assistant's part in the chain of public relations starts when a patient opens the door to the office. First impressions made on the patient because of office or staff appearance and behavior are lasting impressions that will ultimately be conveyed to others.

A first in-office public relations function is to make the office comfortable, appealing, efficient, and professional in every respect. Another important task is to develop an ability to make friends, gain the confidence of patients quickly, work efficiently, and act professionally. These qualities must become second nature to every member of the staff. A third important public relations effort should be one of public education. To be effective, health education must be centered in the office and then expanded in scope to every contact with all personnel.

People tend to generalize and stereotype. Remember, you represent all chiropractic assistants, the chiropractic profession, and especially your office outside the office, at work, or at play. You have a responsibility not only to your doctor-employer, but also to yourself, to be a good courier of public relations.

Your every act as a professional chiropractic assistant, your every word, your every letter, your touch and gentleness, and your every contact with the public should convey a sense of prestige, restraint, good manners, and professionalism. This is the image you should want to build and strengthen. It starts in the morning when you wake up; and it stops when you go to bed at night.

Thus, to many patients and acquaintances, you represent the office. Since you are building an image every minute of every day, your responsibility to yourself and your profession is to build an image of friendliness; sincerity; compassionate, professional knowhow; and respect. Your image should be one of pride in accepting a responsibility and fulfilling a need. Be recognized as a community-minded citizen who aids in the health and welfare of human beings. You will soon find that it's a giant step toward a positive self-image and success.

Summary

In this chapter, we briefly discussed the meaning and philosophy involved in the study of chiropractic and its relationship to the study of medicine. We also talked about the various members of the chiropractic team, including the education, training, and role of the doctor of chiropractic and the chiropractic assistant.

Review Questions

1. Briefly explain the philosophy of chiropractic.
2. What is the name of a physician who specializes in the study of chiropractic?
3. What does the abbreviation *CA* mean?
4. Identify at least three clinical duties of a chiropractic assistant.
5. Identify at least three administrative duties of a chiropractic assistant.
6. Briefly explain the concept of *health maintenance.*
7. In what year, and by whom, was chiropractic first discovered?
8. What is the name of the organization responsible for licensing chiropractors?
9. Briefly explain the philosophy of the *doctor-patient relationship.*
10. Who is responsible for certifying chiropractic assistants?

13

The Role of the Chiropractor

Performance Objectives

Upon completion of this chapter, you will be able to:

1. Briefly discuss the role of the doctor of chiropractic.
2. Explain how the chiropractor uses diagnostics to care for patients.
3. Describe how the chiropractor uses therapeutics to determine what is wrong with a patient.
4. Identify and briefly discuss rehabilitative modalities used by the chiropractor in treating and caring for the patient.
5. Briefly discuss counseling and how it is used by the chiropractor as a preventative therapy.
6. Discuss the role the chiropractor plays in general medical practice.

Terms and Abbreviations

Diagnostics determining the cause of a patient's complaint by using inductive and deductive logic.

Rehabilitation the process by which certain modalities, such as physical therapy, nutrition, and posture and physical fitness are used to aid the body in its natural healing process.

Therapeutics the process by which certain methods, such as dietary and nutritional supplementation, physiotherapeutic measures, and professional counseling are used to correct a medical problem.

Unfortunately, most people do not fully understand the role of the doctor of chiropractic, and therefore, many believe that the only function this professional health caregiver provides to patients is to "make them feel better" by manipulating their back. Not so. Today, the role of the chiropractor is quite varied, and as such involves many aspects of health care, including diagnostics, therapeutics, nutrition, rehabilitation, and patient counseling.

The Art of Diagnosing

The art of *diagnostics,* which is used by the chiropractor to determine what is wrong with the patient, is a process which begins by recording and interpreting the patient's medical history. Thus, the initial interview and consultation with the patient is extremely important, since it will be used to direct the examinations and tests that are to follow. Every measure of observation that will substantially profile the patient is employed and recorded. A systematic and thorough physical examination is conducted using the methods, techniques, and instruments that are standard with all health care professionals. In addition, the doctor of chiropractic will also include a postural and spinal analysis, a process which is an innovation in the field of physical diagnosis and examination.

Obtaining Background Information

The chiropractor uses the standard procedures and instruments of physical and clinical diagnosis, and he or she is well acquainted with the need for differential diagnosis. Diagnostic radiology, especially as it relates to the musculoskeletal system, is a primary clinical diagnostic aid to the chiropractor, and has been since the early 1900s.

In addition to being knowledgeable in diagnostic radiology, the chiropractor must also understand standard and special clinical laboratory procedures and tests which are used in modern diagnosing. These often include radiology, thermography, electrocardiography, and electromyology.

After completion of a diagnostic evaluation by a chiropractor, many patients report that it was the most thorough examination of their lifetime. The reason for this is that the chiropractic physician views each patient as an individual who has been subjected to both unique outside and inside forces, who is interested in both correction and prevention, and who is interested in the preservation of life. Thoroughness, therefore, to the chiropractor, is a necessity in order to achieve such goals.

The Diagnostic Process

Any professional therapy administered ethically, legally, and professionally by the chiropractor must be based upon the doctor's proper diagnosis of the patient's condition. That is, the diagnosis must direct the treatment. By understanding why the chiropractor does what he or she does during the diagnostic process, you will be in a better position to answer patient questions.

Diagnosing, which is used to determine the cause of the patient's complaint, involves the use of inductive and deductive logic. It is a process which can be divided into two major categories: gathering data and interpreting data (Table 13-1).

Table 13-1
Elements of Diagnostic Logic

Data Gathering: Collecting the facts

- clinical history
- physical examination
- orthopedic examination
- neurologic examination
- laboratory data
- ancillary examinations
- progress reports
- periodic reexamination

Data Interpreting: Analyzing the facts

- critical evaluation of the data
- identification of reliable signs and symptoms and findings in order of importance
- exclusion of disorders that might produce similar data
- selection of disease(s) or disorder(s) that best fit facts at hand
- continually verifying current diagnosis

After the initial collection of data is complete, the patient's complaint often tends to fall into one or more of the 13 general etiological classifications. These include intrinsic or extrinsic traumatic, inflammatory, neurological, vascular, endocrine, metabolic, neoplastic, degenerative, deficiency, congenital, allergic, autoimmune, or toxic. Each of these general classes or categories contains scores of specific disorders and diseases. The suspicions obtained at this point will then be either confirmed or rejected by the results or further examination and test data until only one likely cause remains.

The diagnostic process is further aided by determining whether the patient's symptoms are being caused by physiological, structural, or mental and emotional changes. This process is often referred to as problem group analysis.

A physiologic, or functional, disorder is a pathophysiological disease process without overt structural changes. Symptoms resulting from physiological changes often arise from increased function, such as hypertrophy, spastic paralysis, or pain, edema, and articular instability; decreased function, such as atrophy, flaccid paralysis, numbness, and articular fixation; and altered function, such as convulsions, tremors, various visual disturbances, and aberrant articular movement.

A structural dysfunction is one which is an organic disorder, with or without signs of overt pathology. Symptoms resulting from structural changes may arise from bone and joint infection, which can result in soft-tissue reactions, subperiosteal calcification, and bone destruction; congenital anomaly; deformity, which can be witnessed as abnormal changes in angularity, displacement, or loss of continuity; degenerative process; endocrine and metabolic imbalances; trauma; and malignant or benign tumors.

Symptoms which are classified as mental or emotional generally involve a neurosis or psychosis, or a predominantly psychosomatic or somatopsychic disturbance. Symptoms resulting from these types of changes may be the result of either physiologic or structural lesions.

Using Therapeutics to Determine What Is Wrong

Chiropractic *therapeutic* methods are determined by the scope of practice authorized by individual state law. In all areas, however, these methods do not include the use of prescription drugs or major surgery, thus avoiding the possible dangers therein. Most treatment methods include the chiropractic adjustment when indicated and, according to the doctor's judgment, such ancillary services as necessary dietary advice and nutritional supplementation, physical therapy measures, and professional counseling.

The most characteristic aspect of chiropractic practice is the release of one or more fixated and possibly subluxated spinal or extraspinal articular surfaces by making a specific predetermined adjustment. Often referred to as manipulation, the purpose of this correction and its determination is to normalize the dynamic relationships of segments within their articular range and thus associated neurologic, muscular, and vascular disturbances.

Using Physical Therapy Measures

Physical therapeutic methods and modalities are often used as adjunctive therapy to enhance the effects of the chiropractic adjustment. Such procedures may include the use of diathermy, infrared and ultraviolet light, galvanic current, ultrasound, hot or cold compresses, paraffin baths, hydrotherapy, and other commonly used modalities. Taping, strapping, and other forms of minor surgery are also sometimes used in injuries of the spine or extremities. Neck, lower back, elbow, knee, and ankle injuries may require supportive collars or braces to enhance the effects of corrective treatments during recuperation to help tissue heal and become strengthened.

In addition to using physical therapy as a means of increasing the effects of adjustment, many chiropractors often recommend changes and supplements in the patients' dietary needs. The adequate intake and assimilation of essential nutrients is necessary to maintain health, and tissue demands increase during illness and stress. The chiropractor may use vitamin, mineral, enzyme, and tissue supplementation, if professionally supervised, to help the patient prevent the onset or lessen the existence of some types of dysfunction of the nervous system and other tissues.

Rehabilitative exercises, as a physical therapy, make up an important aspect of professional counsel to aid patients in their recovery and thus prevent further strain. In your role as a chiropractic assistant, you may be asked to record in a patient's entering data a few words that would describe the patient's common exercise level. These descriptive terms are defined in Table 13-2.

Often the chiropractor counsels the patient by providing him or her with advice such as dietary regimens, physical and mental attitudes affecting health, personal hygiene, occupational safety, lifestyle, posture, rest, work, and many of the other activities of daily living that would enhance the effects of chiropractic health care. Chiropractic is truly concerned with the total individual, and that includes the patient's health, welfare, and survival.

Using Rehabilitation to Aid the Natural Healing Process

The human body is a complex, integrated organism, and spinal disorders may cause or contribute to disease processes affecting the body. While the nervous system influences the glandular system, for example, hormones in turn have a great influence on the nervous system. A digestive disturbance may result in spinal pain, and a spinal disorder may result in digestive problems. A heart condition may send shooting pain down the patient's arm, and a spinal or rib joint disorder may mimic a heart condition.

The name which has been given to a disease process does not necessarily cancel the chiropractor's responsibility to correct the anatomical disrelationship and/or the neuromechanical disorders that may be causing, maintaining, or associated with the disease process. Through the ages, the musculoskele-

Table 13-2
Terms Used in Recording a Patient's Level of Exercise

Light:	light means light office work, driving an auto, desk work, slow walking, cooking, playing a piano, and using a golf cart when playing golf.
Light–moderate:	light–moderate includes working in light construction trades, such as welding, truck driving in traffic; it also includes fast walking, playing golf without a cart, sailing, bowling, cleaning the house, and pushing a light lawn mower.
Moderate–heavy:	moderate–heavy means performing tasks such as splitting wood, playing a game of tennis, riding a bicycle, cross-country skiing, and square or disco-dancing.
Heavy:	heavy means taking part in tasks such as aerobic dancing, jogging, playing basketball, weight lifting, and being involved in other activities requiring much energy.

tal system has been heated, cooled, massaged, injected, and cut into, yet these modalities were never truly considered of primary importance until the birth of chiropractic medicine. Today, however, this is changing. Just look at the publicity that is reflected in the chiropractic care of various athletes that has enabled several world records to be broken.

The idea that mechanical spinal disorders such as subluxation-fixations may cause functional abnormalities is the basis of chiropractic thought and one of its major contributions to generic medicine. Continuous research in this area must be made since this principle promises to answer many unsolved problems facing health science today.

Components of the Rehabilitation Process: Nutrition, Posture, and Physical Fitness

Nutrition

In addition to the correction of localized biomechanical faults, the development of good posture habits, and the necessity for regular exercise, nutrition also plays an important role in the rehabilitative process. Nourishing food that builds bone and muscle and maintains nerve and blood integrity is essential to good health and repair mechanisms.

Too often in our society, a well-balanced diet has been replaced by manufactured sweets, snack foods, and other junk foods. While four-fifths of our daily foods should consist of alkaline-forming vegetables, raw salads, and fresh fruits, most American tables display four-fifths acid-forming concentrated proteins, starches, and sugars. By altering our food habits and ridding our body of toxins found in manufactured foods, we can help the rehabilitative process by allowing the natural healing process to occur.

Posture and Physical Fitness

Sadly, most members of our society lag behind their counterparts of other countries throughout the world in physical fitness. Much of this is a result of easier living reflected by space-age developments which have encouraged a lifestyle of minimal physical effort. A society of button pushers neglects its physical fitness, however.

Since its inception, the chiropractic profession has offered national and community leadership toward encouraging parents and teachers to support physical fitness programs in schools. Youngsters should also be encouraged by their parents to develop good fitness and health habits at an early age. Fitness should be a family affair.

From birth, we as human beings have enjoyed a type of existence which has allowed for agility, leverage, mobility, and balance against gravity's constant pull. When biomechanics are disturbed through stress and strain even slightly, distortion can result. This is because of the close interrelationship of our structural and functional systems: the body is a whole. Posture not only has a direct bearing on comfort and work efficiency; it is also a factor which determines resistance to disease or disability.

The chiropractic profession is unique in paying attention to the importance of nerve integrity and body mechanics for good health. The doctor of chiropractic is most concerned with the effects of and prevention of spinal defects which affect physical fitness. He or she has been trained and is skilled in treating health problems, and all treatment is aimed at maintaining joint integrity by correcting spinal and extraspinal mechanical defects and postural distortions.

The need for good posture is far more significant than an attractive appearance. To assure health, our bodies must be free from structural distortions and our functions must operate at peak efficiency. Any activity in which the structure of the human frame is thrown out of its normal balance can cause distortion of the spine. The spine not only supports the weight of the entire body above the pelvis, it also protects the spinal cord which connects the higher brain centers with nerves to and from the vital organs.

When disorders occur to our normal musculoskeletal system, we see the rise of sore backs and stiff necks, aching joints and easy fatigue, headaches and nervous tension, and scores of other complaints which are so common to the times we are living in. Such structural abuses and their frequently painful effects are an important area in chiropractic counsel and care for both prevention and treatment.

Using Counseling as Preventative Therapy

We live in an era of rapidly advancing technology, and as such, we have attempted to adapt to both mental and physical stresses which were unknown by our forefathers. While many medical professionals agree that emotional disturbances may cause structural disorders, clinical observations verify that the reverse is also true. Structural faults may lead to a low stress threshold which can result in a variety of emotional illnesses. Thus, the structural neurologic approach of chiropractic may often benefit associated behavioral disorders.

Increasing evidence of the serious consideration now being given to the chiropractic somatopsychic approach to many emotional illnesses is to be found in the scientific literature. Several authorities have shown a distinct relationship between mental illness and vitamin deficiencies; others between mental illness and overconsumption of refined sugar or food additives. And still others show a definite relationship between the ingestion of lead or copper and zinc deficiency. With these dietary factors removed and treatment directed to somatopsychic structural correction, we are beginning to see promise toward the reduction of our nation's increasing mental health problem.

The Role of the Chiropractor in General Medical Practice

While chiropractors emphasize the importance of the correction of spinal and extraspinal mechanical lesions, no medical practitioner believes that these are the sole causes of disease. However, clinical chiropractic has shown us repeatedly that neurologic aberrations which have originated from mechanical lesions are a contributing or inducing factor in many more dysfunctions than commonly realized. When combined with poor nutrition, physical and emotional overstress, germs, trauma, drug-related weakness, poor habits, and other common debilitating factors, such mechanical lesions become an important consideration far too often overlooked.

Pain and Prevention

The chiropractor, like the medical doctor, understands that warning signals matter a great deal. Pain is often considered to be just such a warning. As nature's early warning signal, it is a message that tells us that our body is not functioning properly, that something serious may be wrong with our health. Pain of any kind is an alarm that nature uses in order to signal where there is a health problem that deserves attention. It is just as foolhardy to do no more than kill the pain with a pill or injection as it would be to silence a fire alarm and fail to seek its cause. To effect proper care, the cause must be treated, not just the symptoms.

Headaches are one of the most common complaints of pain encountered in the healing arts today, and a common cause of headaches originates from a vertebral articular disorder in the spine. It is important that such mechanical lesions be recognized by a trained chiropractic physician. Unfortunately, sufferers of headaches are too often offered a generalized diagnosis, such as sinus trouble, migraine, or cluster headaches. Because chiropractic care is attentive to the neurologic implications involved, people suffering from headaches frequently find relief under chiropractic care, where other forms of therapy may have failed.

The second most common complaint of pain is that of backache. Here again, lumbago, sacroiliac strains, and disc injuries are usually of a musculoskeletal nature having neurologic overtones. It is important that the cause be recognized and cared for before permanent damage is done. Because chiropractic care recognizes the structural and functional relationships involved, the profession has earned a respected reputation in handling cases of both acute and chronic back pain.

It's important to remember that many pains remote from the spine originate from a spinal disorder. In the same manner, many pains that appear to be located within the spine may also originate in some distant tissue. Differential diagnosis in such conditions requires a thorough holistic approach, that is, an approach which is demonstrated under modern chiropractic care.

Prenatal and Postnatal Chiropractic Care

During pregnancy, there is a natural change within the mother's pelvic structure along with an accompanying change in weight distribution. Health disorders such as headache, backache, leg pains, and lower extremity circulation disturbances often can be attributed solely to the strain on the neuromusculoskeletal system involved. It is for this reason that many women undergo periodic chiropractic spinal analysis and adjustment in association with regular obstetrical care throughout the course of their pregnancy.

Spinal examination and necessary correction after delivery is also a positive step toward preventing potential lower back and sacroiliac disorders that may have been initiated during pregnancy or delivery. Correction of these often minor disorders at this time may serve as a positive deterrent against possible structural and functional gynecologic problems during later years.

Pediatric Chiropractic Care

The strain of delivery plus disproportionate weight of the child's head upon yet-to-be fully developed neck structures often results in the child suffering from problems in the upper cervical vertebrae. It is for this reason that many chiropractors recommend a spinal examination of the child shortly after birth so that proper corrections can be made if problems exist. Only a chiropractic physician has been trained to make such determinations. By performing early examinations on the child, there appears to be a reduction in the possibility of colic, digestive sensitivities, allergies, and other common dysfunctions in the newborn. Early detection of predispositions toward common childhood diseases also seems to have a direct relationship toward early chiropractic examination of the child.

Summary

In this chapter, we briefly discussed the role of the doctor of chiropractic. We explained how the chiropractor uses diagnostics and therapeutics to care for patients. We also identified and talked briefly about rehabilitative modalities used by the chiropractor in treating and caring for patients, and how counseling can be used by the chiropractor as a preventative form of therapy. Finally, we discussed the role the chiropractor plays in general medical practice, including pre- and postnatal chiropractic care and pediatric chiropractic care.

Review Questions

1. What is the name of the process by which certain methods are used to correct a medical problem?
2. What is the name of the process by which certain modalities are used to aid the body in its natural healing process?
3. What is the term given that uses inductive and deductive logic to determine the cause of a patient's complaint?
4. What are the two categories used by chiropractors and physicians to help them determine the cause of a patient's complaint?
5. Briefly explain the process of *problem group analysis.*
6. Identify at least five therapeutic modalities which are used in chiropractic.
7. Briefly explain the four levels of exercise.
8. What are the four components of the rehabilitation process?
9. Chiropractic is unique in that it pays particular attention to the importance of ______________ ______________ and ______________ ______________.
10. Briefly explain how counseling can be used as a preventative therapy.

14

The Clinical Chiropractic Assistant

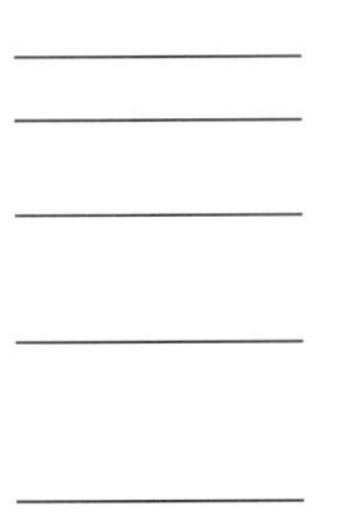

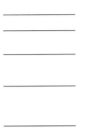

Performance Objectives

Upon completion of this chapter, you will be able to:

1. Briefly discuss the basic functions of the clinical chiropractic assistant.
2. Identify general characteristics of the clinical chiropractic assistant.
3. Identify the classification of clinical procedures performed in the chiropractic office.
4. Briefly explain how accidents can be prevented in the chiropractic office.
5. Identify the most frequently encountered functions of the clinical chiropractic assistant.
6. Identify and briefly discuss some of the more advanced functions of the clinical chiropractic assistant.

Terms and Abbreviations

AP abbreviation for anterior-posterior (front to back); used in radiology to designate that the X-ray beam enters the front or anterior portion of the patient and exits at the posterior or rear of the patient.
Body mechanics the coordinated use of body parts to produce motion and maintain balance.
Chiropractic physiotherapy the therapeutic application of forces and substances that induce a physiologic response and use and/or allow the body's natural processes to return to a more normal state of health.
Chronic disease a continuous or recurrent persistence of a disease.
L abbreviation used in radiology to designate the left side of a patient or part being examined.
LAO abbreviation used in radiology to designate that the left anterior portion of the part being examined is closest to the film; the opposite of RAO.
LPO abbreviation used in radiology to indicate that part being examined is positioned obliquely to the central ray and film with the left posterior portion of the part closest to the film.
PA abbreviation for posterior-anterior (back to front); used in radiology to designate the opposite of an AP view.
Posture the relative position of body parts standing, sitting, lying, or participating in any other type of activity; body alignment.
R abbreviation used in radiology to designate the right side of the patient or part being examined.
RAO abbreviation used in radiology to designate right anterior oblique; indicates that the right anterior portion of the part examined is closest to the film, and the whole of the examined part is positioned obliquely to the central X-ray beam.
RPO abbreviation used in radiology to indicate that the part being examined is positioned obliquely to the central ray and film with the right posterior portion of the part closest to the film.
Sign objective evidences that can be detected by one of the senses, such as sight, hearing, touch, smell, or taste, and which can be noticed either by an observer or by the individual experiencing them.
Symptom pertains to functional rather than structural evidence, which may be objective and noticeable by an observer, as well as by the individual experiencing them, or may be subjective by the individual's own sensations.

The scope of practice for chiropractic physicians is determined locally and may vary from state to state. The same is true for the chiropractic assistant. Therefore, as a professional member of the chiropractic team, you must check with your local or state department of consumer affairs or the agency which governs the practice of chiropractic in your individual state for statutory enactments and judicial determinations and their relationship to your scope of practice as a chiropractic assistant. Because the scope of practice may differ from state to state, most of the clinical duties and procedures we will discuss in this chapter are considered general in nature, that is, they may or may not be applicable in the particular state where you are employed.

Basic Role of the Clinical Chiropractic Assistant

Many of the basic tasks and duties you will perform in the chiropractic office are very similar to those practiced by other allied health care professionals. They revolve around maintaining a professional relationship with your patients, your co-workers, and your employer.

Maintaining Interpersonal Relationships in the Clinical Environment

Developing healthy interpersonal relationships is not always easy. As a matter of fact, they are often much easier to describe than they are to achieve. To deal with others effectively, there are three basic concepts you should understand. The first deals with having a good understanding of yourself. Self-understanding and self-acceptance are based on a realistic self-image and a genuine feeling of self-esteem. The second basic concept in relating and communicating with others is knowing who your line of authority is. This can only be accomplished by gaining a clear understanding of your role and responsibilities as a member of the chiropractic team. Finally, to relate best to your patients, you must first gain an understanding of your patients' needs. Since most patients experience a distinct feeling of loss of control over what is happening to them during health care, all members of the health care team who are required to have direct contact with them should be considerate of the emotions involved. In addition to their need for treatment by competent professional caregivers, patients also need kindness, a bit of sympathy, and simple courtesy. Remember, if a patient knows what is expected from the health care provider, he or she will be less apt to become apprehensive, critical, or demanding.

Working Within Your Scope of Practice

Members of our society have a special trust and confidence in the healing and health care professions and the people who provide health care and treatment. Since laws are written primarily to safeguard the public welfare, those that apply to the provision of health services have special significance.

Any action involving curative or restorative treatment of a patient is a medical act, and many paraprofessional activities are conditioned or dependent on the order and direction of your chiropractor-employer. While the practice of chiropractic is strictly controlled by licensing, the chiropractor may allow his or her assistant to carry out certain activities, as long as specific conditions or guidelines have been met. These guidelines include:

- The assistant must show evidence of proper training, skill, and understanding of the cause and effect of the act to be performed.
- The act being performed must be on the order of a chiropractor-physician.
- The act remains under the direction and supervision of the chiropractor-physician, who maintains overall responsibility for the actions of his or her assistant.

Avoiding Clinical Negligence

While there is no uniform code of health care law, there are laws that have special significance in the care and treatment of patients. A basic rule of law which applies to the provision of health services is the rule of negligence. Most simply put, negligence results from failure to have done something that ordinarily ought to have been done, or doing something that ordinarily ought not to have been done.

The practice of law, particularly as it relates to members of the health professions, holds every individual responsible for his or her own acts of negligence. Negligence is commonly held to be an unintentional injury, but once an act has been performed and injury results, the performance of the act and the consequences of the act are facts. Thus, negligence is one of the most common causes for lawsuits against health care providers.

The law of negligence applies in almost all medicolegal problems which may arise when, in the course of providing a patient treatment, something is done that interferes with the rights and privileges of the patient. However, there is a built-in protection for unforeseeable, unavoidable, or inevitable accidents. Responsible authority provides for investigation in order to establish the facts of an accident or incident, and the facts are generally obtained when five questions are asked: who, what, when, where, and how? These questions are not asked to establish a person's guilt or innocence, but rather, to establish what the facts are, in order to make a correct legal decision.

Laws Governing the Practice of Chiropractic Assistants

A practice act is a law which controls the practice of a legally recognized profession. In chiropractic, the purpose of such an act is to protect the public from persons who are unqualified to practice. In general, this act defines the chiropractic profession, provides standards which control the preparation for the practice of chiropractic, provides for licensure within the profession, and through licensure, defines who shall be licensed to practice and under what terms.

At the present time, there is no federal licensure or laws governing the practice of chiropractic assistants, so requirements for licensure under professional practice acts vary from state to state. This is because, under the Constitution, each state is responsible for passing its own laws regulating the control of professions, trades, and occupations.

Characteristics and Attributes of the Clinical Chiropractic Assistant

The clinical chiropractic assistant may perform any of a number of duties common to the provision of paraprofessional care for sick or injured patients. However, in order to function effectively in this role, he or she must possess basic personal qualities. Many of these characteristics and attributes are inherent; others must be cultivated and improved on; and all are interdependent. To be an effectual member of the chiropractic team, the CA should possess:

- a good aptitude for learning and performing the tasks required of a chiropractic assistant.
- interest in the tasks required of the chiropractic assistant.
- a positive attitude which leads to cooperation, understanding, concern, consideration, and a sense of satisfaction in knowing one's job.
- good personal hygiene habits.
- good self mental health and a sense of tolerance and respect for others.

Basic Technical Functions of the Clinical Chiropractic Assistant

The basic technical functions and responsibilities of the clinical chiropractic assistant are classified into three categories: diagnostic assistance, therapeutic assistance, and patient relations.

Diagnostic Assistance

Tasks which require the CA's assistance in obtaining certain pertinent data and information about the patient are considered diagnostic. They include:

- assisting the chiropractor in diagnostic procedures.
- recording the chiropractor's findings.
- recording general body measurements, such as height, weight, vision, and vital signs.
- collecting specimens and conducting in-office laboratory tests.
- preparing patients for X-ray examinations and conducting X-ray film processing.

Therapeutic Assistance

Tasks which require the CA's assistance in conducting and applying certain therapeutic measures on the patient are considered therapeutic. They include:

- conducting certain physical therapy applications.
- conducting massage and muscle therapy.
- explaining diet and exercise regimens.
- teaching the patient about routine home therapy and rehabilitative procedures.

Patient Relations

Tasks which require the CA's assistance in helping the patient to better understand what is expected of him or her are classified under patient relations. They include:

- orienting patients to pertinent equipment and procedures.
- explaining the necessity of patient cooperation for optimal recovery.
- teaching the patient about good health habits and hygiene.
- performing assigned counsel to patient's family members when necessary.

Classification of Clinical Procedures

Many of the procedures performed in the chiropractic office are clinical in nature, and as such, may require your assistance. Therefore, it is very important that you have a good understanding of how these procedures are classified.

Procedures may be classified into one of three categories. The first are routine procedures, which are performed on a repetitive basis, and which require little or no modification to meet the individual needs of a patient. Basic procedures are procedures which meet hygienic, comfort, and therapeutic needs of patients. Some of these involve direct patient care, such as positioning and measuring the patient's blood pressure, temperature, pulse, and respiration. Others involve indirect patient care, such as ensuring cleanliness, preparing equipment and supplies, and maintaining clinical records and reports.

The third classification is called simple and complex procedures. To determine which procedures fall into this category, you must first understand what the term simple means. Simple, as it is used here, must be considered in relation to the total situation. Four factors decide whether a procedure is simple or complex. It is a simple procedure if (1) abilities required to perform the procedure are based on a limited knowledge of scientific facts; (2) it can be performed by following a defined protocol step by step; (3) it is performed for a patient whose clinical state is relatively stable; and (4) the instructional needs of the patient are minimal.

Any modification or variation of these four factors contributes to the complexity of a procedure. For example, preparing a patient for physical therapy can be a routine, basic, simple procedure, or it can be an exceedingly complex procedure, depending on the condition of the patient. In a simple situation, the CA would be assigned to carry out the procedure with minimal assistance and supervision. However, in a complex situation, the CA would be assigned to help the chiropractor or another CA with some phases of care and would carry out other phases with supervision and direction.

Obtaining and Reporting Clinical Information Through Observation

The manner in which a patient has been received in the examination or treatment area of the office is an important contributing factor to his or her attitude and therefore toward his or her recovery. A feeling of confidence must first be established. And since entering an office often stimulates a considerable amount of dread and apprehension in a patient, you should try to make the admission procedure as brief and reassuring as possible.

The patient's clinical record—which includes the forms recording the medical record of a patient during one current, continuous episode of a disease, injury, or other condition—is prepared and maintained according to office policy. The accumulation of these forms is often referred to as the patient's clinical record file, or chart. It serves as a basis for planning the patient's care, providing communication between the chiropractor, his or her staff, and members of other professional groups, and presenting documentary evidence of the course of illness and treatment.

All clinical records remain in the custody of their owner, the chiropractor, while the patient is under his or her care, and should always be handled so that only authorized persons officially concerned with the patient's care and treatment will have access to them. As a chiropractic assistant, you may have the occasion to enter certain information, or assemble the forms in the prescribed order in the chart holder. You may also be responsible for making sure that all diagnostic and test reports are attached or inserted in the record file on receipt, after these reports have been seen by the chiropractor. When you are required to do this, you must also make sure that each form is placed in its appropriate sequence. As further laboratory reports, consultations, or other forms are completed, they must also be added to the record.

Observing the Patient

The term observation, as it is used in the health care environment, means the process of taking notice of the specific signs and symptoms presented by a patient, which might suggest his or her physical or mental condition. This process is an essential part of providing the appropriate care and treatment for the patient. As a member of the clinical staff, the chiropractor will depend on you to observe, recognize, report, and record the patient's condition accurately during your contact. Meeting these objectives will help to enhance the chiropractor's own observations, as well as aid him or her in making a proper diagnosis and in prescribing the suitable treatment.

When determining the patient's *signs* and *symptoms,* we are actually looking for some type of clinical indication of a patient's condition or disability. Signs are objective evidence which can either be noticed by the observer, or by the patient, and can only be detected by one of our senses, such as sight, hearing, smell, touch, or taste. One example of a sign you might encounter is a swollen area which can be seen or felt.

Symptoms differ from signs in that their evidence is considered functional as opposed to structural. They can either be objective, meaning that they are noticeable by the observer or by the person experiencing them, or they may be strictly subjective, in that they are evidenced by the individual's own sensations. Examples of classic subjective symptoms often include pain, itching, nausea, and dizziness.

There are two main groups of signs and symptoms which you should become knowledgeable about. The first are those caused by a disease or injury, and the second are those which relate to health care, that is, those caused as a result of some type of therapy.

Developing Your Skill in Observation

In order to increase your skill in observing the patient's condition and to determine his or her needs through your own awareness of their signs and symptoms, it's important that you expand your own knowledge base. You should also take an active interest in the patient, as well as develop a sympathetic understanding of the patient as a whole person. Also, you should always strive to be a good listener, attentive and accurate. You can increase and augment your knowledge by being conscientious and accurately using all of your senses by accumulating a fund of information from books and from the chiropractor concerning specific signs or symptoms which can be expected in various patient conditions. You can also try to anticipate the patient's emotional and physical needs and discomforts and do what can be done appropriately to relieve such discomforts. Finally, you can be accurate and conscientious in your performance of procedures that may uncover signs of illness such as noting the patient's pulse and respiratory rates and rhythms, and blood pressure levels.

Reporting and Recording Your Observations

If at all possible, in order to reduce the patient's level of anxiety or any misunderstandings, detailed reporting should be done away from the patient and out of his or her sight and hearing. And any comments made in the patient's presence should be appropriate to what he or she needs to know or hear about the medical condition. It will be helpful if you learn to use plain, everyday, factual language in reporting and recording. And remember, always identify the patient by his or her name, and the time the observation was made.

Any clinical measure taken should be reported, including a statement whether the measure seemed to help or not. Any complaints or signs of pain should be reported as precisely as possible. Such things as location, and any comments from the patient as to the pain being sharp, dull, aching, throbbing, constant, or knife-like, are all important. If the patient is quoted, you must use his or her exact words. And you should ascertain how long the patient has had the pain.

During your observation of a patient complaining of pain, always try to pay particular attention to any position assumed to relieve the pain. Look to see if the patient is bent over. Is he or she unwilling to take a deep breath or to straighten an arm or leg? Ask the patient if a measure previously used to relieve the pain helped? Or did a specific therapy or a change of position relieve the pain for a period of time? Remember, whenever you are required to report and record your observations of the patient, it is important to note signs of health, and any indications of returning strength. You should also note any statements by the patient about his or her feelings of well-being, as well as any evidence or statements by the patient regarding signs of disabilities and progressing distress.

Typical Clinical Functions of the Chiropractic Assistant

The role of the clinical chiropractic assistant generally involves assisting the chiropractor in the assessment, care, treatment, and follow-up of the orthopedically disabled patient. Depending on your training and the needs of your employer, your responsibilities, while always directed and supervised by the chiropractor, may be quite varied, and may be as basic as taking and recording the patient's vital signs, or as advanced as assisting in the X-ray department.

Working with Disabled Patients

Chiropractic offices are carefully designed and planned to meet the needs of the practice, especially if the chiropractor anticipates a large number of orthopedic cases. Patients affected with orthopedic problems often find it difficult to support themselves and move about because musculoskeletal disorders affect the locomotor and structural systems of the body. Therefore, most chiropractic offices employ devices to help the patient support him- or herself and move about the facility. These may include hallway handrails, grab bars by toilets, cushioned chairs with armrests, and so forth.

Understanding Applied Biomechanics

Working within the field of chiropractic means gaining an understanding of how we use our own muscles to instruct patients on how to use theirs. The combination of good posture and the use of proper body mechanics benefits members of the chiropractic team and the patients. This includes making the most efficient use of muscles, promoting optimal biomechanics, and avoiding strain and fatigue.

Posture is defined as body alignment; that is, the relative position of body parts standing, sitting, lying, or participating in any other type of activity. Posture also determines the distribution of body weight and the consequent pull on muscles and joints. It affects the size and shape of our body cavities, which, in turn, affect the position of the viscera. Circulation, respiration, digestion, and joint action are directly affected by posture. Body alignment favoring normal function and requiring the least strain is also reflected by good posture.

Body mechanics has to do with the coordinated use of our body parts to produce motion and maintain balance. The use of biomathematical efficiency promotes the efficient use of our muscles, and thus conserves energy. To understand the concept of body mechanics, you must also understand the principles which apply to any type of moving or lifting activity. These principles include:

- always face the direction of the movement.
- always use the large muscle groups of the legs, arms, and shoulders to lessen the strain on your back and lower abdominal muscles.
- always bring the object to be lifted or carried as close to your body as possible before lifting it; this keeps both centers of gravity close together.
- always bend the knees and keep the back straight when leaning over a work level.
- when kneeling on one knee, or squatting, always keep the back straight, especially when working at floor level.
- always push, pull, slide, or roll a heavy object on a surface to avoid unnecessary lifting.
- always obtain help and work in unison before attempting to move obviously unmanageable weight.

In order to avoid possible back strain, applying the principles of body mechanics will help to provide a safer, more efficient, and more comfortable means of moving and positioning patients who may not be able to assist themselves. Preparation for these procedures often includes the following:

- knowing what the patient can and cannot do, and then encouraging him or her to do what can be done.
- telling the patient exactly what is expected and what he or she can do to assist.
- obtaining necessary equipment and arranging it conveniently near the patient before you begin the movement.
- obtaining necessary assistance before trying to move a difficult or hard to manage patient.

Working in Orthopedics

Orthopedics is a specialty of medicine which includes the investigation, preservation, restoration, and developing for the form and function of the arms and legs, the spine, and associated structures by therapeutic means. The basis for your role in working with orthopedic patients has to do with understanding and applying the principles of biomechanics. However, while the application of these principles is a basic requirement in all health care, additional emphasis is needed for those of you who choose to work with orthopedic patients.

The challenge in caring for the orthopedic patient has to do with developing ways to carry out basic care while at the same time understanding and working with orthopedic mechanical devices, such as braces and traction devices used in aiding and treating the healing process of subluxations, joint disorders, muscle and nerve injuries, and other affections of the neuromusculoskeletal system. The injured part and associated structures must sometimes be immobilized, while at the same time circulation must also be maintained and muscles exercised in order to prevent atrophy.

The average orthopedic patient is a long-term case. Following a period of intensive treatment, he or she generally undergoes a period of supervised convalescence to insure optimum recovery. Often, the patient is expected to resent the necessary restriction imposed, and to become impatient or discouraged. Therefore, every orthopedic patient must be taught and encouraged to become as self-reliant as possible, while at the same time he or she must also understand the limits ordered by the doctor or chiropractor to insure healing and regaining optimal function.

The doctor of chiropractic is likely to encounter orthopedic conditions caused by subluxations, sprains, and strains of either a postural or traumatic nature. Besides injury to bones and joints, there are complicating factors to injury to muscles, tendons, blood vessels, and nerves. Degenerative diseases, congenital deformities, developmental defects, and post-disease or post-trauma paralysis and disorders often respond exceptionally well to chiropractic treatment.

Musculoskeletal and neurologic disorders often present similarities. Both can be long-term illnesses, both cause motion impairment, both require concern to prevent immobility complications, and both require the regaining of or compensation for musculoskeletal impairment or loss.

Innovative orthopedic devices are constantly being used in the field of chiropractic, and they are all directed toward two goals: providing support for the injured part until it heals and preventing deformity and stiffness of injured tissues. Support for an injured part is often provided by bandages, adhesive or elastic strapping, slings, splints, foam supports, braces, and casts.

To prevent stiffness, the patient should be encouraged to use the affected part as much as possible within the limits prescribed by the doctor. Rehabilitative physical therapy generally begins as soon as possible and may be continued for an extended period following the initial healing of the affected part. The patient may also need some type of mechanical support, such as a cane, crutches, sling, or brace for several weeks after he or she becomes ambulatory.

Pain, immobility, and changes in one's self-image can all result when the patient suffers from a musculoskeletal disorder, and becomes discouraged and depressed. Therefore, because of your frequent contact with the patient, it is essential that you be motivated and foster hope, always trying to exhibit a positive influence during periods in which the patient may be distressed. However, rehabilitation cannot be a haphazard process based on hope alone. Successful rehabilitation is not possible without the doctor's planning and scheduling. Therefore, you must be alert to assist the chiropractor in achieving the goal(s) of the patient's treatment plan. Often this involves being called upon to perform periodic muscle strength, joint motion, and neurovascular checks and to monitor traction setups to assure their correct application.

Assisting the Orthopedic Patient

As a professional member of the health care delivery team, it's important that you understand the need for patient confidence in your care. To the orthopedic or chiropractic patient, it's even more important, especially when it comes to helping the patient move about. You must always be safety conscious. When assisting, moving, or supporting a patient, especially one with an orthopedic disorder, you need to keep three things in mind. First, you must always remember to be gentle. Second, always remember to provide adequate support. And third, avoid sudden movements. Tell the patient ahead of time what is expected and how you are going to help. Handle the patient as carefully as you would want to be handled. Keep in mind those movements and positions contraindicated for a specific patient's complaint because adverse movements or positioning can easily produce unnecessary pain or tissue injury and thus interfere with the healing process. If you cause unnecessary or unexpected discomfort, it will be difficult to regain the patient's confidence.

Whenever you are required to help a disabled patient, always remember to offer your help on the affected side, since that is the side where you can best contribute your strength and stability.

Providing Patient Education

As an able-bodied and caring assistant, you can also be a good teacher who helps your patients to learn about their condition, treatment, and how they can most effectively cope during the recovery phase of their disorder. The chiropractic assistant can help the patient learn the correct use of equipment, exercises, procedures to be done at home, and other aspects of self-care. Of course, all of this must be done with the chiropractor's approval and under his or her supervision. Teaching duties may include helping the patient learn proper body alignment during bed rest, range-of-motion (ROM) exercises to maintain joint mobility and strengthen muscles, correct positioning of limbs to prevent deformities and complications, and instructions about personal hygiene and sanitation.

Caring for the Patient Experiencing Pain

Many of the patients you encounter in the chiropractic environment experience pain. And because many painful disorders are often chronic in nature, pain management must be carefully planned by the chiropractor. General measures used to reduce pain and inflammation associated with neuromuscular disorders include resting the affected joint or extremity, such as by bed rest or application of a brace; employing physical measures, such as moist heat, massage, or trigger-point therapy; therapeutic exercise; and professional therapy, such as manipulation, reflex techniques, meridian therapy, and muscle-relaxing procedures.

Severe musculoskeletal pain often causes the patient to be restless and change position frequently. The patient may also attempt to protect the anatomical region or affected part from which the pain arises by splinting the muscle. Muscle splinting is active, often involuntary muscle contraction that immobilizes the part. It differs from muscle spasm in that relaxation of the affected muscles occurs at rest. Prolonged pain in bone, muscle, tendons, and joints with resultant long-term muscle splinting may lead to eventual osteoporosis in affected and possibly adjacent bones. Joint contractures may also develop.

Disorders of the musculoskeletal system frequently feature associated muscle cramps or spasms. These are powerful involuntary muscular contractions which shorten the flexor muscles. The result is extreme, often incapacitating pain stimulated by ischemia or hypoxia of the muscle tissue. These spasms are generally associated with such chronic disorders as myositis, arthritis, and fibrositis.

Pain Fallacies

Since you will probably be involved in caring for patients experiencing pain, you should have a general understanding of the pain phenomenon. First, however, you must realize that there are three commonly held delusions regarding pain. First, it is a fallacy that all persons who are critically ill or gravely injured experience intense pain. Actually, people who are critically ill or who are gravely injured do not inevitably experience pain. Some do; others may not.

The second delusion about pain is that it is a fallacy to think that the greater the pain, the greater the amount of tissue damage. Intensity of pain is not directly proportional to the severity or extent of tissue damage.

Finally, it is a fallacy to think that pain is always symptomatic of an incurable illness. Pain is an important symptom that indicates treatment may be necessary, and most painful conditions are treatable and curable.

Components and Types of Pain

Generally speaking, there are three basic components to the sensation of pain. These include reception of the pain stimulus by pain receptors and conduction of the pain impulses by nerves; perception of pain in the higher brain centers; and reactions to pain such as physical, emotional, and psychologic responses. Pain is a complex mind-body experience which involves the total person rather than only the mind or solely the body. Indeed, the mental and physical experiences of pain are, as many of the early theologians and medicine men told us, inseparable.

There are many ways of identifying or explaining the various types of pain or severe discomfort. For example, pain is often referred to in terms of:

- *time of occurrence:* post-therapy pain.
- *duration or length of time experienced:* chronic or acute pain.
- *intensity:* mild or severe pain.
- *causative agent:* self-inflicted pain or spontaneous pain.
- *mode of transmission:* referred or projected pain.
- *ease of transmission:* inhibited or facilitated pain.
- *location:* superficial, deep, or central pain.
- *source:* sacroiliac pain or headache.
- *manner experienced:* sharp, dull, or burning pain.
- *general causation:* organic, psychologic, or pretended pain.

Classification of Pain

Pain syndromes are often classified into three major groups: superficial pain, deep pain, and central pain.

Superficial pain usually has a prickling or burning quality to it. This is often due to its sudden onset. It is relatively uncomplicated since it is directly perceived and can be readily and precisely localized. Associated symptoms often include hyperalgesia, paresthesia, analgesia, tickling, or itching. It may also be associated with brisk movements, a quick pulse, and a sense of invigoration. The quality of pain is generally a sharp sensation felt near the surface, and its duration is relatively short. Superficial pain is often experienced by the patient as a point, surface, or line.

Deep pain arises from structures far below the surface, and any one of three varieties may occur. The first is true visceral and deep somatic pain, which is felt at the point of noxious stimulation and which may or may not be associated with referred pain. Deep visceral pain arises from a diseased organ, while deep somatic pain is generally characterized by its segmental distribution and its origination from a lesion of vertebra, muscle, or other neuromuscular origin. The second is referred pain, which is pain experienced at a site other than the area of stimulus. It is pain projected from a viscus or other deep structure to the surface of the body. The third is pain from secondary skeletal muscle contractions, which causes pain from spreading excitation within the spinal cord.

Central pain is that for which no peripheral cause exists at the time the pain is perceived by the patient. Causalgias, phantom limb pains, and central pains are sometimes spoken of collectively as central pain syndromes, though their etiologies differ. Causalgia, which is caused by an injury to a peripheral nerve, is sometimes distinguished from central pain, often the result of lesions within the central nervous system that affect pain pathways. Causalgia, phantom limb pain, and central pain are all related because all three are autonomic reflex pain syndromes. The etiology of causalgia is usually a penetrating wound or injury damaging peripheral nerves where the wound or injury does not completely divide the nerves. Phantom limb pain often follows amputation of a limb.

Because a patient's pain has special meaning to him or her alone, the patient may expect that those providing care will intuitively understand his or her subjective view of the situation and respond appropriately. If your view of the pain fails to coincide with that of the patient's, a breakdown in communication occurs. Your response must consider the sociocultural, personality, and psychogenic factors involved.

There are several elements which join together and contribute to a patient's perception of the nature of their pain. Some of the general factors include the integrity of the patient's nervous system, the patient's state of consciousness, previous experiences, training, or conditioning of the patient, the patient's age and racial or ethnic background, and the patient's state of fatigue, debility, or lack of sleep.

When talking with the patient and taking his or her history, use that time to assess the nature of his or her pain. This assessment should record such items as the history of the origin and occurrence of pain; localization of the pain in the body; extension, radiation, and depth of pain; duration of pain; onset or pattern of the pain; and character or quality of the pain.

The chiropractor is fully aware that the cause of a patient's pain must be sought. Pain is a symptom, not a disease itself. However, accurate recording of the nature of a patient's pain is helpful to the chiropractor in seeking its cause. Keep in mind that a patient's description of pain is often influenced by his or her perception of that pain and what it means to him or her individually.

Assisting in Physical Examinations

A physical examination is made by the doctor of chiropractic on the patient's admission to his or her practice. It is the most valuable diagnostic procedure used by the chiropractic physician to obtain vital information regarding the functional and structural state of the patient, and the data gathered can be used by the doctor for a variety of purposes. Physical examinations are performed as a general health assessment measure whenever a person seeks health care attention for an illness or disorder, and are usually required for entry into most schools and for the issuance of insurance policies.

There are five major goals of a physical examination. First, it determines a person's level of health or physiologic function. Second, it helps the physician to arrive at a tentative diagnosis of a health problem or disease. Third, it is used to confirm a diagnosis of dysfunction or disease. The fourth goal is to provide an indication for examining specific body areas or systems for additional examination or testing. And the fifth goal is to provide a tool for evaluating the effectiveness of a prescribed procedure or therapy.

Role of the Chiropractic Assistant During the Physical Examination

Your responsibility as a chiropractic assistant is to assist both the doctor and the patient during the physical examination by obtaining firsthand information about the patient's condition that may be used in reinforcing the doctor's health care plan. In order to meet this responsibility, you must also understand that your role in the physical examination has a dual purpose. First, you should be both patient-oriented and doctor-oriented. This means being concerned with the psychological, social, and physiological needs and responses of the patient prior to, during, and after the examination. Also, your role is to enhance the doctor's efficiency by preparing the patient, providing the supplies and equipment needed, helping the doctor during the actual examination, and conducting some tests and measurements independently.

Whenever a female patient is being examined, a female assistant is expected to be present in the exam room at all times. If a male is being examined, a female assistant leaves the room during the examination of his genitals.

For most physicians, including doctors of chiropractic, there are five methods of examining patients. These include inspection, palpation, auscultation, percussion, and mensuration.

Inspection is the process by which observations of the patient's expression, habits, skin condition, posture, gait, body structure, and presence of scars or swelling are made. Internal surfaces of body openings are observed through instruments such as a speculum or scope. For example, an ophthalmoscope is used to view the posterior area of the eye, and an otoscope is used to view the eardrum.

Palpation is the diagnostic use of touch and feeling. Changes in bone surface quality and position, skin texture, superficial muscle, integrity, and normal body contours, and the detection of masses and enlarged organs not obvious by inspection are often perceived by palpation.

The process of listening for sounds which may indicate changes from the norm is called auscultation. Areas of sound production in the body include the heart, lungs, blood vessels, gastrointestinal tract, and the joints. The doctor may use his or her ears with or without the aid of a stethoscope.

Percussion means tapping body surfaces. This may be combined with auscultation and palpation to differentiate hollow air-containing structures from solid or fluid-containing structures. The doctor often uses a percussion hammer to test the patient's reflexes.

Mensuration means to measure the patient's height, weight, body dimensions, limb circumferences, vital signs, muscle strength, joint ROM, and blood pressure, all of which are common measurements included during a physical examination.

Duties of the Chiropractic Assistant During the Physical Examination

Many of the tasks required of the chiropractic assistant during the physical examination, have to do with preparing for and assisting the chiropractor with the exam. The most common of these include the following:

- assembling the equipment and supplies needed for the examination.
- checking the patient's records, and obtaining his or her cooperation.
- taking any physical or functional measurements of the patient which have been directed by the doctor and then recording the results in the patient's chart.
- preparing the patient for the exam; this often includes having the patient undress and put on an examination gown, positioning the patient on the examination table as required by the physician, and draping the patient to maintain his or her privacy.
- assisting the doctor during the examination, including handing him or her the appropriate equipment and supplies as they are needed.
- assisting the patient during the examination and giving reassurance and comfort.
- changing the patient's position for appropriate examinations.
- providing for the patient's comfort at the conclusion of the examination by removing the drapes, and assisting the patient in dressing, if needed.
- carrying out the doctor's orders for additional tests or examinations.
- collecting, cleaning, and returning used equipment and supplies, and disposing of and replacing all supplies used.

Various routine measurements are part of the patient's physical examination. However, your role and the degree to which you are required to take these measurements and perform specific tests and procedures will depend greatly on the chiropractic office, and the requirements of the chiropractic physician. Some of these measurements and procedures, such as obtaining laboratory specimens and recording an electrocardiogram, may require the skills of a trained medical assistant, while others, such as applying physical and therapeutic measures and taking X-rays, may be performed by the clinical chiropractic assistant.

Assisting the Chiropractor with a Spinal Examination

One area in which the chiropractor almost always requires the aid of a trained chiropractic assistant is in the performance of a spinal examination. In most cases, this particular exam also includes a postural and a spinal analysis. Thanks to the field of chiropractic, the inclusion of analyzing the patient's posture and structure of the spine has become an innovation in the field of physical diagnosing and examinations.

General considerations in the spinal analysis include the patient's body type, occupational and outdoor activities, past trauma, and gross mechanical disorders. Also considered is a detailed differential diagnosis of any mechanical lesions, the presence of pain and tenderness, joint and tissue mobility and locking, bone displacement or subluxation, muscle tone, soft tissue changes, skin changes, reflexes, and associated X-ray findings.

The examination of intervertebral segments include both active and passive tests. Active tests are active movements and axillary tests associated with active movements such as flexion, extension, rotation, and lateral bending. Axillary tests include joint-compression tests and evaluations for vertebral artery insufficiency. Passive tests include palpation, passive range of intervertebral movement, and movement of the pain-sensitive structures in the vertebral canal and intervertebral foramen. These findings are coordinated with other examination findings to arrive at a diagnosis.

Physiologic Therapeutics in Chiropractic

In many cases, the use of physiotherapeutic measures to facilitate the chiropractic adjustment is extremely valuable. These procedures offer the patient specific functional benefits, as well as help to reduce stiffness in joints, relieve tension, relax muscle spasm, enhance circulation, control pain, and excite lazy nerves and muscles.

Physical therapy techniques are used before and after the chiropractic adjustment to normalize function, as well as to prevent and minimize pain and deformities which may have resulted from trauma or disease. It may also be used to maintain what has been gained in the treatment. Superficial heat, cold, diathermy, microwave, ultrasound, meridian therapy, percussion, ultraviolet light, galvanic and sinusoidal currents, traction, hydrotherapy, and therapeutic massage and exercise are among the many common therapies used in chiropractic that may benefit the patient when properly applied.

Chiropractic physiotherapy can best be defined as the therapeutic application of forces and substances that help to induce a physiologic response and use, and thus allow for the body's natural processes to return to a more normal state of health. Physical therapy modalities do not cure a disease, but rather influence functional reactions.

Types of Physiologic Applications

While there are many different types of physiologic applications available to the medical practitioner, some are more common to the chiropractor than others. Those most frequently used in the chiropractic practice include therapeutic baths, cryotherapy, therapeutic exercises, heat, massage therapy, meridian therapy, microwave and ultrasonic diathermy, soft-tissue manipulation, traction, and ultrasound.

In addition to using physical therapeutic applications, oftentimes the chiropractor finds it necessary to use a mechanical support to help rest and protect a part during its healing process. Those most frequently used by the chiropractor include semiflexible knee supports, ankle wrap supports, tennis elbow elastic bandages, and foam cervical collars (Figure 14-1).

The Role of the Chiropractic Assistant in Physiologic Therapeutics

The chiropractic assistant is frequently directly involved and of special help to the chiropractic physician in applying a variety of apparatus and specialized equipment. As we have already discussed, while many forms and designs of equipment are available, only a few forms of application are used in most chiropractic offices. Often the types of applications available greatly depends on the doctor's experience and preference.

Once the chiropractor prescribes the type of therapy or treatment which is needed, he or she will call upon you to administer it under his or her direct supervision. The practitioner is well acquainted with the underlying fundamentals and physics to properly prescribe the appropriate modality, intensity, duration, and technique, as well as to effectively analyze procedures and evaluate treatment. Your responsibility is to make sure you are thoroughly aware and knowledgeable about the application technique, indications, and contraindications that may vary with a patient's age and condition, as well as his or her individual tolerance.

In a few states, the law may require that applications be performed only by a licensed physician or a registered physical therapist. However, even when the doctor begins the therapy, as an assistant you may be called upon to remain with the patient during the therapy and monitor the process. Therefore, as a professional member of the care-giving team, it's imperative that you understand that as a well-trained chiropractic assistant, you have a responsibility to become acquainted with each therapeutic modality within your office.

Caring for Physiotherapeutic Equipment

In addition to being responsible for administering physiotherapeutic applications, it is often customary for the clinical chiropractic assistant to see that all therapy equipment is clean and in good working order. Modalities and their attachments should be wiped clean after each use. Metal should shine, and wooden cabinets should be occasionally polished and frequently dusted. If an apparatus is not working properly, you should notify the doctor immediately. Likewise, any signs of wear, especially of electrical cords, should also be brought to the doctor's attention. Remember, cleanliness and good operating order are a priority when it comes to using therapeutic applications.

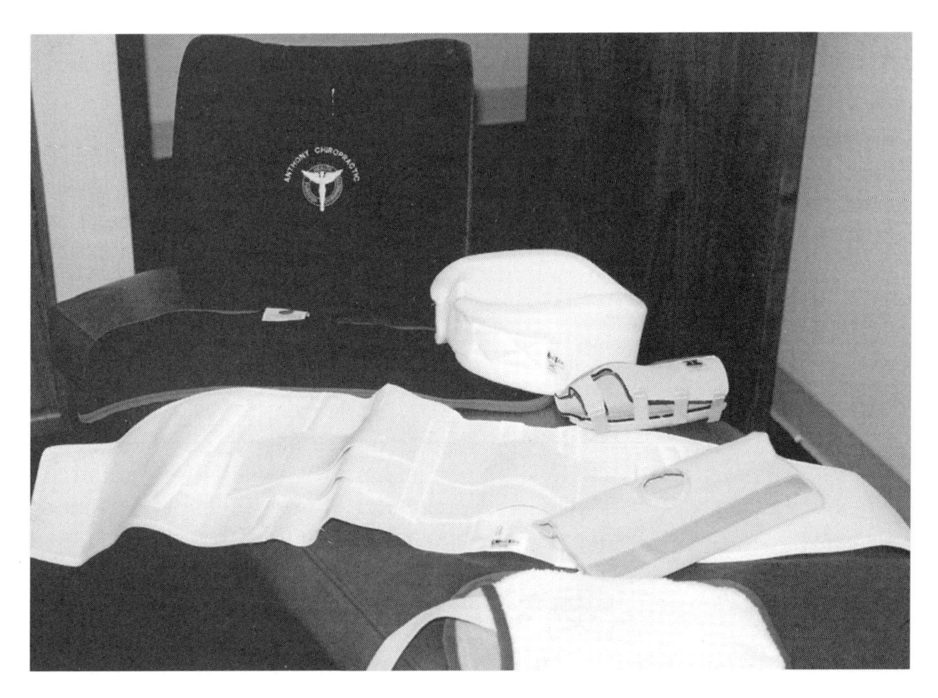

Figure 14-1
Types of physiotherapeutic supports.

Using Roentgenography in Chiropractic

The use of roentgenography, or X-ray therapy, has been a valuable diagnostic resource of the chiropractic profession since the early 1900s. When the doctor of chiropractic uses X-rays for diagnostic purposes, he or she is employing one of the most helpful tools of the health professions.

Diagnostic imaging enables the chiropractic physician to analyze bone integrity and structural balance. A patient's diagnosis is often based in part on roentgenographic findings corroborated by other tests. X-ray films can often reveal the cause, extent, and seriousness of many body ills and degenerative processes as well as traumatic effects. X-ray films are also readily capable of showing skeletal relationships and postural deficiencies.

The use of X-rays as an aid to diagnosing assists the chiropractor in correcting a patient's disorder or disability. At the same time, it also enables the chiropractor to offer the patient sound advice that can help avoid future illness or discomfort. As an aid for accurate diagnosing, X-ray films are studied by the doctor and used as a guide in development of a treatment plan. Accurate and early diagnosis of health problems assures a favorable opportunity for correction.

The Role of the Assistant in Chiropractic Radiology

While your role and responsibilities in chiropractic radiology may vary according to the individual state in which you are employed, in most states the assistant who works in a chiropractic X-ray department must have a general knowledge of anatomy to properly assist in taking films of most parts of the body. You should also be familiar with the principles of exposure and film processing. A chiropractor who is not a radiologist will prefer an assistant who has had training in X-ray technique, but few are available to meet the need. Therefore, most doctors will teach their assistant, within the realm of state laws, how to operate the equipment safely, how to develop films, and how to properly position the patient for those particular procedures necessary. The assistant must also learn the rules regarding protection from harmful exposure, preparation of the patient, and filing and record keeping of films and reports.

Basic Principles of Radiology

In radiology, the goal of the chiropractic assistant is to both ensure the safety of the patient and to provide the chiropractor with quality film production. To meet these goals, you must have a basic understanding of the principles of radiology. If you were to go into an established X-ray laboratory to study X-ray technology, you would learn these principles, and it wouldn't be too long before you could go through the mechanics of making a radiograph. You could get the film and patient ready, place the X-ray tube just so, operate the controls exactly as you had been shown, and develop, fix, wash, and dry the film. But that would not mean that you had become an X-ray technician, for radiography is much more than a series of procedures. It is a science and an art. It is a science in that it embodies the sciences of physics, geometry, and chemistry. It is an art in that it requires practice and experience to attain the desired skill.

Since the study of radiology is very involved and could not possibly be covered in a textbook of this size, for our purpose we will only discuss those areas which the chiropractic assistant should be most concerned with. Emphasis here will be on monitoring exposure absorption, patient safety and preparation, film information, common terms and designations, patient positioning routines, record keeping and filing, and film handling.

The most important principle that you must understand about X-ray production is that X-rays are like light in that they radiate in straight lines in all directions from the focal spot of the tube unless stopped by an efficient absorber. For that reason, an X-ray tube is enclosed in a lead housing that stops most of the X-radiation except useful rays, which are permitted to leave the tube through a window, often referred to as a primary beam. And to produce an X-ray image of lasting value, it must be properly recorded on specialized film, and then processed to provide a visible image.

Protecting the Patient from X-Radiation

Ionizing radiation, which includes X-rays, has been well documented for its potential harmful effects. Included are the influence on the thyroid gland, eyes, testes, ovaries, and fetus. Of these, an embryo and the reproductive organs are of special concern. It has been shown that certain aberrations to cellular structures are caused by excessive ionizing radiation.

The in utero embryo has shown extreme radiosensitivity, particularly within the first 8 to 12 weeks of pregnancy. As a result, it is absolutely necessary that the patient be questioned closely about the possibility of pregnancy. If the patient is pregnant or unsure on this point, find out from the ordering physician if the examination might not be delayed until such determination can be made. This is particularly so should the examination ordered expose the reproductive organs, that is, pelvis, sacrum, coccyx, spine, or lumbar, as part of the routine examination.

A radiograph is unnecessary unless the information gained by such an examination is useful in the total diagnosis of the patient's complaint. Only when a need is shown will the chiropractor order X-ray examination. Careless or needless exposure of a patient to the potentially harmful effects of ionizing radiation is both morally and professionally unethical.

Protecting the Male Patient

In the male patient, protection of the male reproductive organs by lead shielding is always recommended. This is so the male can be protected against any aberration or deviation of the spermatozoa. The extreme radiosensitivity of the testes demands their protection at all ages, whenever possible. This is typically accomplished with a gonad shield, which is a cup-like protective device that surrounds the entire gonads. Placement of the shield is best made by using briefs or underwear specifically designed for holding the shield. In this manner, once the shield is in place, it will afford complete protection in all views, regardless of the position of the patient. The importance of this device is so well documented that in many states its availability for use by the patient, if requested, is mandatory.

Protecting the Female Patient

Unlike the male patient, with females there are no specific measures available for protection. Due to the deeper anatomical location of the ovaries and uterus, even when adequately protected by placing lead directly over the organs, scatter and secondary radiation can still find their way to these structures. While attenuation of the ionizing radiation can be reduced in the male by upwards of 95 percent through the use of gonad shielding, it is estimated that only about 35 percent can be achieved in the female. These figures are applicable when the reproductive organs are in the direct field of exposure.

The problem of protection in the female is not only the anatomical location of the organs. To protect these structures completely, the attenuating device would also obscure the anatomical structures that prompted the need for the radiograph in the first place. Thus, to adequately shield often means the loss of information sought for diagnosis. Therefore, the chiropractor is often faced with seeking a compromise between a clinical need for the X-ray and the patient's absolute safety.

Protecting Yourself and Others

As important as the safety of the patient is, so is the accurate and detailed radiation exposure level toward yourself and other members of the department. It is common knowledge that all people are exposed daily to minute amounts of radiation through the earth's atmosphere or as it is commonly known, background radiation. While in itself not a hazard to health, it becomes more important to people who work with or around other sources of radiation. Radiation has an accumulating biologic effect.

Both federal and state laws require protection for those working with radiation to be monitored for any detectable amounts of exposure received on the job. Most health care facilities meet this requirement by providing their employees with badges to monitor exposure. These badges are provided in many forms, such as clip-ons, pins, or rings. And each is always worn when working in, with, or near the X-ray room. Monthly determination of exposure is afforded so any failure of safe procedures becomes immediately known. Most badges measure primary, secondary, and scatter radiation, despite origin.

Preparing the Patient for X-Ray

Diagnostic roentgenography in the chiropractic office, for the most part, is often confined to examination of the osseous structures, particularly of the spine, with chest examinations the second priority. Some more sophisticated procedures such as gastrointestinal and urological examinations are generally confined to those practices which employ a Diplomat of the American Chiropractic Board of Roentgenology.

For most X-ray examinations in the chiropractic office, your role in preparing the patient will be mostly concerned with gathering and recording the patient's name, age, and sex, assisting the patient to properly disrobe for the examination, providing both physical and emotional support by explaining what is going to take place, and assisting the patient in the proper positioning for a specific X-ray examination.

Obtaining Patient Information

Each radiograph must have specific information permanently affixed to it to meet medicolegal requirements concerning identification of the patient and where the radiograph was taken. The doctor's name or that of the facility where the procedure was performed is also necessary. The patient's name or case history number and the date of the exposure are also essential. For females, the inclusion of the age and date of the last menses (DLMP) is also highly recommended.

There are two methods of patient film identification. The first is by using lead letters and characters which are held in place by a master letter holder. The lead letter holder usually has the doctor's or facility's name and location preset, and merely the addition of the patient's name, age, case number, and DLMP are needed. This is done by handloading the master holder with the appropriate letters and numbers into the channels provided. As the characters are lead, they will attenuate the X-rays, and the finished film will show all information which has been fed into the holder.

The second method of patient film identification is by using a semiautomatic card imprinter (Figure 14-2). A card imprinter is a device that allows light, set from a switch, to pass through a card with information typed or written on it that is then transferred directly to a pre-exposed film. The pre-exposed film requires that a lead blocker of the same size used by the card imprinter be placed in the cassette to prevent that portion of the film from being exposed. This portion of film will then be exposed by the light emitted from the card imprinter.

Identifying the X-Rayed Part and Position

In addition to identifying whose image is being X-rayed, it will also be necessary for you to identify what part of the patient is being visualized on the finished film. This information is essential, oftentimes even critical, to ensure for proper film interpretation by the chiropractor. A cardinal rule is to always mark the part closest to the film, and be certain that all designations such as right and left are referring to the patient's right or left.

Every film must have at least the designation of the patient's right or left. Other designations, such as LPO, LAO, RPO, or RAO should be used when patient oblique views are taken. The film is marked by placement of the appropriate marker on the cassette before exposure. These characters can be taped to the cassette with adhesive tape and then be removed prior to reloading or reusing the cassette. Remember, each film must show the patient's right or left, and on oblique views, what part is closest to the film at the time of exposure (Figure 14-3).

Positioning the Patient

When positioning the patient for a specific type of X-ray, there are three general factors which must be considered, and which may vary according to the preference of the doctor and the limitation of the equipment. The first is the use of an upright or recumbent position. The second is the focal-film distance and/or central ray angle used. And the third is the film size.

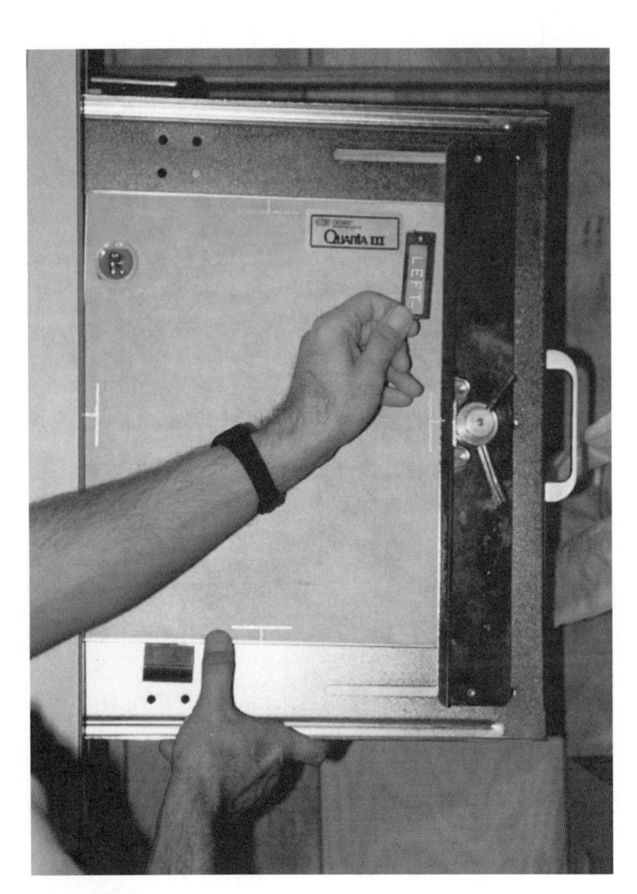

Figure 14-2
Photographic method of imprinting data.

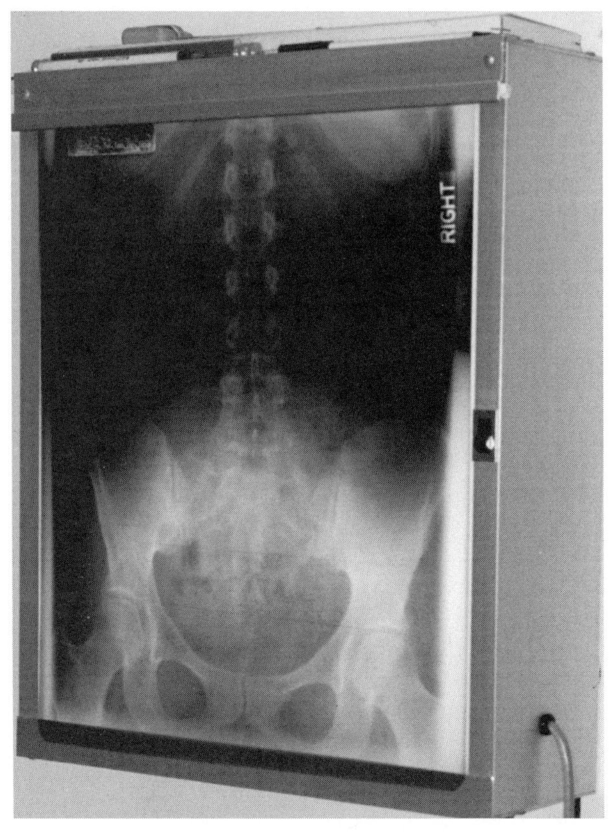

Figure 14-3
Radiograph showing proper identification and markings.

The minimum film focal distance (FFD), or the source image distance (SID), of 72 inches should be used along with an upright position for chest films, lateral cervical films, and, under most circumstances, oblique cervicals. Full spine films should use no less than a 72-inch distance; however, in most cases, 84 inches is recommended. An acceptable film focal distance for recumbent films and for most upright studies except those specified otherwise is 40 inches. Variation to a longer distance than this is acceptable, but less than 40 inches should only be used for specific reasons, such as a magnification technique.

Film size, as we have already stated, is another important factor. Good radiological practice mandates that only those areas showing clinical necessity should be exposed to X-rays. In addition to that, the smaller the film size and the tighter the collimation, the sharper the radiographic detail and the less there is scatter radiation. This will lower patient dose and decrease scatter fog to the film. It is therefore recommended that the smallest film size compatible with clinical needs be used. The X-ray beam should be centered over the area to be exposed.

Film Handling and Processing

X-ray film is highly sensitive, especially to light, heat, moisture, and some gases. It is also easily damaged, and because of the delicate chemically-coated surfaces of X-ray film, unless it is handled properly, it can easily be marred.

Film Packaging and Storage

Protection of X-ray film begins in the factory where it is manufactured and where its packaging is rigidly controlled. After the film is enclosed in individual paper folders, each lot of 25, 75, or 100 sheets is inserted into a moisture-proof container that is hermetically sealed and then boxed. The paper folder protects the film from any possibility of abrasion during shipment as well as during its removal from the box. The sealed inner container provides additional protection against any moisture and fumes. As long as the seal has not been broken, the film retains its ideal moisture content.

Once you have received the film from the factory, you should pay special attention to the way it needs to be stored in the office. Film should always be kept in a cool place that is well protected from radiation. The supply should also be adequate, yet small enough to provide a reasonably rapid turnover of stock. This is necessary to ensure its freshness. Proper turnover is easily controlled because each package of film is dated. Always remember to use the oldest film first.

Handling Film Prior to Exposure

There are several types of film manufactured for X-ray use. The choice often depends on the part to be examined, the type of equipment which is used, and its capacity. Despite type, X-ray film must be handled carefully to avoid physical strains due to pressure, creasing, buckling, and friction (Figure 14-4 on p. 134). Never draw film rapidly from cartons, exposure holders, or cassettes, or handle it in any manner that would produce static electric discharges. And when removing the film from a carton, always remember that the paper wrapper should be withdrawn with it to protect the film surface from any possible abrasion.

Use of Film Containers and Cassettes

There are two types of containers in which sheet films are held during exposure. The first, which is called a cassette, houses a pair of intensifying screens between which the sheet of film is placed. When holding a cassette, you must place the film without its inter-leaving wrapper in the cassette on the front screen (Figure 14-5 on p. 135). Always handle the film between your thumb and one finger. This will prevent the film from kicking. Close the lid carrying the other screen gently, and then lock it with the back springs.

The second container which is used to hold film during its exposure is called an exposure holder. It is a hinged cardboard folder which contains a light-tight envelope to enclose the film for direct exposure techniques.

Processing Exposed Film

Processing exposed film consists of developing, stop bath, rinsing, fixing, and washing. While a few years ago this was considered to be a very tedious, smelly chore, in which the assistant was cramped into a small darkroom working over large tanks of chemical solutions, today most offices use automated temperature-controlled units for film processing and drying. Past problems with film fog, preparing and maintaining developer, rinse, and fixer solutions, and visually determining development have been virtually eliminated through technological advances.

Protection of the Skin

Because anyone can become sensitized to processing solutions, contact with these solutions and chemicals should be kept at an absolute minimum. Avoid getting developer solution on your skin. And if your fingers happen to be occasionally dampened, remove the solution immediately by rinsing your hands in a stop bath solution. Rinse them again with tap water and then dry them off as quickly as possible. If your office uses cloth hand towels, they should

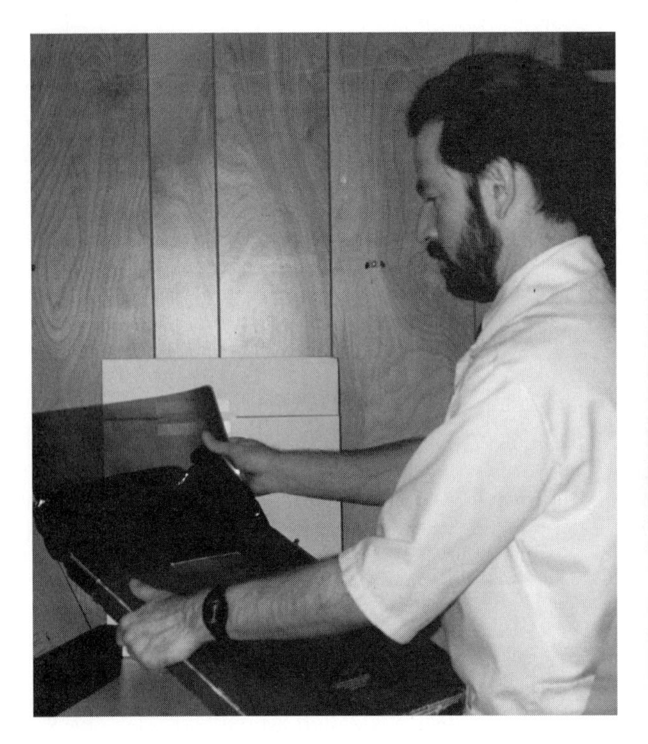

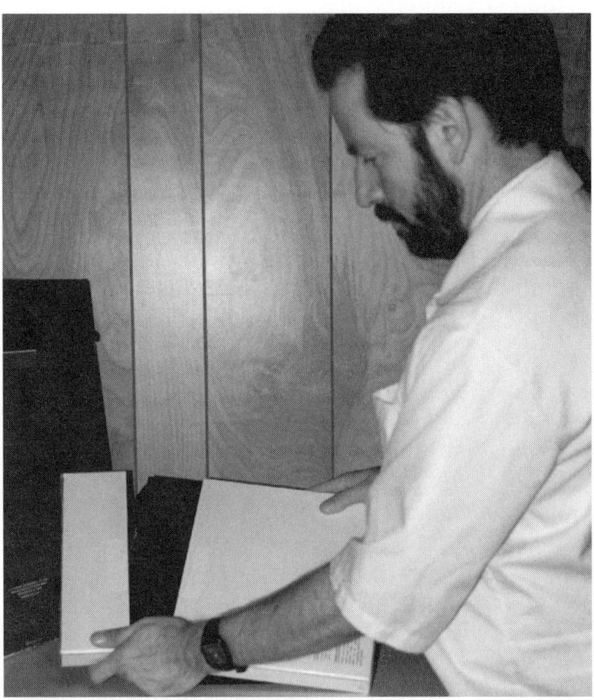

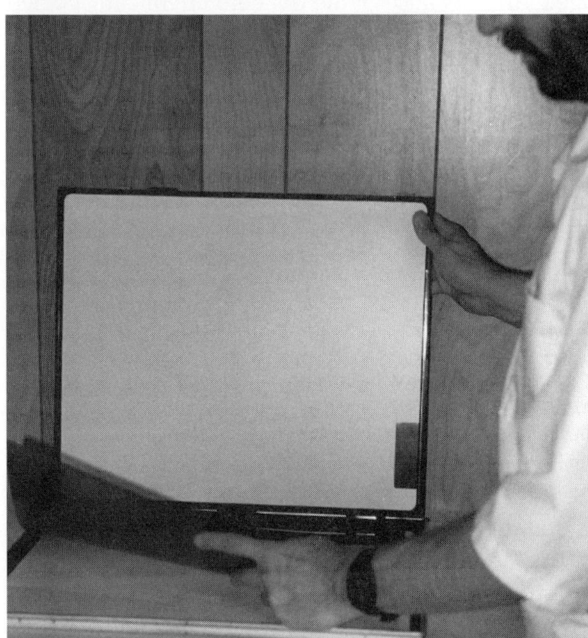

Figure 14-4
Removing film from its packaging.

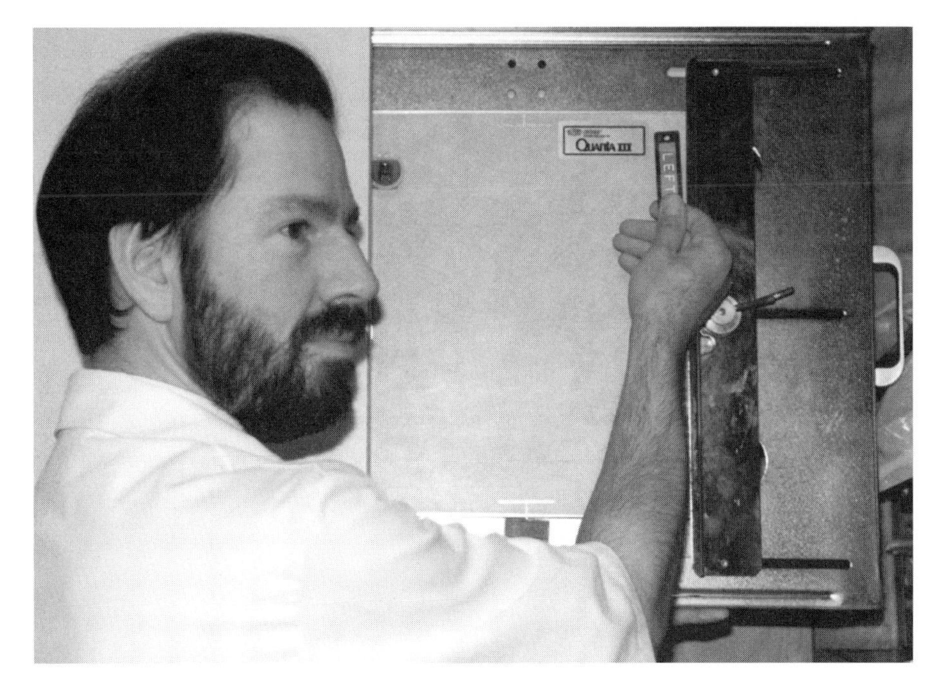

Figure 14-5
Loading the film cassette.

be changed frequently to avoid them from becoming contaminated with chemicals and accidentally transferring them to the skin.

If your skin happens to become stained with developer, a helpful remedy is the application of a potassium permanganate solution, followed by a rinse, first in sodium bisulfate solution, and then in warm tap water. The first solution consists of one-quarter ounce of potassium permanganate dissolved in 32 ounces of water. The second is made of 10 ounces of sodium bisulfate which is dissolved into 32 ounces of water. Both solutions should be kept in labeled bottles ready for use when needed.

Summary

In this chapter, we discussed both the basic and the typical functions of the clinical chiropractic assistant. We identified the various clinical procedures performed in the chiropractic office, as well as the role of the chiropractic assistant in aiding with these procedures. We also talked about those tasks which were most frequently encountered by the clinical CA, such as assisting in physical therapeutics and radiology, and identified and briefly discussed some of the more advanced functions of the person in the capacity of a clinical chiropractic assistant

Review Questions

1. Briefly explain the difference between *signs* and *symptoms.*
2. A ______________ disease is one which is continuous or recurrent.
3. What does the abbreviation *RAO* mean?
4. What does the abbreviation *RPO* mean?
5. What is the name of the study that deals with the coordinated use of body parts in order to produce motion and maintain balance?
6. What does the abbreviation *AP* mean?
7. What does the abbreviation *PA* mean?
8. What is the name of the study that deals with the therapeutic application of forces and substances that induce a physiologic response, thus allowing the body's natural processes to return to a more normal state of health?

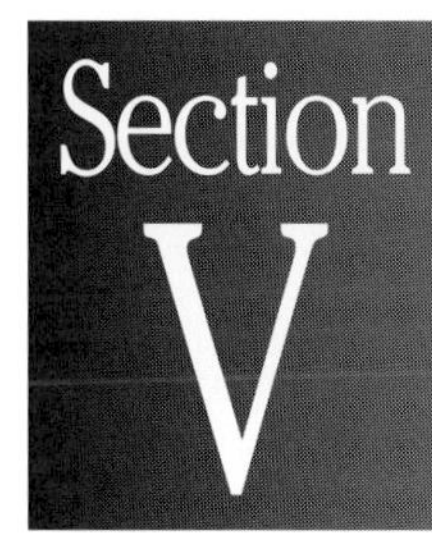

Massage Therapy: Basic Concepts and Applications

15

Introduction to Massage Therapy

Performance Objectives

Upon completion of this chapter, you will be able to:

1. Briefly discuss the history of massage and its usefulness as a therapeutic modality.
2. Identify individual forms of massage and their relationship to helping the main body systems.
3. Explain the purpose and function of aromatherapy.
4. Explain the purpose of using oils for massage and briefly define the properties of essential oils.
5. Briefly explain the types of touch used in massage therapy.
6. Discuss how the massage therapist prepares for a therapeutic session.

Terms and Abbreviations

Centering a way in which one focuses by gathering energy into a point so that one can channel it more easily into any activity one chooses.

Effleurage a gentle rhythmical massage stroke used all over the body.

Hara a Japanese word which means belly or abdomen, and which refers to the source of vital energy and strength in the lower abdomen, more precisely, to a point a few inches below the naval called the Tan-Den.

Homeostasis the physical balance and equilibrium of the body.

Petrissage a type of massage stroke in which kneading, wringing, and rubbing are used.

Massage has been used as a therapeutic modality throughout history, both as a form of relaxation and as a treatment for enhancing one's beauty. It was particularly popular with the ancient Romans, who used base oils mixed with essential oils and herbs to regenerate and beautify the skin, especially the skin of the face. For them, it was a real treat to spend all day at the Roman baths, indulging themselves with hot vapors, swimming, and then being massaged with aromatic ointments.

After the fall of the Roman empire, the Western world adopted a more righteous view of life, and any so-called pampering of the body was viewed as sinful. As a result, massage, both as a form of relaxation and as a form of medicine, was ostracized. It remained that way for many centuries. In Europe, it was not until the end of the eighteenth century that the relaxing and therapeutic effects of massage witnessed a true revival.

The Art of Massage

The art of massage is as ancient as touch itself. Both humans and animals have always been endowed with the intuitive knowledge that stroking and caressing with a caring, loving attitude brings comfort, relaxation, and a general sense of well-being. In our scientifically minded age, studies have overwhelmingly confirmed that a loving touch can also relieve pain, soothe sorrows, promote health, and ensure the growth and development of healthy, happy offspring, for both humans and animals.

The essence of massage is a loving, caring touch, and whether it is applied in a family, between friends, or in a therapeutic environment, it has become a structured part of the healing arts. Massage also brings people together. Where there is conflict and misunderstanding, it calms tensions and creates unity by engendering feelings of closeness and tenderness.

How Massage Helps the Body

A good massage affects you on all levels of your being. Physically, its benefits include relaxation and toning your muscles; assisting the venous flow and oxygenation of the blood; and stretching the connective tissue of joints. On a mental level, massage not only relieves stress and anxiety, but it also helps you to become more conscious of your body as a whole, of the parts that you are in touch with and those that you may feel "cut off" from. Once you are aware of where your own energy blocks lie, you can begin to integrate your body, and, in developing a more positive self-image, take responsibility for your own happiness and health.

A caring massage creates feelings of well-being, trust, and joy. It can also release a great deal of energy which was previously wasted in tension, and by transforming chronic habits of acting and reacting, can effect a profound change on posture and facial expression. The emotional aspect of massage is all-important.

On a spiritual level, the benefits of massage are hard to describe, for we are talking of something that is intrinsically indefinable, the very essence, the life force, the whole that is more than the sum of its parts. But it is not uncommon during a massage session for both the giver and the receiver to attain a state of heightened awareness, of a presence in the moment, that is akin to the experience of meditation.

Affects of Massage on Individual Body Systems

Our nervous system operates like a vast electrical network which, along with the endocrine system, interconnects and harmonizes all the individual parts of our body. Our blood pressure, the rate at which we breathe, and how our food is digested are all directed by our brain, which, in turn, transmits signals through nerve pathways in order to keep our body in balance. The nervous system also regulates the relationship with the external environment by relating information to the brain through our five senses—sight, hearing, taste, smell, and touch—and then receiving instructions on how to act.

Massage and bodywork, with their great variety of healing strokes, can be very effective in balancing the nervous system and restoring *homeostasis.* The skin and muscles contain many nerve endings and connections, and the soothing, balancing, and healing touch of massage is relayed by them to every part of the body, which in turn brings relief and promotes a sense of well-being.

By contracting and extending, the skeletal muscles create movements in various parts of our body. They can, however, become painful and contracted with spasms and abnormal tissue. In certain conditions, they can waste away, and become weak and flaccid. Such conditions can make some movements difficult, painful, or in some cases even impossible.

Massage can be used to stretch and regenerate the muscles, restoring them to a state of normal elasticity and strength. People involved in sports, for example, can benefit greatly from massage treatment. And so can everyone else: the young, to grow up with healthy muscles; and the old, to avoid weakness and the wasting away of muscle.

Freeing the Body and Improving Circulation

All bone movements occur at joints, as in the shoulder, neck, hip, knee, and spine. Many schools of healing, such as yoga in the East and osteopathy in the West, believe that long-lasting youth and good health depend greatly on the flexibility of our joints. Massage techniques and bodywork concentrate on releasing the joints and thus contribute to keeping our bodies upright, agile, and as free as possible from arthritic conditions.

Most nerves, arteries, and veins pass through the joints and muscles and, as a result, abnormalities and restrictions within the muscular and skeletal system can drastically hamper the healthy functioning of our body's metabolism. The vagus nerve, for example, which originates in your skull, passes into the neck from an area which is located at the base of the skull and the first cervical vertebrae. Muscular and joint restrictions around this area can disturb the vagus nerve, which in turn can contribute to the dysfunction and deregulation of a wide range of organs and functions, such as the pharynx and most of the organs of both the thoracic and abdominal cavities. When obstructed, it can also disrupt some of the vital functions involved in breathing and respiration. This example is a good illustration of how massage work on our neck can improve our respiration and digestive process.

Massage can also improve the body's circulation by exerting a beneficial pumping action on the circulatory system. It does this by gently squeezing and then releasing the muscles and circulatory vessels that pass through it. This improves blood circulation by favoring the exchange, at a cellular level, of fresh nutrient-filled blood, to blood that is carrying toxins away from the cells.

It works in the same way on the lymphatic system by favoring the passage of lymph fluid into the bloodstream and thus promoting detoxification. In this way, massage exerts an important influence on the regenerative and cleansing capabilities of our body.

Forms of Therapy

Because of the major improvements in global communication and international travel, we have all become more and more attracted to one another's cultures and ways of life. This interest has encompassed most spheres of human life. At first it seemed that it was mainly the West which was exporting its unique ways abroad and from the early 1920s the whole world seemed to adopt the Western ways of medical science. In recent years, however, there has been a dramatic change.

The West has discovered aspects of Eastern traditions that have greatly improved our quality of life, physically, emotionally, and spiritually. Acupuncture, shiatsu, Chinese herbal medicine, yoga, and many other healing traditions are now part of our awareness and way of life, and we have all benefited from this very integrated vision.

When this realization is applied to massage and bodywork, it contributes a great deal to broadening and improving the scope and efficiency of manual therapy. For example, Western forms of bodywork are good for working with the body in an anatomical and muscular way, while Eastern forms are good for working at a more vital energetic level. Used together, they compliment one another, and thus improve health and our sense of well-being.

Swedish Therapy

Swedish therapy, considered by most massage therapists to be the forerunner of all massage and bodywork therapies, was first developed in Sweden by Henrik Ling. A devoted and enthusiastic massage therapist who dedicated his life to the development and acceptance of this healing, Ling realized that it was advisable for the person giving the massage to have a certain knowledge of anatomy and physiology. With this aim in mind, Ling created training centers which taught Swedish massage and exercise. He introduced, among others, such terms as *effleurage* (Figure 15-1 on p. 142), which is a gentle rhythmic stroking used everywhere on the body to improve one's circulation, and *petrissage,* which is a type of kneading, wringing, and rubbing used to squeeze toxins and tensions out of the body's muscles.

The main goal of Ling's method, which was based upon many ancient traditional massage practices combining therapeutic massage with exercises for muscles and joints, was to improve circulation, manipulate joints, and stretch and release muscles throughout the body to create a variety of beneficial effects. Since the nineteenth century, Swedish massage, combined with the use of base oils and their life-enhancing qualities, has become increasingly popular both in Europe and in the West.

Eastern Massage Therapy

In order to best explain the Eastern forms of massage therapy, such as acupressure and shiatsu, let's first review some of the information covered in our discussion of the basic concepts of Chinese medicine which we talked about earlier in this textbook. To begin with, as you recall, in the East, medicine is part of an all-encompassing philosophical and religious vision of one's life. The universe is viewed as a unity where opposites complement one another and always seek a level of harmony. Disease occurs only when this harmony is broken. Western thought, however, differs from Eastern philosophy, in that it has had a tendency to separate the material from the spiritual levels.

Qi, as you recall, is the subtle and vital force of energy so often referred to in oriental therapy, that runs through our body in meridians. These are clearly defined channels which are connected to, and influenced by major organs of the body. When the vital Qi force flows freely, there is health and well-being; when the flow of Qi is disrupted, there is a blockage leading to problems.

Meridians are best seen as flowing rivers where, at certain key points, the current and power of the river is stronger and even visible from the surface. These points along the meridians of the human body are defined as acupoints. Through these points, which are used in acupressure, acupuncture, and shiatsu, the energy can be contacted in order to maintain or to restore a life-and-health enhancing flow.

Osteopathic Therapy

Osteopathy is a therapeutic method which uses physical manipulation of joints and bodywork. First introduced into the United States in the later part of 1870 by Dr. Andrew Still, osteopathy, which follows principles that have actually been around for cen-

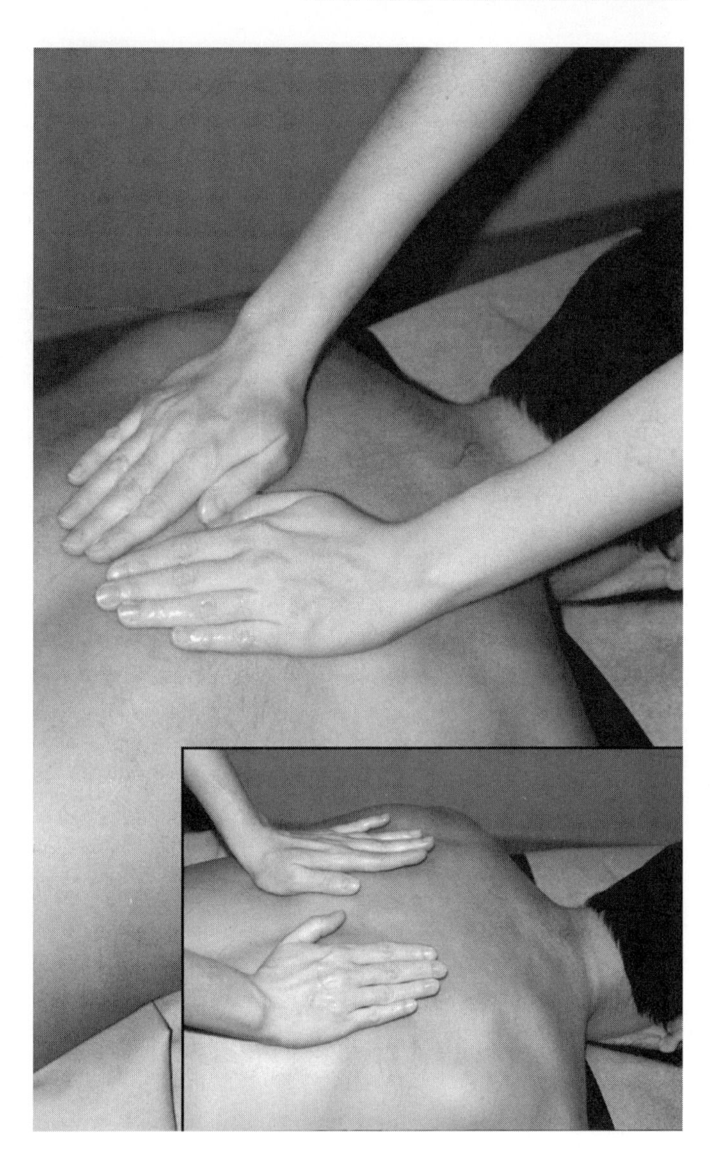

Figure 15-1
Using effleurage techniques.

turies, has only recently become a widely practiced part of the medical mainstream.

Dr. Still perceived that most health problems arose when part of the body's main frame structure of bones, joints, muscles, and ligaments got out of alignment, and that manipulation could bring about release, restore mobility, eliminate congestion, and ultimately, dramatically improve health-related problems. For example, when a joint is impaired and/or deviates from the norm, arteries and nerves can become pinched and obstructed, and thus give rise to trouble. Freeing the joints through manual manipulation results in better circulation and enables the various body structures and organs that were formerly starved of fresh blood to regenerate themselves and thrive again (Figure 15-2). Muscle agility and lymphatic drainage can also be improved in this way.

Chiropractors are somewhat similar to osteopaths, in that they generally treat a wide range of disorders through the manipulation of joints, muscles, and especially the spine. Chiropractors, however, make much greater use of X-rays and conventional diagnostic techniques than do osteopaths.

Osteopathy is best known as an effective system for treating problems of the musculoskeletal structure, such as back pain, and many modern osteopaths tend to concentrate their energies on manipulating and freeing spinal column restrictions.

While Dr. Still concentrated on safe ways to stretch and mobilize the musculoskeletal system, many of his followers later turned toward techniques involving high velocity. These techniques, which have since come to be known as cracking, can be very effective in freeing joint restrictions.

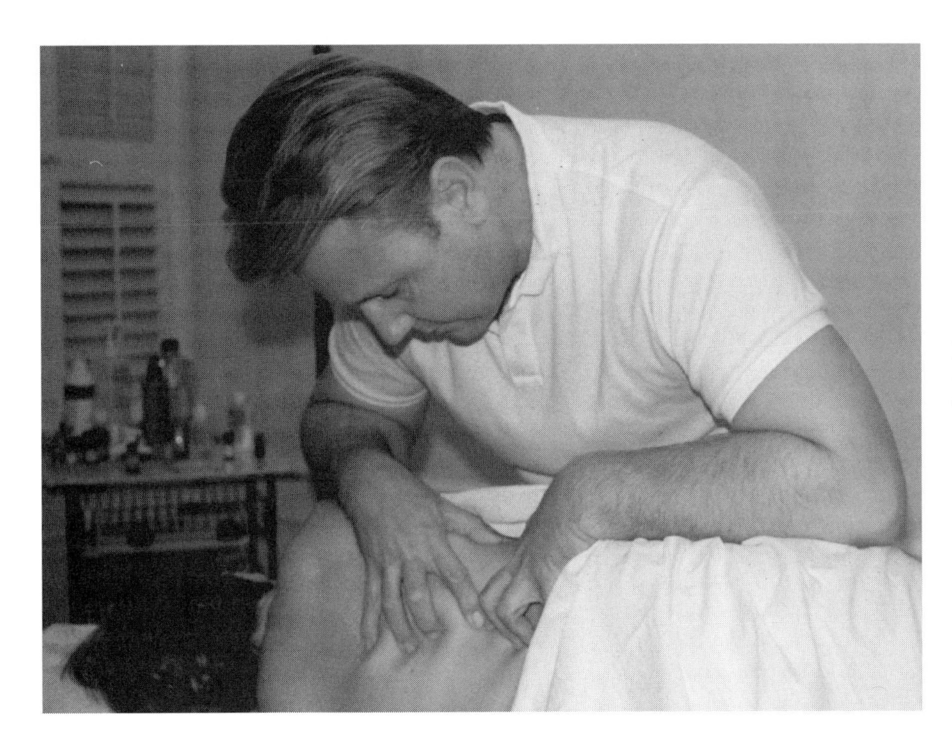

Figure 15-2
Using osteopathic techniques.

Neuromuscular Massage Therapy

Neuromuscular massage, which concentrates on releasing muscular contraction and tension, was first developed by Stanley Lief. Lief, who was a chiropractor and naturopath, took this approach to treating illnesses by combining bodywork techniques and natural cures. Ultimately, this form of massage gained its largest following in England.

Neuromuscular techniques tend to use friction and pressure techniques which are often applied with the thumbs. The technique can be applied to most muscular areas of the body; however, it is most frequently used to free rib restrictions. Working, for example, on the intercostal muscles increases respiratory capability and thus improves lung function. If the lungs are restricted, they will not be able to expand properly in order to fill with the cleansing and revitalizing oxygen that is so essential to the health of the body. Thus, a chain reaction is caused which prevents the lungs from fully eliminating carbon dioxide.

Aromatherapy

There are many types of plants, flowers, and wood resins which contain volatile aromatic oils. These are referred to as essential oils. By volatile, we are talking about an oil that quickly evaporates on contact with air, in contrast to one which is fatty, meaning that it sinks in and remains in the place that it penetrates.

The essential oil in a plant gives it a unique fragrance or personality. While research into understanding the function of these volatile oils is still under way, we do know that one of their main functions is defensive. With their many highly antiseptic properties, they are able to repel harmful germs and insects which might endanger the survival of the plant. Laboratory experiments have also shown scientists how essential oils are capable of killing certain bacteria. This makes the oils useful in fighting skin infections, grazes, and cuts and lacerations. They have also been used throughout the ages in creams and perfumes.

Some essential oils, which are added to a base oil (Figure 15-3 on p. 144) for massage, have antibacterial qualities that preserve skin tissue and thus are able to block the spread of infection. Some, such as lavender, also have an analgesic action, which are helpful and are often used to reduce pain.

Properties of Oils Used in Aromatherapy

Because essential oils are used as an adjunct to healing in massage therapy, it's important that you have a basic understanding of some of the most frequently used oils. The following information provides a brief description of the healing properties of these oils, and what they are generally used for.

- *Aniseed:* acts as a sedative on the nervous system, and also aids in digestion, relieving flatulence, and in nervous indigestion; it also calms coughing spasms and helps in expectoration.
- *Benzoin:* improves the respiratory system by aiding expectoration, while at the same time calms coughing spasms; also useful for flu-like symptoms, colds, and sore throats.

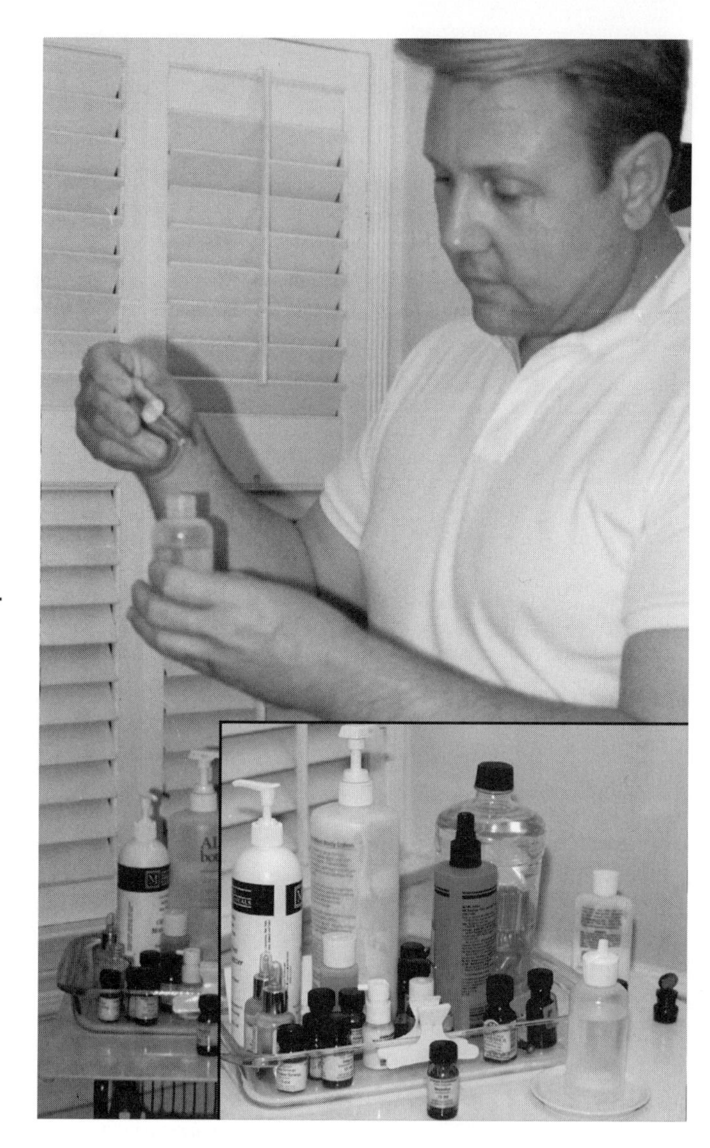

Figure 15-3
Adding an essential oil to a base oil.

- *Bergamot:* benefits the nervous system by acting as an antidepressant; may also be diluted as a douche to treat urinary and vaginal infections.
- *Chamomile:* has a marked effect on the nervous and digestive systems, particularly when indigested because of stress and worry; may also be used as a good remedy for pain and as a useful anti-inflammatory agent; often used for skin irritations which are characterized by redness, and for restlessness and insomnia.
- *Clary sage:* because of its pronounced action on the respiratory and nervous systems, this oil is often used on people who have a weak chest, tire easily, and suffer from shortness of breath.
- *Cypress:* mainly used to improve the functioning of the circulatory system; strengthens the valves of the veins, helps in conditions such as varicose veins, and promotes the flow of blood throughout the body.
- *Eucalyptus:* most frequently used for respiratory problems and infections, such as colds and flu, where mucus is present, and in bronchitis.
- *Fennel:* used primarily for improving digestion by alleviating flatulence, abdominal swelling, and discomfort; also helpful in relieving constipation and irritable bowel syndrome, and considered to be a good diuretic.
- *Geranium:* promotes relaxation, while leaving the person alert and fresh; also useful as an excellent anti-inflammatory oil, and in helping skin conditions characterized by redness and dryness, and as a mild astringent.
- *Ginger:* used to warm the body and mind, and recommended for people who suffer from cold symptoms; also used to treat poor circulation, and for coughs and bronchitis.
- *Jasmine:* enlivens the heart, opens the chest and lifts depression; increases vitality without

overheating the system, and, at the same time, encourages joy and enthusiasm.

- *Lavender:* considered one of the most popular oils, because of its multi-usefulness; used to regulate the nervous system, acting as a sedative for anxiety, insomnia, and hysteria; also calms pain and often used for complaints such as neuritis and neuralgia associated with sciatica; may be used as a disinfectant to help heal cuts, bruises, abrasions, skin irritations, and bee stings; improves circulation and muscle cramps.
- *Mandarin peel:* decongests the liver, and is useful for pain and discomfort in the right flank accompanied by a bitter taste in the mouth; also helps in digestion, alleviating flatulence and belching; has a mild astringent quality, and as such is helpful in alleviating diarrhea.
- *Marjoram:* highly regarded for its action on the respiratory and nervous systems because of its ability to combine tonic and calming actions; used to increase stamina while calming tension; also soothes coughing spasms, strengthens the lungs, and promotes expectoration; may be used for treating muscular aches and pains associated with arthritis.
- *Neroli:* considered one of the best calming and relaxing oils that can be used without sedating or creating drowsiness; generally recommended for insomnia, anxiety, and alleviating stress.
- *Orange peel:* helps to regulate liver functioning and good for digestion, especially when abdominal discomfort is accompanied by constipation; also has a calming effect without acting as a sedative.
- *Peppermint:* acts primarily on the digestive system by stimulating the digestive processes; also alleviates flatulence, belching, and abdominal swelling; provides the body with a stimulating and refreshing effect; also widely used for colds and flu.
- *Rose:* relaxes, creates trust, and opens the heart to love; also helps irregular and painful menstruation; anti-inflammatory and astringent properties make it useful in ridding skin problems; may be used to alleviate anxiety and encourage relaxation and cheerfulness.
- *Rosemary:* stimulates poor circulation and weak blood flow to the brain, and often used to alleviate poor memory and low concentration; also stimulates the liver and increases appetite; may be used to treat people who suffer from colds, lethargy, and arthritis made worse by cold weather; should never be used on people suffering from hypertension.
- *Sandalwood:* promotes peace of mind, meditation, and spiritual thoughts, and encourages clear thinking in difficult situations; because of its anti-inflammatory and soothing nature, may also be used for urinary infections and diarrhea.
- *Thyme:* because of its very strong, hot and pungent properties, should only be used in very small amounts (one drop added to a bath or to 30 ml of massage oil is more than enough); very powerful action on the respiratory system; may be used to eliminate harmful microorganisms of the respiratory tract, as an expectorant, and often used to treat bronchitis; should never be used in cases of hypertension.
- *Ylang-ylang:* promotes serenity and joy; because of its sweet scent, is considered highly popular as a relaxant and aphrodisiac; often prescribed for sexual inadequacy which has been caused by anxiety and apprehension.

Guidelines to Working with Oils

Now that you have an understanding of some of the properties of essential oils used in massage therapy, you are ready to begin using these oils as therapeutic tools. However, because many of these oils have very specific uses, there are some important points that we need to go over before you start using them. The following are some simple guidelines that will help you when working with oils and aromatherapy:

- Be aware that some people may be allergic to certain essential oils, so always try a small amount to test the skin's reaction.
- Never use essential oils when there is a possibility that your client may be pregnant, is breast-feeding, or for massaging babies or children under the age of 12, except under the guidance of a qualified aromatherapist.
- Never allow your client to take oils internally, except under strict medical supervision.
- Since essential oils tend to deteriorate and evaporate rapidly, always store them in dark glass bottles or metal containers with airtight lids or stoppers, kept in a cool, dark, dry place. If stored correctly, an essential oil which has been diluted in a base oil will last for two to three months.
- Before beginning a massage, always remember to pour the diluted oil into the palm of your hand, and then gently rub your hands together so that the oil becomes warmed. Once the oil is warm, you should then oil the body before you begin to massage.

Herbal Medicine

Herbal medicine, often regarded as an extension of nutrition, is one of the pillars of natural healing, and its therapeutic value is as old as humanity itself. As one of the most ancient systems of natural treatment, herbal medicine has the advantage of having been enriched by the experience of countless practitioners throughout time. Many of these practitioners from ancient Egypt, Greece, Rome, India, and China relied on a sophisticated system of plant healing. This ancient knowledge has been, and continues to be, enriched by present-day scientific research. Today's pharmaceutical companies continue to search for new compounds that can be extracted from plants, and many existing medical prescriptions are plant-based.

Using Herbal Preparations

Although there are many ways in which herbal preparations can be administered, two of the most frequently used methods are infusions and tinctures. When using infusions, you must remember to thoroughly mix the chosen herbal mixture before using it. Once it has been mixed, infuse 5 mg (one teaspoon) in a cup of hot water. Cover the mixture and then let it stand for 5 to 10 minutes. Once it has been strained, the person may drink it slowly while it is still warm.

Tinctures are generally sold in herbal or health food stores in bottles containing 50 to 100 ml (two to four ounces). Once you have added 7 to 10 drops of the solution into a glass of cold or warm water, you should instruct the person to drink it very slowly.

An important point to remember whenever you are using herbal preparations is that they should never be given to babies or children under three years of age without expert supervision. However, for children between the ages of three to six years, you can add three drops of the tincture, and for children seven to ten years old, you may add as much as five drops.

Using Touch as a Therapy

Now that we have identified the individual types of massage therapy, and have discussed some of the preparations and oils used in massage, we are ready to begin talking about the specific types of touch which are used in therapeutic massage.

Massage involves movements which are loving, caring, comforting, relaxing, soothing, invigorating, energizing, and healing. In order to achieve these effects, we use various techniques to massage in a variety of ways, depending on how we use our hands, the size of the area that is to be massaged, and the depth of stroke. Some techniques encourage circulation and stretching, while others are used to pump toxins out of muscles; still others are used to relax the body.

Some types of touch are used more frequently than others. These include effleurage, petrissage, percussion, pressure, acupressure, and articulations.

Effleurage

Effleurage is derived from the French word *effleurer,* which means to touch lightly or skim over. It is a wide-area stroke performed with the palm of the hand and the fingers (Figure 15-4). The goal of effleurage is to massage in a rhythmic, smooth, flowing, gliding, stroking way. It is enhanced by the use of oil, and is often an excellent way to begin and end a massage. Among its many benefits, effleurage creates an immediate sense of trust and relaxation between the person who is giving and the person who is receiving the massage.

Light effleurage promotes relaxation, alleviates pain, and encourages sleep. Deep effleurage improves circulation, stretches and relaxes tense muscles, helps lymphatic drainage and the elimination of waste products, and improves the elasticity of the skin.

Although effleurage is mainly performed with the flat palm of the hand in long regular strokes, it can also be practiced with a cupped hand, by placing one hand on top of the other, and by using the tips of the fingers for feathering, a very calming and soothing technique.

Petrissage

The main goal of petrissage is to stretch the muscles in a deeper and more stimulating way than effleurage. It is a form of kneading, wringing, and firm rubbing (Figure 15-5 on p. 148) that can be practiced with both hands together, with alternate hands, or with one hand on top of the other. The movements, used mainly on fleshy parts of the body like the thighs, can be slow and deep or quick and energizing, and gentle or firm. They relax tense muscles, releasing deep muscular contractions, revitalize tissues, improve circulation, and help to eliminate wastes.

In kneading, you use both hands alternately. The movements are rhythmic squeezing which flow toward and away from each other. Wringing, which is most effective on the thighs and calves, adds a twisting-like action to the kneading. You must remember to keep your thumb close to your fingers. Push in opposite directions with each hand, squeezing the flesh between them. It is a flowing movement, but is deeper and more stimulating than kneading.

Percussion

There are three main types of percussion used in massage. These are referred to as hacking, cupping, and pummeling (Figure 15-6 on p. 148). The main goal of percussion is to increase circulation, break down fatty deposits, and revitalize tissues. The movements, which are mainly brisk and stimulating, but can also be soothing if performed slowly, are most commonly used on fleshy muscular areas, such as

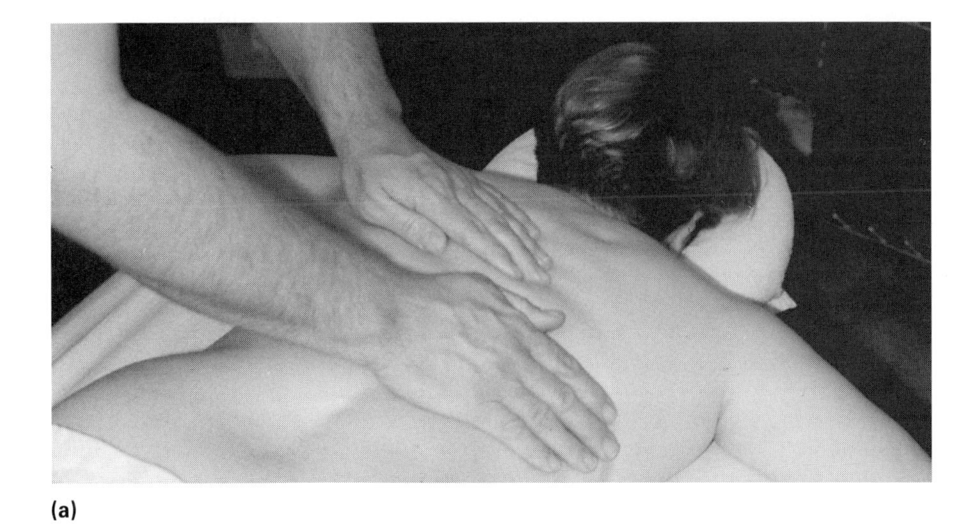

(a)

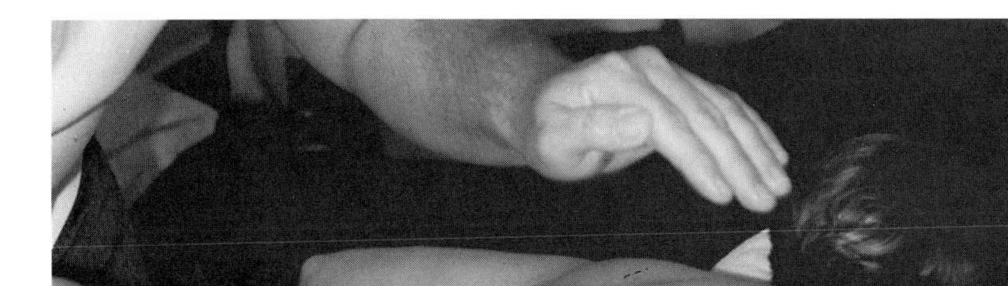

(b)

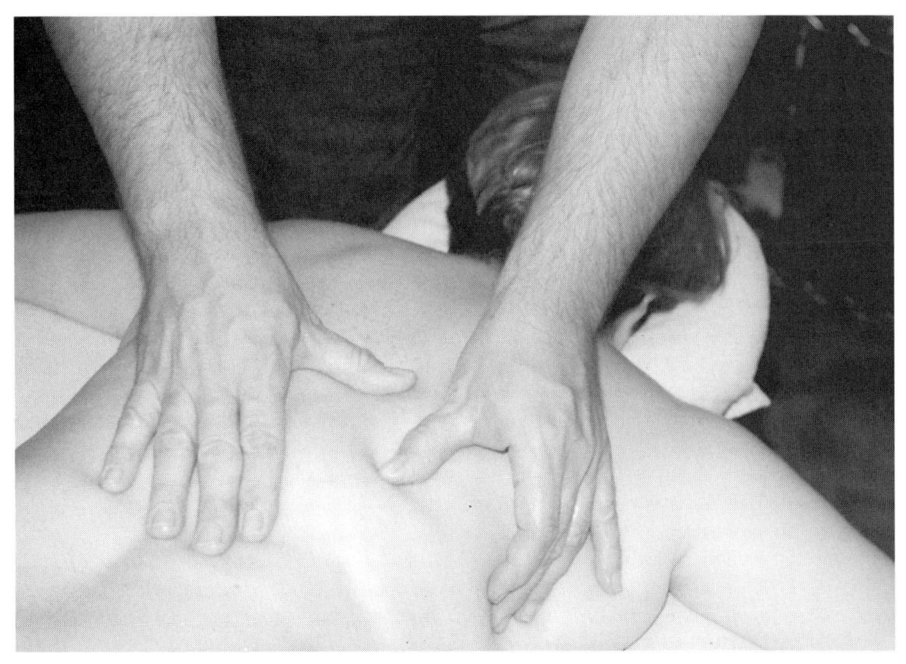

(c)

Figure 15-4
(a) Fat-hand effleurage;
(b) cupped-hand effleurage;
(c) feathering.

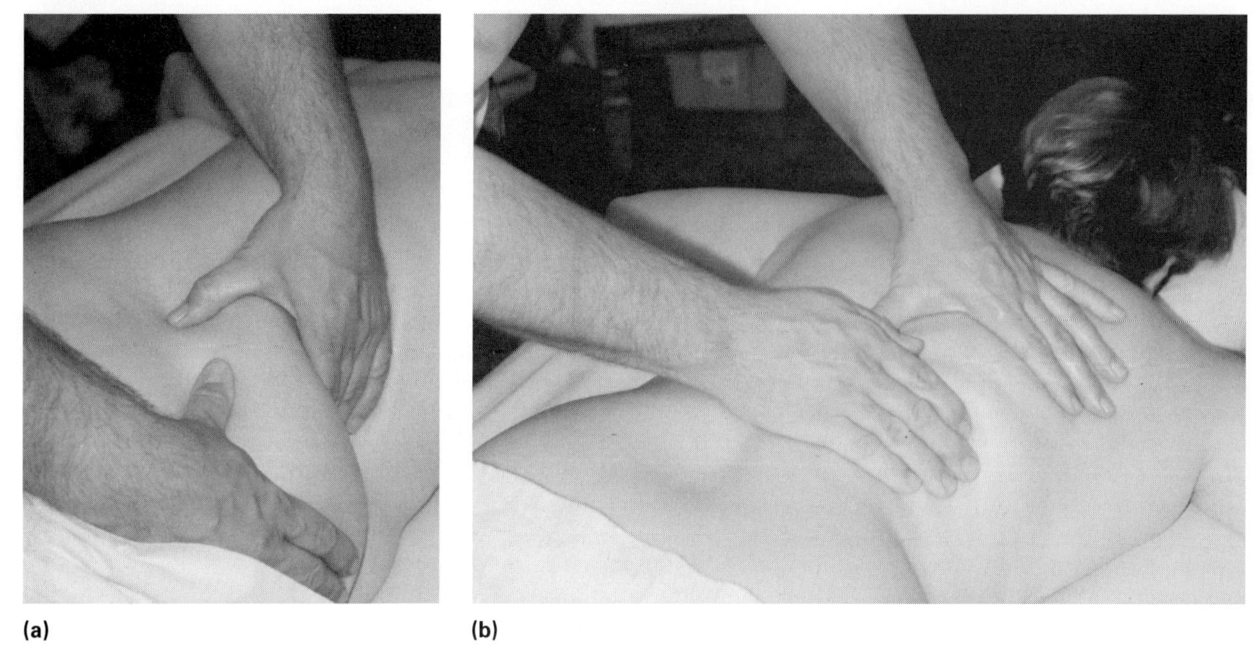

(a) (b)

Figure 15-5
(a) Kneading; (b) wringing.

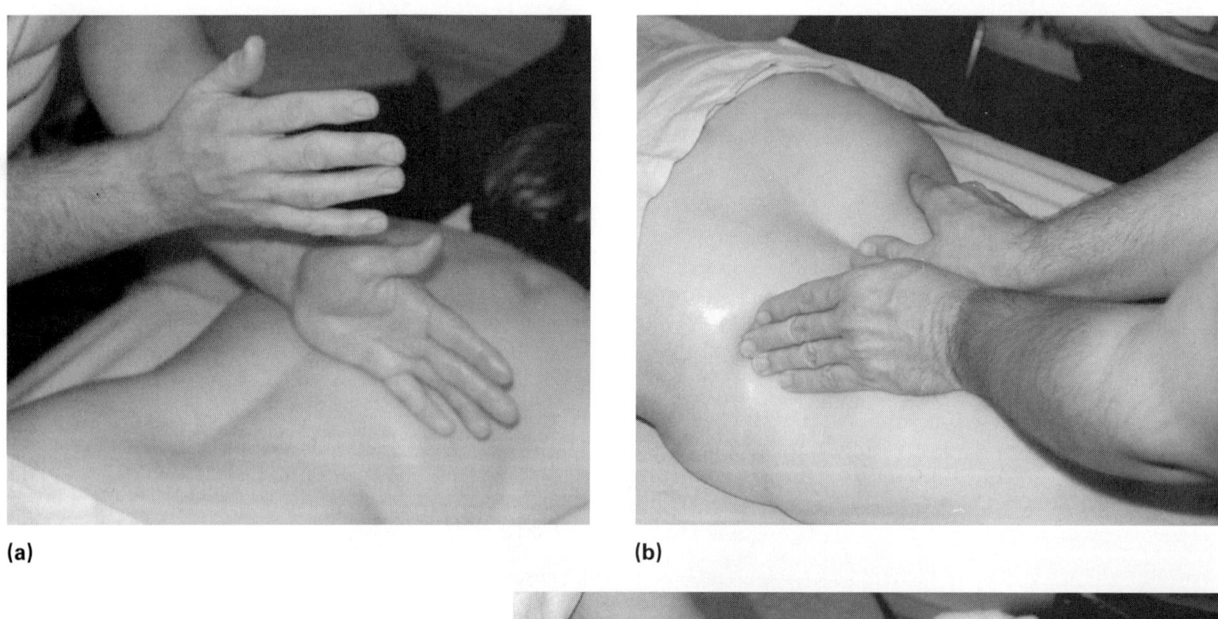

(a) (b)

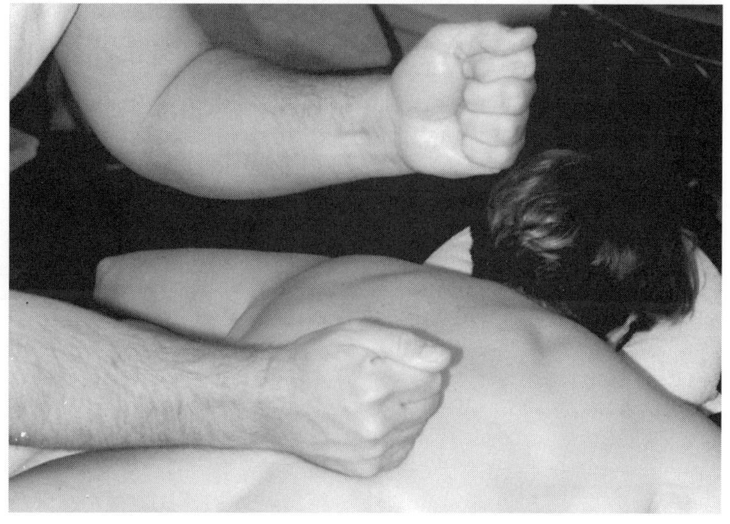

(c)

Figure 15-6
(a) Hacking; (b) cupping; (c) pummeling.

the buttocks and tops of the thighs. They should never be used on bony, injured, or painful areas.

When using percussion, you must always remember to keep your hands relaxed, and maintain a gentle flowing rhythm, using light springy movements. Also, watch for any discomfort in the person you are massaging. Remember, if a movement hurts, do not repeat it.

Pressure

Pressure techniques are used for massaging smaller areas of the body, most notably the muscles along the side of the spine and around the shoulder and buttock areas.

Thumb circling (Figure 15-7) is achieved by tucking the fingers into the palm, or spreading the fingers for support, using the pads of the thumbs to press directly on the underlying muscles for a few seconds before releasing. In order to improve the flow of energy and circulation, the thumbs are used for applying a rolling circular pressure. Pressure with the hands is used in the same way as pressure with the thumbs, but here the palm is used, rather than the heel of the hand.

Acupressure

Meridians and the acupressure points located on them are treated with thumb pressure (Figure 15-8 on p. 150). Here, the pressure is applied using either a toning or sedating method, depending on whether you wish to add to or disperse energy from a particular area.

To tone or increase energy, take a slow deep breath and as you breathe out, press down with your thumbs for a few seconds. Remember to keep the pressure firm and constant without hurting. Repeat this three to five times. To sedate or disperse energy, rotate your thumb in a clockwise direction in a gentle but constant manner for two or three minutes.

Articulations

The main goal of using articulation techniques is to stretch and free any impeded joints and related structures, such as ligaments and adjacent muscles (Figure 15-9 on p. 151). By keeping the body supple, mobile, flexible, and youthful, the onset of rigidity that is so common in aging and all health problems related to the body's main structure of bones, joints, muscles, and ligaments is hopefully delayed or even avoided altogether. Oriental body therapy techniques and osteopathy make excellent use of articulations.

Preparing to Work as a Massage Therapist

Before you actually begin working as a massage therapist, there are some important points that you must first go through.

To start with, you should understand that when functioning as a massage therapist, creating the right state of mind, surroundings, and atmosphere is as vital as the massage itself. Therefore, there are several key preparations you must make prior to using

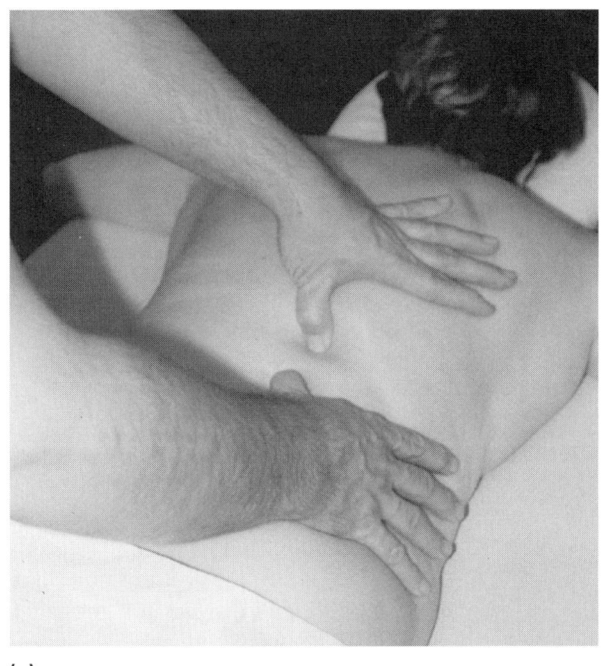

(a)

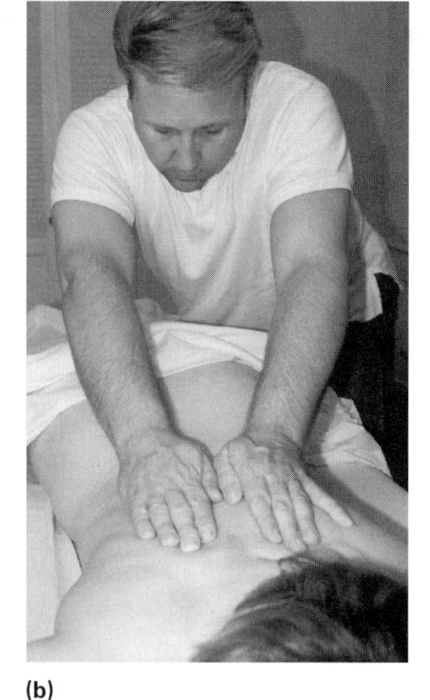

(b)

Figure 15-7
(a) Thumb-circling pressure; (b) palm press.

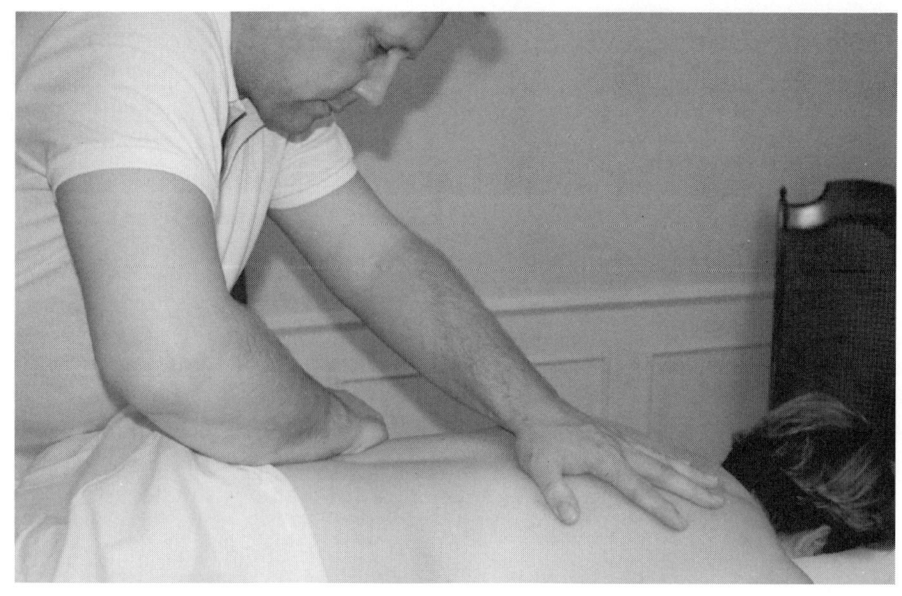

(a)

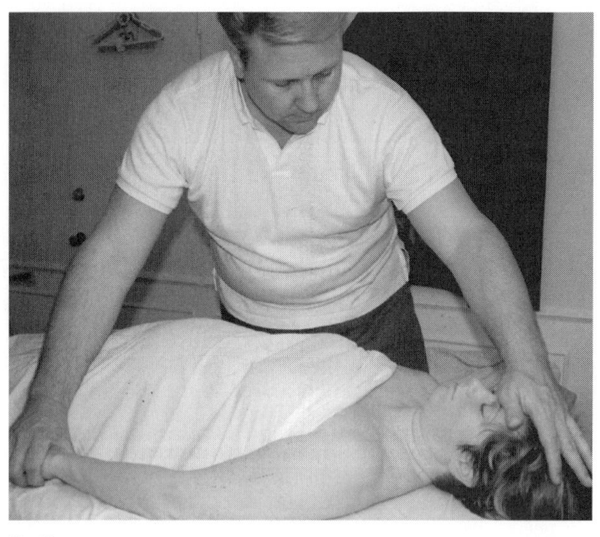

(b-1)

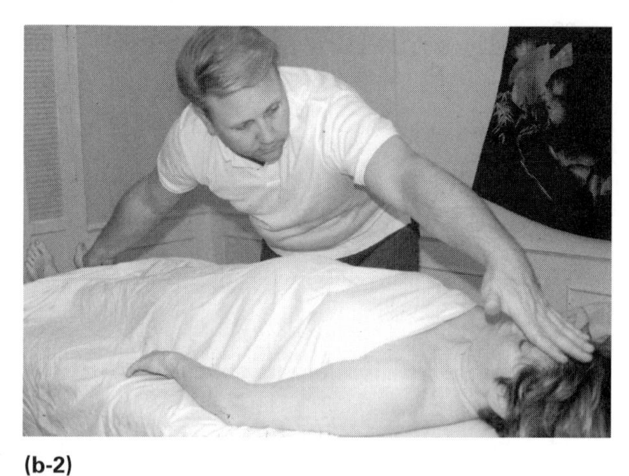

(b-2)

Figure 15-8
(a) Using acupressure to tonify; (b) using acupressure to sedate or disperse energy.

therapeutic touch to soothe and heal your client. These preparations involve ensuring the correct mood of the room, and creating the right frame of body, mind, and heart, both on the part of yourself and the client.

Preparing the Room

The room which you will be using should be clean and spacious, with a decor and ambience that is calming to the senses. The colors used in the room should be neutral, with natural daylight or soft lighting used in the area. The playing of soothing, unobtrusive background music is also often used because of its beneficial effects on both the therapist and the person receiving the massage. It is also important to make sure that the room is warm, yet not stuffy, since chilled muscles may contract and tense up if the person is too cold.

The table or surface which you will be using to work on should be firm, but not too uncomfortably hard. A mattress or futon may be used, however, some therapists prefer to place a folded blanket, covered by a towel, directly onto the floor, in order to

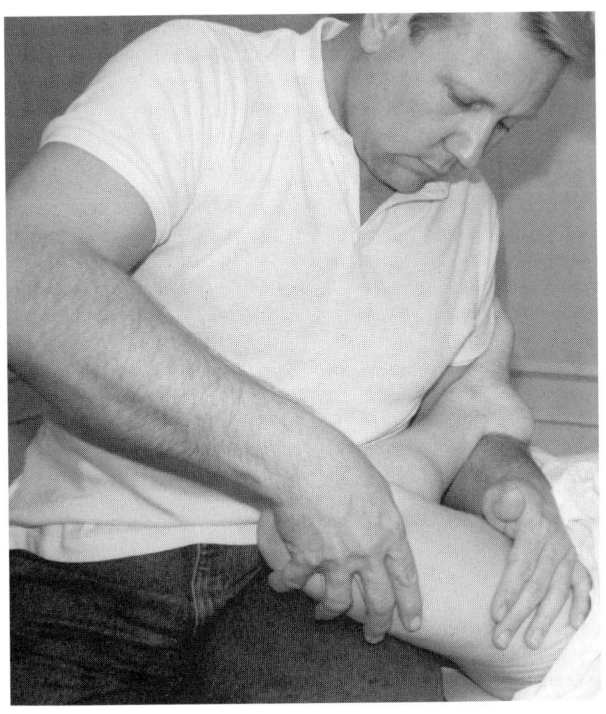

Figure 15-9
Supporting the leg while applying pressure to stretch and articulate the part of the body that is being treated.

perform the massage. If at all feasible, a massage table is generally the best surface to work on.

Preparing Yourself

Since giving and receiving a massage is usually considered to be an intimate activity between yourself and the person receiving the massage, practicing good personal hygiene before and after the session is extremely important. This applies both to the person receiving the massage as well as yourself. And since your hands are the most important tools in this therapeutic modality, it is also important that you care for them correctly. This includes making sure that your nails are also kept short to avoid any scratching or digging of them into your client.

Because much of the time you spend in providing the massage is spent in a standing or bending-over position, it is also important that you make sure you properly care for your back. Always aim to keep your back fairly straight but not rigid, and make sure you turn from your waist, rather than twisting your body in awkward positions. It is also very important that you learn how to properly relax and breathe deeply, since doing so will help you to avoid tiring, and thus will enhance the effectiveness and sensitivity of your touch.

During the session, try to keep your conversation to a minimum. This is a time to relax; you can always talk before or after the massage.

Finally, always try to use your own senses to monitor what your client may be experiencing, and never repeat an action that appears to be hurting the recipient. Remember, your actions should always be guided by the receiver's expressions and experiences.

Preparing Through the Art of Centering

Centering is a process in which one focuses and gathers his or her energy into a point so that it can be channeled more easily into any activity one chooses. It is a state of balance, quietness, strength, and presence in one particular moment. More specifically, centering means focusing on the *hara,* or the center of energy in the abdomen. For any form of massage, being centered in the hara is of primary importance, since it enables you to be flexible, yet at the same time resilient, so that you can work with your intuition rather than with your mind. When your energy is channeled, you need less muscle power and thus can give even a series of massage treatments without becoming tired or drained. Being centered also involves having the correct posture; with your spine erect and your neck and shoulders relaxed; and remaining grounded, or aware of your contact with the ground, through your legs and your feet.

Before you give any form of touch therapy, whether it is massage, shiatsu, or reflexology, you should spend a few minutes centering yourself and connecting the energy between your hara and your hands. To do this, you can either sit cross-legged or kneel down on the floor. If necessary, put a cushion under your buttocks to ease any strain on your legs. If you are still uncomfortable, you may sit on a straight-backed chair with both of your feet flat on the floor. Now close your eyes and direct your attention inward (Figure 15-10). Feel the strong foundation of your buttocks, legs, and feet as they make contact with the cushion, chair, or floor. From this firm base, allow your spine to float gently upward, without strain. Let go of any tension in your shoulders, neck, and face. Now begin to focus on your breath. Allow it to find its own rhythm. Imagine, as you begin to inhale, that your breath is filling your lower abdomen or hara. After a few breaths, begin to visualize that as you exhale, your breath flows up your torso from the hara, through your shoulders, down your arms, and out of your hands. If it helps, you may visualize the breath as a stream of energy or white light flowing up your body and out of your fingers.

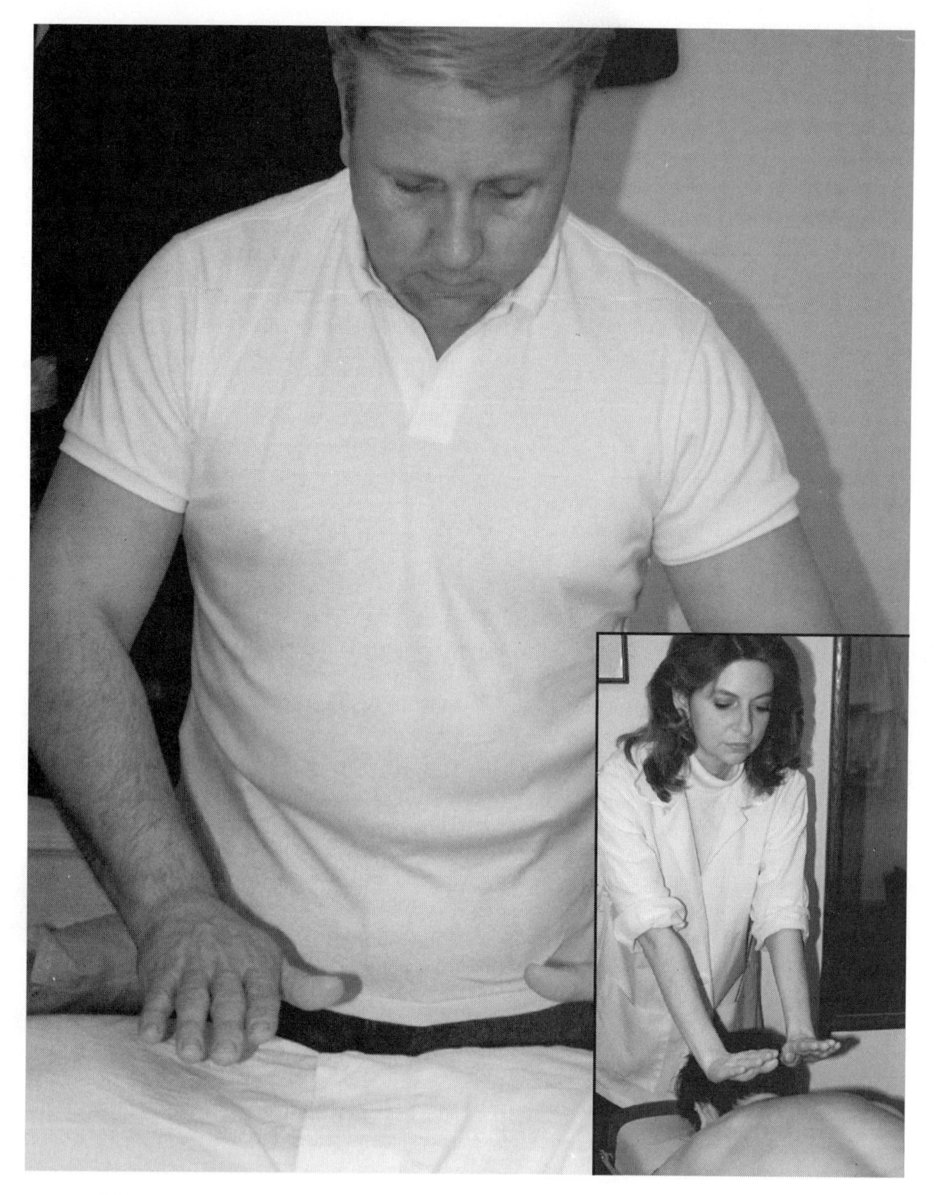

Figure 15-10
One form of centering in which the therapist and the patient become "at one" with each other.

Summary

In this chapter, you were introduced to massage therapy and its usefulness as a therapeutic modality in the study of physical medicine. During the chapter, we briefly discussed the history of massage, as well as identified some of the individual forms of massage and their relationship to helping the main body systems. We discussed the purpose and function of aromatherapy, and talked about how various oils can be used as part of the therapeutic session. We also talked about the different types of touch used in massage therapy. Finally, we discussed the role of the massage therapist, and how he or she prepares for a therapeutic session.

Review Questions

1. Briefly explain the concept of *centering*.
2. What does the term *hara* mean?
3. What is the name of a type of massage stroke that uses gentle rhythmical massage stroking, and which can be used all over the body?
4. What is the name of a type of massage stroke that uses kneading, wringing, and rubbing movements?
5. What does the term *homeostasis* mean?
6. Briefly explain how massage can help the body.
7. List at least three effects of massage on individual body systems.
8. Briefly explain the difference between *Swedish therapy* and *osteopathic therapy*.

16

Caring for the Body Through Massage

Performance Objectives

Upon completion of this chapter, you will be able to:

1. Define the basic massage sequences that are used on the back, the legs, the arms, the shoulders, neck, and scalp, the front of the torso, and the face.
2. Define the basic massage sequence for connecting.

Terms and Abbreviations

Long stroke a broad, fluent, and soothing movement which is used on each part of the body to apply oil and to warm and relax the area.

As you begin to learn how to care for the body through the use of massage therapy, the first thing you must understand is that each individual part of our body is seen as a separate entity, each capable of causing us joy as well as pain and sadness. Therefore, each of these parts must be treated differently. Ultimately, your goal should be to memorize the sequence of strokes which are used to massage each of the individual sections of the body.

When defining the basic sequence of massage, we begin at the back of the body, working our way down from the head to the feet. This is followed by turning the person over and massaging the front of the body, once again working down from the top.

The sequence consists of seven separate areas: two on the back of the body, and five on the front. Individually, they are identified as the back, the back of the legs, the shoulders, neck, and scalp, the face, the arms and hands, the front of the torso, and the front of the legs. You should understand that it makes little difference which area you are working on, as long as you follow the same order of strokes.

Preparing to Begin the Massage Sequence

Once you have determined which area you are going to work on, you begin by oiling that part thoroughly, and then work from lighter, broader strokes to the deeper, more specific ones, eventually ending once more with the lighter ones. When giving a full massage, you will be affecting many of the body's systems, including the lymphatic and venous circulation and the nervous system. Traditional massage always works toward the heart, and thus aids in venous circulation. However, since the purpose of the massage is often more concerned with relaxing and balancing a wide range of processes, the sequence of strokes you will be using generally adheres to this rule only where it is particularly appropriate. For example, if you are working on the arms and legs, you should use firmer strokes toward the heart and lighter ones away from it. By doing this, you help to assist the flow of blood back to the heart.

The Basic Massage Sequence

You should start your massage with the back, first working broadly over the whole area, then concentrating on the smaller portions: the shoulder blades and upper back; the lower back, buttocks, and sides of the torso; and finally, the spine itself. Next, you come to the back of the legs. Begin by oiling them both together, then massage each individually. First you work up the leg, draining it. Then knead your way down, and finally, massage the foot.

After the person turns over to expose the front of his or her body, you begin with the shoulders, working on both front and back at the same time. Next, turning the head to one side, you should work on each shoulder separately. The area is completed by massaging all over the scalp. You should then move to the face. Here you start on the forehead and make your way down to the chin, working outward from the center to the sides. The eyes, nose, jaw muscles, and ears should all receive special attention.

Once you have completed the face, you are ready to work with the arms and hands. Each is massaged individually. As on the leg, you should first work up the extremity, draining it, then knead downward again, ending by massaging the wrist and hand. Then move to the front of the torso. After you have focused on the rib cage and sides of the torso, move down to circle around the abdomen. Then work your way up from the belly in long sweeping strokes. You are now ready to work on the front of the legs. After you have applied oil to both legs, concentrate on each one individually, working up the leg to drain it, circling the kneecap on the way, then kneading down the leg again, and ultimately ending on the feet.

After you have completed working on each individual area, you are ready to link all the parts of the body together. This is done either by connecting strokes or by resting your hands briefly on two separate parts of the body.

Massaging the Back

The back is the main structure of support for our body, and as such, is a great source of mobility and strength. Since it is more protected than the softer front of the body, it is also the best place to begin a massage. And by starting at this point, by the time you come to work on the more vulnerable front part of the body, the receiver of the massage often feels more trusting and relaxed.

The back is also the single largest area you will be massaging and as such, often requires more time and attention than any other part. Also, because you will be reaching nerves on the back that spread to every part of the body, most people feel a deep sense of release after the completion of a thorough back massage.

When massaging the back, it is extremely important that both the receiver and you are comfortable. This is so you can reach down and across the back easily. To avoid tiring yourself, remember to use your whole body, and not just your arms. Since the massage begins with the back, it is here that the receiver not only becomes accustomed to your touch, but also, with the feel of his or her own body.

Oiling and Stroking

To massage the back, lay the person down on his or her stomach, with the arms by their sides. If necessary, you may pad the ankles and upper chest with a small cushion or pillow. Now position yourself at the receiver's head and spend a few minutes centering yourself before beginning the long oiling stroke (Figure 16-1 on p. 156). This stroke spreads the oil and warms the back; it also allows you to become familiar with the receiver's body.

Bring your hands down gently onto the upper back; then begin to travel down the center along the spinal column. At the base of the spine, allow your hands to separate and curve around to the sides of the buttocks. Then pull slowly up the sides and across the shoulders. Repeat the movements until the back is thoroughly oiled.

Massaging the Individual Sections

You are now ready to massage the individual sections of the back. This will include working the shoulder from the head, the shoulder from the side, the lower back and buttocks, and the spine.

Working the Shoulder from the Head

After you have completed oiling the back, you are ready to begin on the shoulders, one at a time. Start with the shoulder away from the direction the receiver's head is facing. First, circle around the shoulder blade and up the side of the rib cage. Then start to work more firmly, kneading all the fleshy parts of the shoulders (Figure 16-2 on p. 157). Gradually

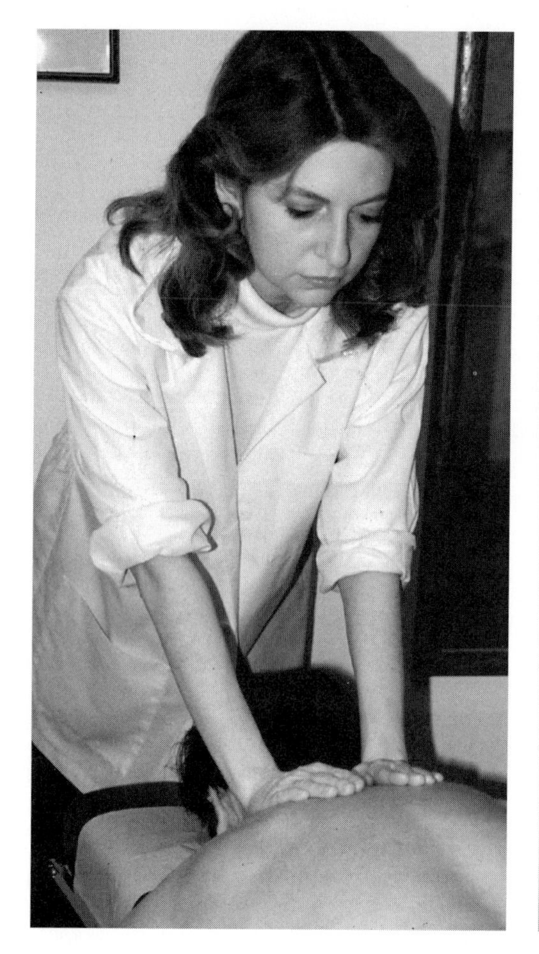

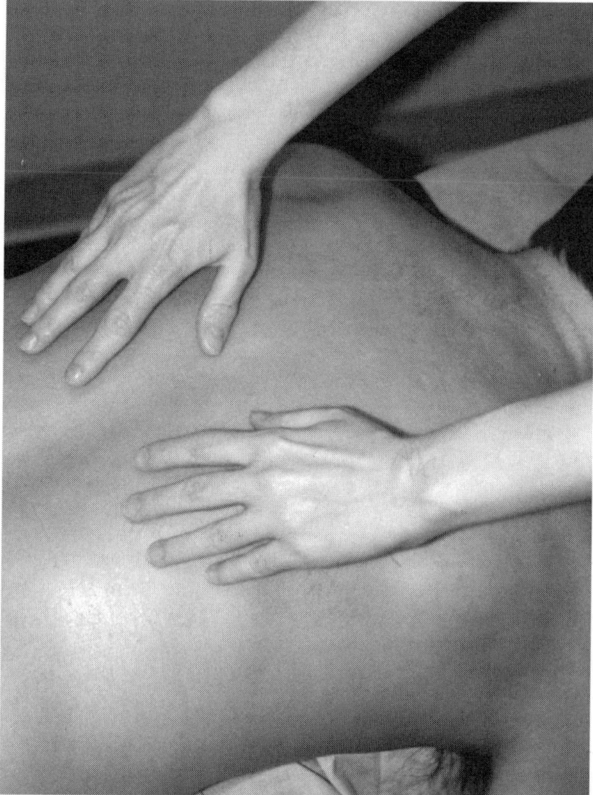

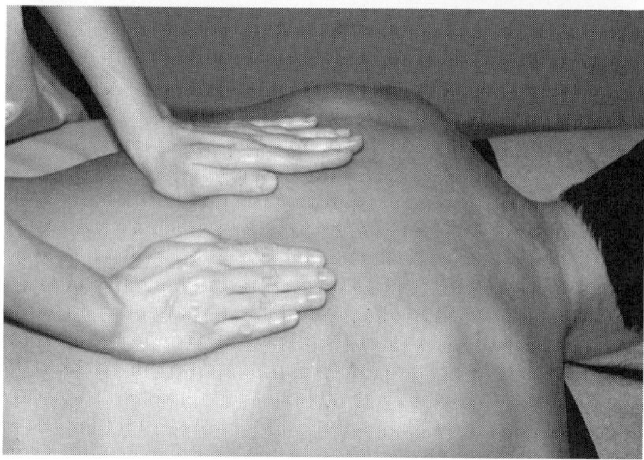

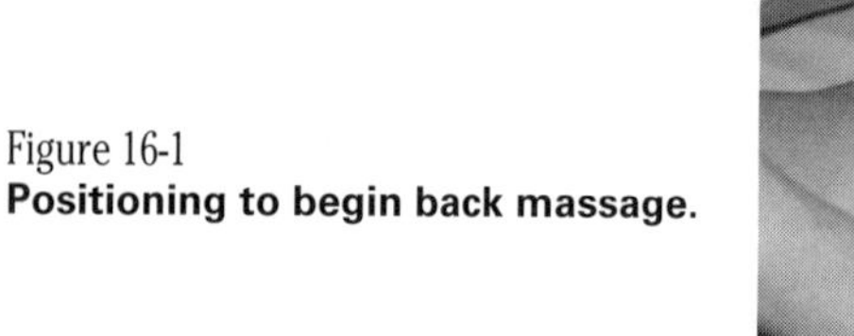

Figure 16-1
Positioning to begin back massage.

begin to use more pressure, applying the thumb-rolling stroke around the base of the neck and the trapezius muscle (Figure 16-3). Try to spend some time on any little knots of tension you may find, interspersing this more concentrated work with soothing broader strokes. Finish with deep alternate thumb strokes along the side of the spine (Figure 16-4 on p. 158).

Working the Shoulder from the Side

You are now ready to shift your position to work on the same shoulder from the side, facing the receiver's head. Gently lift the forearm onto the lower back, as shown in Figure 16-5 (on p. 158). Anchoring the arm on the back, cup your other hand under the shoulder joint (the left hand under the left shoulder

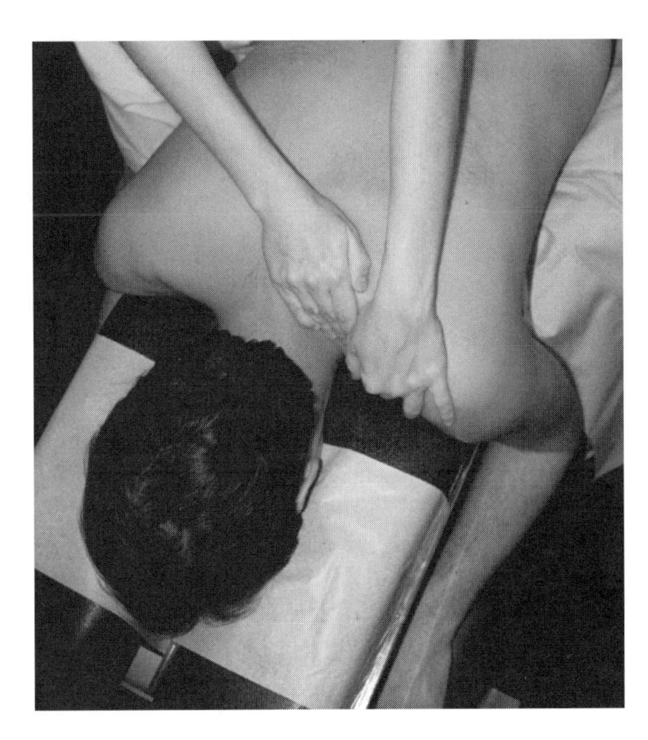

Figure 16-2
Kneading the shoulder.

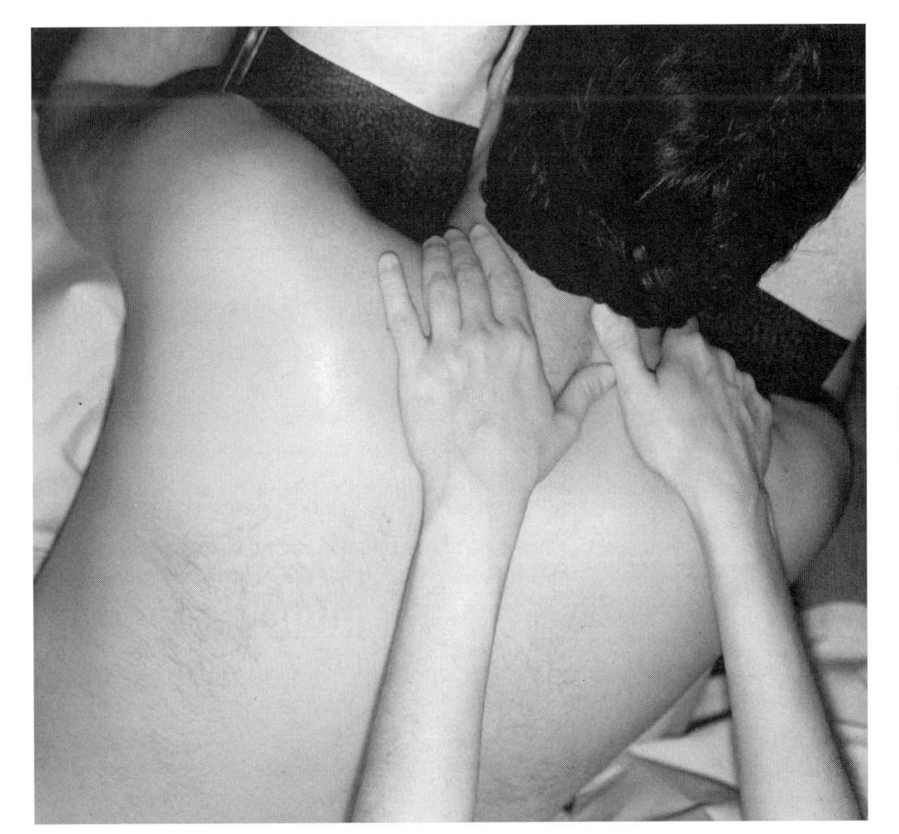

Figure 16-3
Using thumb-rolling stroke at the base of the neck.

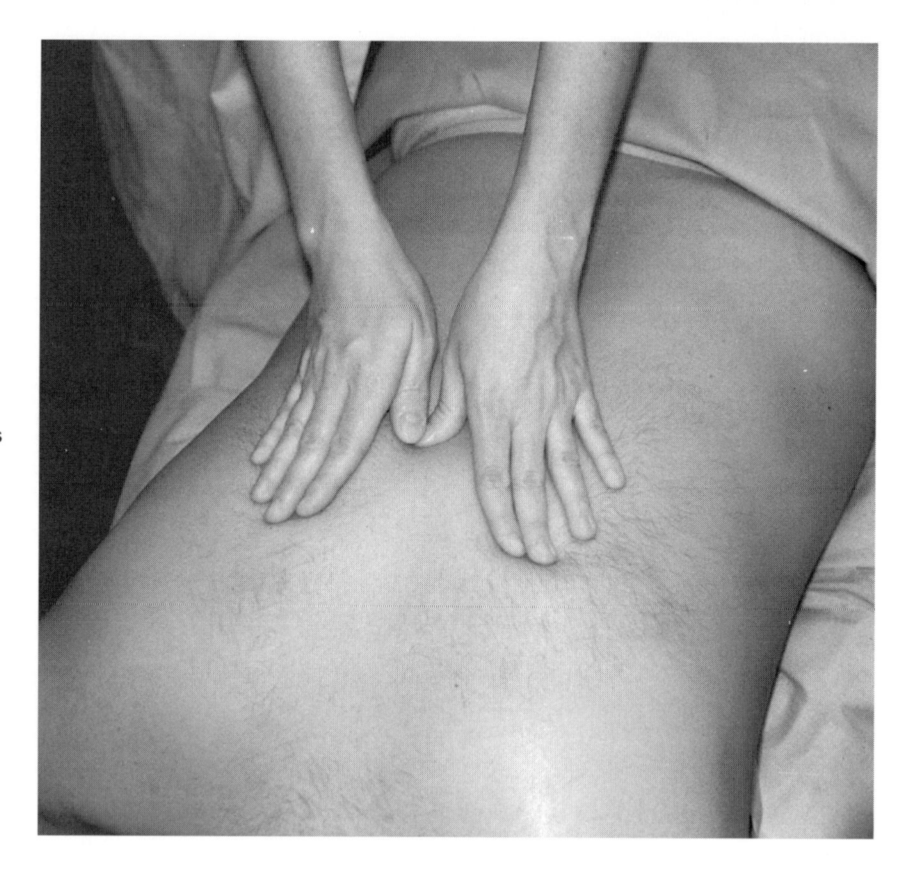

Figure 16-4
Using alternate thumb strokes alongside the spine.

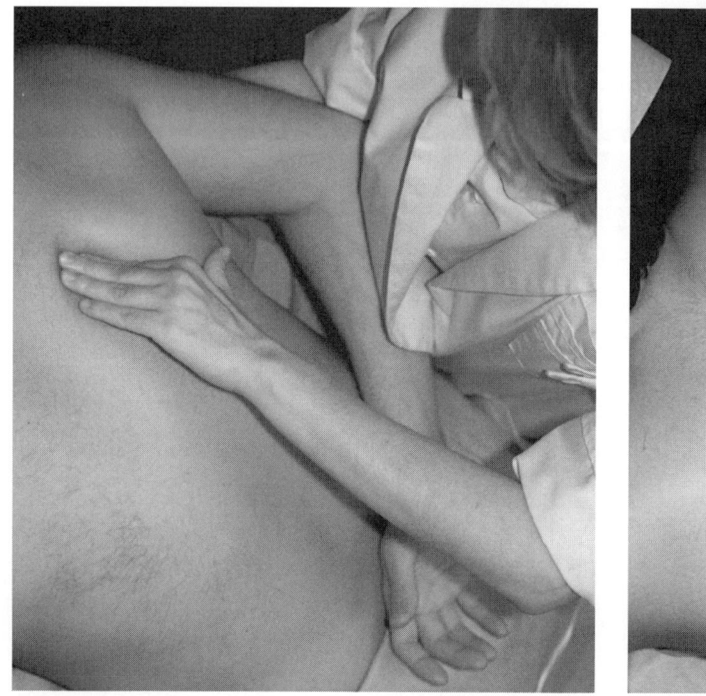

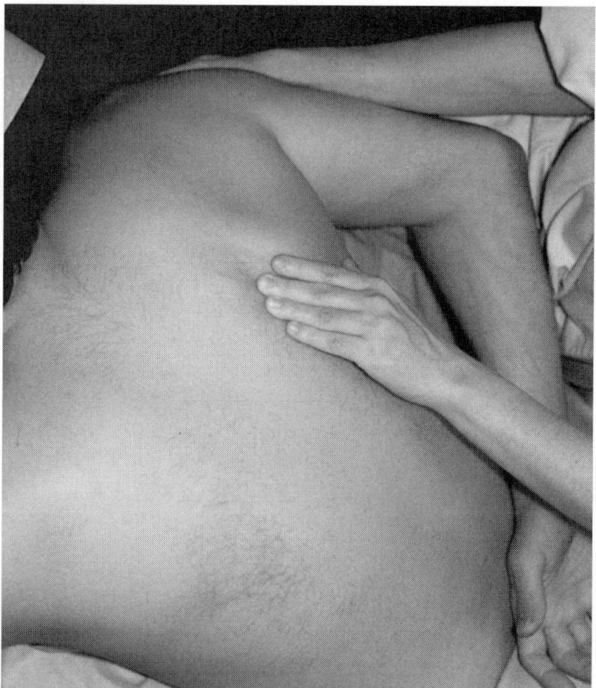

Figure 16-5
Working under the rim of the shoulder blade.

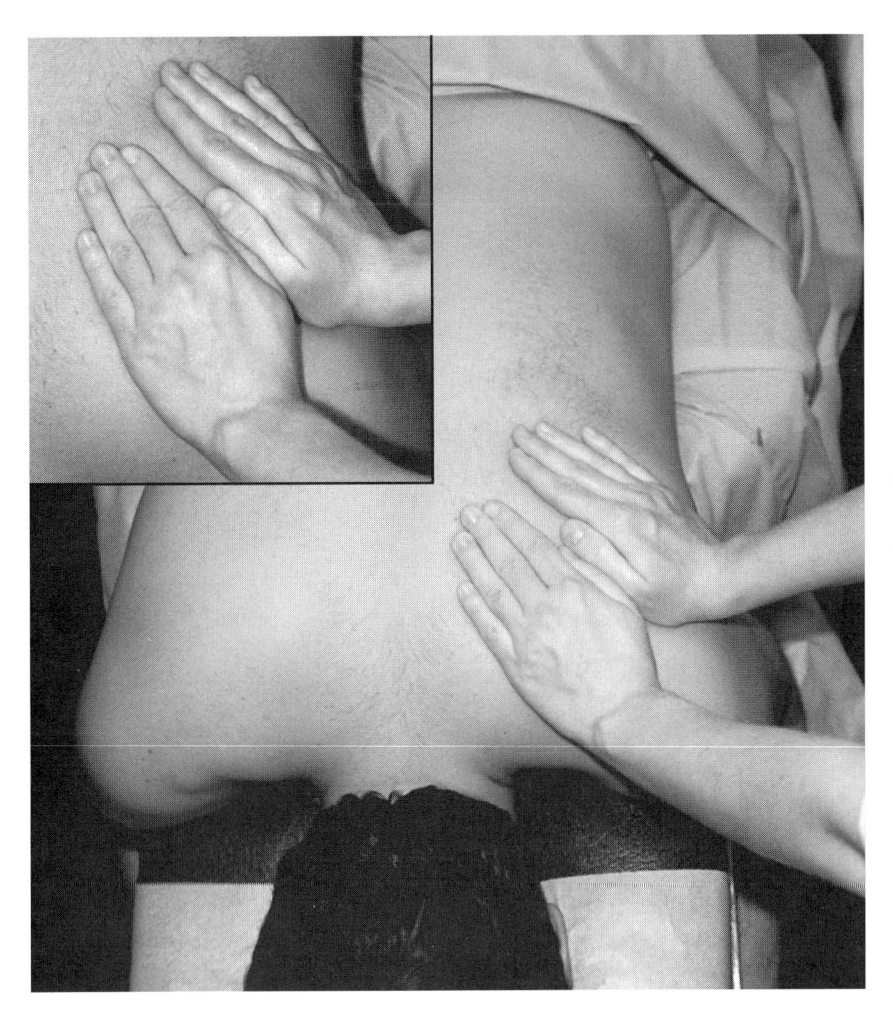

Figure 16-6
Pressing the flat of the shoulder blade.

and vice versa). Having isolated the shoulder blade by raising it, use your free hand to begin to work around and across it (Figure 16-6). Once you have squeezed along the spine of the blade and kneaded the back of the neck (Figure 16-7 on p. 160), gently slide the receiver's arm down off the back and reposition yourself at the head. When ready, ask the receiver to turn his or her head the other way. Then repeat the sequence on the other shoulder.

Working on the Lower Back and the Buttocks

To work on the lower back and the buttocks, you must first position yourself at the receiver's side again, level with the thighs. After you have thoroughly kneaded the lower back using circling strokes (Figure 16-8 on p. 161), you must then massage one buttock, before pulling up that side of the torso (Figure 16-9 on p. 161). After pulling up the sides of the buttock (Figure 16-10 on p. 162), complete the sequence by using a gliding stroke down the body from the shoulders to the foot. Now move to the other side of the receiver and repeat the sequence on the opposite buttock and side.

Working on the Spine

Yoga tells us that the condition of our spine affects us at every level: physically, emotionally, and spiritually. The spinal nerves link our brain with all the other parts of our body and since they lie close to the surface of our back, massage can have a profoundly relaxing effect. Spinal massage is divided into three main strokes. The first is a broad stroke, called a rocking horse (Figure 16-11 on p. 162). It is made up of two parts; one that is soothing, and the other more stimulating. The second stroke is a deep friction stroke used to ease tension around the vertebrae (Figure 16-12 on p. 163). And finally, use a connecting stroke with your forearms, which imparts a feeling of wholeness to the entire back (Figure 16-13 on p. 163). In this third stroke, you should avoid pressing directly on the vertebrae while working on either side of the spine.

Text continued on page 164

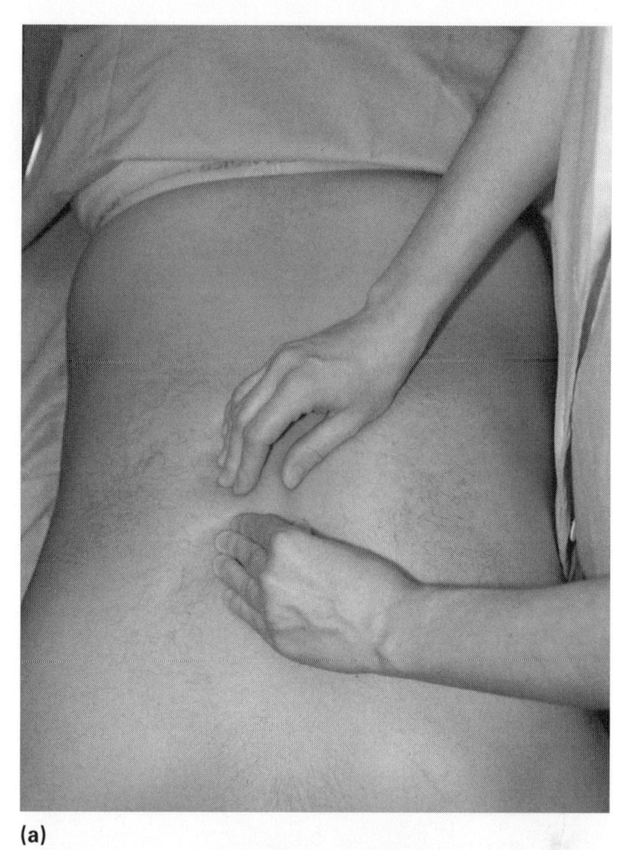

(a)

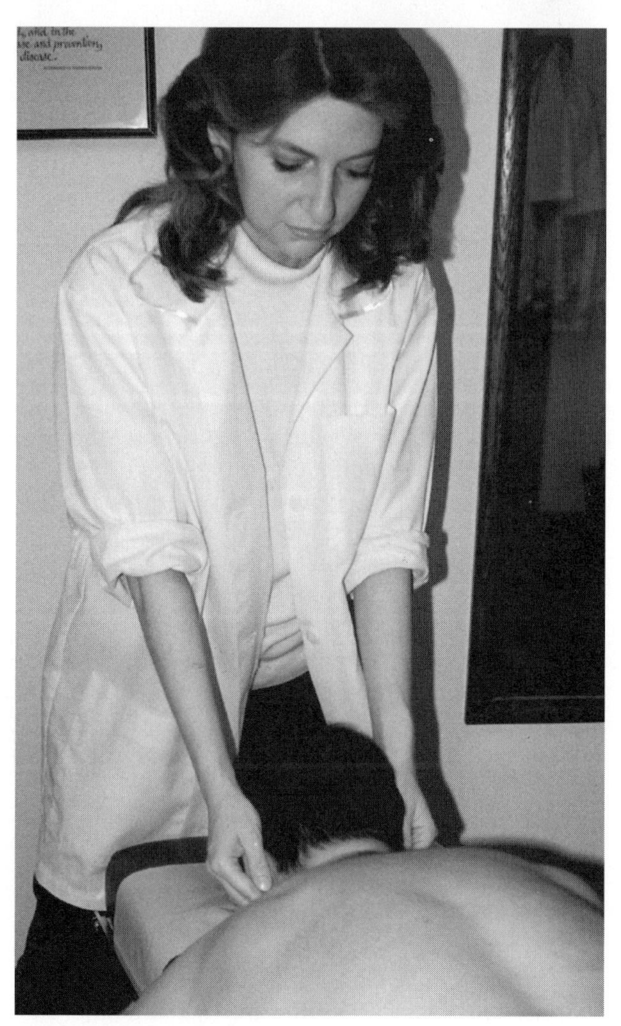

(b)

Figure 16-7
(a) Squeezing the spine; (b) kneading the neck.

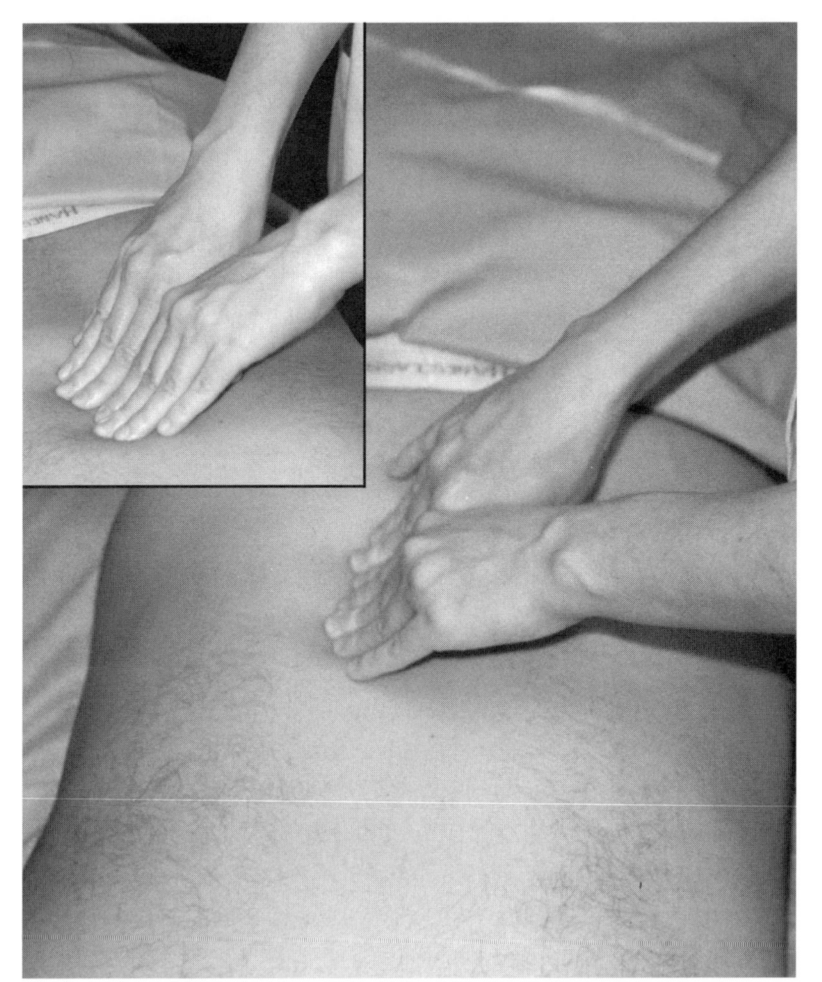

Figure 16-8
Kneading the lower back using circling strokes.

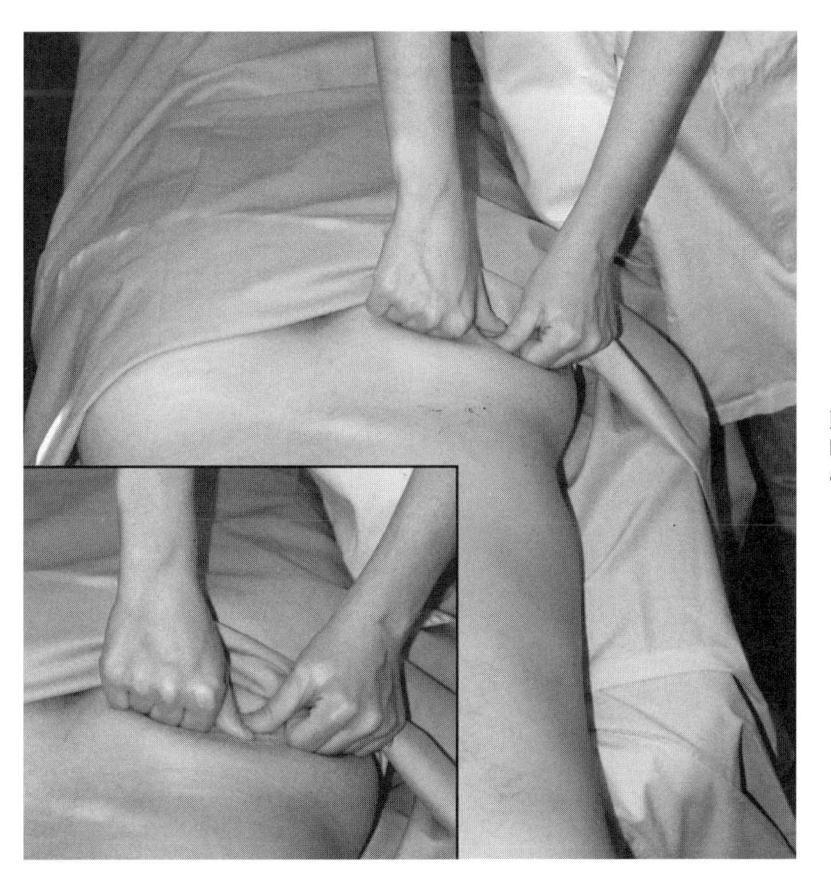

Figure 16-9
Massaging the buttock using kneading and plucking strokes.

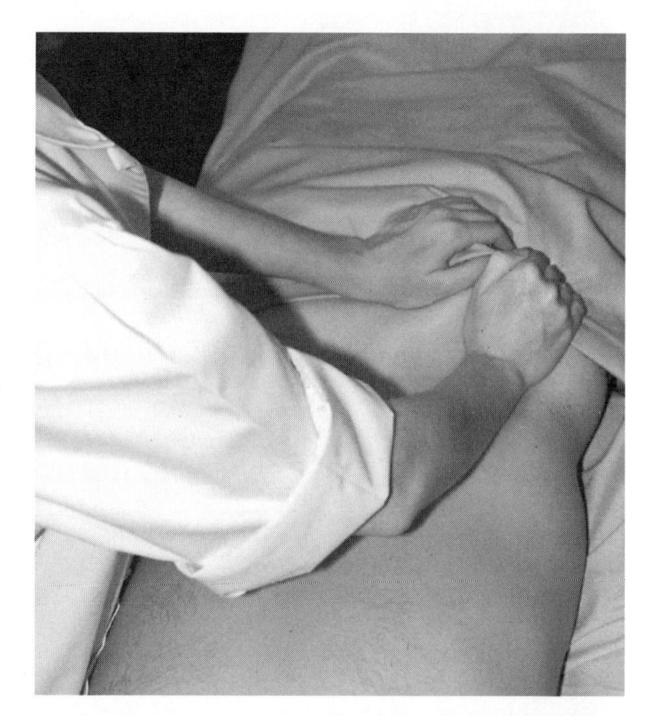

Figure 16-10
Pulling up the sides of the buttock.

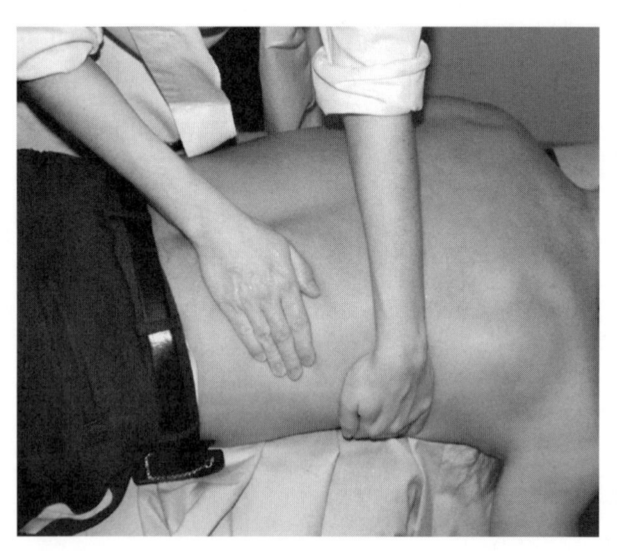

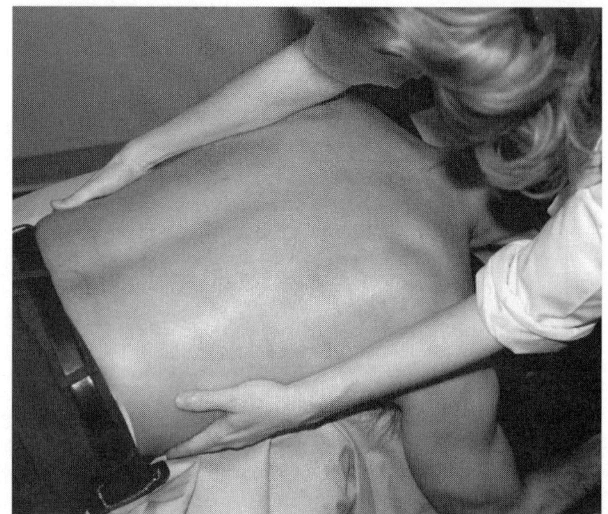

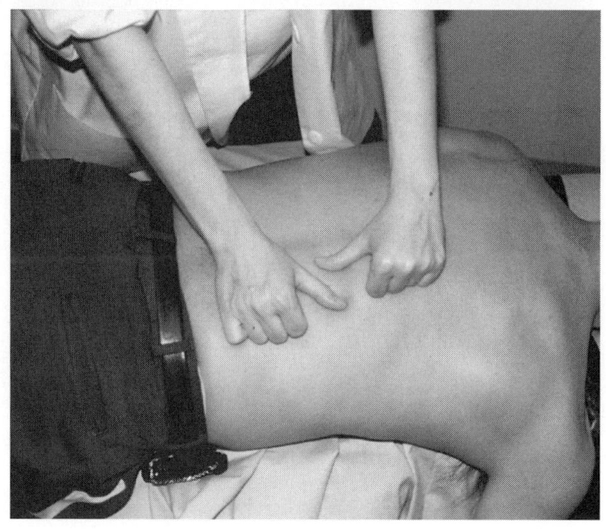

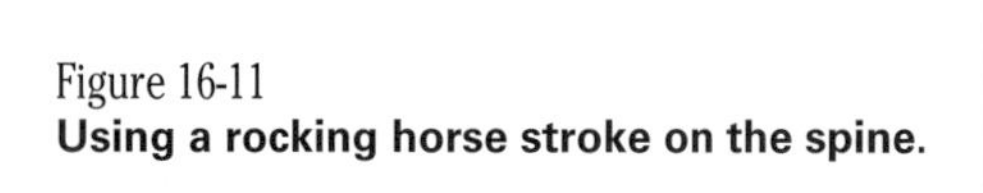

Figure 16-11
Using a rocking horse stroke on the spine.

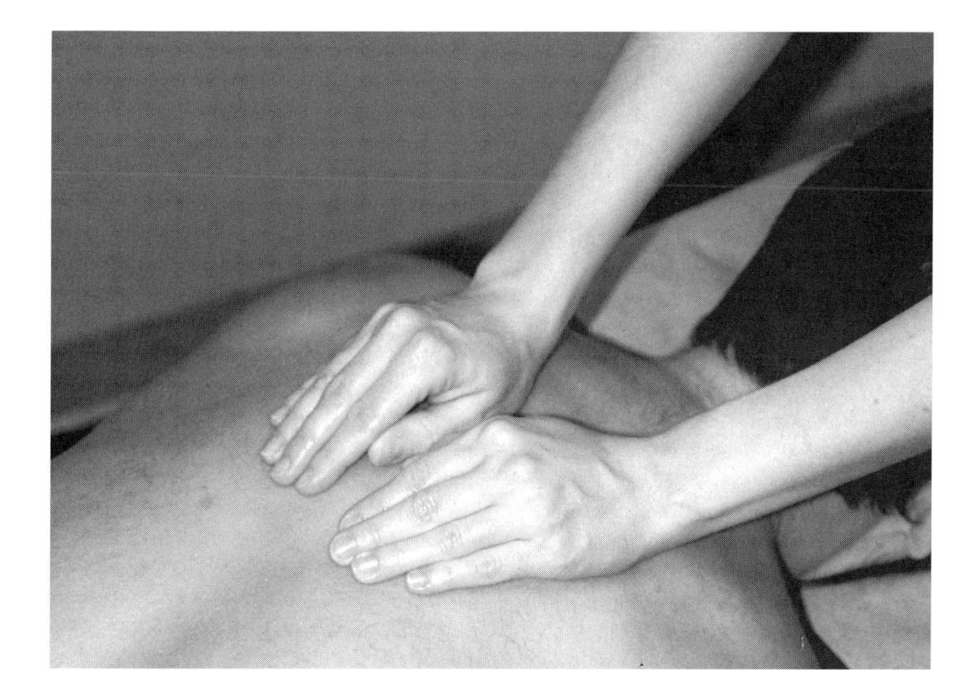

Figure 16-12
Using friction along the spine.

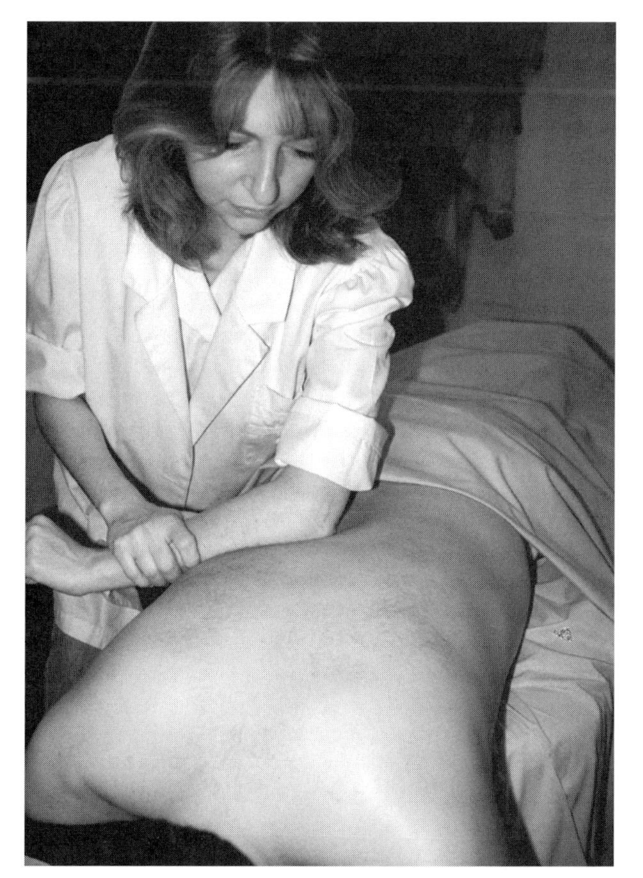

Figure 16-13
Using forearm pressure while working on the spine.

Massaging the Back of the Legs, the Ankle, and the Foot

To complete your massage on the back of the receiver's body, you will work on the legs, and finally on the feet. By bringing energy down to the legs and feet, you will be helping the receiver to feel more grounded and stable. The soft, fleshy backs of the legs are ideal for kneading and wringing strokes.

If the area along the backs of the legs is especially sensitive or painful, you may find that the receiver suffers from low back problems, since the sciatic nerve runs from the base of the spine right down the back of the leg to the heel. Massaging the back of the leg will not only relieve some of the tenderness experienced and felt there, but also, will help to alleviate pain or stiffness felt in the lower back.

Oiling and Stroking

Place yourself between the receiver's feet and start by oiling both legs at the same time, one hand on each leg (Figure 16-14). If you are working from a kneeling position, you may need to come up on your knees to reach the hips, especially if the receiver is tall. After you have chosen which leg you are going to

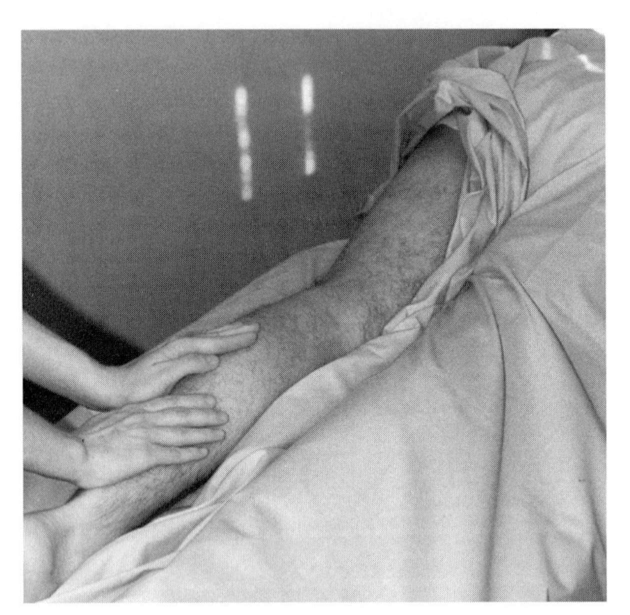

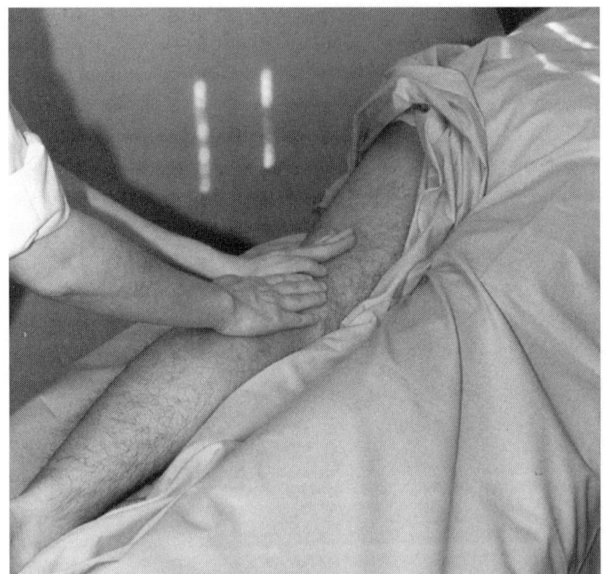

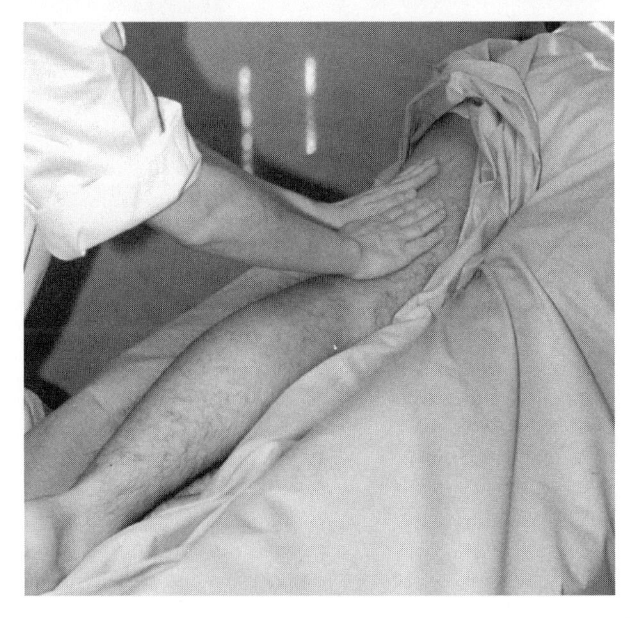

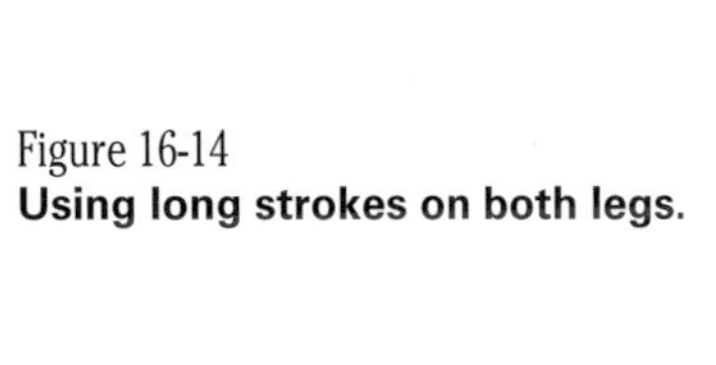

Figure 16-14
Using long strokes on both legs.

work on first, position yourself at the foot. To spread the oil thoroughly and warm the leg before massage, you can either use the long stroke with your fingers pointing straight up the leg, or with cupped hands, as shown in Figure 16-15.

Massaging the Leg

In addition to using basic strokes to massage the receiver's leg, you may also incorporate various passive exercises into your session. One example of such an exercise is called the half lotus leg lift (Figure 16-16 on p. 166), which helps to mobilize the joints and stretch the muscles. This particular exercise gets its name because the movement imitates the half lotus position in yoga. Because of the benefits brought to both the hip joint and the muscles of the front of the thigh, it is extremely useful during a leg massage.

Draining and Working Down the Leg

When massaging the leg, there are certain strokes that will help with the circulation and assist the flow of blood back to the heart. After you have positioned yourself either at the receiver's foot or by the side of his or her leg, you begin to work up from the ankle, first with your thumbs, then with the heels of your hands (Figure 16-17 on p. 166). When you come to the back of the knee, your strokes should be much broader and lighter. If you press too hard, the kneecap will be pushed uncomfortably against the working surface. The draining stroke with the heels of the hands is most effective on the back of the thigh and buttocks, where there is a generous amount of flesh; however, you can also use it on the calves.

Once you have drained the leg up to the hip, you are ready to move down again toward the foot, using a kneading stroke on the thigh and the calf (Figure 16-18 on p. 167). After thoroughly massaging the entire leg, you can either pull down along the inside of the leg in overlapping strokes or wring your hands along the leg (Figure 16-19 on p. 167). The backs of the legs are particularly suitable for wringing work since there are no protruding bones to interrupt your path.

Massaging the Ankle

Like other joints in our body, the ankles are often a great storehouse of tension, blocking the free flow of energy between our feet and our legs. People who experience stiffness in their ankles may suffer from cold feet and thus may find themselves not being grounded, that is, being at a loss between their connection with the ground and with reality. Massaging the ankles will not only help to restore flexibility and assist energy flow; it will also relieve any build-up of fluid in the tissue.

There are three types of movements most often used to massage the ankles. They are rotation, flexing, and pushing (Figure 16-20 on p. 168). Rotating the ankle gives one a sense of flexibility of the joint. Flexing the foot tests the tension in the muscles and tendons. If the hamstrings are tight, you will not be able to push the foot far forward. If the extensor muscles at the front of the lower leg are too tight, pushing the foot backward will be painful.

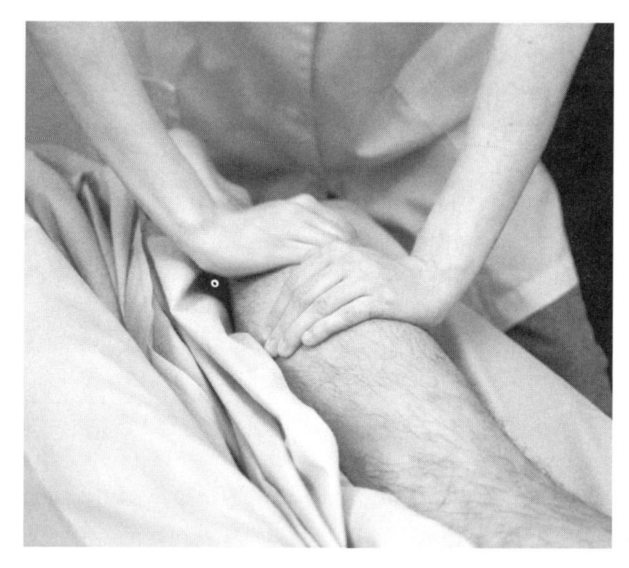

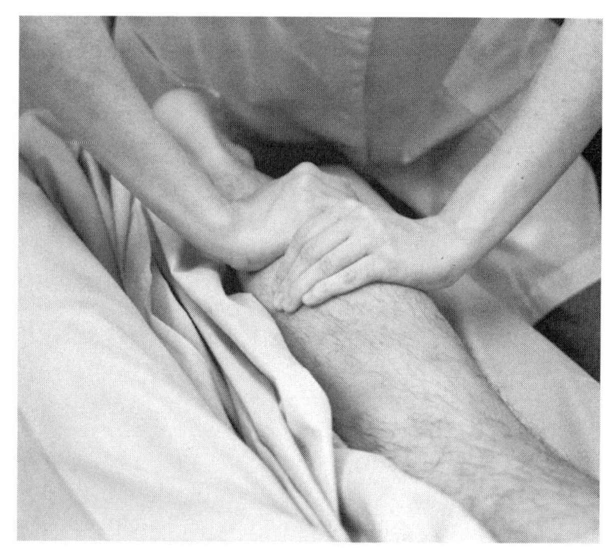

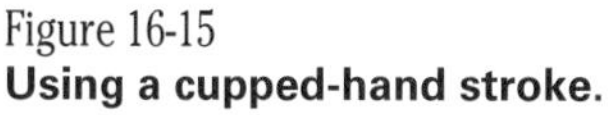

Figure 16-15
Using a cupped-hand stroke.

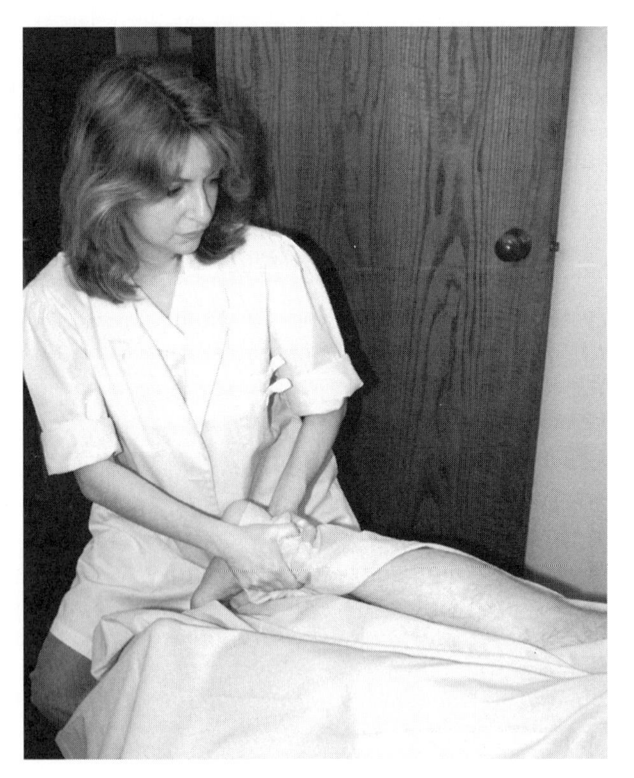

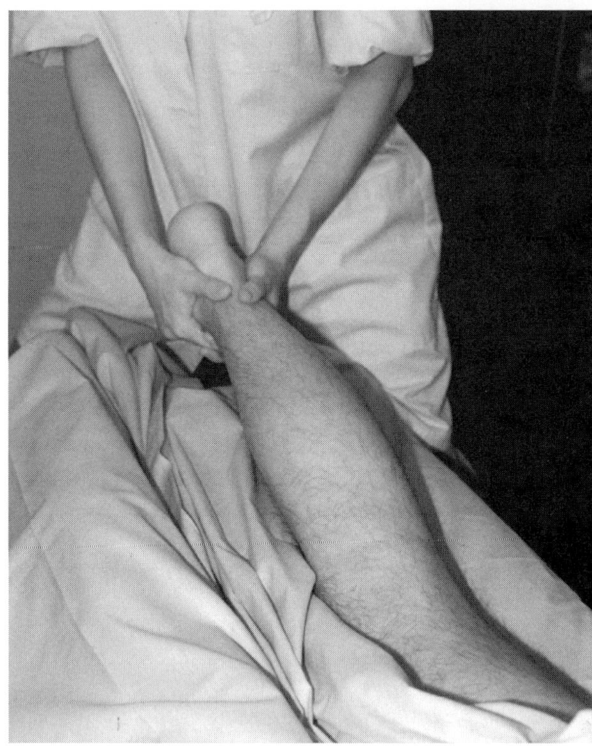

Figure 16-16
Leg lift using the half lotus technique.

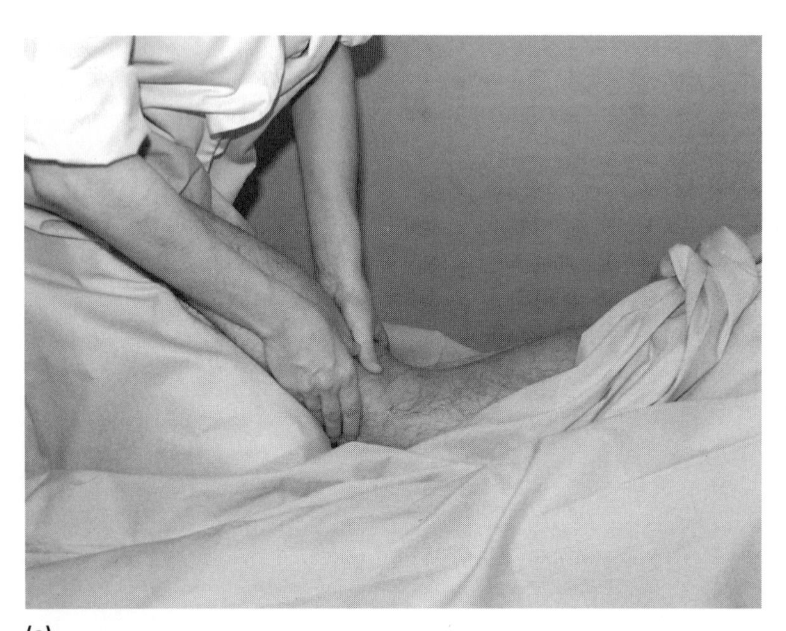

(a)

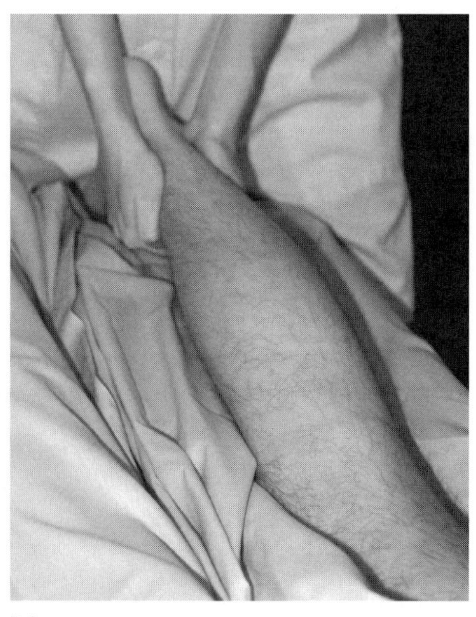

(b)

Figure 16-17
(a) Draining the leg using the thumbs; (b) draining the leg using the heels of the hands.

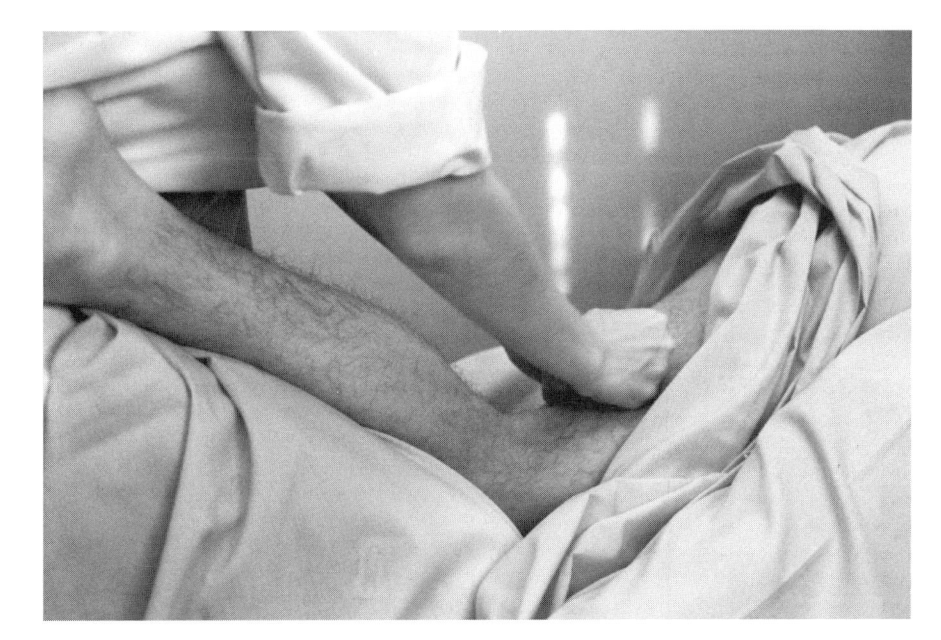

Figure 16-18
Working down the leg using a kneading stroke.

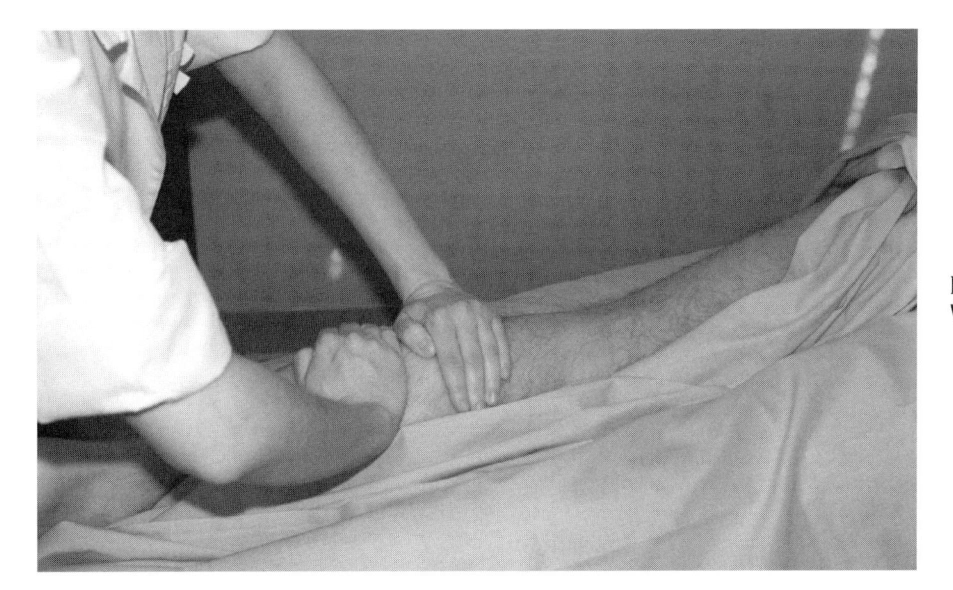

Figure 16-19
Wringing down along the leg.

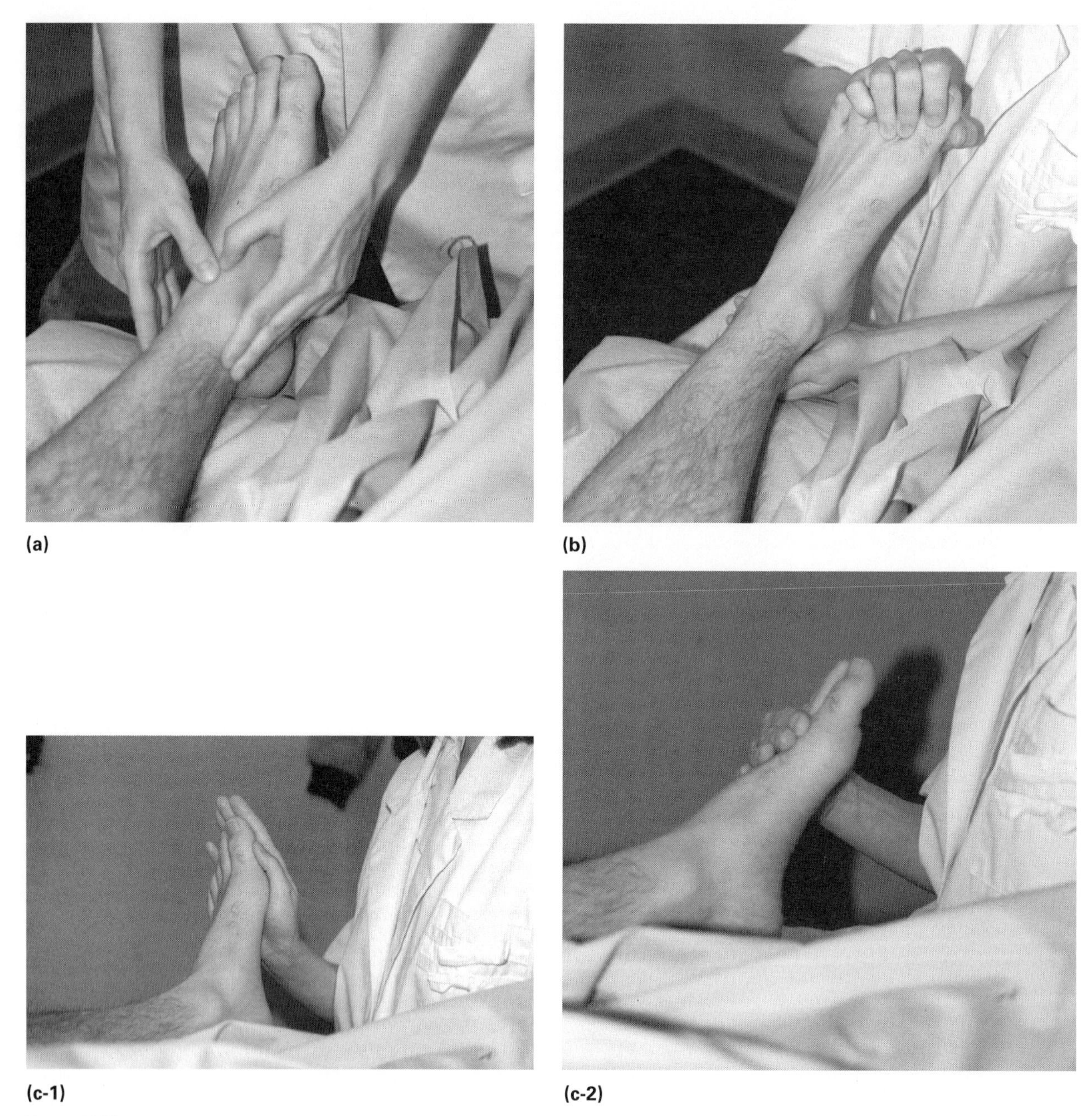

(a) (b) (c-1) (c-2)

Figure 16-20
(a) Working around the ankle; (b) rotating the ankle; (c) pushing the foot down and up.

Massaging the Foot

The human foot has evolved into a highly complex structure, made up of 26 small bones, some of which form the two large supporting arches. In addition to carrying the entire weight of our body, our feet serve as shock absorbers. The soles of our feet also contain thousands of nerve endings, with reflex connections to the rest of our body. Therefore, when the feet are massaged, the entire body is affected. For this reason, many massage therapists concentrate on a foot massage when there is not enough time for a full body massage.

There are four steps to massaging the foot (Figure 16-21). The first step involves cleaning between the tendons. With one hand, hold onto the sole of the foot, making sure that the toes are pointed upward. Use your thumb or fingers of your other hand to press slowly along each channel between the tendons that link the base of the ankle to the toes. Thumbing the sole, which is the second step, involves the supporting of the foot with one hand, while working across

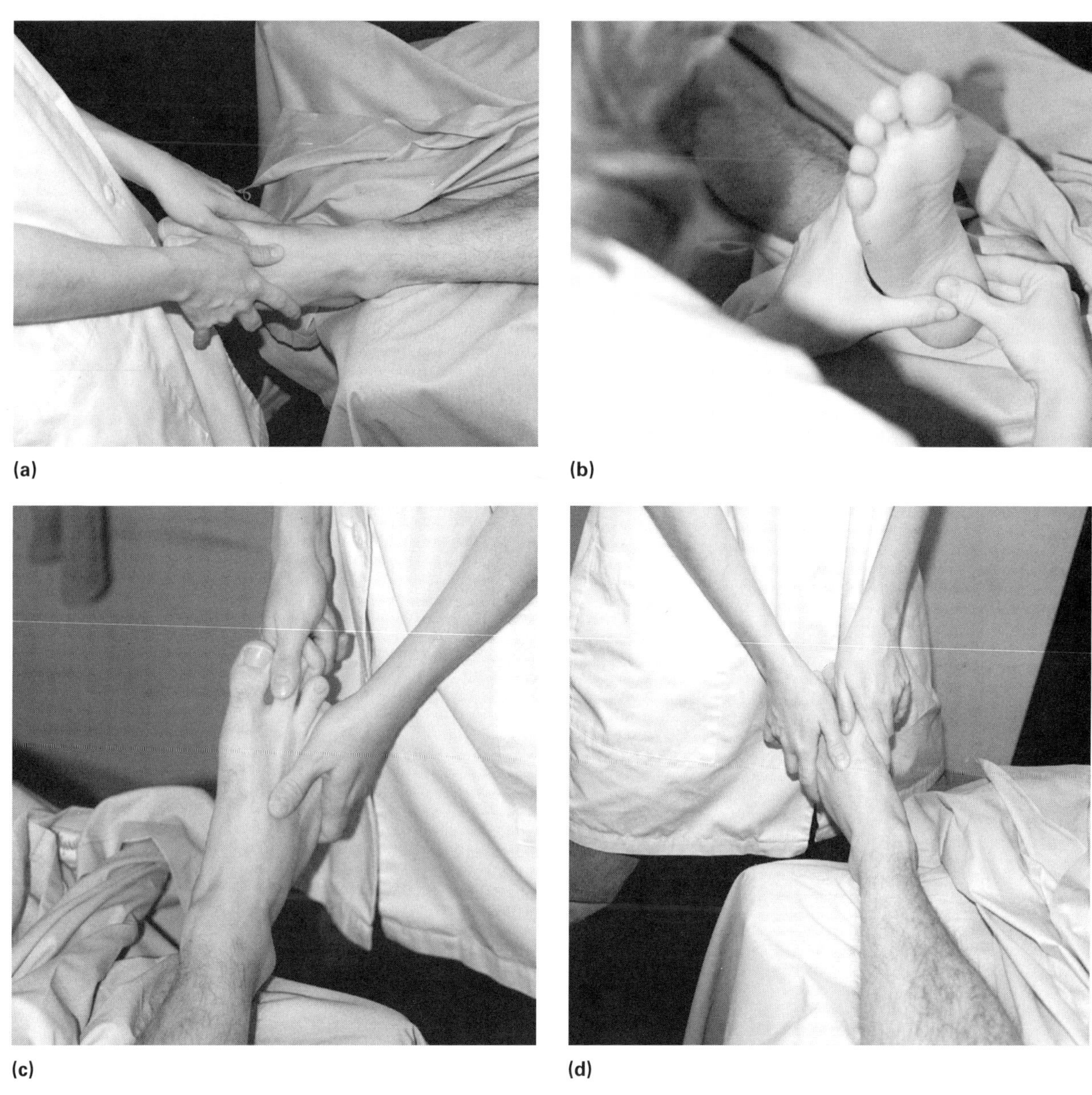

Figure 16-21
Four steps to massaging the foot: (a) cleaning between the tendons; (b) thumbing the sole; (c) stretching the toes; (d) wringing the toes.

the whole of the sole with the thumb of the other hand. It is best to start at the heel and end at the ball of the foot, just under the toes. The third step is to stretch the toes. Working systematically along the toes, first stretch them apart sideways, then stretch each toe backward and forward. Be sure that you check with the receiver as to how far you can stretch the toes, since it is often farther than you can imagine. The fourth step in massaging the foot is wringing the toes. One at a time, hold each toe at the base between your thumb and fingers and tug steadily, twisting it a little from side to side as your fingers slide to the tip and off. As you come off each toe, shake your hand, ridding yourself of any negative energy.

Once you have finished massaging one foot, you are ready to move over to work on the back of the other leg and foot, starting from the beginning of the sequence. Treating the feet ends the massage on the back of the body. After you have completed massaging both legs, instruct the receiver to rest for a few moments; then suggest that he or she turn gently over, ready for massage to the front of the body.

Massaging the Shoulders, the Neck, the Scalp, and the Face

Once the receiver has turned over, you are ready to begin your massage on the front of the body by returning to the shoulders. The shoulders are considered to be one of the principal storehouses of tension in the body. In a healthy person, feelings that arise at one's gut level are often expressed physically through the arms and hands, or verbally, through the throat. However, many of us are forbidden to express our emotions freely as children, and, as such, learn to suppress feelings of anger or sorrow by tightening up in the shoulders and throat. It is for this reason that special attention is often paid to both the back and the front of the shoulders.

The main advantage of working on the shoulders from the front is that the receiver's own weight presses down onto your hands under the back, giving extra impact to the strokes. The sequence of strokes may seem somewhat complex at first, since it happens out of sight, between the receiver's back and the working surface. But once you have learned it, you will find it a most rewarding part of your massage session, and one that feels especially good to the receiver.

Oiling, Stroking, and Stretching

After the receiver has turned over, check to see whether he or she needs a cushion. Then sit down at the head end and begin to apply oil in one continuous long stroke to the whole upper chest, shoulder, and neck area.

Using Long Strokes

To use *long strokes,* you must first place your hands on the upper chest just below the collar bone, fingers pointing toward one another. Slowly draw them apart, heels leading out toward the shoulders (Figure 16-22a). Next, as you reach the shoulders, curve your hands around the joints, then slide them along the tops of the shoulder, until you come to the back of the neck (Figure 16-22b). Complete the sequence by continuing the stroke up the back of the neck to the base of the skull, then up the back of the head and off the crown (Figure 16-22c). After you have completed all three steps to the sequence, you should repeat the entire process over again.

Using Neck Stretches

Neck stretching movements lead on naturally from any of the long strokes. Instead of bringing your hands off the top of the head, you simply stop at the base of the skull and, holding the head securely, gently pull it toward you (Figure 16-23 on p. 172). You can also stretch the neck forward, backward, and to one side. This stretches right along the top of the shoulder and side of the neck.

Massaging the Shoulders

Now that you have loosened the whole neck up a little, you are ready to begin massaging the shoulders. You must remember that when massaging the shoulders, it is important to focus on one side at a time. Laying the head on its side on one hand, you use the other hand to work the whole upper back and neck area on the opposite side, using a three-part sequence (Figure 16-24 on p. 173). Begin the sequence in the same manner as you did for the long stroke, but instead of going up the neck, push down alongside the spine, as far as you can comfortably reach. Then pull your curved fingers very slowly up the groove at the side of the spine and up the back of the neck to the base of the skull. Now use your fingers to make tiny arches all along this side of the base of the skull, working just under the rim of the bone.

The second part of the sequence begins as your hand reaches the shoulder joint, with your fingers curved around under the shoulder and pushed down along the receiver's side. When you reach the waist, pull diagonally across the back and shoulder blade, with your fingers slightly curved, and continue until you come back to the neck and base of the skull. After circling as before at the base of the skull, repeat the movement.

Once your hand has circled the shoulder joint and pulled along the top of the shoulders and up the side and back of the neck, you should already be into the third part of the sequence. The inside edge of the index finger and the web of the thumb should create a taut band. After circling as before at the base of the skull, repeat. Then leave the receiver's head in your hand so you can start to work on the scalp.

Massaging the Scalp

Surprisingly, the scalp can get tense and contribute to both tension headaches and hair problems, such as dandruff and hair loss. Massage helps to relieve this tightness and also aids in the circulation. In the process, it also improves the health of the hair.

The technique involved in massaging the scalp is a three-part sequence (Figure 16-25 on p. 174). The first step is to rotate the scalp. To do this, spread your hand over the receiver's head and rotate it, moving the scalp against the bone. Then "pull off" the hair. Taking a bunch of hair at a time, gently pull from the

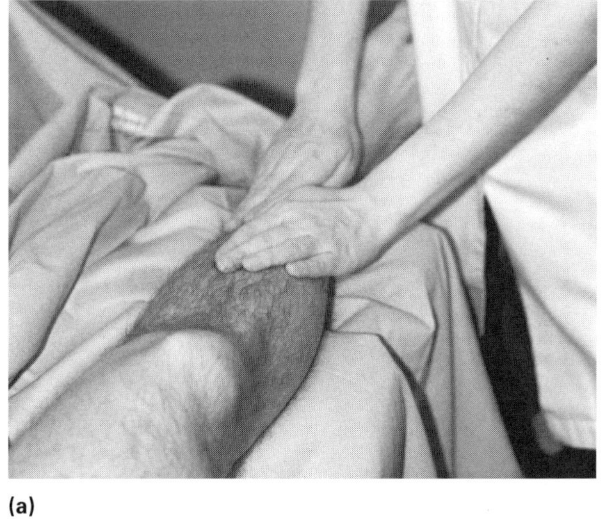

(a)

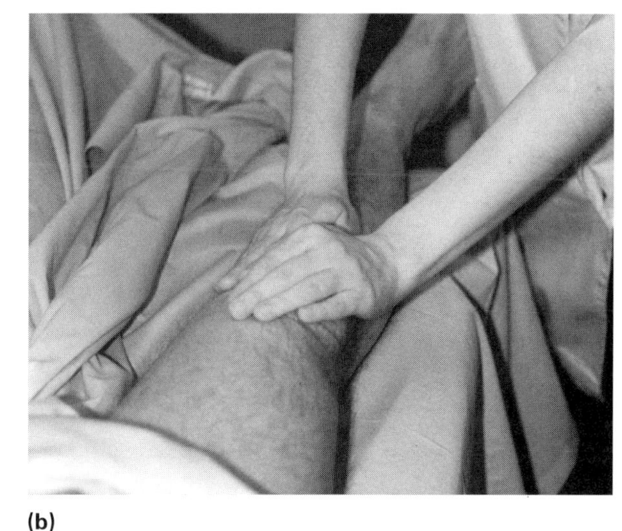

(b)

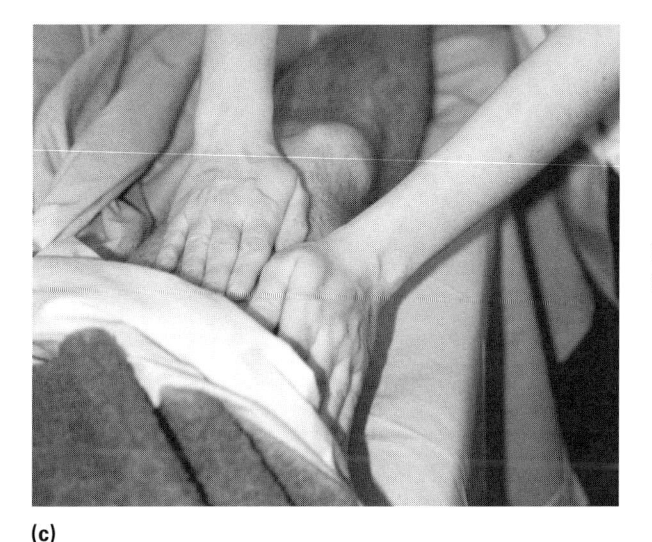

(c)

Figures 16-22a, b, and c
Sequence of using long strokes.

roots and slowly slide your fingers off. Repeat this four or five times on the other side. Finally, you are ready to "shampoo" the hair by rubbing vigorously all over the scalp with your fingertips. Once you have completed the three strokes shown in Figure 16-25, cup your free hand over the receiver's ear and very gently turn the head to the other side.

Performing a Spinal Stretch

Whenever you are working with the shoulders and neck, a spinal stretch is often used, since it is the one stroke which provides the entire spine with a wonderful stretch that helps the receiver to feel remarkably good.

The spinal stretch is the only stroke in the front of shoulders and neck sequence that requires the cooperation of the receiver, who must lift up his or her head to enable you to reach under it with your hands. You may need to practice a little before you can use this stroke effectively. But you should be able to manage it, unless the receiver is very heavy or much larger than you, in which case, you can omit it from the sequence. If you do choose to use it, always make sure to pull from the hara and pelvis, not just from the shoulders.

To execute the spinal stretch, you must first ask the receiver to raise his or her back a little so that you can push your hands as far under it as possible, placing your palms up alongside the spine, as shown in Figure 16-26 (on p. 175). Ask the receiver to relax onto your arms. Once you feel that they have fully let go, start to pull your hands up along the grooves beside the spine, fingertips curved up a little. Travel very slowly along the whole length of the spine, up the neck and back of the head, and end by "pulling off" the hair.

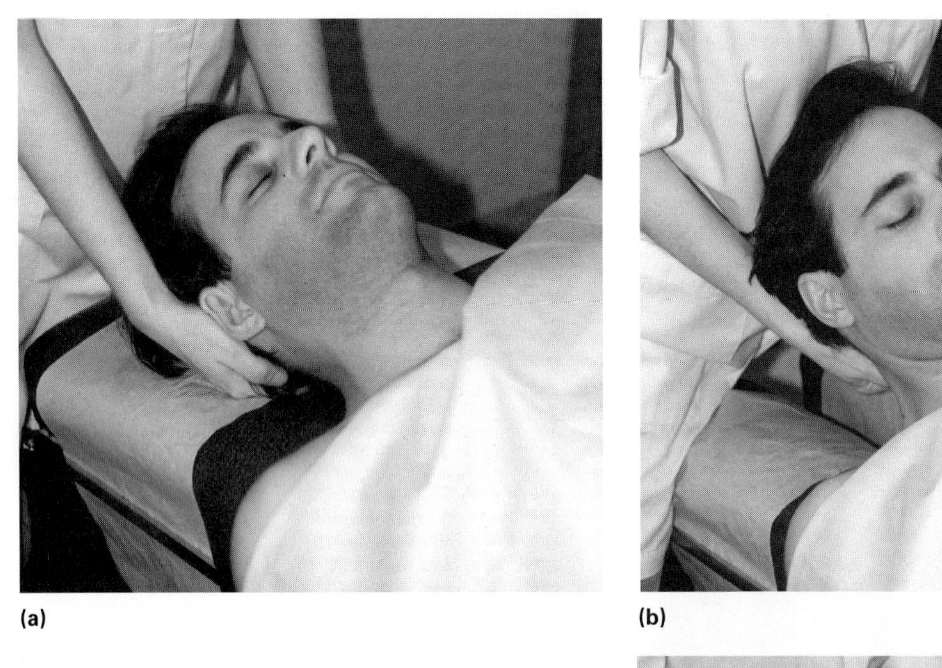

(a) (b)

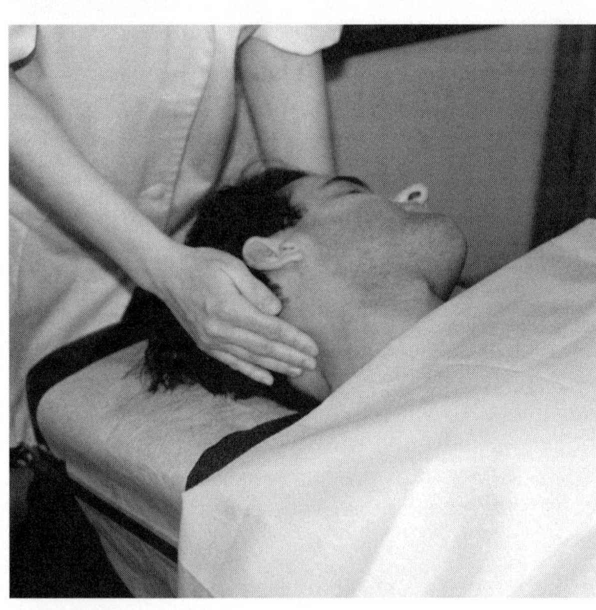

(c)

Figure 16-23
(a) Stretching the neck; (b) stretching the neck up and down; (c) stretching the neck from side to side.

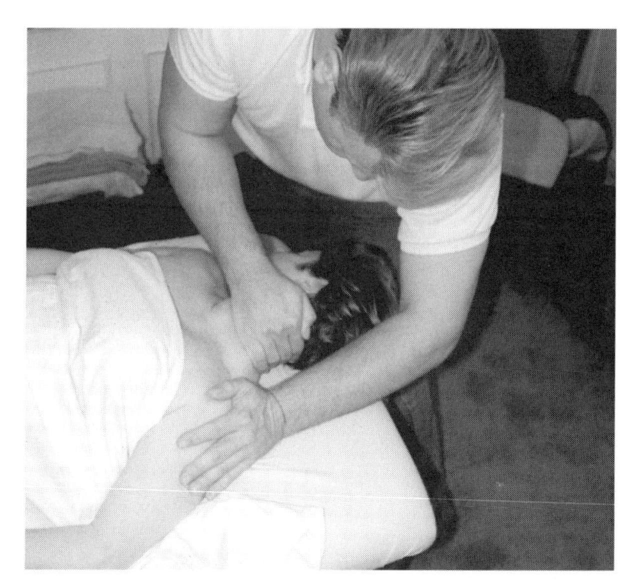

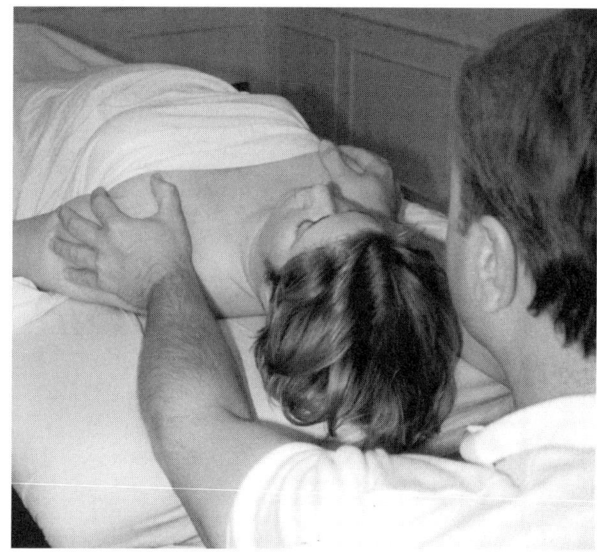

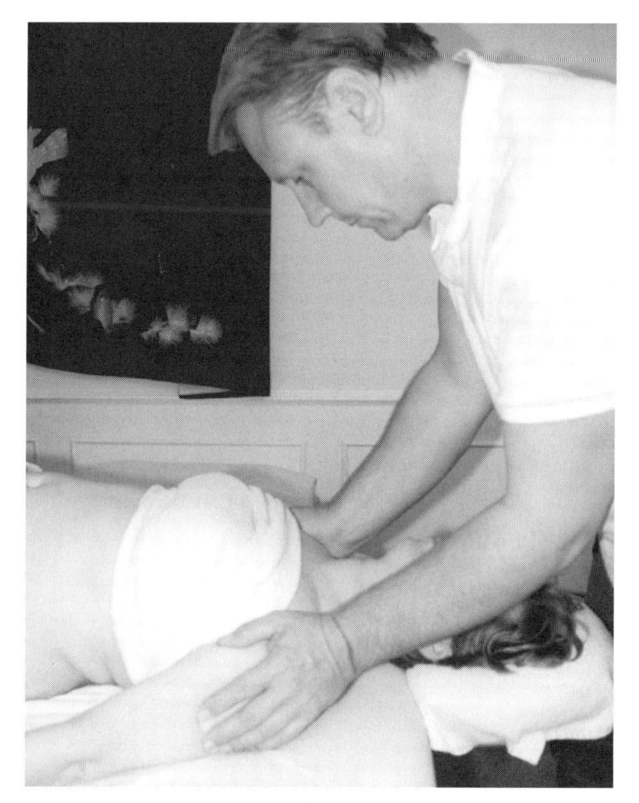

Figure 16-24
Massaging the shoulder using the front and back sequence.

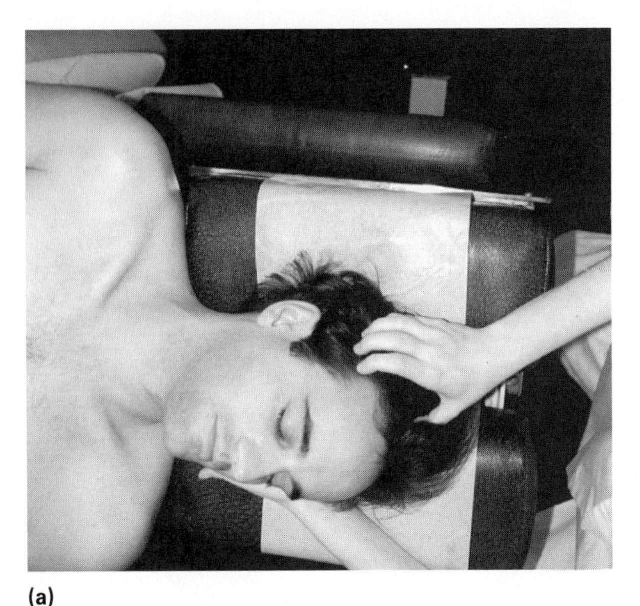

(a)

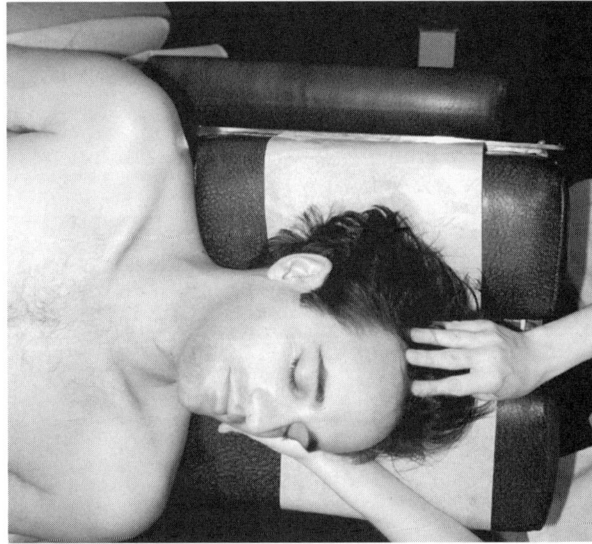

(b)

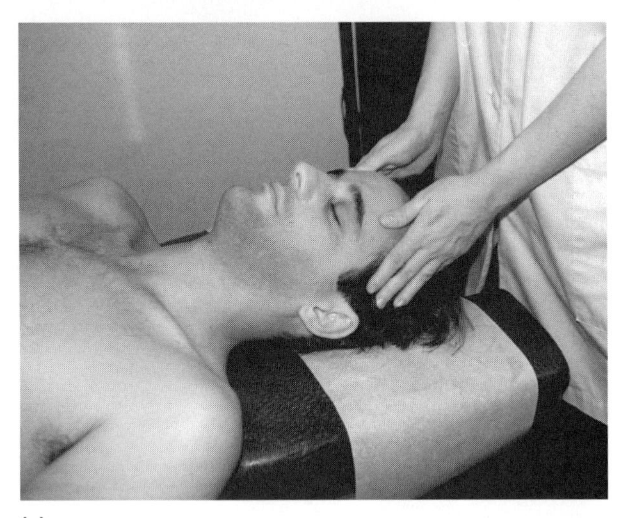

(c)

Figure 16-25
(a) Rotating the scalp; (b) "pulling off" the hair; (c) "shampooing."

Massaging the Face

For most of us, the face is usually the part of a person that we notice first. It is uncovered, exposed, and often the part of the body which tells us the most about the history of its owner. Its character is sculpted by the many tiny muscles that give us the mobility to make facial expressions. Stress and tension are reflected in our face, often noticeable in the tightness around the brows, jaw, and eyes. Joy and serenity, on the other hand, are often viewed by an open, relaxed expression. And whether we wear a mask that shows a smile or a look of surprise, the patterns frozen onto our faces help others to understand our attitudes and character. By enabling us to let go of some of our masks, a caring face massage can lead to a sense of deep relaxation and contentedness throughout our whole body.

You do not need to oil your hands to massage the face, since you probably will already have enough on your fingers to massage this relatively small area. However, because the structure of each face is different and is much bonier and less fragile than it looks, before you begin the massage on the receiver for the first time, it's important that you practice on your own face to see how it feels.

Sequence for Massaging the Face

Once you are ready to begin the massage, you must position yourself sitting or standing at the receiver's head (Figure 16-27). You will remain in this position throughout the sequence of the massage. Make sure you keep your pressure even as you work down from the forehead to the chin.

The first part of the sequence begins with the forehead (Figure 16-28). Place your thumbs at the center of the forehead, just above the brows, anchoring your hands on the sides of the head. Moving up a

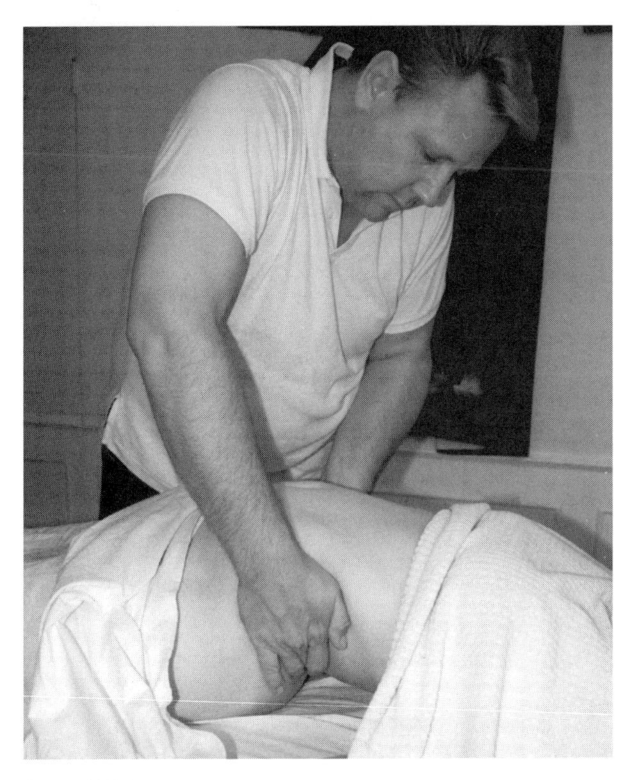

Figure 16-26
Executing a spinal stretch.

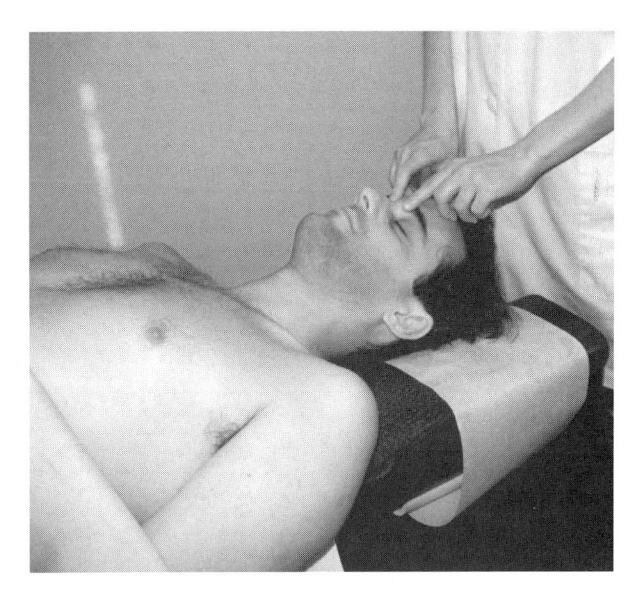

Figure 16-28
Massaging the forehead.

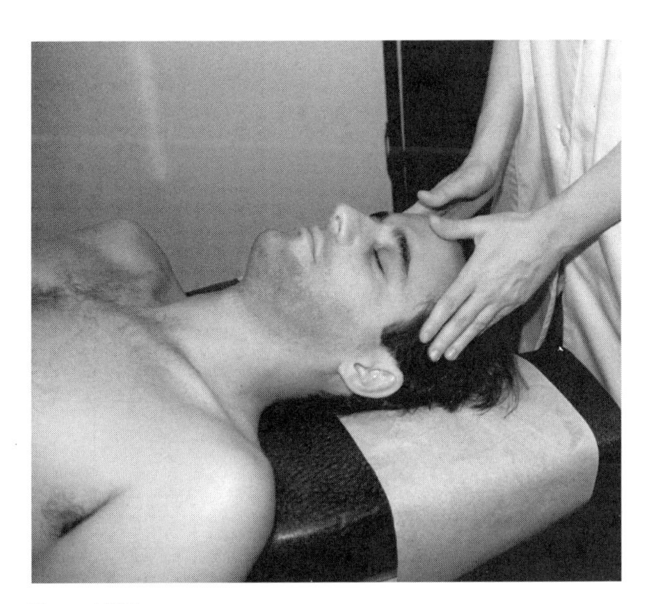

Figure 16-27
Position for massaging the face.

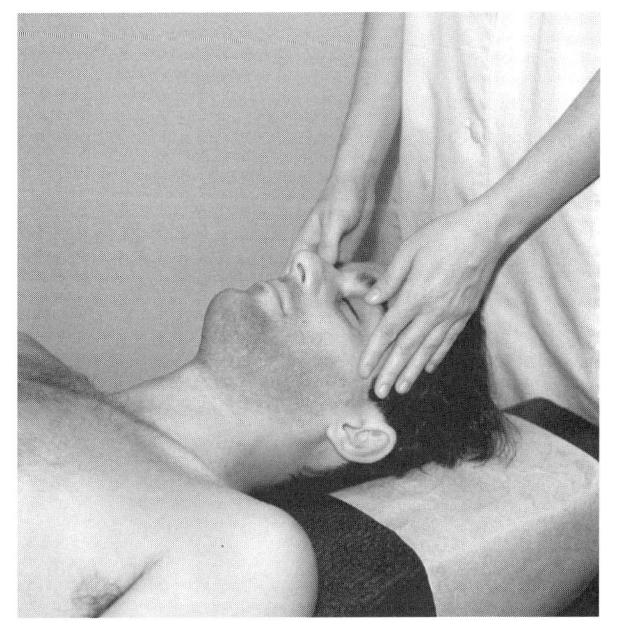

Figure 16-29
Massaging the eyebrows, eyelids, and eyes.

strip at a time, draw your thumbs apart slowly, coming out over the hair and off the sides of the head. Cover the whole forehead in this way, traveling up as far as the hairline.

Continuing to move down the face, you should begin to work over the eyebrows, eyelids, and nose to the chin (Figure 16-29). Working around the eye, eyebrows, and temples in particular often helps to soothe away stress, relieve headaches, and clear the sinuses.

The technique involved in massaging the eyebrows and eyes starts at the inner end of the eyebrows. Draw your thumbs firmly out of the sides over the hairline and off the head, and smooth the entire browline. Next, draw your thumbs smoothly and gen-

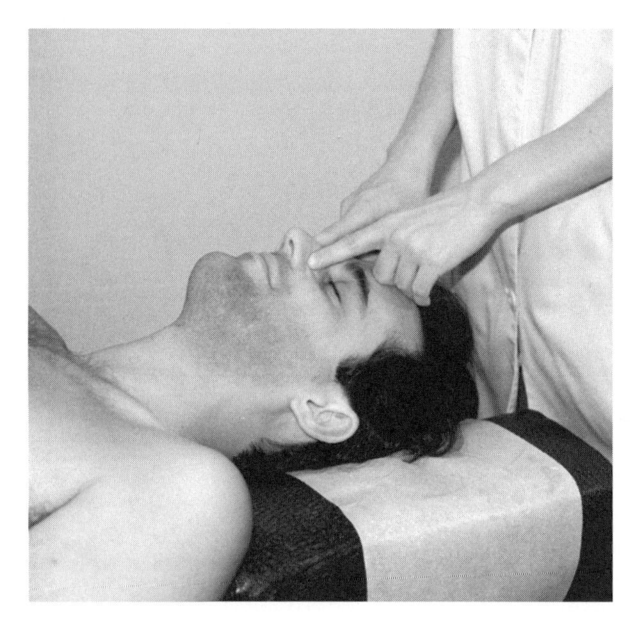

Figure 16-30
Massaging the nose.

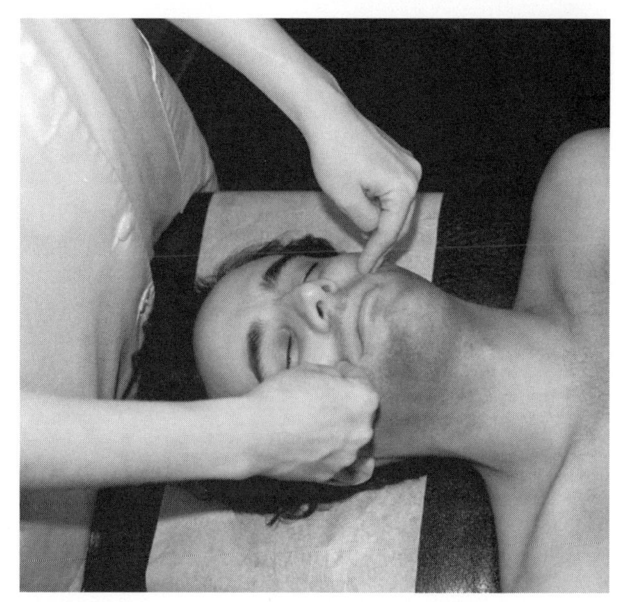

Figure 16-31
Massaging the cheeks.

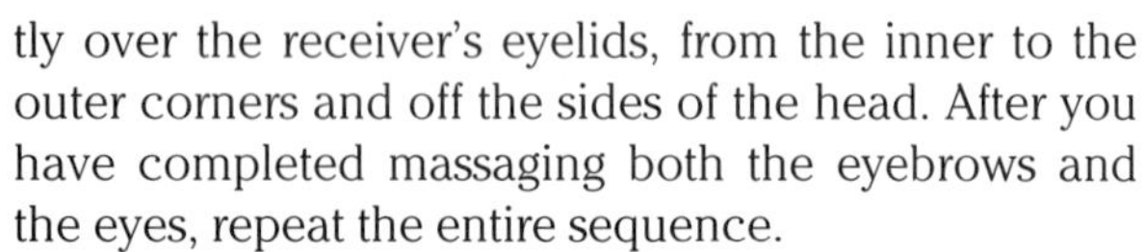

tly over the receiver's eyelids, from the inner to the outer corners and off the sides of the head. After you have completed massaging both the eyebrows and the eyes, repeat the entire sequence.

You are now ready to massage the nose, cheeks, chin, and jawline. Using your thumbs alternately, stroke down the bridge of the nose from the top to the tip (Figure 16-30). Then gently squeeze the tip of the nose between your thumbs and index fingers. Carefully moving your fingers down the face, beginning just under the inner corners of the eyes, stroke your thumbs across the cheekbone to the hairline above the ear and off the head (Figure 16-31). Repeat the stroke in strips as you travel gradually down the face, below the cheekbone, and above the upper lip and below the lower one. When working near the nose, always be careful not to close the breathing passage.

Massaging the Chin and Jawbone

When massaging the lower part of the receiver's face, you will be using a squeezing technique. Begin by squeezing the chin, working along the jawbone and then circling over the chewing muscles (Figure 16-32). If you find it difficult to locate these muscles, place your fingers on the person's cheeks and ask him or her to clench their teeth. By doing this, you will be able to feel the muscles rise up and harden as they contract in the face.

After you have completed massaging the chin, hold the rim of the jawbone at the chin, and then draw your hands slowly apart, gently squeezing right along the jawbone as far as the ear lobe (Figure 16-33).

Massaging the Cheeks and Ears

Massaging the cheeks and ears involves a two-part sequence which begins with a broad stroke across the cheeks, and ends with stretching and squeezing the ears (Figure 16-34). Gently place the heels of your hands on either side of the nose, with

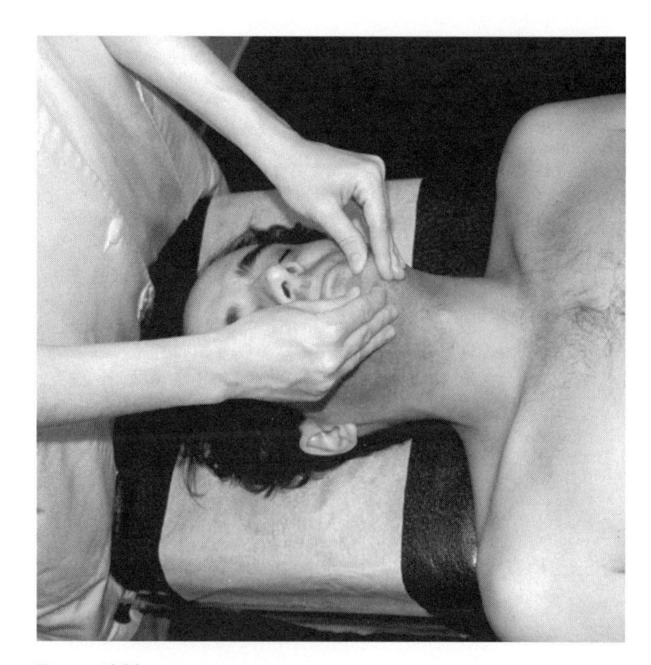

Figure 16-32
Massaging the chin.

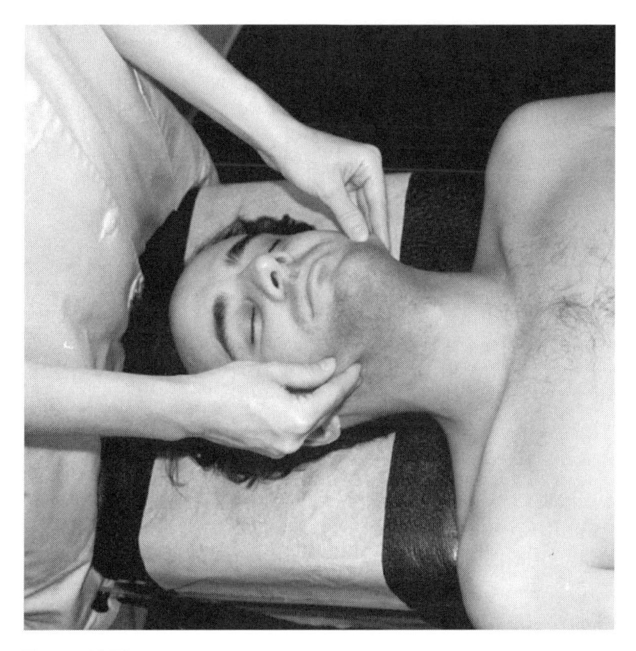

Figure 16-33
Massaging the jawbone.

your fingers pointing toward the ears. Now, slowly part your hands, carefully gliding them firmly over the cheeks toward the ears. Grasp the ears between your fingers and the heels of your hands and very gently stretch them away from the head. Complete the sequence by squeezing all around the ears with your fingers and thumbs.

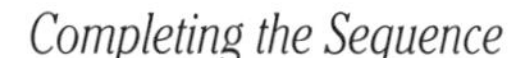

Completing the Sequence

Once you have finished massaging the cheeks and ears, you are ready to connect the face to the head. This involves using a long stroke which is completed in three parts (Figure 16-35 on p. 178). First, cup your palms over the receiver's eyes with your thumbs on either side of the nose. Remain there for a moment, allowing the eyes to rest within the darkness of your hands. Then, using your fingers first, begin to slide your hands smoothly down over the face, across the cheeks, and under the ears to the back of the neck. Without stopping, pull your hands up the neck and, cupping your hands under the back of the head, draw them toward you, coming slowly off the top of the head and then into the air.

Massaging the Arms and the Hands

Our arms and hands are intimately involved in how we relate to one another, and with the world as a whole. They are instruments we use to "do" and to express. And out of these instruments, feelings can flow freely, without tensions. Through our arms and hands, we express our most powerful emotions, showing love by embracing, giving, protecting, or stroking; rage or anger through hitting, shaking our fists, or punching. An arms and hand massage is, therefore, a wonderfully liberating and relaxing experience, especially for those of us who tend to bottle up our feelings and emotions.

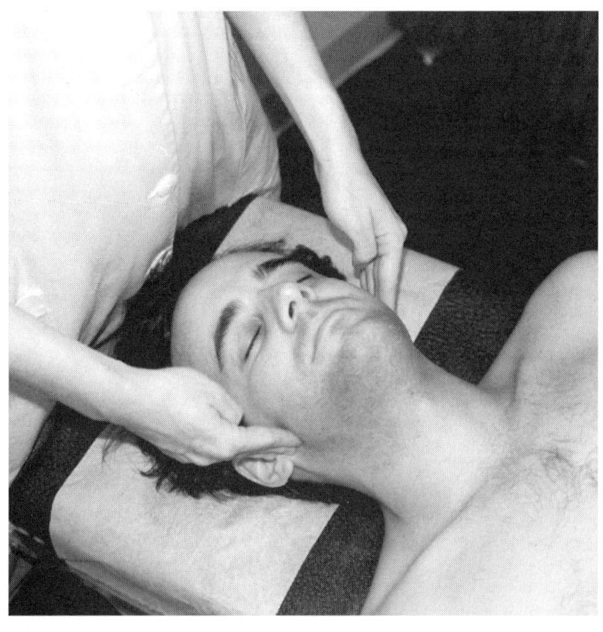

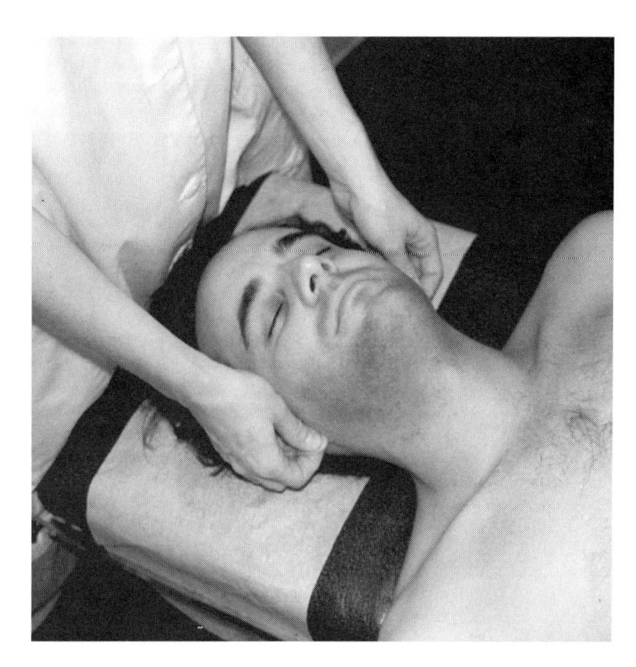

Figure 16-34
Massaging the cheeks and ears.

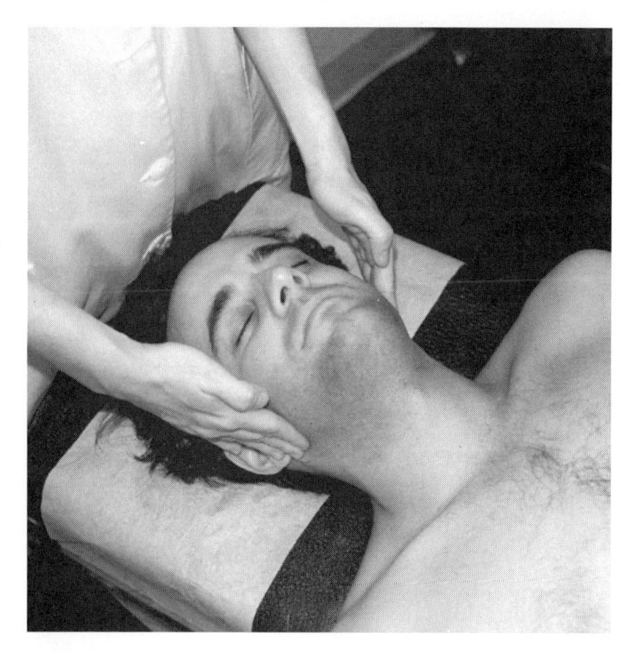

Figure 16-35
Connecting the face to the head.

Oiling and Stretching

To work on the arms and hands, you will have to position yourself to the receiver's side, level with his or her hand and facing the head. Start by oiling and warming one of the arms, using the long stroke. Always remember to keep these initial strokes slow, helping the receiver to become aware of each new part of the body.

To begin the long stroke, rest your oiled hands on the receiver's wrist, fingers pointing up the arms. Then glide your hands up the arm, undulating over the contours, as shown in Figure 16-36a. Just before you reach the shoulder joint, let your leading, or outside, hand curve over the joint while your other hand curves down onto the inner arm, just below the axilla (Figure 16-36b). Embracing as much of the arm as possible, pull your hands down the arm to the wrist. Complete the stroke by wrapping the receiver's hand into your two palms as you slide them down and off the fingertips.

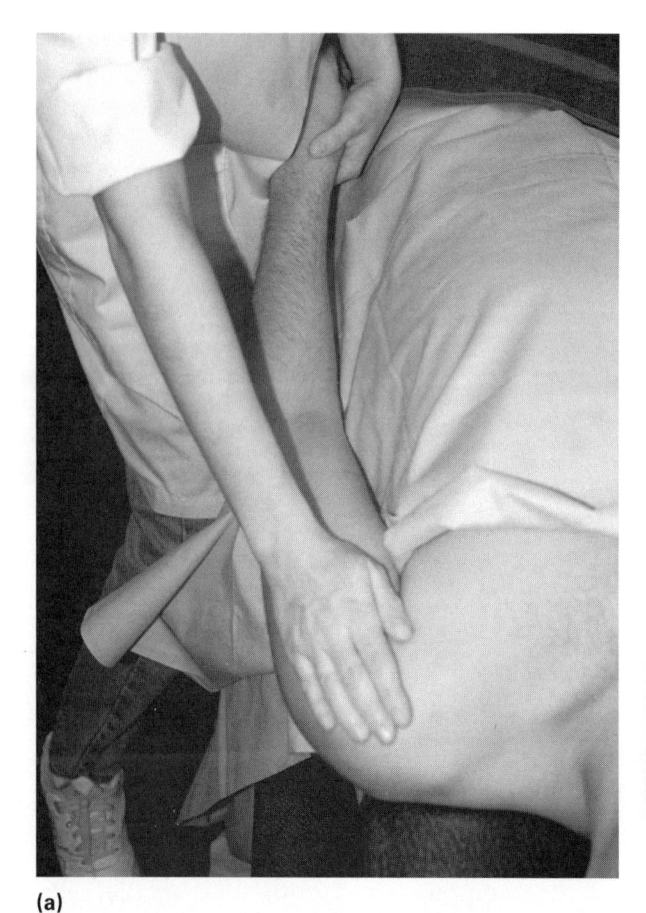

(a)

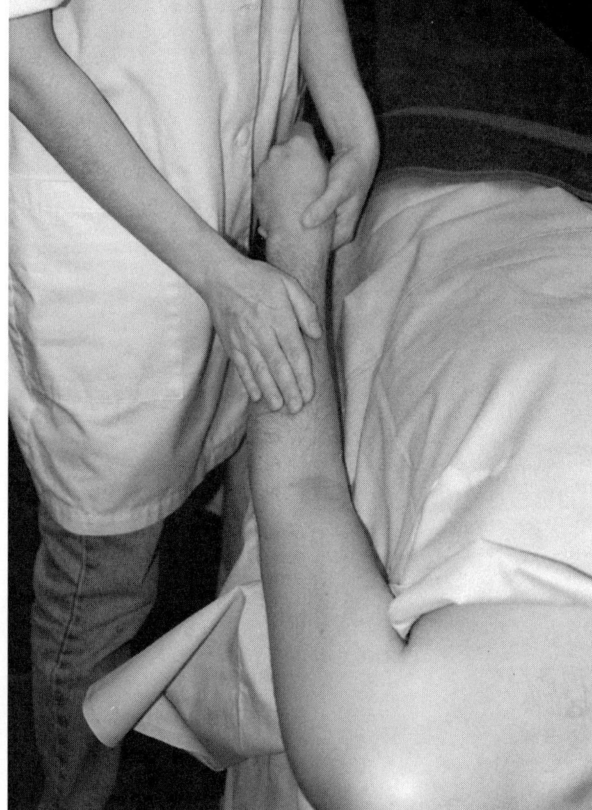

(b)

Figure 16-36
(a) Using the long stroke to massage the arm and hand; (b) completing the long stroke used to massage the arm and hand.

Draining and Stretching the Arm

The four-step sequence used to drain and stretch the arm involves working with the circulation of the blood and lymph. Its purpose is to assist the lymphatic flow and the blood's venous return to the heart. Since veins are located closer to the skin's surface than are the arteries, they respond more readily to external pressure.

Start the sequence by first draining the forearm, then work systematically along the upper arm (Figure 16-37). While squeezing down the forearm, you may notice that the receiver's fingers are opening and closing. This is because muscles controlling the fingers are in the forearm.

After you have drained the forearm, lift the receiver's arm and let it bend at the elbow with the hand hanging down on the other side of the neck, so that the upper arm rises vertically. Grasp it near the elbow between both hands and pull down toward the shoulder joint, squeezing firmly. Then, kneeling at the receiver's shoulder, link one arm under the elbow joint, making sure that the crooks of your arms are together. Take hold of your own opposite forearm near the elbow, and with your free hand, anchor the receiver's wrist. Now use your body to lift the arm, stretching his or her shoulder up off the floor. Then bring it down gently. The sequence is completed by first taking hold of the receiver's wrist and lifting the arm above the head, and then pulling gently on the wrist to stretch the arm. At the same time, run your other hand firmly down the side of the rib cage from the axilla so that you stretch all the way along the arm and side.

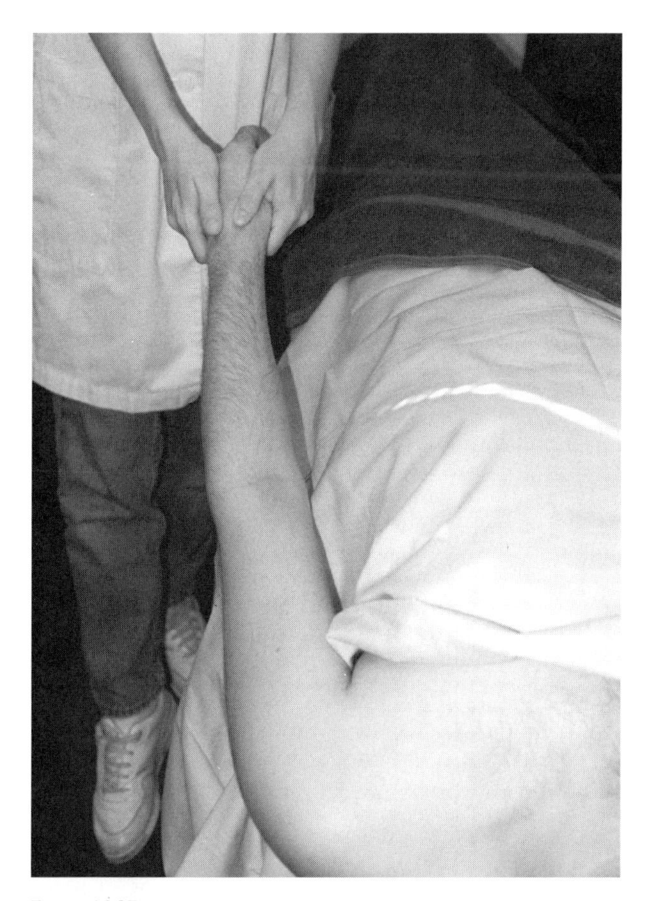

Figure 16-37
Draining and stretching the arm.

Massaging the Shoulder Joint and Arm

Once you have stretched the arm and shoulder joint, place it back by the receiver's side and work around the shoulder girdle and down the arm. Begin with a stroke that squeezes from the center of the upper chest and back out to the shoulder joint; then continue with some medium depth work down the whole arm to the elbow and the wrist.

Squeezing the Shoulder Joint and Kneading the Arm

To squeeze the shoulder joint, first place one hand on the middle of the receiver's upper chest, below the collarbone, and the other under the middle of the upper back, just below the neck. Sandwiching the body between your hands, draw them slowly toward the shoulder joint, leading with the heels of your hands, as shown in Figure 16-38. When both hands reach the joint, curve them around the top of the arm and work deeply around the joint.

After you have squeezed the shoulder joint, massage down the arm, using a kneading stroke, and then wring the whole limb until you reach the wrist (Figure 16-39). Try to pay particular attention to the elbow, carefully exploring around the joint with your thumb and fingertips.

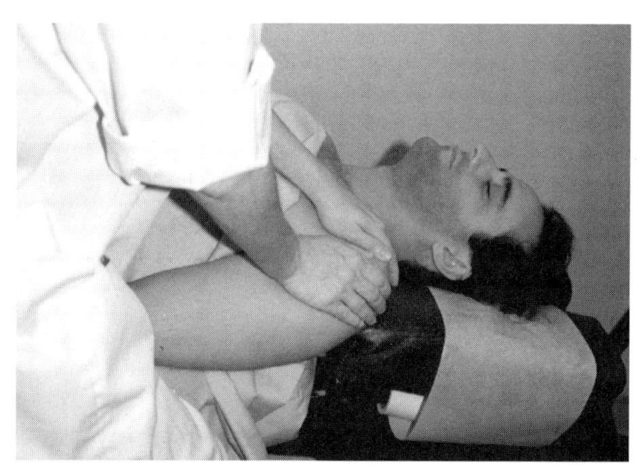

Figure 16-38
Squeezing the shoulder joint.

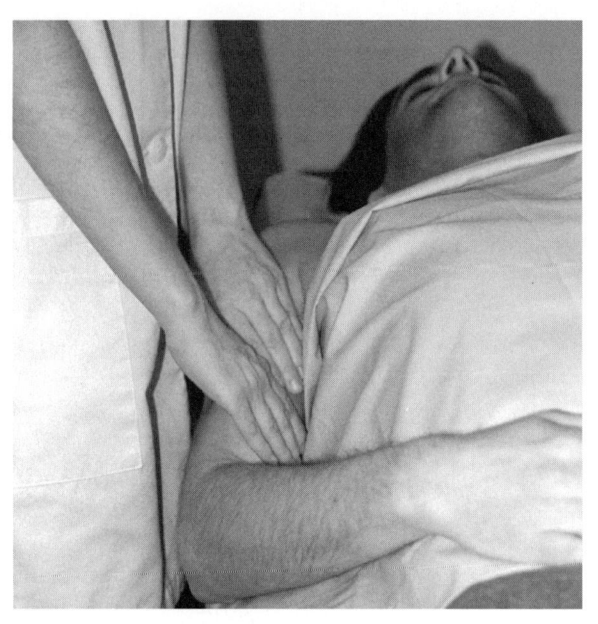

Figure 16-39
Kneading the arm.

Massaging the Wrist and Hand

Massaging the hand is especially relaxing, both because our hands are so accustomed to being touched and because, like our feet, the hands have reflex connections with the rest of our body.

Sequence for Massaging the Wrist and Hand

The sequence for massaging the wrist and hand involves four parts: working around the wrist, opening the palm, cleaning between the bones, and wringing off the fingers.

Begin by lifting the receiver's forearm and resting it on the elbow. Now use your thumbs to work in small circles over the whole wrist area, holding the wrist between your thumbs and fingers (Figure 16-40a). Grasp the hand with your fingers on the palm and the heels of your hands on the back. Then squeeze and stretch the hand open by drawing your fingers away from one another while pressing the heels of your hands down (Figure 16-40b). Hold the receiver's wrist to support the hand. Now use the thumb and index fingers of your free hand to work along each of the grooves between the bones of the hand, from the wrist to the webs between the fingers (Figure 16-40c). Complete the sequence by enclosing the thumb and each of the fingers in turn in your hand and gently pulling them, then stretch and twist them as you slide your hand down and off the tip (Figure 16-40d). Move over to the other side and repeat the sequence on the other arm.

Massaging the Torso

When we massage the torso, we are exposing the receiver's most unprotected and vulnerable part of his or her body. The front of the torso is often related to how we feel and the way we relate to others. It is also the part of the body which contains many of our most vital organs, such as our heart and lungs. Therefore, prior to starting the massage process, try to take a few moments to observe which part of the torso moves when the person takes a breath. Our breathing pattern is intimately connected with our vitality and our emotional health. If the person is trusting, having this area massaged can be a profound experience for both yourself and them, since it establishes a deep contact between the two of you.

Oiling and Stroking

To correctly oil and use long strokes on the front of the torso, you must position yourself to the receiver's head. Always go gently over the solar plexus and belly, until you have a sense of how trusting they are. Now rest your hands gently on the middle of the upper chest (Figure 16-41a on p. 182). Then let them slowly glide down the center of the torso, allowing them to mould to the forms. Just below the navel, let your hands divide and curve out to the sides. Then pull them back up the body along the sides.

If you choose, you may use a broad circle stroke to massage the torso. To do so, start from the same position as you did when you used long strokes. But when your hands divide on the receiver's abdomen, let them describe large overlapping circles as you travel smoothly up the sides (Figure 16-41b).

Massaging the Rib Cage and the Chest

In addition to protecting the vital organs located in our upper chest, the rib cage also plays an important role in the breathing process. While we often tend to think of our rib cage as a fixed and static object, when breathing correctly, the ribs rise up, pushing the mediastinum, or breastbone, forward, and thus open up the chest cavity, causing air to be drawn into our lungs. The muscles which are used in the act of breathing are the large diaphragm muscle that crosses our body horizontally just below the rib cage, and those connecting the ribs themselves. To allow proper breathing, the diaphragm must be relaxed and the rib cage flexible. Therefore, massaging this area helps to loosen these muscles and thus increases the mobility of the ribs. In this way, it helps the receiver to breathe more deeply.

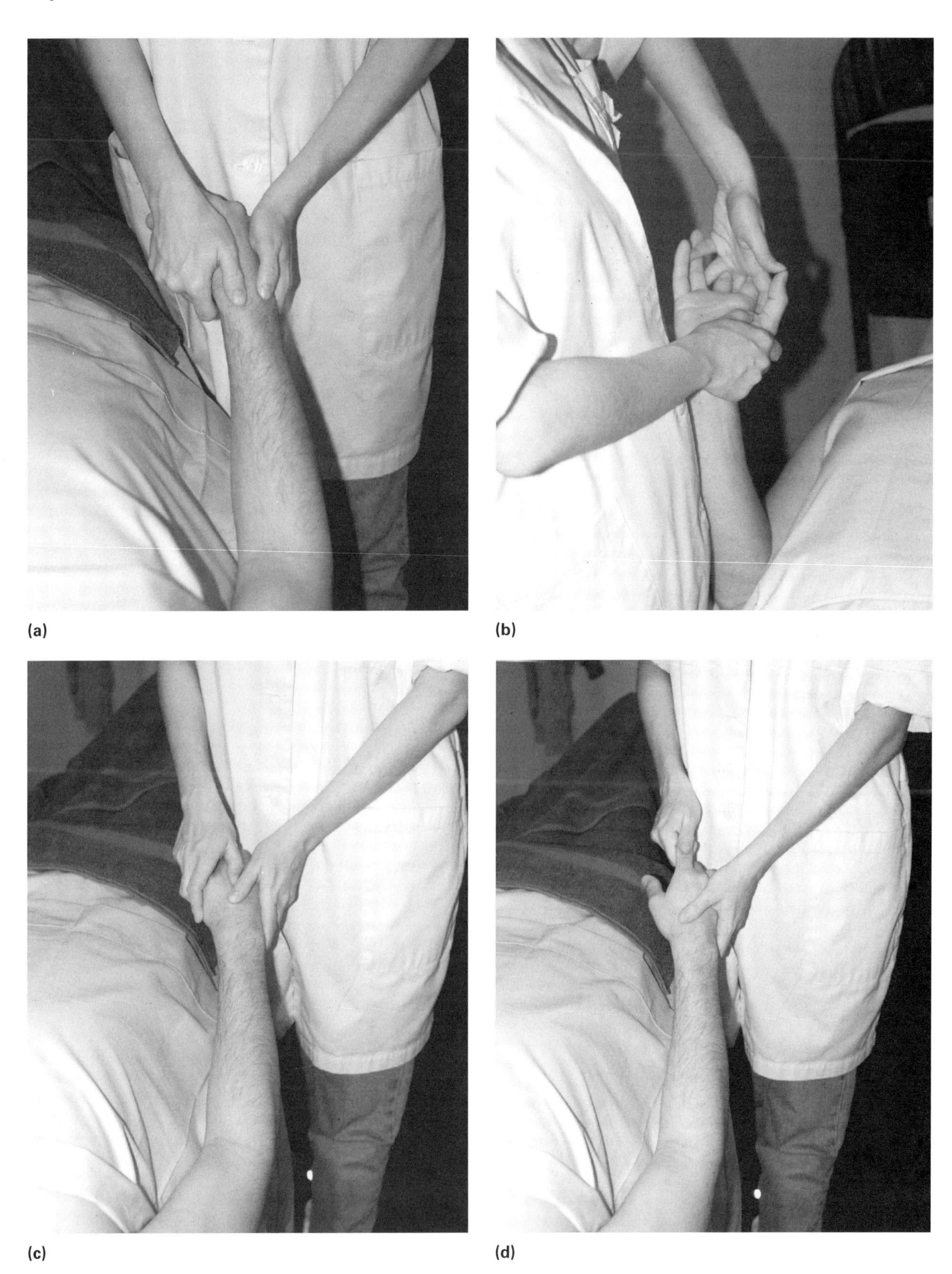

(a) (b) (c) (d)

Figure 16-40
(a) Working around the wrist; (b) opening the palm; (c) cleaning between the bones; (d) wringing off the fingers.

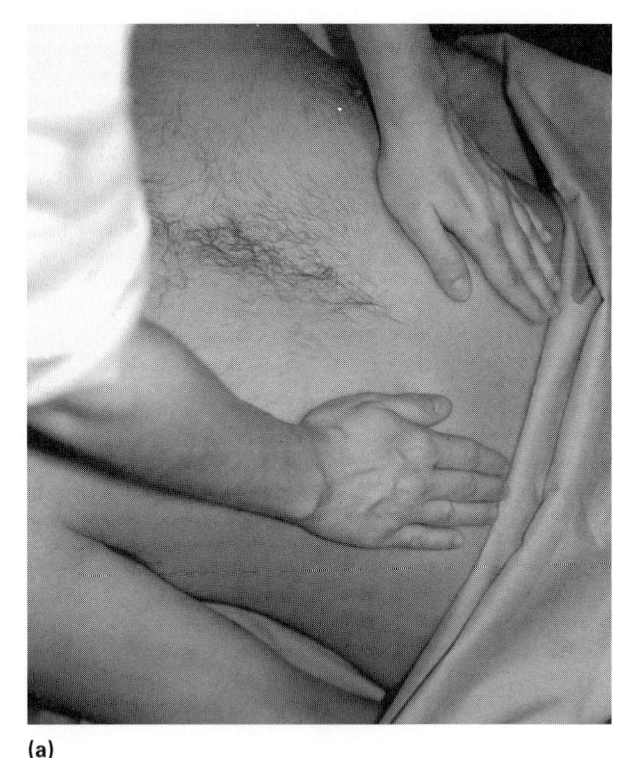

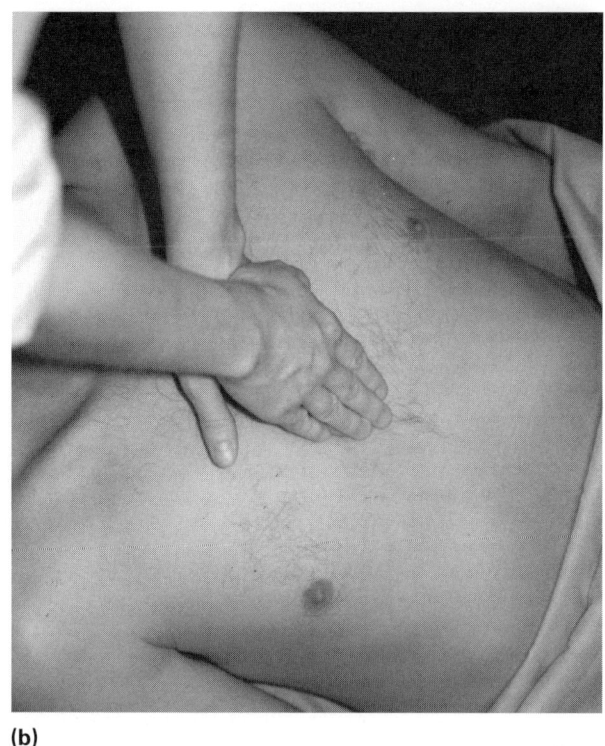

(a) (b)

Figure 16-41
(a) Using long strokes to massage the front of the torso; (b) using broad circling strokes to massage the front of the torso.

Sequence for Massaging the Rib Cage and Chest

Massaging the rib cage and chest involves a three-part sequence. These include working between the ribs, pulling up on the sides, and kneading the pectoral muscles.

After you have positioned yourself at the receiver's head, place your first two fingers of both hands at the center of the upper chest, in the grooves on either side of the topmost rib. Pressing firmly, draw your fingers out to the sides and off the body. Repeat, moving down to the grooves on either side of the rib below. Continue right down the rib cage in this way, as if you were tracing the rungs of a ladder. When you reach the bottom of the mediastinum, you will find that the ribs no longer start at the center. Therefore, you must curve your hands around to work along them, as shown in Figure 16-42a. If the receiver is a female, you should avoid working on the ribs that lie directly under the breasts. When you reach the breasts, press along the grooves for a short distance only, and then move down to the next rib. Do not press into the soft tissue of the breasts themselves. Continue the full stroke once past the line of the breasts.

Leaning over the receiver, use alternate strokes to pull up one side of the rib cage from the waist to the axilla (Figure 16-42b). When working on a female, remember to work around, and not directly across, the breasts. While you are still working on the same side of the body, thoroughly knead the pectoral muscle, that is, the muscle that forms the "pit" of the arm and supports the breast (Figure 16-42c). Then slide your hands across the body and repeat the pulling-up and kneading strokes on the opposite side.

Massaging the Abdomen

To massage the abdomen, you should first position yourself to one side, level with his or her belly (Figure 16-43 on p. 184). The abdomen is highly sensitive, so in the beginning, gently let your hands come down and then pause for a moment before you start. Begin by moving your hands in clockwise circles around the belly. It's important that you travel clockwise, since this echoes the direction of the large intestine. After you have rotated your hands over the belly in a broad circle, using smaller circles, gradually increase the depth of your pressure. End the massage on the front of the torso by working with the rhythm of the receiver's breath. While the receiver breathes slowly and deeply, you should be gliding your hands over the torso in a long circulatory stroke; up from the belly to the chest on an inhalation, and

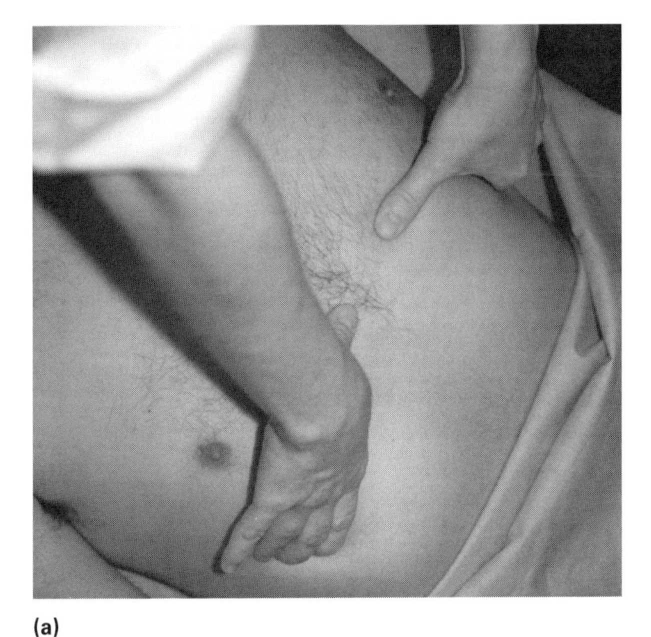

(a)

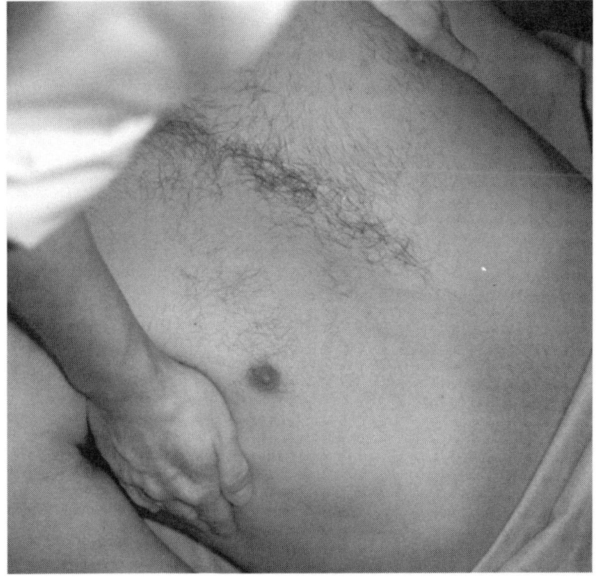

(b)

(c)

Figure 16-42
(a) Massaging between the ribs; (b) pulling up on the sides; (c) kneading the pectoral muscle.

down the sides on an exhalation. Remember, it's up to you to follow the receiver's breath with your hand, and not vice versa.

Sequence for Massaging the Abdomen

Massaging the abdomen involves using broad circling, spiraling, and long stroking movements. Begin by letting your hands come to rest very gently on the receiver's belly and then remain there for a moment or two. Then move both hands clockwise around it, letting them flow over the contours. One hand can complete whole circles, but the other will have to break contact each time the hands cross (Figure 16-44a on p. 184).

Still moving in a clockwise direction, divide your broad circles into smaller ones, making sure that you let your hands spiral around as they travel over the belly. Then ask the receiver to breathe slowly and deeply. Facing the head, rest your hands on the belly, fingers pointing up the body. As he or she inhales and the chest rises, slide your hands up the center of the torso; as they exhale and the chest contracts, circle your hands around the shoulders and pull down the sides of the torso (Figure 16-44b). Bring your hands back to the belly and repeat from the beginning, two or three times. When you pull your hands down the sides for the last time, continue down over the hips and off the toes.

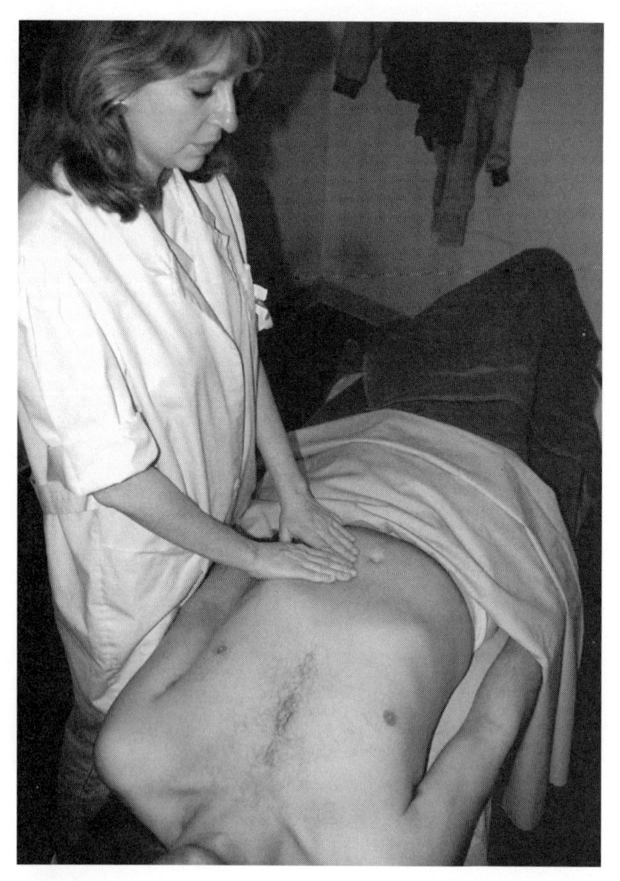

Figure 16-43
Positioning to massage the abdomen.

Massaging the Front of the Legs

A whole body massage ends on the front of the legs. This is so we can bring the receiver's awareness right down to the toes, and he or she leaves the session feeling grounded and at one with the universe. The sequence for massaging the front of the legs is similar to the one you used on the backs of the legs. However, here the terrain is a little different. You are working with the soft muscle area of the thigh, on the bony areas of the shin, and the knee. Knees that are continually braced or pulled back can often indicate that the person is insecure, or that he or she is striving to maintain a hold on life and stand their ground. Massage can help to release the energy which has been blocked in the legs, thus allowing the person to move more freely as he or she goes through life.

Oiling and Stroking

Start by positioning yourself between the receiver's feet. After you have applied the oil to your hands, you can begin by oiling both legs. Rest your hands on the ankles, and then slide them all the way up the fronts of the legs to the top, around the hip joint, and back down to the feet again (Figure 16-45). Repeat this stroke several times, then choose which leg you will work on first and position yourself on ei-

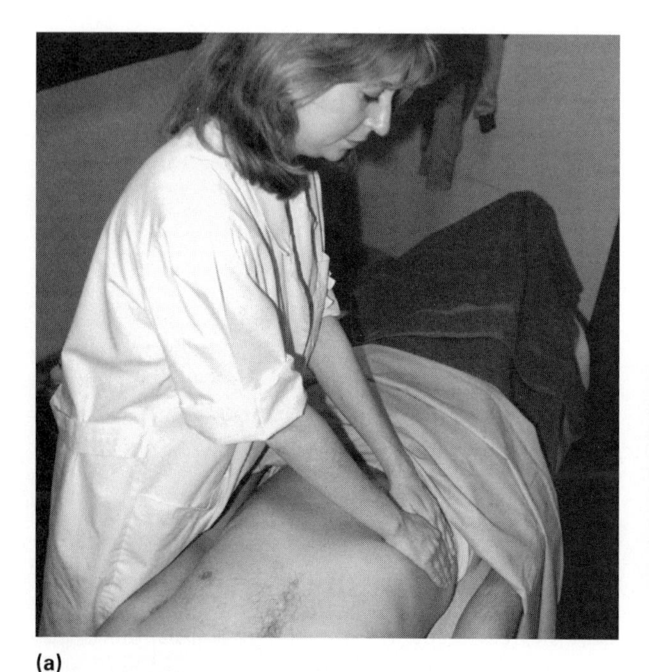

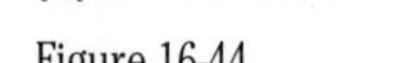

(a)

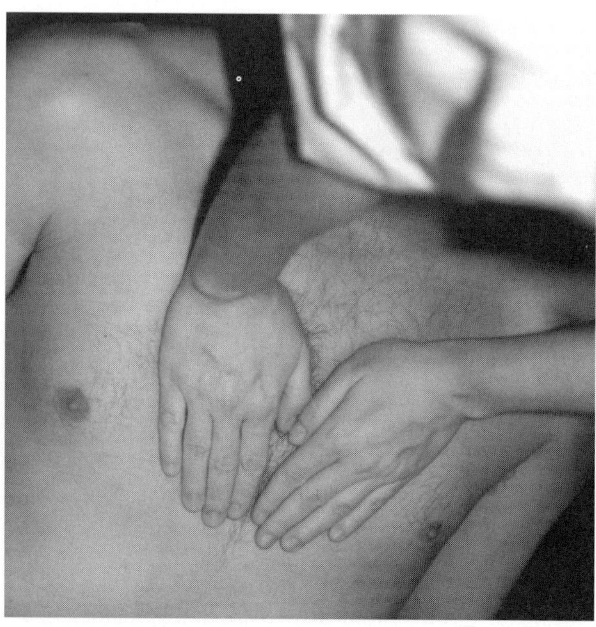

(b)

Figure 16-44
(a) Using broad circling on the belly; (b) spiraling and using long strokes for breathing.

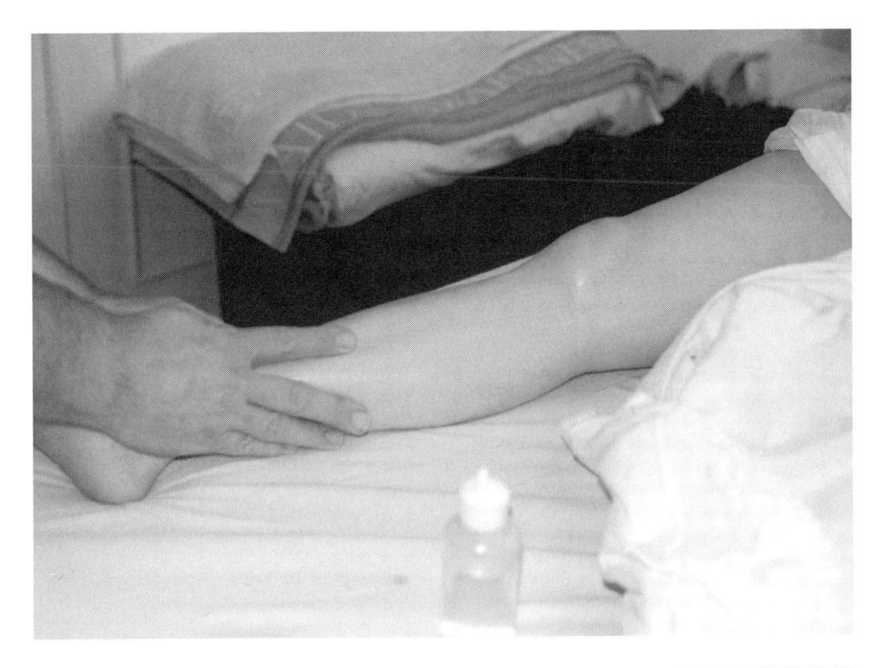

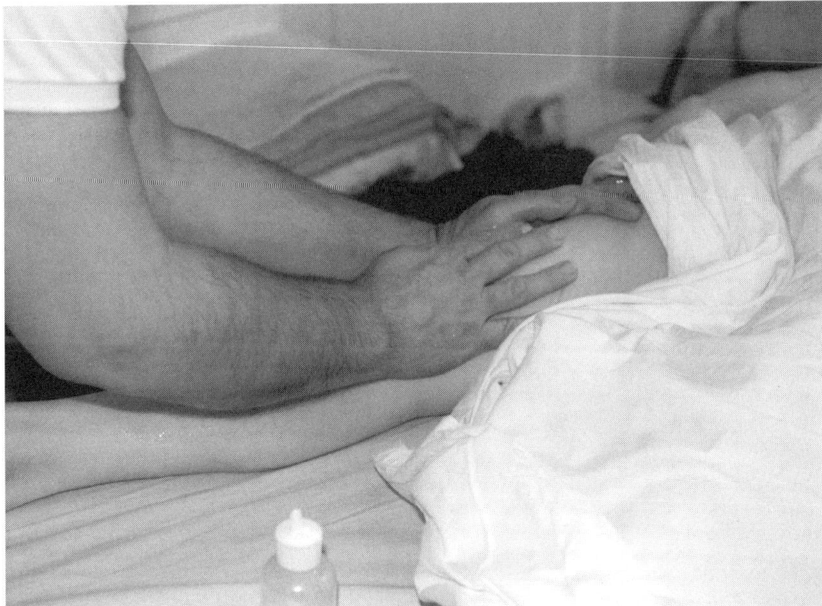

Figure 16-45
Oiling and using long strokes to massage the front of the legs.

ther side of the foot. Now use both your hands to spread the oil and warm the leg, either with your fingers pointing up the leg or with your hands cupped across it. Make sure you also take care to respect their privacy when working on the inner thigh.

Stretching and Working up the Front of the Leg

Most people say that when receiving a massage, it feels unexpectedly good to have your limbs passively exercised. It's almost like having someone else doing an exercise for you, without your having to make any effort. When stretching the leg, you are actually exercising three joints: the ball-and-socket hip joint, and the hinge joints of the knee and ankle. As the person giving the massage, you will find it much more effective and less tiring if you pull with your whole body, not just your arms.

Sequence for Stretching and Draining the Leg

To stretch the leg, you must first cup one hand around the person's heel, and place the other across the top of the foot. Lean back until your arms are taut like ropes. Now raise the foot a few inches off the floor, and lean back from your pelvis, shaking the leg slightly as you pull. Release slowly and then repeat (Figure 16-46a).

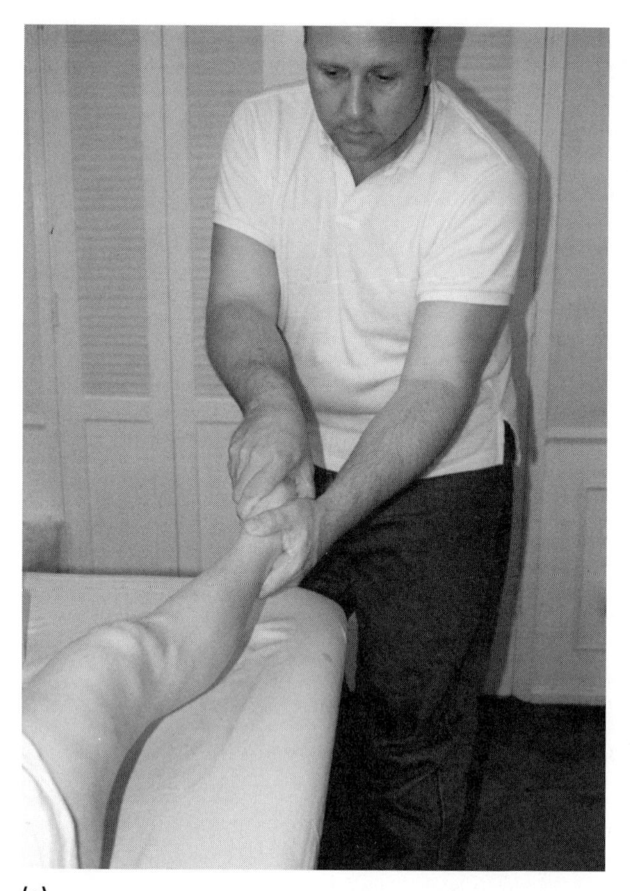

(a)

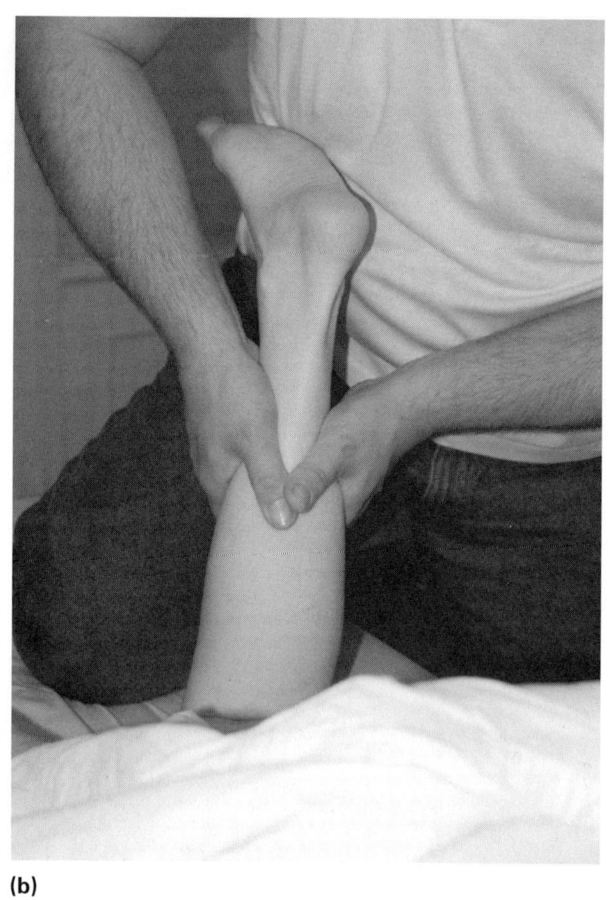

(b)

Figure 16-46
(a) Stretching the leg; (b) draining the lower leg.

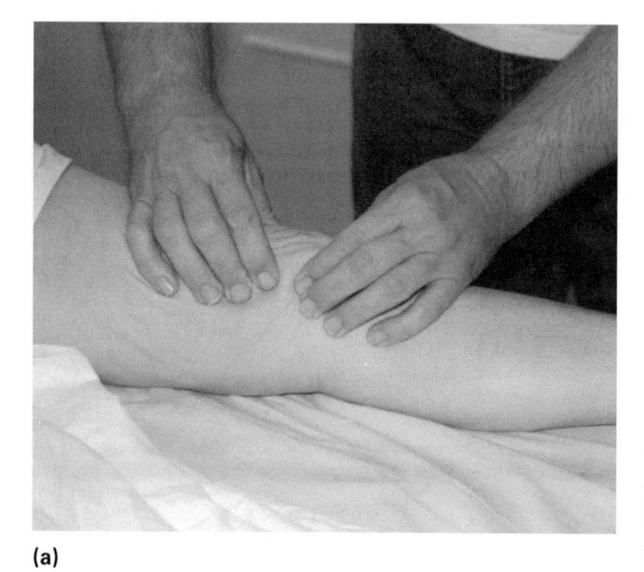

(a)

Figure 16-47
(a) Circling the kneecap; (b) draining the thigh.

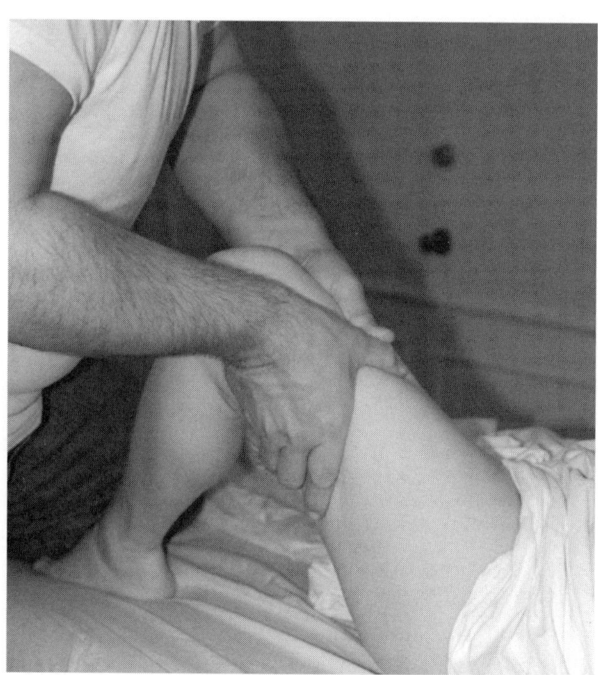

(b)

Use the "V" between your thumbs and fingers to press firmly along the muscles on either side of the shinbone. Carefully move your hands alternately, letting one follow the other rhythmically up from the ankle to the knee (Figure 16-46b).

Sequence for Working up the Front of the Leg

The sequence used to work up the front of the leg involves draining strokes to aid the circulation, interspersed with some additional precise work around the kneecap. On the lower leg, you must be sure to work on the muscles on either side of the shinbone, though direct pressure on the shinbone can be painful. On the thigh, make sure you use broad, fairly deep strokes to push upward, assisting the venous and lymphatic flow. If the person is long-legged, you may find it next to impossible to reach the thigh unless you move to the side.

Start by overlapping your thumbs just above the kneecap, anchoring your fingers on the side of the knee. At the same time, begin to draw your thumbs away from each other to circle around the bone from opposite directions, letting them cross above and below the kneecap. Circle several times (Figure 16-47a). Using both hands to push alternately on the thigh from the knee to the top of the leg, let your

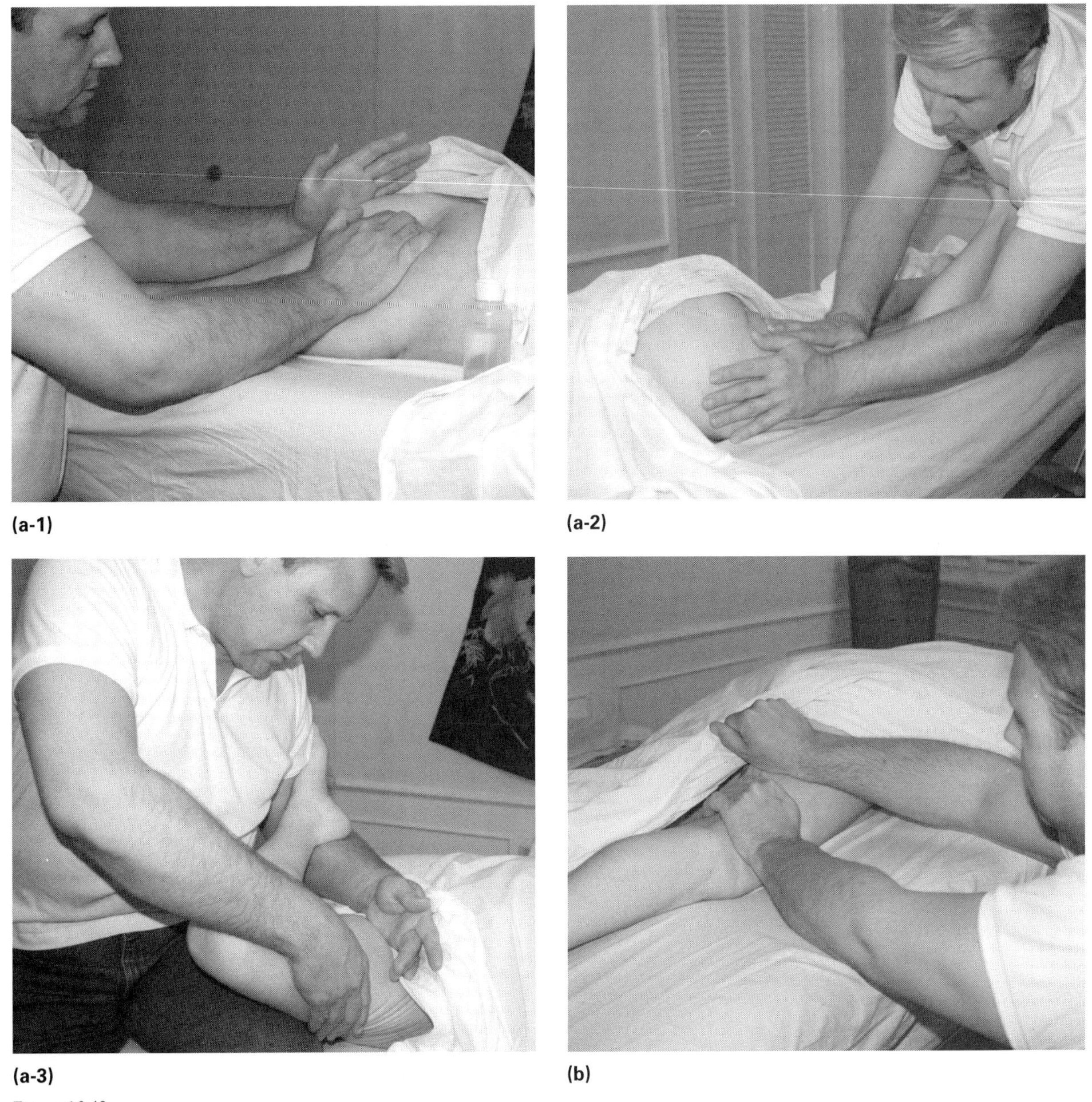

(a-1) (a-2) (a-3) (b)

Figure 16-48
(a) Working around the hip joint; (b) working down the leg.

thumbs circle up and outward as you gradually move up the leg (Figure 16-47b).

Massaging the Hip Joint, Moving Down the Leg, and to the Front of the Foot

The hip joint is a large ball-and-socket joint which links the top of the leg to the pelvis. It has a wide range of movement and is packed in firmly by the surrounding muscles. Thus, it may be difficult to find at first. Press in under the rim of the pelvis to locate the bony protuberance at the top of the thigh bone. If you go a little deeper around this bone, you will be working on the connections of the hip joint. Having pressed around the joint thoroughly, begin to work down the leg, using broad strokes on the thigh, and more precise finger strokes around the kneecap. Finish the sequence by squeezing down the shin muscles to the ankle. As you work down the leg, you will need to move. If you are working on a massage table, it is generally easier to move more smoothly; however, if you are working on the floor, you will probably have to break contact, change your position, and then resume the massage.

Sequence for Massaging the Hip Joint and Moving Down the Leg

Facing the receiver's hip, place both your thumbs on the side of the buttocks, two to three inches below the rim of the pelvis. Now knead around the joint, pushing in deeply with alternate thumbs. Use the rest of your hands to anchor yourself (Figure 16-48a on p. 187). To work down the leg, gather and squeeze large bunches of flesh down the thigh, and then wring or pull along it. Work around the knee with your fingers, then continue down the lower leg, squeezing alongside the shinbone to the ankle joint (Figure 16-48b).

Sequence for Massaging the Foot

The massage session is rounded off by paying special attention to the feet. Since you have already massaged them thoroughly while the receiver was lying on his or her back, the strokes which you will be using now are only intended to help "ground" them, and bring their energy level right down. After first opening and stretching the foot, enclose it in both of your hands and pull it smoothly off the toes. After you have completed one foot, reposition yourself on the other side to work on the other leg.

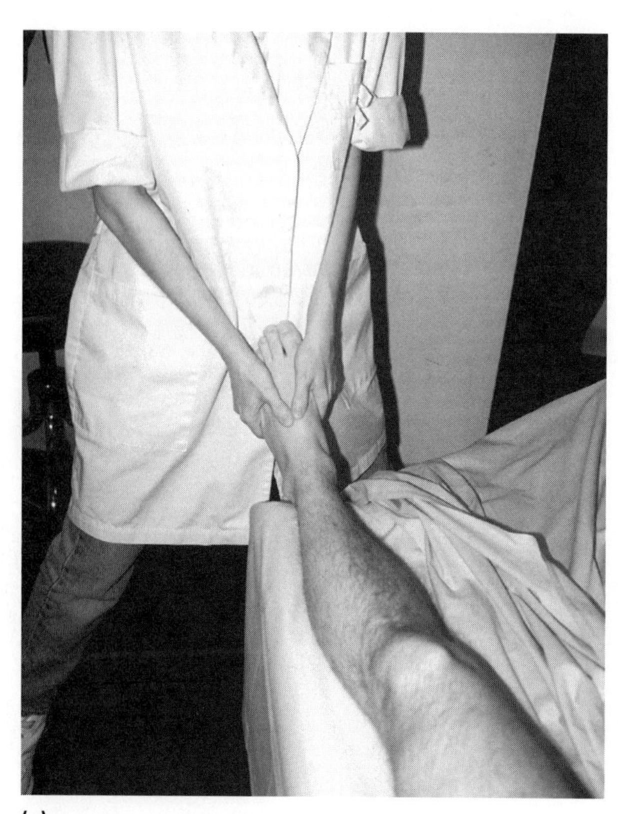

(a)

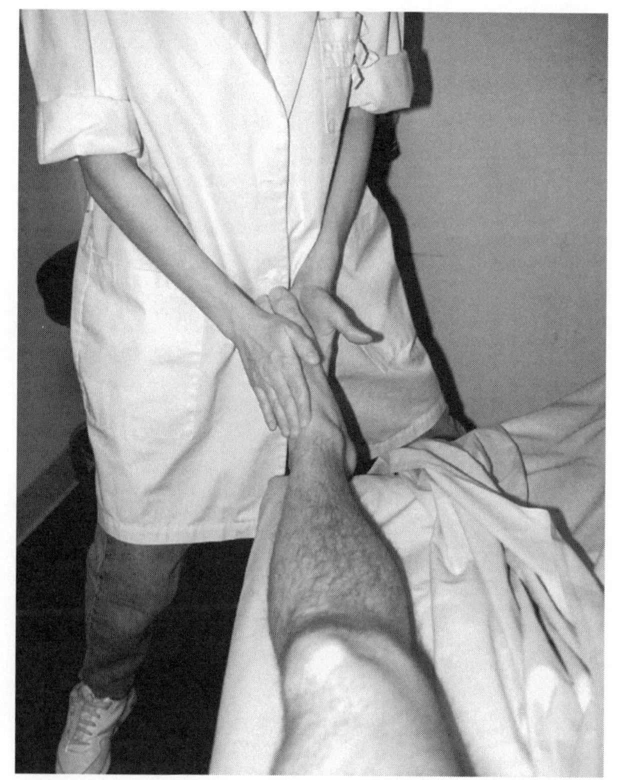

(b)

Figure 16-49
(a) Opening the foot; (b) stroking the foot.

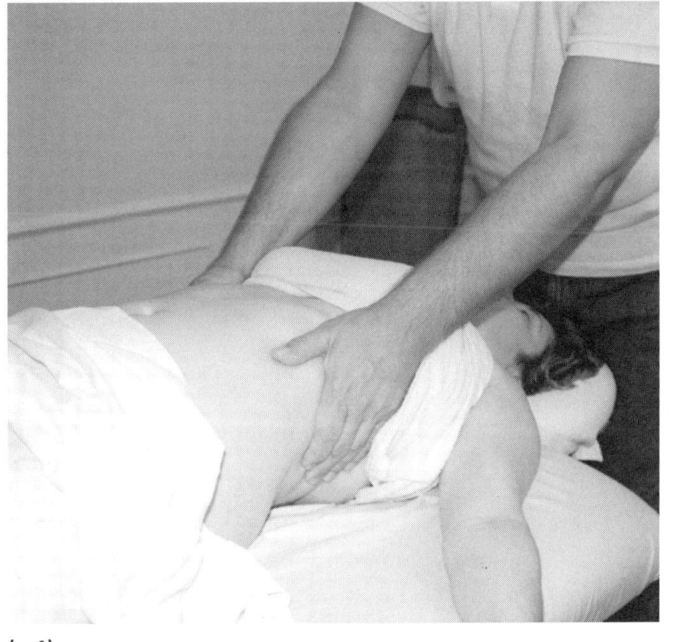

(a-1)

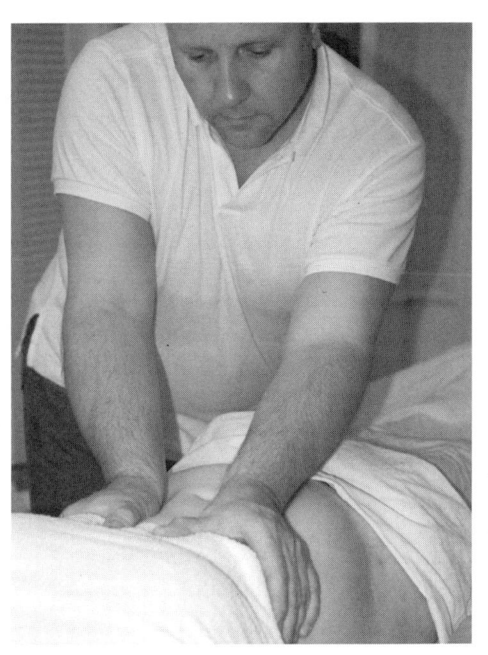

(a-2)

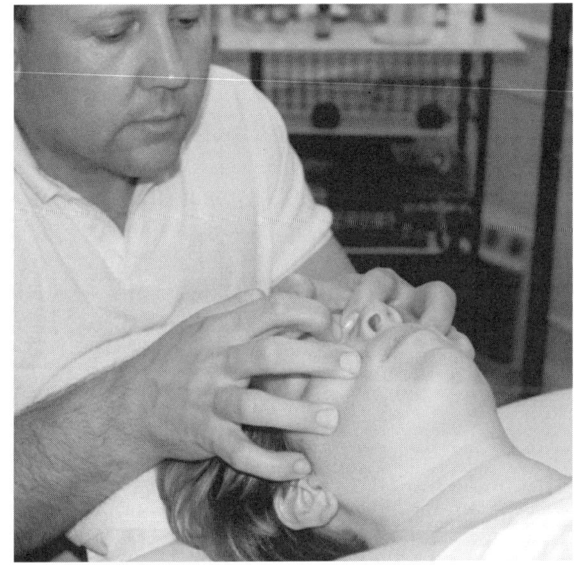

(b-1)

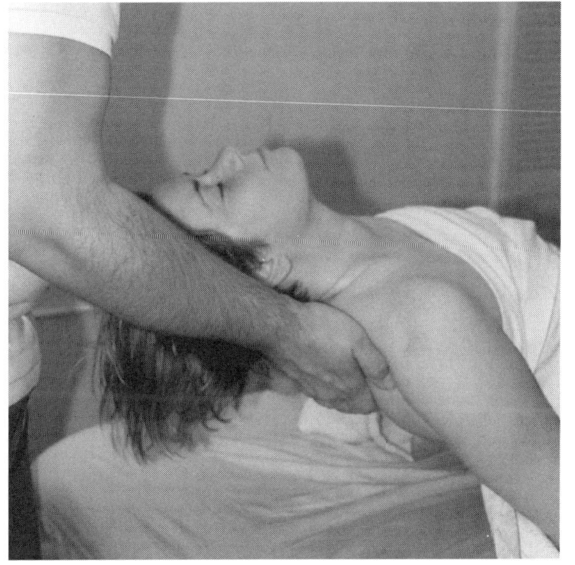

(b-2)

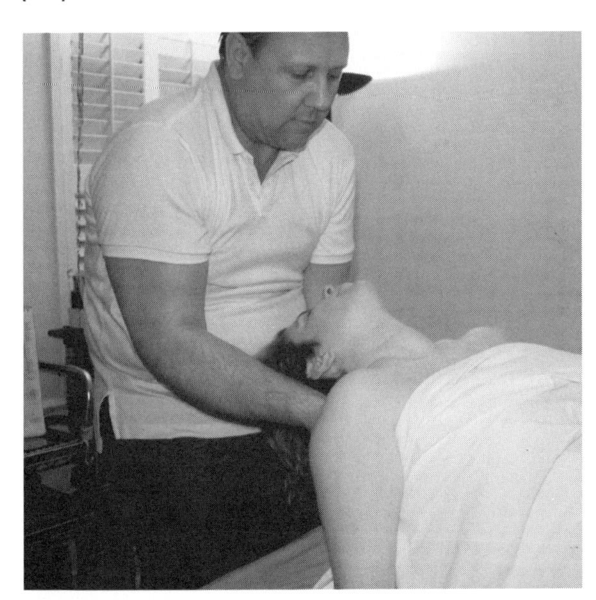

(b-3)

Figure 16-50
(a) Connecting from the belly to the leg and arm;
(b) connecting from the head to the hands and feet.

To open the foot, clasp it with your fingers under the sole and your thumbs alongside one another on the top. Squeezing the foot firmly, draw the lengths of your thumbs away from each other, opening the foot and stretching the bones apart (Figure 16-49a on p. 188). Then sandwich the foot between your hands, with your fingers pointing up the leg. Draw them slowly toward you and slide gently off the toes (Figure 16-49b). Repeat the sequence on the other leg.

Providing a Sense of Wholeness

Having worked on each individual part of the body, you are now ready to connect the various parts and give the receiver a sense of their own wholeness. We call this process connecting.

There are two ways of connecting the body: either by using long strokes which flow over the person's entire body, from one end to the other; or by simply resting your hands on different parts of the body for a few moments.

Using Long Connecting Strokes

To complete the final connecting strokes, you can either position yourself at the receiver's side, at hip level or at the head. This is so you can easily reach both ends of the body at the same time. You can either do just one of the strokes shown in Figures 16-50a and b (on p. 189), or all three if you wish. Whichever stroke you choose to end with, you must make sure that your fingers rest for a moment before breaking contact with the receiver. Then, gently release both of your hands together, at the same time.

Sequence for Connecting from the Belly to the Leg and the Arm

Start by resting both of your hands on the person's belly. Then, slowly move one hand down one leg and off the foot and the other up to the opposite shoulder, down the arm, and off the hand. Bring the hands back to the belly and repeat the stroke along the other leg and arm.

Sequence for Connecting from the Head to the Hands and Feet

Begin by resting your fingertips on the receiver's forehead, and then move lightly up over the top of the head, down the back of the neck, down the arms, and off the middle fingertips. Repeat, but at the base of the neck, come around to the front and down the torso. At the navel, separate your hands and come down the legs and off the big toes.

Summary

In this chapter, we discussed how the body can be cared for through the use of massage therapy. To do this, the first thing we learned is that each individual part of our body is seen as a separate entity, each capable of causing us great joy, as well as pain and sadness. Therefore, each of these separate parts must be massaged in a different manner, using specific sequences. Because of that fact, we identified the basic individual massage sequences which are used on different parts of the body. These include the sequences for massaging the back, the legs and arms, the shoulders, neck, and scalp, the front of the torso, and the face. We also talked about the process of connecting all the parts of the body together, and by doing so, defined the basic massage sequence used for connecting.

Review Questions

1. What is the term given by the Japanese to describe the belly or abdomen?
2. Explain the basic massage sequence.
3. What part of the body often requires more time and attention to massage than any other part of the body?
4. Briefly explain why it is important to *oil* before beginning a massage.
5. Explain the difference between *kneading, wringing,* and *hacking.*
6. What philosophy tells us that the condition of our spine affects us at every level?
7. Briefly explain what a *half lotus* leg lift is.
8. During a massage session, why is it important to drain and work down the leg?

17

Understanding the Art of Shiatsu

Performance Objectives

Upon completion of this chapter, you will be able to:

1. Briefly define the concept of *shiatsu* therapy.
2. Briefly explain the concept of *ki.*
3. Briefly discuss the ancient philosophy of health.
4. Identify the various techniques used in *shiatsu* therapy.
5. Identify the sequence used in basic *shiatsu* therapy, and briefly explain the various massage sequences used to massage the back, hips, legs, shoulders and neck, head and face, and arms and hands.

Terms and Abbreviations

Shiatsu a form of physical therapy which involves the use of pressure applied to the acupuncture points of the body to help balance energy and promote good health.

Shiatsu is a type, or form, of physical therapy which involves the use of pressure applied to strategic acupressure points on the body in order to balance the body's energy and promote good health. Originally used in Japan, shiatsu may be applied using the hands, elbows, and knees.

While the word shiatsu is actually used to describe many variations of techniques, both the ancient Japanese and many of today's holistic practitioners believe that all of these techniques are linked together by a common thought; that is, their belief in a vital force known as ki. Ki, as we discussed earlier in this book, has to do with the flows of energy connected by channels, or meridians, throughout our body. Each meridian is linked to an individual body organ or function, and its ki can only be contacted at specific points along its path. These paths are identified as acupuncture points known to the Japanese as tsubos. In the ideal state of health, or homeostasis, a balanced condition prevails, and the ki flows smoothly along the meridians, like fuel through a gas line in an automobile, supplying and maintaining all parts of our body. But when our body has been weakened, as in the case of an injury, emotional stress, or change in lifestyle, the ki can no longer flow smoothly, and thus becomes deficient in some areas and excessive in others. The final outcome ultimately results in a state of disease.

Preparing to Use Shiatsu as a Therapy

Shiatsu as a form of massage therapy is easy to learn and requires no special equipment or oil. All that is needed is a warm and airy room, loose and comfortable clothing for both yourself and the patient, and a floor which has been carpeted to work on. However, before you do begin, it's important that you first understand the basic premise behind this form of ancient massage; that is, that your ultimate goal should not only be to treat the symptoms, but also their cause. If, for example, you were to treat only a person's back for pain, and disregarded the rest of the supporting system of interconnecting meridians which makes shiatsu so effective, you would be ignoring one of the most basic fundamental principles of oriental medicine; that is, that our body and mind are an inseparable and organic whole.

Meridians, Tsubos, Kyo, and Jitsu

As we have already stated, meridians are channels along which ki flows through our body. The best known are the 12 meridians of acupuncture (Figure 17-1). All 12 meridians are bilateral, making 24 in all. The paired meridians run close to each other and their functions are complementary. Each meridian is associated with a specific organ or function, but in its effect it extends far beyond the activity of the organ. For example, the meridian associated with our nails, muscles, and tendons is also associated with our liver, reproductive system, and our emotion of anger. When you press a point on a meridian, you are not only stimulating the local nerves and tissues; you are also influencing the flow of ki throughout the meridian and hence, through others. And if an area is too painful to touch, you can help by working on other areas located further along the meridians which cross the painful area.

The Tsubos

Acupuncture points, or tsubos, are located on the meridian where the ki can be most easily reached and manipulated. Acting a little like amplifiers, passing through the ki from one point to another, these points are proven to have a lower electrical resistance than surrounding areas.

Many of the tsubos are what we in the Western world refer to as trigger points, which stimulate the muscles so they can contract or relax. However, according to ki, the tsubos have a much more subtle effect. According to oriental medicine, some connect

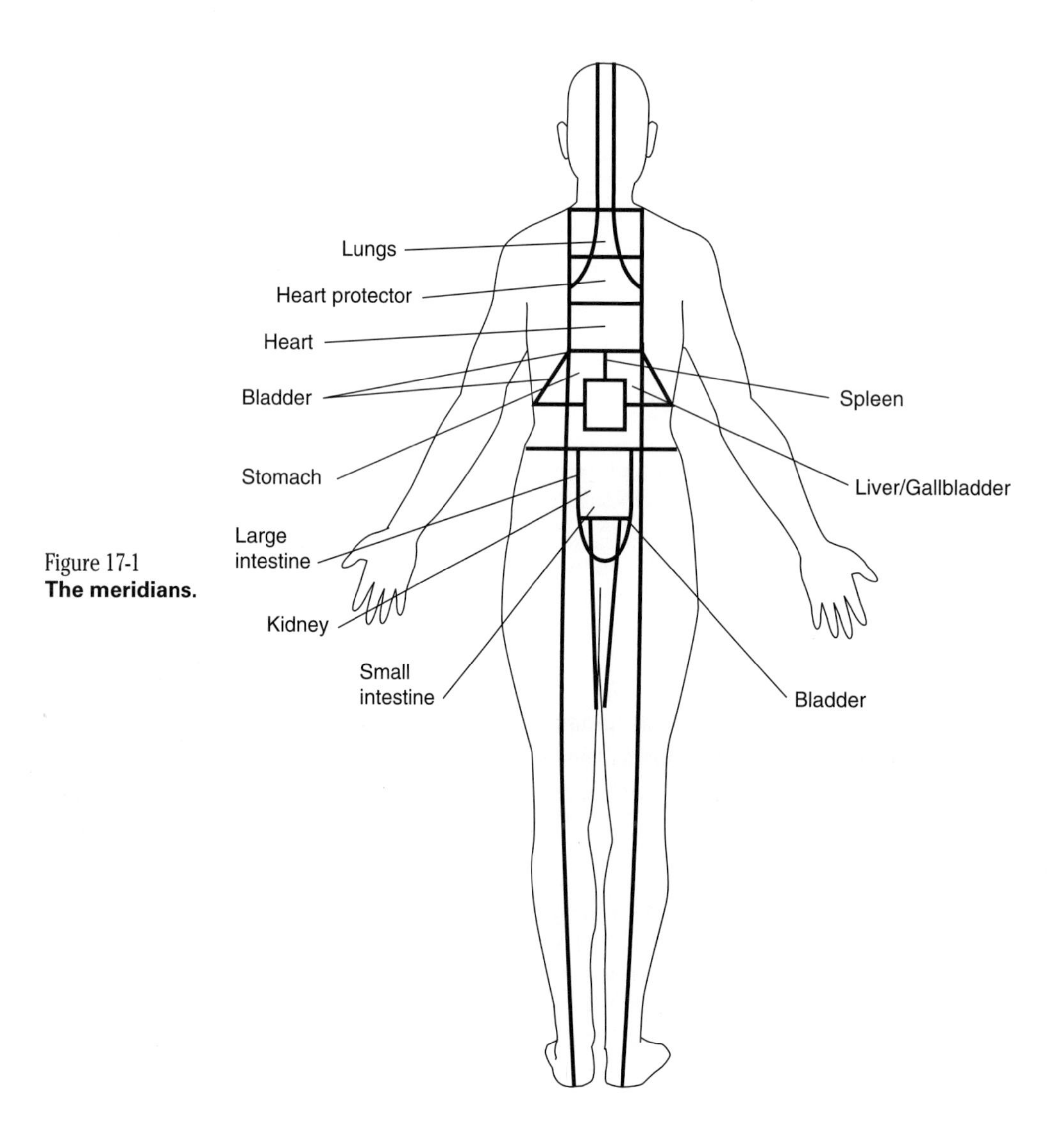

Figure 17-1
The meridians.

with other meridians, some influence the balance of elements, and others may calm the mind or reduce fever. If you learn the locations of the meridians, you will become familiar with the passageways of ki within the body, and thus will be able to develop a more instinctive understanding of where the tsubos are. (Table 17-1.)

Kyo and Jitsu

In an unbalanced meridian, the ki is either deficient or excessive. If it is deficient, it is known as kyo; if it is in excess, it is called jitsu.

Areas which are deficient often look and feel slightly hollow and generally yield to the touch. When you press a kyo meridian, it usually feels good to the receiver, as you are supplying ki energy to a deficiency. Jitsu areas are much easier to locate, since they are usually hard or tense. They may be spontaneously painful, or they may only feel painful when pressed. The pain is often sharp, whereas kyo pain is usually dull and gives relief when pressed.

Understanding the Basic Massage Sequence for Shiatsu

Before you begin using shiatsu, you must first understand the basic massage sequence. You should begin the sequence with the patient lying prone, with his or her arms at the sides. Working down the body, start

Table 17-1
Pressure Points Used in Shiatsu Massage

Back of Body	
Back:	located on each side of the spine between the vertebrae; balances all of the internal organs.
Hips:	located on the sides of the buttocks; relaxes the pelvis and unlocks ki to the legs; also relieves menstrual problems in the female.
	Sacral holes: relieves pelvic congestion.
	Center of buttock crease: relaxes muscles of lower back and hips.
Ankles:	located on both sides of the Achilles tendon; at once, stimulates water function; also relieves back pain.
Feet:	located under the center of the ball of the foot; calms and relaxes.
Front of Body	
Neck and Face:	
	Neck: located on both sides of the spine at the back of the neck and at the seam between the two muscles; relieves still necks, tension headaches, and eye problems.
	Face: (a) in the area of the eyes: located in the inner corner of the eye socket, just above the corner of the eye; at the inner end of the eyebrow; in the hollow outside of the eye socket, level with the outer corner of the eye; (b) around the mouth: located just below the widest part of the nostril; halfway down the "laugh line;" in the center of the chin groove; and in the center of the upper lip.
Shoulders:	located one and one-half inches below the hollow at the outer end of the collarbone; stimulate lung function.
Arms and Hands:	
	Great Eliminator: located on the large intestine; eliminates colds, headaches, and toothaches.
	Center of palm: calms mind and emotions.
	Outside of elbow at outside end of crease when arm is bent: tonifies large intestine and relieves arm and shoulder pain.
Hara:	located about three inches on either side of the navel; stimulates intestines and thus relaxes tension.
	Tan-Den: located in bladder region and connects with the muscles supporting the spine; when pressed deeply with the flat of four fingers, stimulates the whole body.
Legs:	
	Stomach 36: located at the top of the shinbone, in the curve where the bone widens toward the knee; promotes general energy and well-being.
	Four fingers up from the inner anklebone next to the shin: calms; relieves menstrual pain.

by treating the back, then the hips, the back of the legs, and then the feet. Before returning to the head, give shiatsu to the back of the shoulders. On the front of the body, start with the shoulders and neck, then the head and face, the arms and hands and the hara, and finish with the front of the legs.

Basic Sequences for the Back, the Hips, the Back of the Legs, and the Back of the Shoulders

Begin by stretching the back. This is so you can loosen it and establish your own rhythm. Next, stimulate all of the body's functions by applying pressure down both sides of the spine with your palms, then your thumbs. Next, move down the hips. You can press the points in the sacrum, then squeeze the sides of the buttocks, and use your elbow on the upper curve. When you are ready, you can begin to work on one leg at a time. Start by pressing down the center with your palm, then your knees. Once you have pressed the ankle points, you should stretch the leg three ways, then crook it outward to press down the side. Next you "walk" on the patient's soles, then treat each foot. Your work on the back of the body should end with the shoulders. Press along the top of each shoulder, then rotate the shoulder blades. Now you treat the area between the spine and the shoulder blades and finish by loosening the shoulder muscle with your feet. When you have completed the shoulders, ask the patient to turn over.

Basic Sequence for the Front of the Shoulders, the Head and Face, the Arms and Hands, the Hara, and the Front of the Legs

Once they have turned over, you are ready to begin working on the front of the shoulders, the head and face, the arms and hands, the hara, and the front of the legs. Begin by "opening" the chest. This is done by first leaning on the front of the shoulders, and then pressing along the spaces between the ribs to relieve congestion in the chest. Resting your elbows on your knees for leverage, you can work on the meridians on the back of the neck from below, and then circle the sides of the neck to loosen the muscles. Stretching the neck completes the sequence for the shoulders. Then, starting with the top of the head, run your fingers through the patient's hair and gently pull it. After massaging the ears, work systematically down the points on the face, around the eyes, on the temples and jaw, near the nostrils and mouth, and then back along the midline of the head.

To initiate the sequence for the arms and hands, taking one arm at a time, begin by treating the inner surface with the arm palm up, then the forearm with the hand palm down. Now pull the fingers and treat the point between the thumb and forefinger, ending by shaking the arm to loosen and relax it. Now, using both hands, work clockwise around the lower hara, then press gently under both sides of the ribs and down the midline to the navel. Relax the hara by rocking it. Working down toward the feet, press down the inside of the leg, then the front of the thigh. After rotating the kneecap, use one thumb to press the point below the knee, the other to press down the inside shin. To complete the entire sequence, stretch the foot forward and back, and then repeat the sequence on the other leg.

Treating the Back, the Hips, the Back and Outside of Legs, and the Shoulders

To use shiatsu as a massage therapy, we begin the technique on the patient's back. During the treatment, we will be using a diagonal stretch (Figure 17-2) followed by a lumbar stretch with pressure applied down the spine (Figure 17-3).

Sequence for Performing a Diagonal Stretch

Start by placing one hand on the patient's shoulder blade, and the other on the opposite hip, with the arms straight and fingers pointing in opposite directions. Now bring your hips up and forward so you can stretch their back. After you have repeated the technique, change your hands over to rest on the other hip and shoulder blade, and perform the same diagonal stretch on this side. If you find it easier, you may cross your arms.

Sequence for Performing a Lumbar Stretch

The lumbar stretch is an excellent movement to use on someone who suffers from lower back prob-

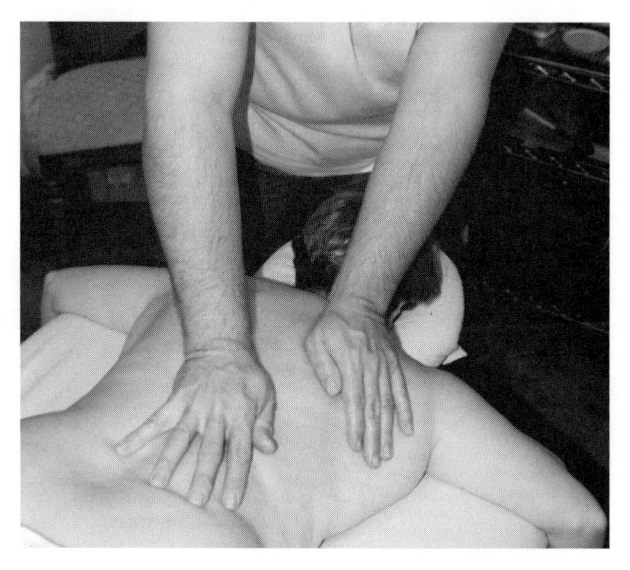

Figure 17-2
The diagonal stretch.

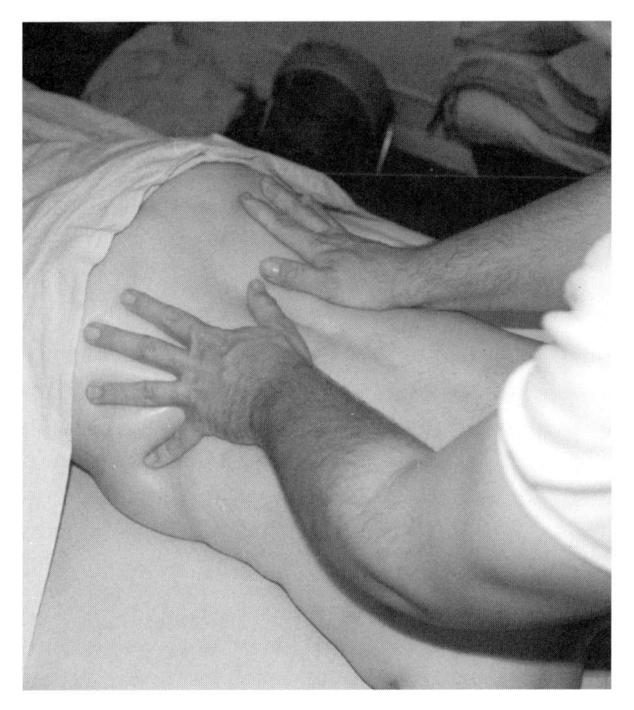

Figure 17-3
The lumbar stretch.

lems, since it stretches the whole lumbar region. Start by crossing your arms and placing one hand in the center of the hips and the other on the spine, halfway down the back, just above the lumbar area. Now, bring your entire weight forward and stretch the lower back. After you have repeated this sequence, place your hands on either side of the patient's spine, halfway down the shoulders, heels alongside the spine and palms on the ribs. Bring your hips up and forward, transferring your weight through straight arms to their back. Sit back and move your palms down an inch or so, and then repeat. Keep inching your way down until you have reached the slope of the hips. Complete the sequence by applying thumb pressure down the spine. To do this, rest your fingers on the ribs and place your thumbs on either side of the spine, halfway down the shoulders, making sure that they are not lying painfully on a bone. Supporting most of your body on your thumbs, allowing your fingers to take a little of your weight, proceed by moving down an inch at a time, applying pressure by bringing your hips forward, and then releasing it by moving them back.

Sequence for Treating the Hips

To treat the hips, you must begin by applying pressure on the four pairs of holes through the sacrum, then squeeze the hips, and finally, conclude by applying elbow pressure down the hips (Figure 17-4 on p. 196). Begin by kneeling astride the patient's legs. Locating the upper pair of holes with your thumbs, bring your hips forward and lean into the holes. Moving your weight back, locate the pair of holes about an inch below. Then, leaning forward, press into these holes. The two lowest pairs are harder to find, so you will have to use your intuition and lean into where you think they are. Now you are ready to squeeze the hips. Begin by kneeling astride the person's knees. Then, with the heels of your hands, locate the hollow in the side of the buttock muscle, slightly above and behind the point where the hip juts out. With your fingers turned in and lying relaxed on the patient's body, lean forward while pressing inward with the heels of your hands. To complete the sequence, apply elbow pressure down the hips. Starting with your knees wide apart, place one hand on the small of the back for support. Keeping the other hand relaxed, lay your open elbow on the meridian line close to the division of the buttocks. Leaning forward, bring the weight of your upper body onto your elbow. Proceed in this way down both meridians on both sides.

Sequence for Treating the Back and Outside of the Legs

There are two methods which you may use to treat the back and outside of the legs. The first is by applying palm pressure to the back of the leg, followed by knee pressure onto the back of the leg, and finishing with pressing the ankle tsubos (Figure 17-5a on p. 197). The second method is by using the three-way stretch (Figure 17-5b).

To use the pressure method, start by kneeling parallel to the patient's leg. Then, using your entire weight, press down the center of the leg with your palm. Keeping the other hand on the buttock, lightly press on the back of the knee and moderately on the calf. As you approach the ankle, apply gentle squeezing and pressure to it. To begin the second part of the sequence, applying knee pressure to the back of the leg, start by supporting yourself with your hands at the top and bottom of the leg. Squatting on your tiptoes, and keeping your knees slightly above the leg's midline, lightly "bounce" your knees up and down the center of the leg, always making sure that you avoid the knee area. Complete the sequence by pressing the ankle tsubos. To do this, lift the foot of the same leg and press both sides of the hollow area between the ankle bone and the Achilles tendon for about three to five seconds.

To use the three-way stretch method for treating the back and outside of the legs, you must first understand that this sequence works on the meridians at the front and sides of the leg, although you will only be applying shiatsu from the back. Also, remember to stretch the leg in each direction as far as it is comfortable for the person. And, after completing the three

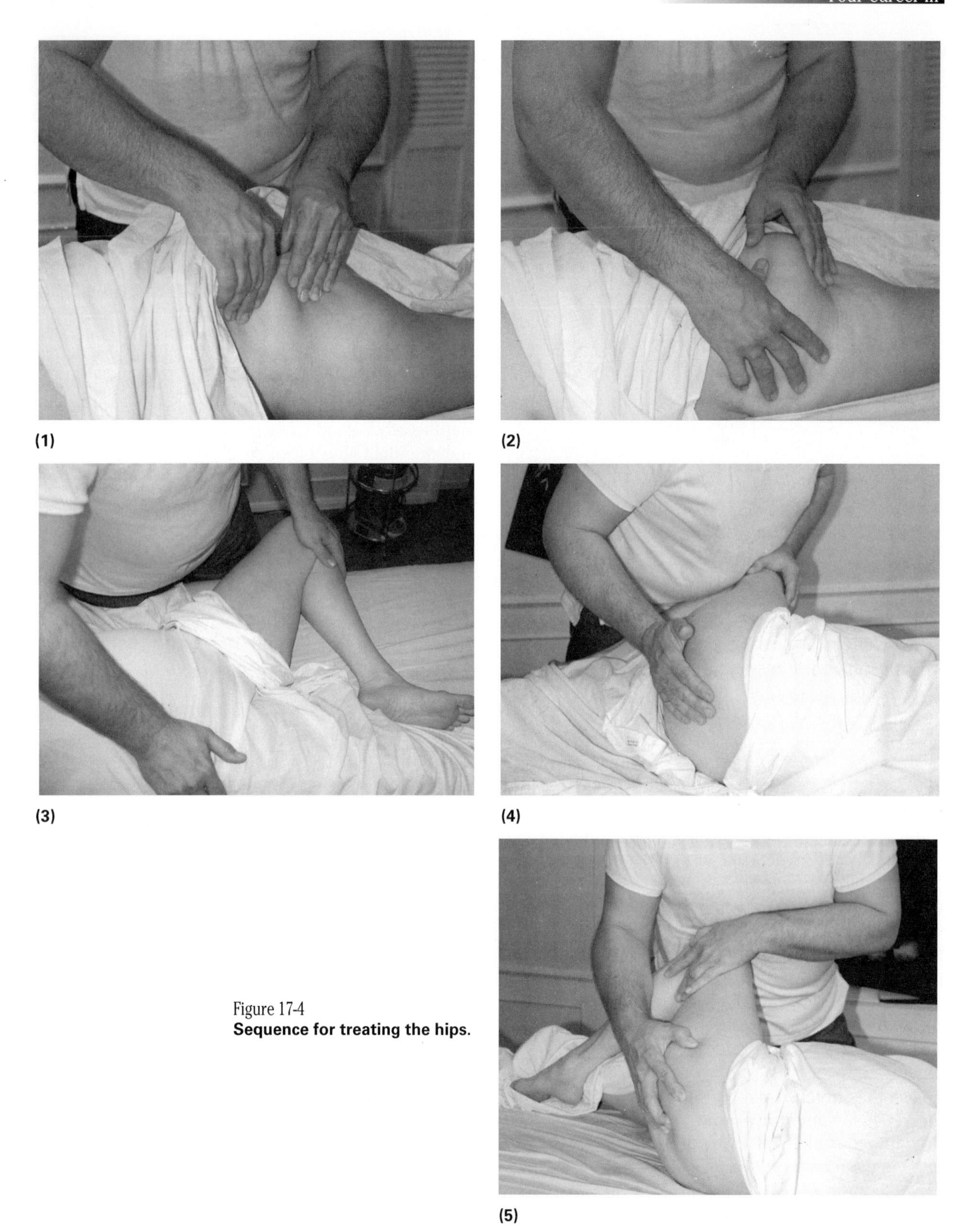

(1) (2) (3) (4) (5)

Figure 17-4
Sequence for treating the hips.

movements involved in the sequence, rearrange his or her position so that you can go straight to work on the side of the leg.

Begin the sequence by first placing one hand on the small of the back, and use the other to bring the foot back toward the buttock. Holding the foot under the toes for a maximum stretch, bounce the foot a little at the point of maximum tension. Now take the foot halfway back to release the knee. Then bring it over to the opposite buttock, as far as it will comfort-

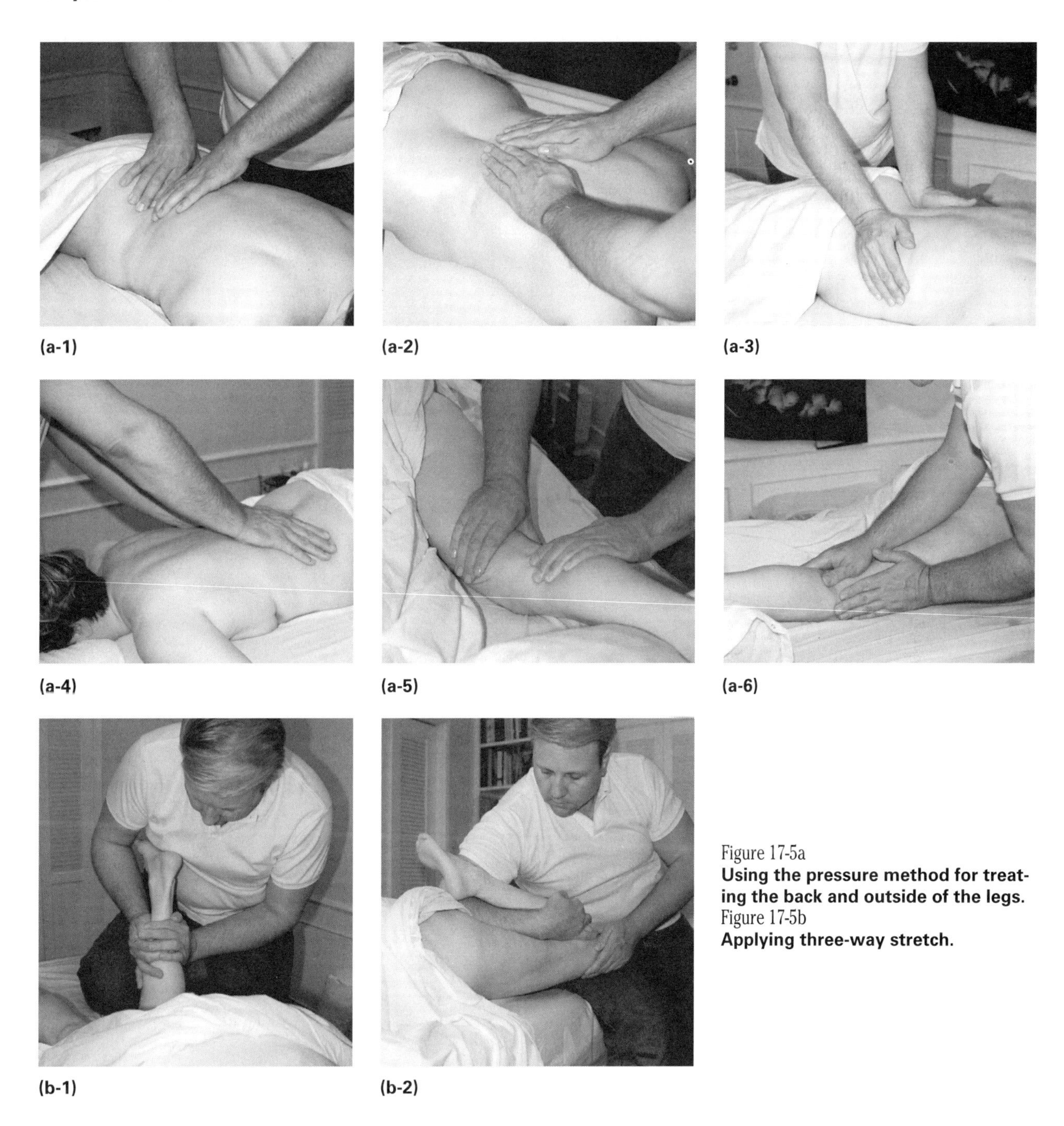

(a-1) (a-2) (a-3)

(a-4) (a-5) (a-6)

(b-1) (b-2)

Figure 17-5a
Using the pressure method for treating the back and outside of the legs.
Figure 17-5b
Applying three-way stretch.

ably go, and bounce it up and down a little to increase the stretch. Take the foot halfway back once more. Then bring it over toward you as far as it will go, and bounce it up and down again. Now take it halfway back without releasing the foot. With your other hand, pick up the inside of the knee and crook the leg outward. You are now ready to begin applying palm pressure down the side of the leg (Figure 17-6 on p. 198).

Kneeling nearest the person's feet, place your hand on the hip. With the palm of your other hand, work down the center of the side of the leg, swaying your weight back and forth. Now, using your thumb, press the ankle tsubo, by pressing the sensitive hollow just below and slightly to the front of the outside anklebone for three to five seconds (Figure 17-7 on p. 198).

You are now ready to begin working on the soles, the heel, and toes of the feet (Figure 17-8 on p. 199). Begin by massaging the sides of the heel with a circular movement, thumb on one side, fingers on the other, for at least five to ten seconds. Now pinch along the outside edge of the foot. Then, using a firm tugging movement and holding the side of the foot, pull each toe. Keeping your wrist relaxed so that your hand can easily flap up and down, slap the sole repeatedly in a fast, forceful rhythm. To complete the

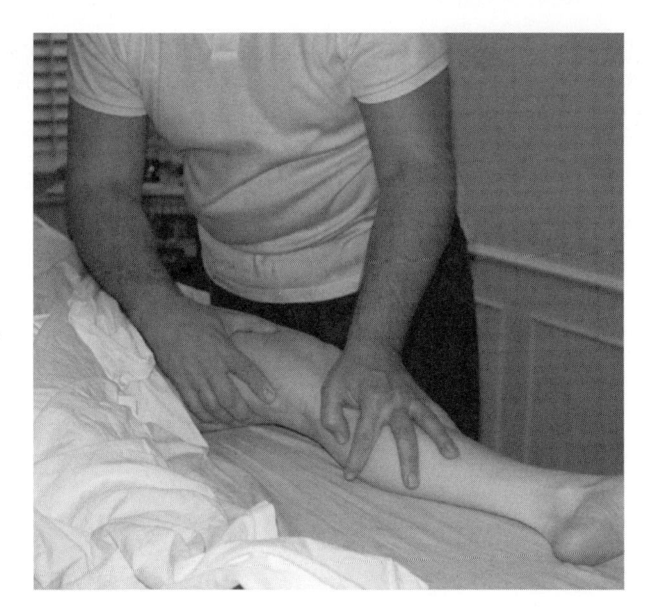

Figure 17-6
Applying palm pressure down the side of the leg.

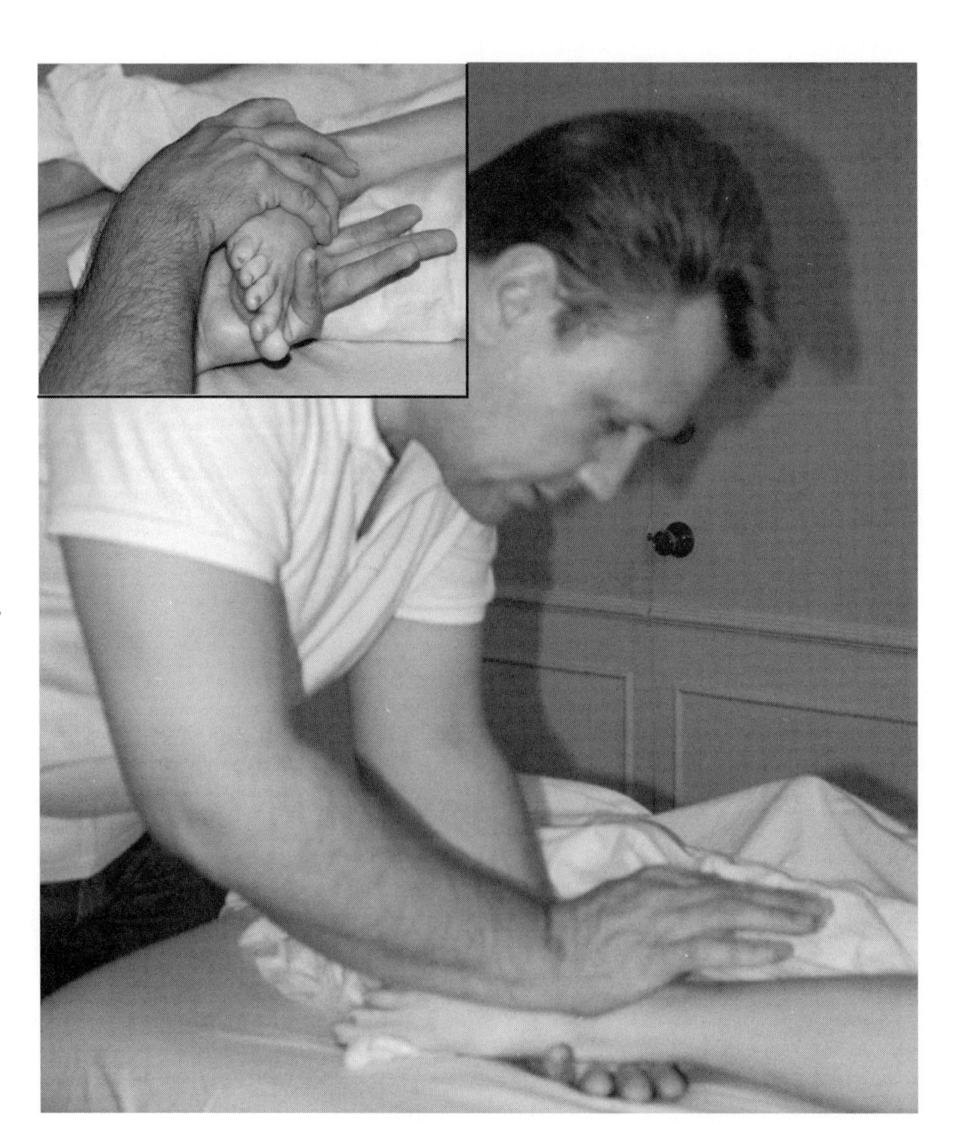

Figure 17-7
Pressing the ankle tsubo.

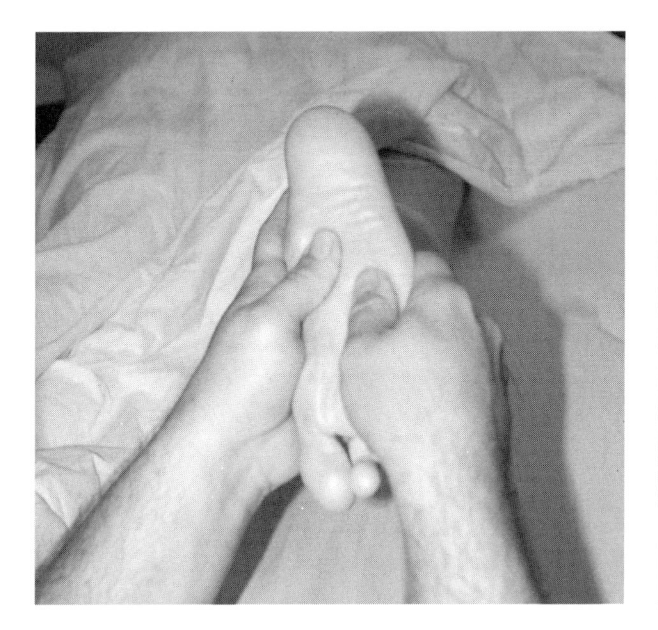

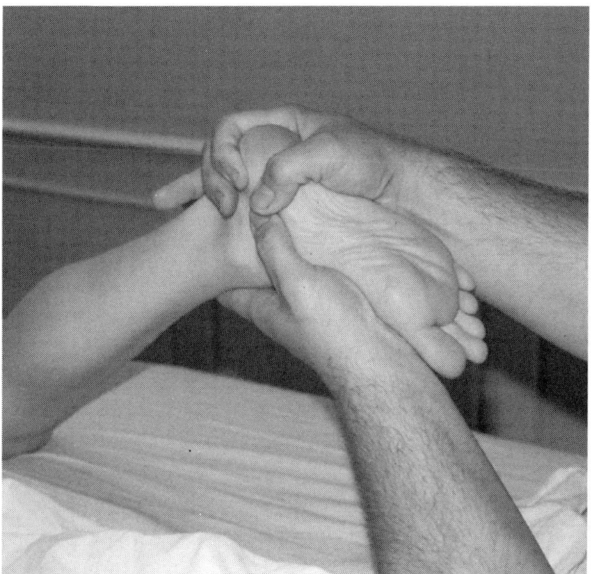

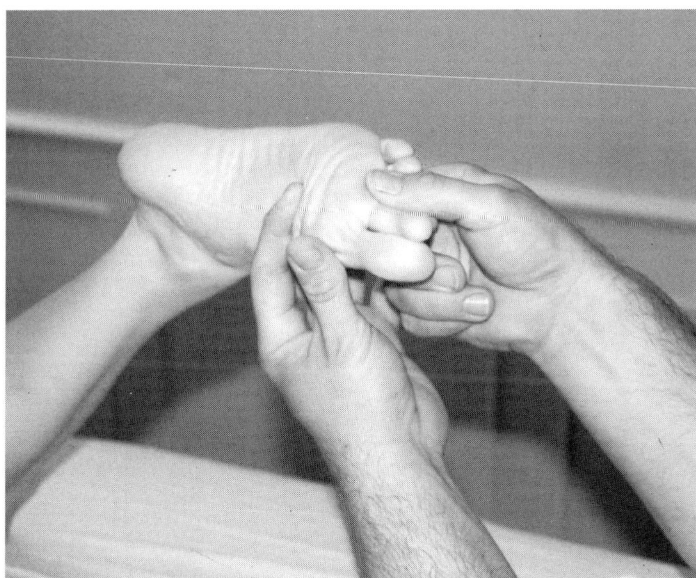

Figure 17-8
Sequence for working on the soles, heels, and the toes.

sequence, with your hand poised in a relaxed fist, gently pound the sole of the foot for a few seconds, then stroke the foot to soothe it.

Sequence for Treating the Back of the Shoulders

There are four steps involved in treating the back of the shoulders: applying thumb pressure on the top of the shoulders, elbowing between the shoulder blades, rotating the shoulder blades, and applying foot pressure to the shoulders (Figure 17-9 on p. 200).

Start the sequence by first placing one hand on one shoulder blade. Lay the length of the thumb of the other hand along the top of one shoulder. With your elbow resting on your thigh for support, lean forward and press gently out from the neck to the notch in the shoulder joint. Now, with your hand on one shoulder, lean your open elbow into the groove on the other side of the patient's spine, and using steady pressure, work gradually down from the base of the neck. Work thoroughly down the entire area between the shoulder blades. Then switch hands and elbows and work on the other side. Next, placing both of your hands on the shoulder blades, spread your fingers to gain a better grip, then curl your fingers under the outside of the blades and rotate them firmly, making sure you move the shoulder blades themselves, as well as the muscles above and below them. Complete the sequence by applying foot pressure to the shoulders. To do this, first sit back, and place your hands behind you so that you can support yourself.

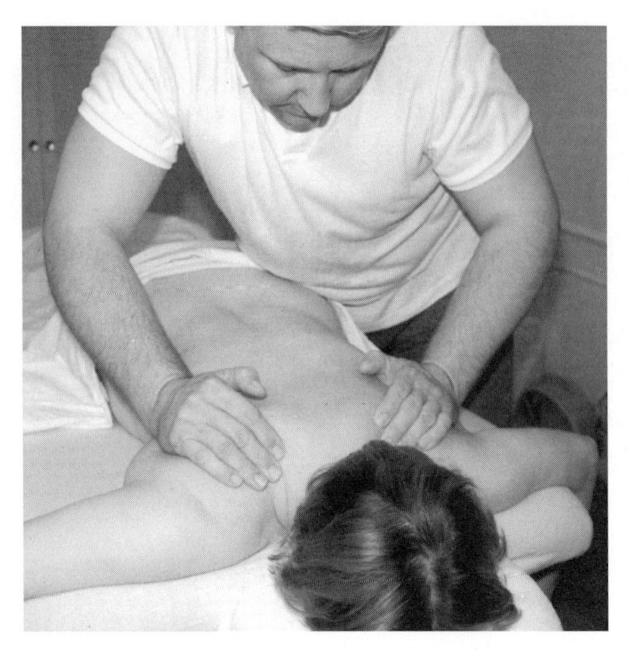

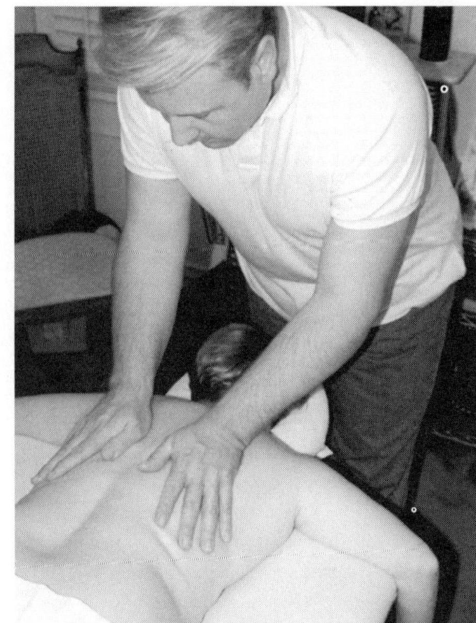

Figure 17-9
Sequence for treating the back of the shoulders.

Then, after you have placed your feet on top of the patient's shoulders, gently but rapidly use your feet to tread all over the shoulders for about a minute.

Treating the Shoulders, the Neck, the Head, and the Face

Sequence for Treating the Front of the Shoulders and the Neck

After the patient has turned over, you can resume your kneeling position on either side of the head, and begin the sequence for treating the front of the shoulders and the neck. Start by placing the heels of your hands in the hollows between the person's chest and shoulder joints, with your fingers turned outward, and enclosing the rounded part of the shoulders. Now bring your hips up and forward and lean on the shoulders as shown in Figure 17-10a. Placing your hands so that the palms face down the sides of the body and the thumbs are resting along the front of the chest in a space between the ribs, lean forward slightly and gently press with the whole length of your thumb outward from the breastbone (Figure 17-10b). Now move to the space between the next two ribs and cover the whole upper chest. If you are working on a female, remember to use caution and avoid the breasts.

Sequence for Treating the Neck

Treating the neck involves a three-step method: initiating the sequence, circling the sides of the neck, and stretching the neck (Figure 17-11a, b, and c on p. 202). Start by positioning yourself on your knees, on either side of the head, with your elbows resting on your thighs. Lean forward from your hips, as you press upward with your fingers. Then, using your middle fingers, press on either side of the spine at half-inch intervals from the base of the neck upward to the base of the skull. Now move your fingers to the outer edge of the large muscles at the back of the neck. Press at half-inch intervals from the base of the neck up, applying more pressure in the hollows at the base of the skull. Then go back to the midline of the neck and with your middle fingers on top of one another, press in the sensitive hollows located between the vertebrae. Separate your fingers and press firmly outward along the base of the skull toward the ears at half-inch intervals.

Now you are ready to begin circling the sides of the neck. Start by laying your fingers close together on the sides of the patient's neck. Now circle slowly several times, moving the flesh over the underlying muscles. Then, sitting on your haunches with your fingers clasped lightly under the neck and the thumbs pointing toward the collarbones, and the heels of your hands placed under the person's jaw with your inside forearms lying along the cheeks, lean backward, and with your arms straight, stretch the neck.

Sequence for Treating the Head and the Face

When using shiatsu to treat the head and face, you will be using a six-point method (Figure 17-12a, b, and c on p. 203). It includes running your hands through the person's hair, pulling the hair, massaging

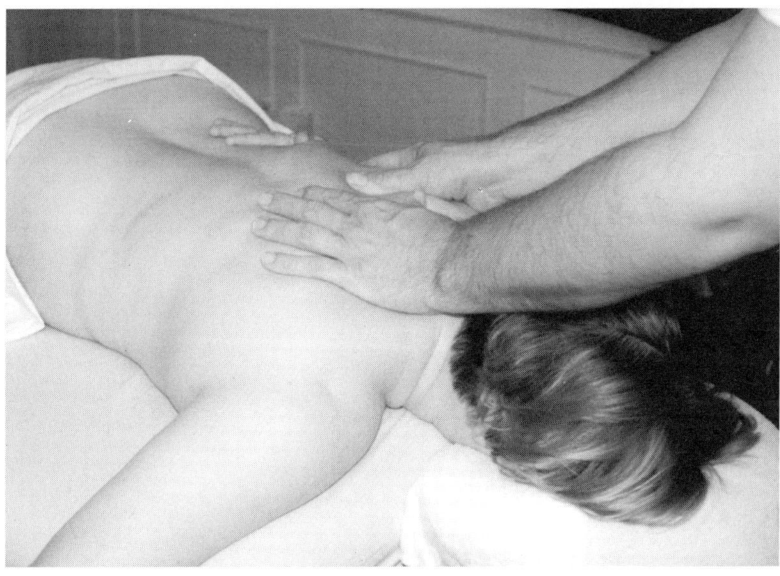

(a)

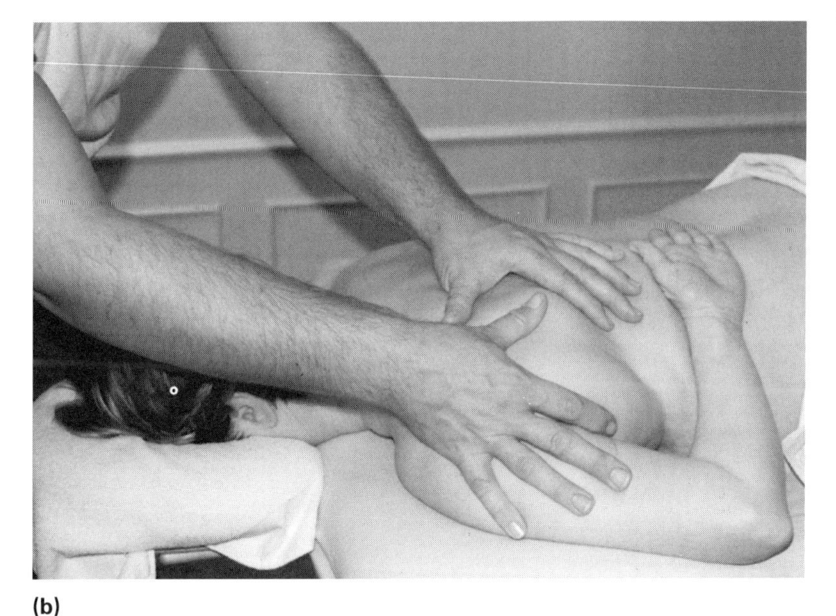

(b)

Figure 17-10
(a) Leaning on the shoulders; (b) pressing along the ribs.

the ears, pressing the top of the head points, treating the eyes, and treating the temples. The sequence also involves treating the nose and mouth.

Begin by running your hands through the hair a few times, so that your fingers brush the whole scalp, working back from the hairline. Then, taking one section of hair at a time, gently tug each section. After you have pulled lightly over the entire head, massage the ears between your thumbs and forefingers, carefully moving up from the lobes to the tops of the ears. Cover the whole ear twice. Gently holding the patient's head at his or her temples and overlapping your thumbs on the midline of the head, press at one-inch intervals back toward the crown as far as you can go.

After you have completed working on the head points, you are ready to begin the sequence for treating the eyes, temples, nose, and mouth. Start by pressing the points at the inner corners of the eye sockets for three to five seconds. Then, lightly pinch along the length of the eyebrows. Press the points located just outside the bony ridge at the outer end of each eyebrow. From the eyebrows, move up and out to the points on the temples. Remember not to press too hard. Move down in a straight line to the point located just under the cheekbones and press gently. Now move down in a single line where the muscle meets the inside of the jaw and carefully feel for the point in the center. Because of the sensitivity of this location, the person will let you know just when you have found the right spot. You are now ready to move to the nose and mouth.

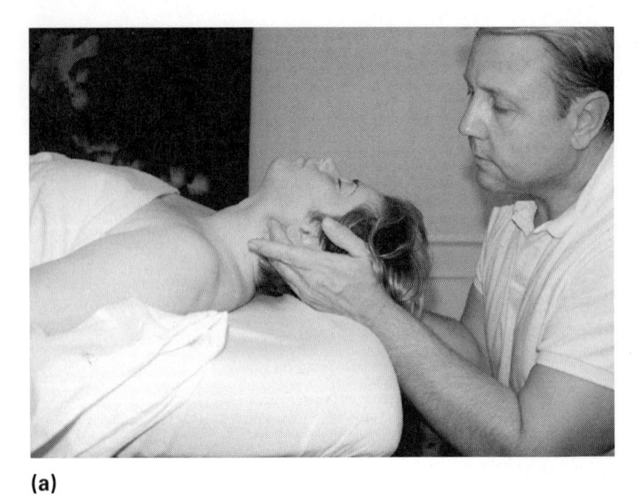

(a)

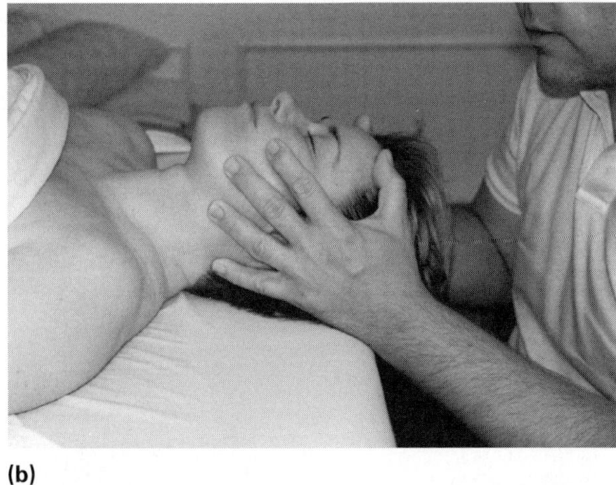

(b)

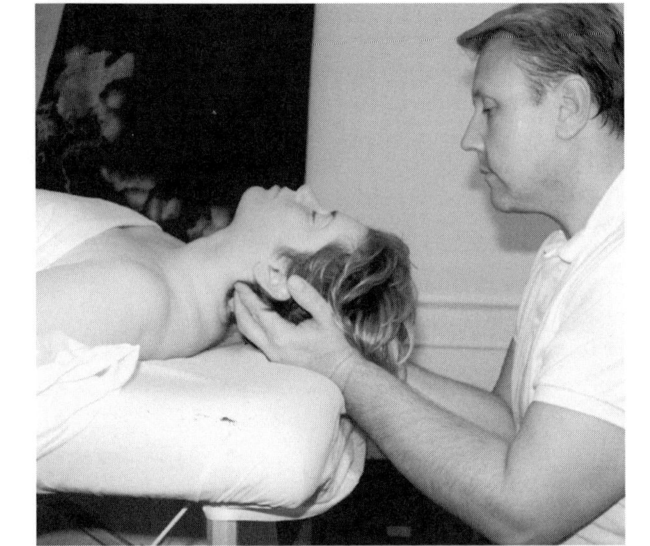

(c)

Figure 17-11
(a) Initiating the neck sequence; (b) circling the sides of the neck; and (c) stretching the neck.

With the edge of your thumbs, gently press into the grooves beside the lower edge of the nostrils. Then, press the line of points along the "laugh lines," being very careful to direct your pressure upward under the bone. Complete the sequence by cupping your hand under the receiver's chin and pressing the points in the center of the groove of the chin and the center of the upper lip.

Treating the Arms and Hands, the Hara, and the Front and Inside of the Legs

When treating the arms and hands, the sequence is performed in six steps. These include applying palm pressure along the inner arm, grasping the upper arm, applying palm pressure down the forearm, pulling the fingers, pressing the great eliminators, and shaking the arm (Figure 17-13 on p. 204).

Position yourself by kneeling at the patient's hips, laying his or her arm out horizontally from the shoulder, with the palms facing up. Then place one hand on the pectoral muscle and apply palm pressure down the inner arm from the shoulder to the wrist. Mould your hand to the contours of the arm. Now, lay the person's arm down by your side, with the palm also facing down. With one hand on their shoulder, gently grasp the upper arm and apply pressure to the back of it with your fingertips, from the shoulder to the elbow. Next, apply direct downward pressure to the forearm, from the elbow to the wrist. Reposition yourself by sitting back and taking his or her wrist in one hand. With the other hand, gently pull and shake each finger, from base to tip, being very careful to hold the finger at its sides. After you have treated each finger, for each one press the point in the middle of the web of flesh located between the thumb and forefinger for at least five seconds. Complete the

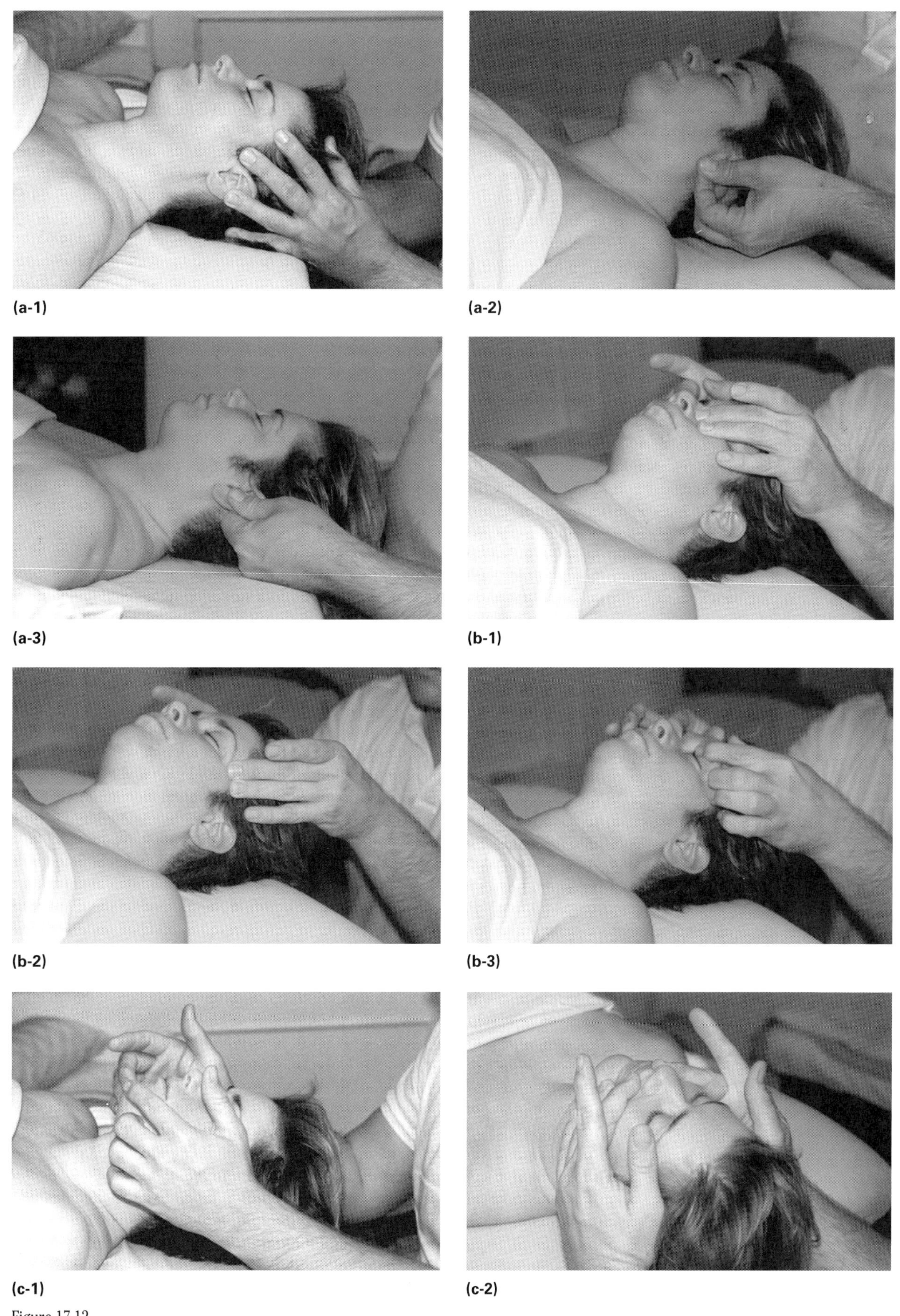

Figure 17-12
(a) Treating the head and massaging the ears; (b) treating the eyes and the temples; (c) treating the nose and mouth.

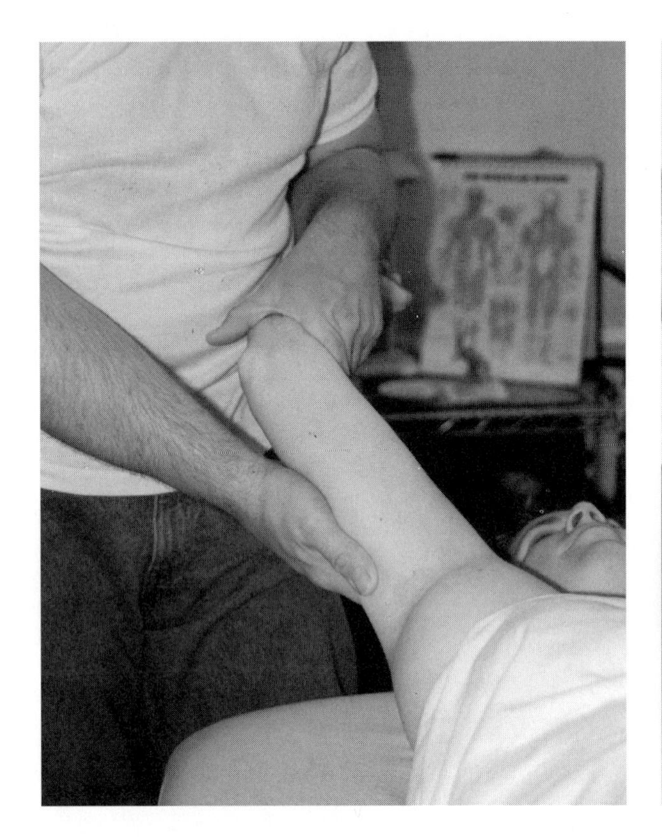

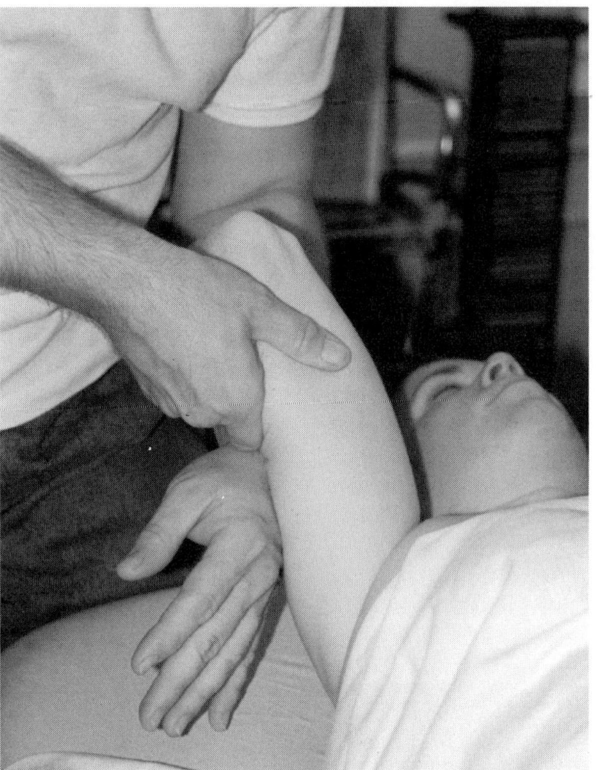

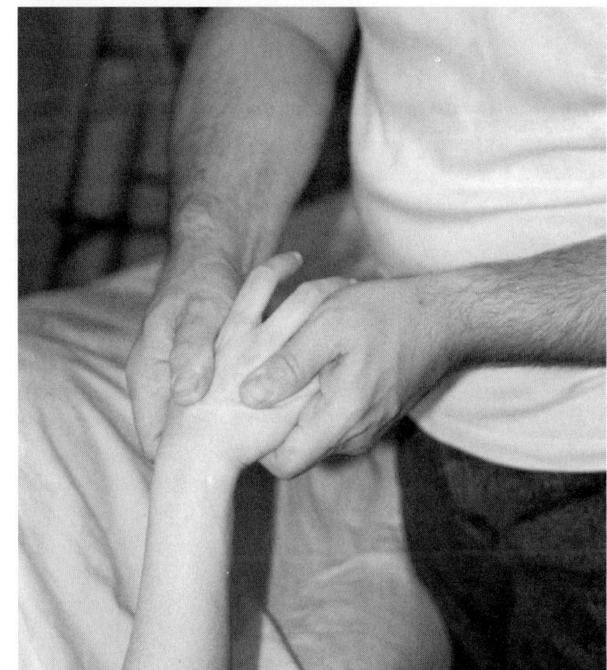

Figure 17-13
Treating the arms and hands.

sequence by holding the hand firmly in both of your own, and carefully lean back until the arm is slightly stretched. Shake the arm fast, but not too hard. Repeat the sequence on the other arm.

Sequence for Treating the Hara

Because the hara is seen as the storehouse of the body's energy, and is responsible for housing many of our vital organs, it demands great respect. Therefore, the pressure you exert on the hara should be very smooth and gradual. And always remember to work in a clockwise direction around the hara, since this strengthens the hara's weaker areas.

Begin the sequence by positioning yourself by giving ampuku, or shiatsu, to the hara. To do this, sit by the receiver's side, with your thigh lightly touching the receiver's (Figure 17-14).

Now, you must identify the two sections of the hara: the lower section and the upper section. When working on the lower section (Figure 17-15 on p. 206), use the edge of your hand as though it were a knife to go in beside the bones of the hip and the area of the large intestines. With three fingers laid flat, press at one-inch intervals clockwise around the outer part of the lower hara. This will treat the part of the hara where the bladder is located. Work in the same way along the central abdominal muscles, with longer pressure on the midline point. Here you are tracing the area in which the kidney is located. You are now ready to begin working on the upper hara. Begin by gently, yet deeply, pressing with the full length of your thumb under the left side of the ribs, working from the top to the bottom. Remember to keep your palm and fingers in relaxed contact with the patient. Now, using your fingertips, press inward in the hollow below the lowest point of the ribs. This is where the lung region is located. Work in the same way down the right-hand side, ending with the same inward pressure under the ribs. Finish the sequence by lightly pressing with one finger under the central meeting of the ribs; then, with three flat fingers on the solar plexus, halfway to the navel; and finally on the navel area itself (Figure 17-16 on p. 206).

After you have completed your sequence on the upper hara, you must rock it. To do this, reposition yourself by moving up and kneeling, facing the person's hara. With one hand on top of the other, gently rock the hara with a wavelike motion, making sure

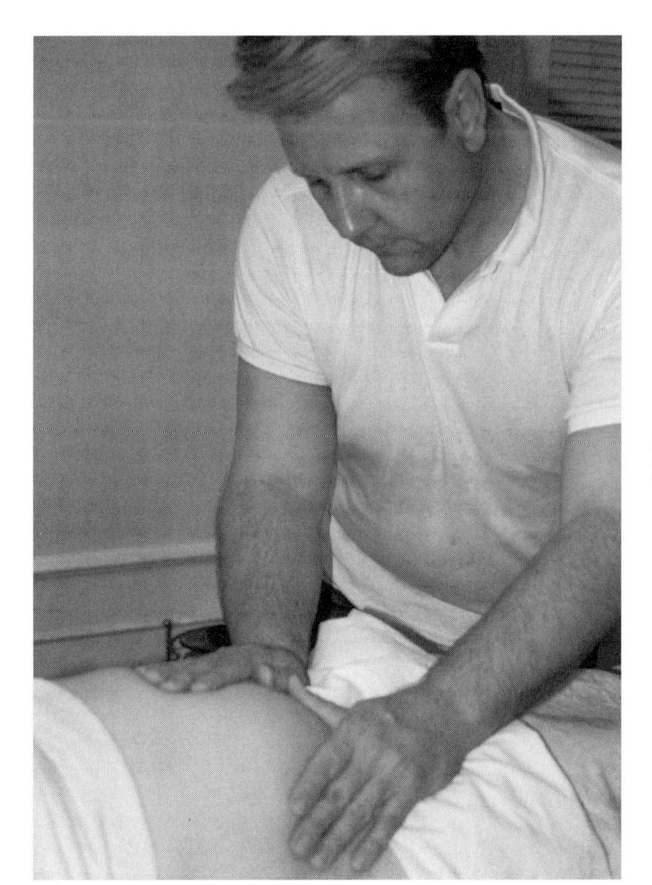

Figure 17-14
Position for treating the hara.

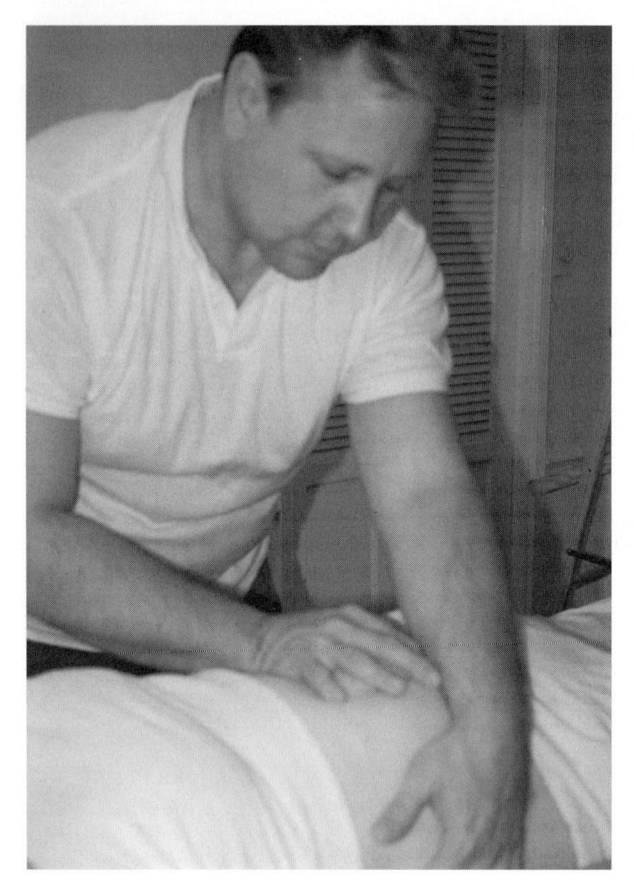

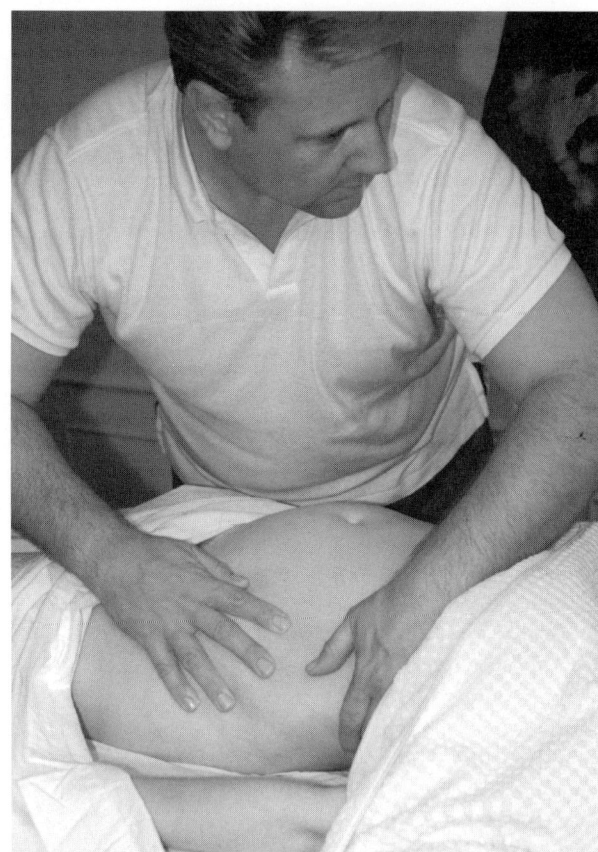

Figure 17-15
Treating the lower hara.

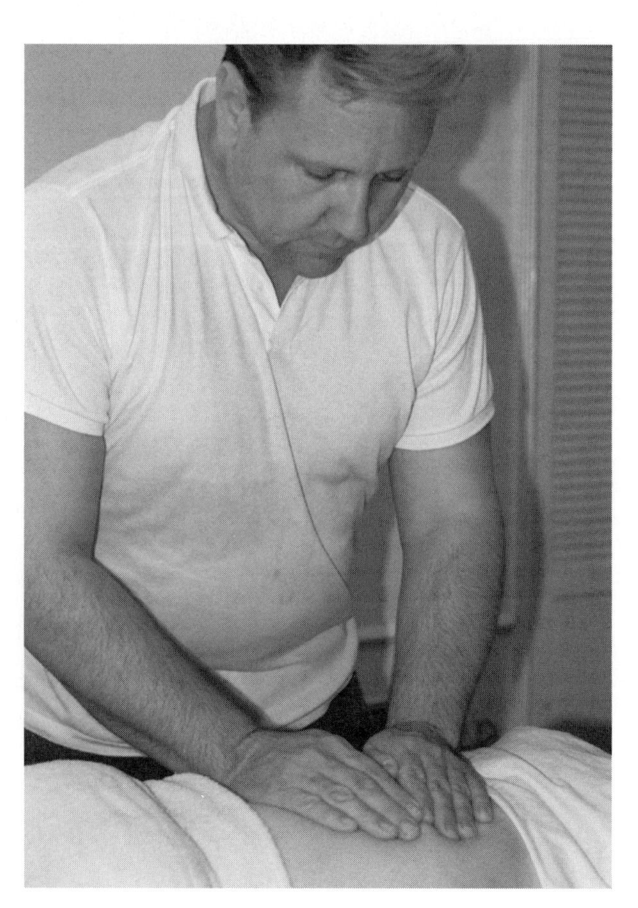

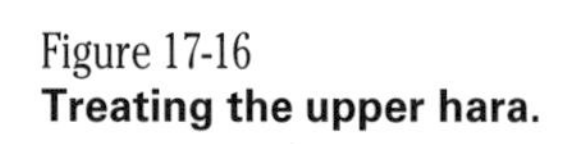

Figure 17-16
Treating the upper hara.

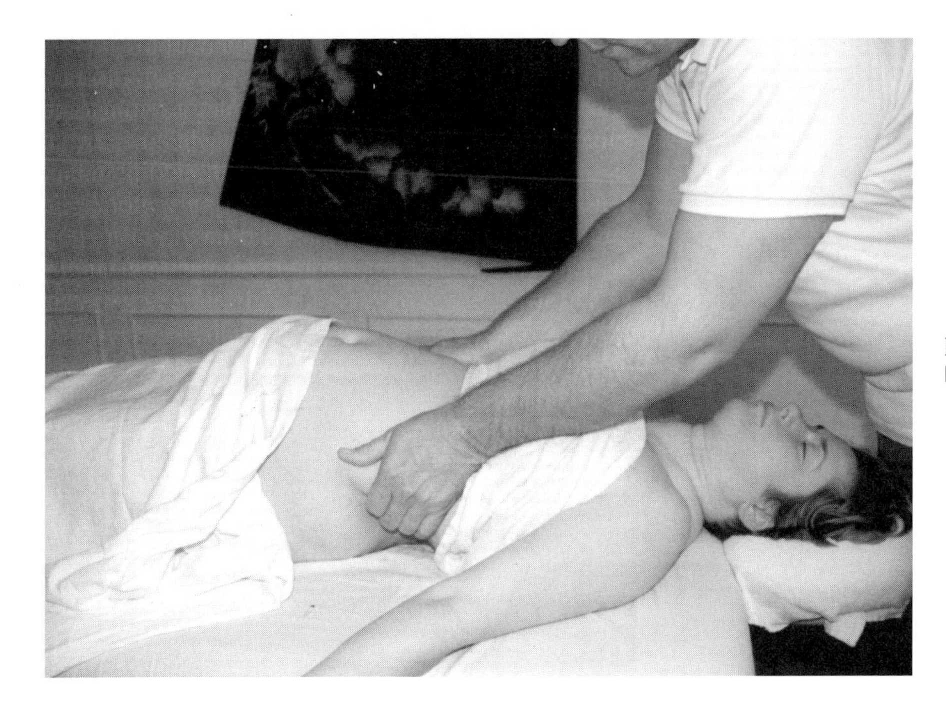

Figure 17-17
Rocking the hara.

that you push with the heel of your hand and pull toward you with the fingertips in one continuous movement (Figure 17-17).

Sequence for Treating the Front and Inside of the Legs

When treating the front and inside of the legs, you will be working on the meridians which are most concerned with digestion, so the most natural place to start is with your hand positioned on the person's hara (Figure 17-18). The patient should be positioned on his or her back, with one leg bent outward and the other fully extended. After you have bent the leg outward, bringing the foot beside the other knee, use the palm of your hand which has been placed atop the hara to hold down the inside thigh.

As you continue down the leg, turn your hand when you pass the knee and use the heel of your hand to gently press down on the groove beside the shinbone. Now press along both sides of the big muscle at the front of the thigh. Still working on the same leg, use one hand to support it nearest the knee and the other to grasp the kneecap. Gently rotate it two or three times in each direction. Working your way down the leg, use the thumb of one hand to press down the outside of the shinbone. To complete the sequence by stretching the foot forward, you must first adopt a "racing start" position. Now, holding the foot firmly, lift it off the ground and lean forward to stretch the leg. Still holding the foot, take your weight back onto your haunches and bring the foot back toward you (Figure 17-19 on p. 208). Repeat both movements, and then move to the other side of the receiver.

Summary

In this chapter, we discussed the art of shiatsu, and the role it plays as a therapeutic modality in massage therapy. We also talked briefly about the concept of ki, as well as the ancient philosophy of health. Finally, we identified the various techniques used in shiatsu, as well as the individual sequences used to treat the back, hips, legs, shoulders and neck, the head and face, and the arms and hands.

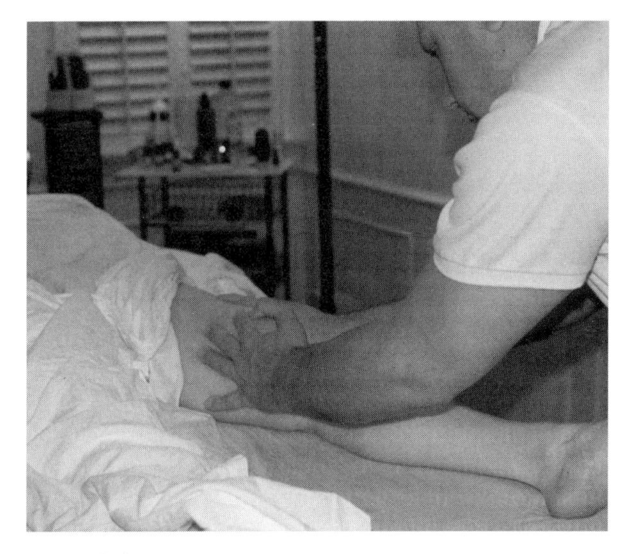

Figure 17-18
Position for treating the front and inside of the legs.

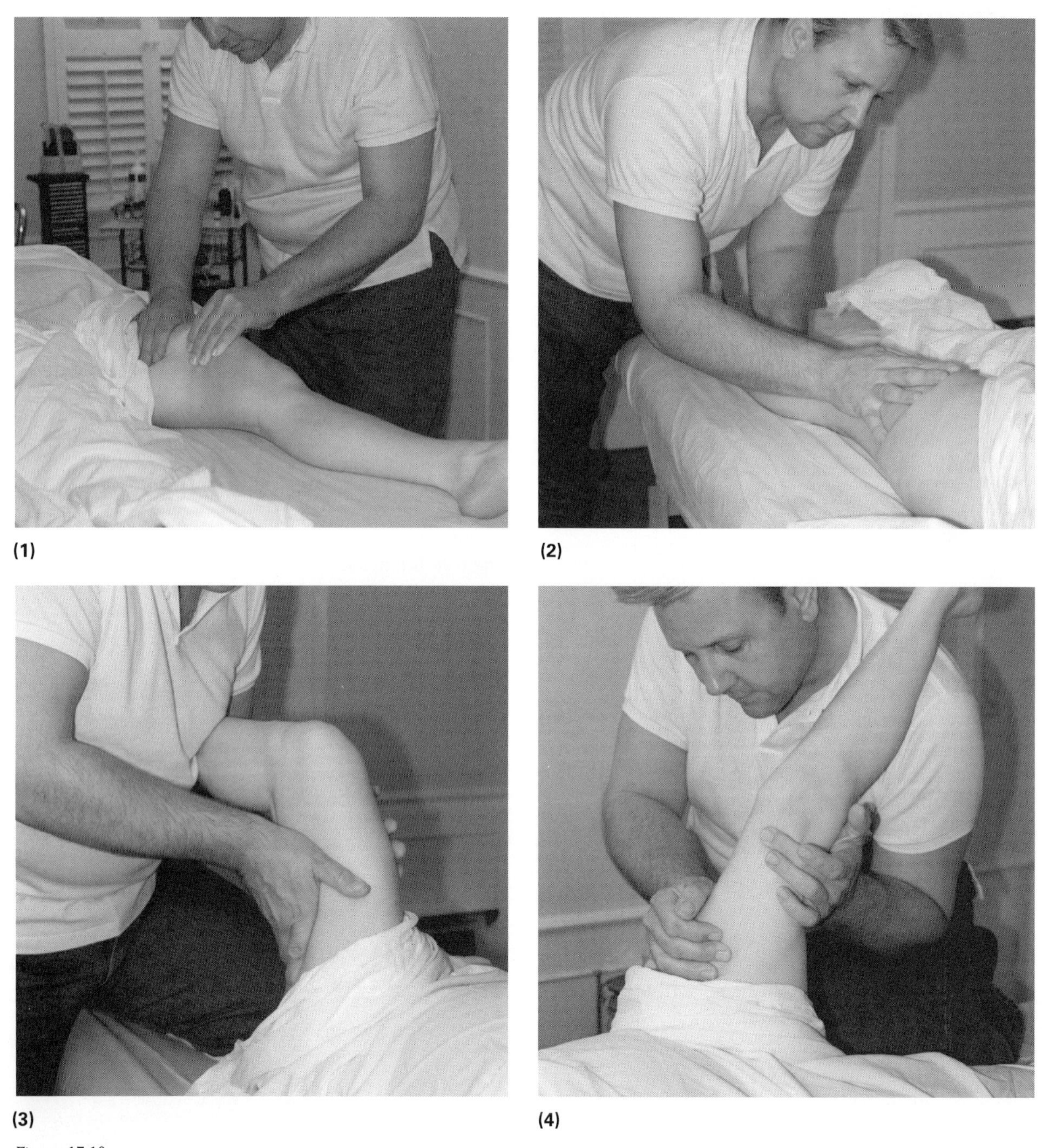

Figure 17-19
Sequence for treating the front and inside of the legs.

Review Questions

1. Briefly explain the philosophy of *shiatsu.*
2. Briefly explain the concept of *ki.*
3. What does the term *tsubos* mean?
4. What does the term *meridian* mean?
5. Briefly explain the difference between *kyo* and *jitsu.*
6. Explain the basic massage sequence used in *shiatsu.*
7. Briefly explain the sequence for using shiatsu to treat the hips, the back and outside of the legs, and the back of the shoulders.
8. Briefly explain the sequence for using shiatsu to treat the front of the shoulders, the neck, and the head and face.
9. What is the sequence for using shiatsu to treat the hara?
10. What is the sequence for using shiatsu to treat the front and inside of the legs?

18

Understanding Reflexology

Performance Objectives

Upon completion of this chapter, you will be able to:

1. Briefly describe the theory and principles involved in reflexology.
2. Explain the role of the foot in the study of reflexology.
3. Discuss the various techniques involved in reflexology.
4. Explain the role of the hand in the study of reflexology.
5. Identify and briefly explain the sequences involved in treating the hand and foot when using reflexology.

Terms and Abbreviations

Reflexology theory based upon using various techniques to stimulate *reflex points*, which, when properly touched, help to reduce tension throughout the body.

Zone theory the theory holds that there are zones, or channels of energy, which run up the body from feet to head; these may be stimulated by points on the feet.

Reflexology is a hands-on technique often used in conjunction with massage therapy. While the precise origins of reflexology are not known, we do know that it is based upon the principle of reflex points, located on our hands and feet, that correspond to each individual organ, gland, and structure in our body. By applying pressure to these specific areas, the practitioner can greatly reduce tension all over the body.

Because it is believed that the foot contains reflex points for our entire body, reflexology is also used for diagnosing weaknesses and health-related problems in any one of our body systems, as well as the individual organs. The caregiver can accomplish this by detecting crystalline deposits located under the skin at the many reflex points of the foot. The goal of reflexology is to use massage to disperse these deposits and thus encourage the body's ability to heal itself.

In addition to enhancing the body's ability to heal itself, reflexology is also used as a way to free us of the stress and tension suffered during our everyday life. This is accomplished through techniques used to relax and improve the body's circulation and nerve functioning. Therefore, one of the greatest benefits reflexology brings to the body is its ability to establish a sense of harmony or homeostasis among all body functions.

Understanding the Principles of Reflexology

Before you use reflexology as a therapy, it's important that you first understand the basic principles which it is built upon, particularly the zone theory and the use of reflex charts.

The *zone theory* proposes links between the reflexes located on our feet and the parts of the body to which they correspond. According to this theory, there are ten individual zones, or channels of energy, which run longitudinally up the body from the feet to the head; five on each side, one for each finger or toe, as shown in Figure 18-1. Any organ, gland, or part

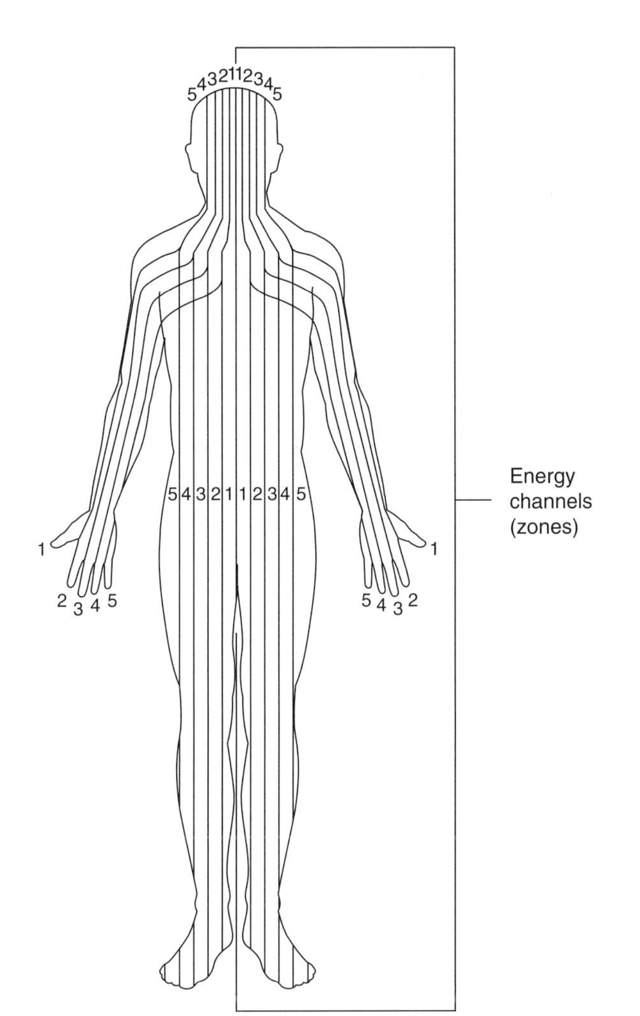

Figure 18-1
Individual zones of the body.

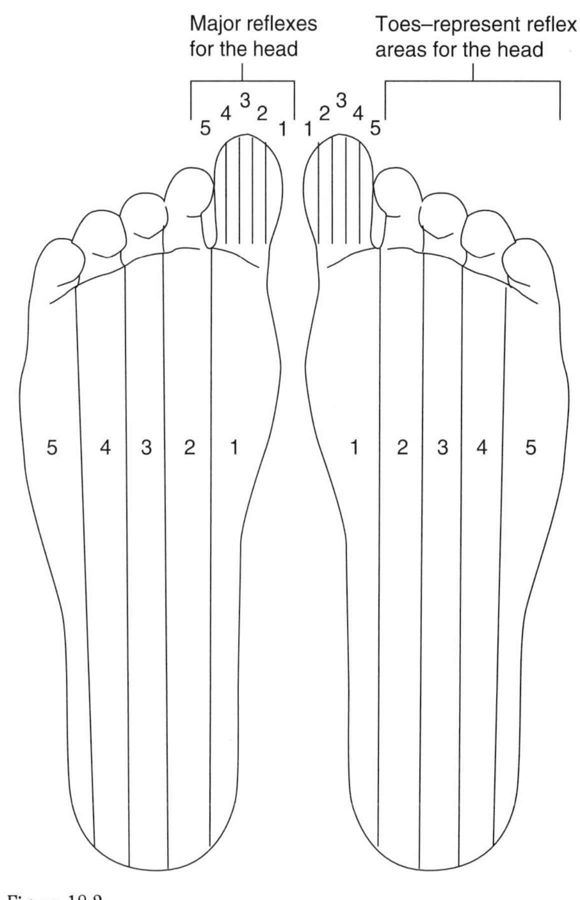

Figure 18-2
The zones of the feet.

of the body that is located within a specific zone will have its reflex in the corresponding zone found on the foot or hand. For example, the reflex of the spine runs along the inside of both feet (zone one), and the reflex of the liver lies across the outer four zones of the right foot, or zones two, three, and four.

The Zones of the Feet

Each of our toes represents an individual zone which travels the length of our body. All the toes are reflex areas for our head; however, the major reflexes for the head are located in the big toes, which subdivide into five separate zones (Figure 18-2).

Reflexology and the Feet

Before you can begin to use reflexology correctly as a modality for caring for your body, you must first acquire an understanding and working knowledge of the feet, since they are the very basis of this treatment. A good way to start is by using your hands to explore your own feet to see and feel how each of the bones is arranged.

Guidelines for Working on the Feet

It is almost impossible to work on an unfamiliar pair of feet simply by referring to a foot chart of reflexes. After all, feet, like the people to whom they are attached, come in all different shapes and sizes. Therefore, to find your bearings on each individual pair of feet, you will first need to locate individual landmarks, or guidelines. Using these guidelines will help you to hone in on the reflexes more accurately.

There are three guidelines which run laterally across the foot: the diaphragm line, the waist line, and the heel line (Figure 18-3). The diaphragm line runs across the feet just below the ball of the foot, and the heads of the metatarsals. The waist line can be located by drawing an imaginary line across the foot from the protrusion on the outside of the foot, the fifth metatarsal. To find the heel line, look for the point just above the heel, where the lighter softer skin of the arch area changes into the darker and thicker

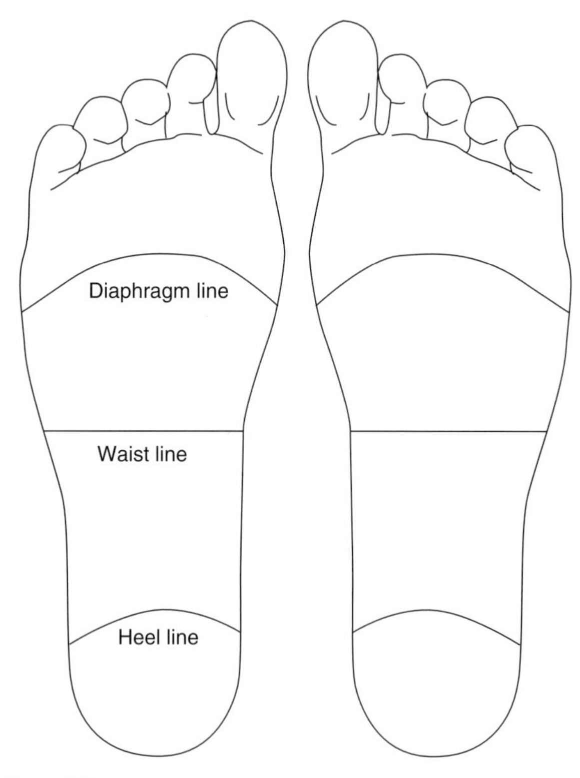

Figure 18-3
Guidelines of the foot.

skin of the heel. Once you have located these three guidelines, you will be able to better determine the exact position of the reflex that lies above and below them.

Using the Foot Reflex Chart

The foot reflex chart shown in Figure 18-4 indicates the exact location of the reflexes for the various parts of the body, as they are seen on the soles and outside of the foot. As you can see, the reflexes on the two soles are very similar; however, they appear on one foot only, because the organs to which they correspond lie on one side of the body. The heart, for example, is on the left sole, while the liver is on the right.

Basic Techniques Used in Reflexology

The basic techniques used in reflexology are unlike any other strokes or movements used in massage therapy or the natural healing arts. Therefore, they often take some time to master. Most reflexology treatments are done using both hands, with the basic thumb and index finger techniques, and moving forward like a caterpillar across each individual reflex. Hooking and reflex rotation are two specialized techniques which are generally used only on specific reflexes.

Preparing to Begin

The best part about using reflexology is that it can be given anywhere, at any time. All you really need is your hands. The only provision is that both you and the patient be as comfortable as possible. The person's feet should be at about the same level as your lap, so that you will not need to bend over too far. Apart from a couple of chairs, all that is necessary is a little talcum powder or cornstarch if the feet are damp, and a towel to cover your lap. Also, it's important to make sure that your nails are short before you begin a session.

There are two positions considered the best for using reflexology. The first, which uses a reclining chair, provides the ideal position for someone receiving reflexology, since it gives firm support for the head and knees, thus allowing the patient complete relaxation. If you don't own a reclining chair, the second option is to instruct the person to sit on an armchair or sofa with the leg you will be working on supported on a stool of similar height.

Relaxation Techniques Used in Reflexology

In reflexology, the key to an effective treatment is the ability to provide the patient with a sense of total relaxation. Therefore, you should begin your treatment by first relaxing his or her feet.

There are three techniques used to promote total relaxation. The first, called the back and forth technique (Figure 18-5a on p. 214), is done by first placing the palms of your hands on either side of the foot, with your fingers completely relaxed. Now, gently push forward with one hand, while pulling back with the other. Continue this movement, alternately pushing and pulling the foot back and forth fairly rapidly, making sure that you keep your hands constantly in contact with the foot.

For the second relaxation technique, called the diaphragm and solar plexus flexing movement (Figure 18-5b), begin by pressing your thumb firmly into the arch just below the ball of the foot. Your right thumb should be placed on the right foot, with your left hand supporting it. Now grasp the base of the toes with the supporting hand. Gently flex the toes toward you, carefully pulling the foot against the thumb. Beginning at the inside edge of the reflex, slowly inch your thumb across toward the outer edge.

The third relaxation technique, called ankle rotation, starts by you providing support to the heel in the opposite hand, right heel in left hand and vice versa, with your thumb wrapped around the outside of the ankle, just below the ankle bone (Figure 18-5c). Now, grasp the top of the foot in your other hand and gen-

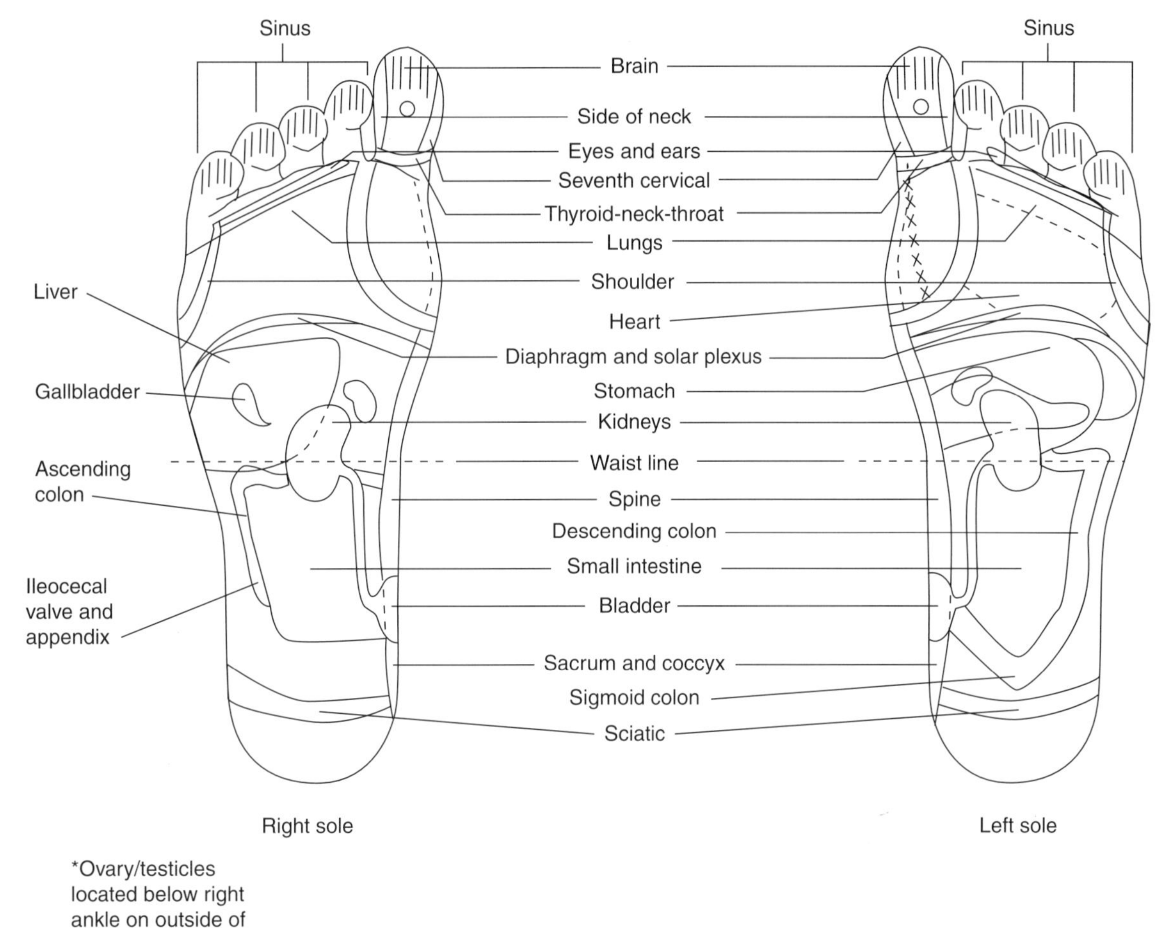

Figure 18-4
Foot reflex chart.

tly rotate it a few times in one direction, then a few in the other.

Using Basic Holding Techniques

To be most effective with reflexology, one of the most important tasks you will have to learn is how to correctly use and coordinate both your hands. The easiest way to do this is through teamwork between your right and left hands. In reflexology, we refer to this process as a holding technique. You can begin by first using one hand to hold the person's foot steady while the other works with the reflex. To work on the right foot, wrap your left hand around the toes, holding them straight without bending them forward or back excessively, and use your right hand for working (Figure 18-6a on p. 215). Now change hands. To work on the left foot, start by using your right hand as the holding hand and then change over.

When you are ready to start working on the soles of the feet, you will use the basic thumb technique. Working with the first joint of your thumb, begin the movement by "walking" forward along the reflex by successively bending and unbending the joint a little way. Remember, too, it is the inside or medial edge of the thumb, and not the tip or the ball of it, that should be making contact with the foot. Once you have made contact, with the thumb at its correct angle, and with the fingers of the "working" hand wrapped around the top of the foot to provide leverage, gently bend the joint forward (Figure 18-6b). When using this technique, always be careful not to bend the joint over too far, since doing so will not only put excessive strain on the joint, but could cause the patient's foot to come into too close contact with your fingernails.

Using Basic Finger Techniques

There are three basic finger techniques you can use in reflexology. The first, called the index finger technique (Figure 18-7a on p. 216), generally comes into play when you are working on the top and side of the foot. As is the case when you use your thumb,

Figure 18-5
(a) Back and forth technique; (b) diaphragm and solar plexus flexing technique; (c) ankle rotation technique.

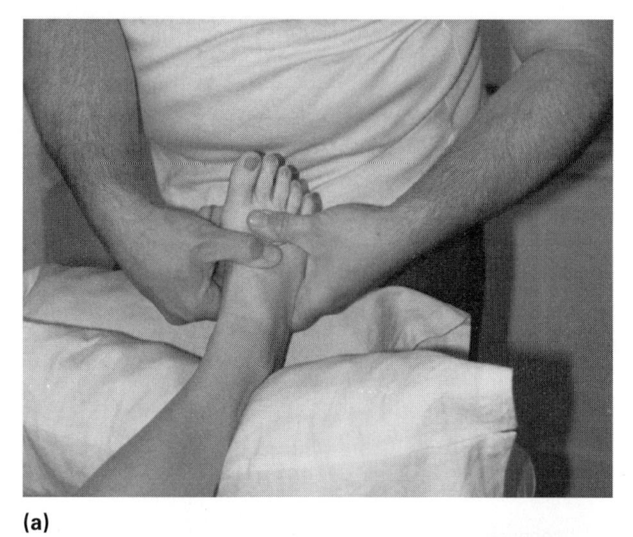

(a)

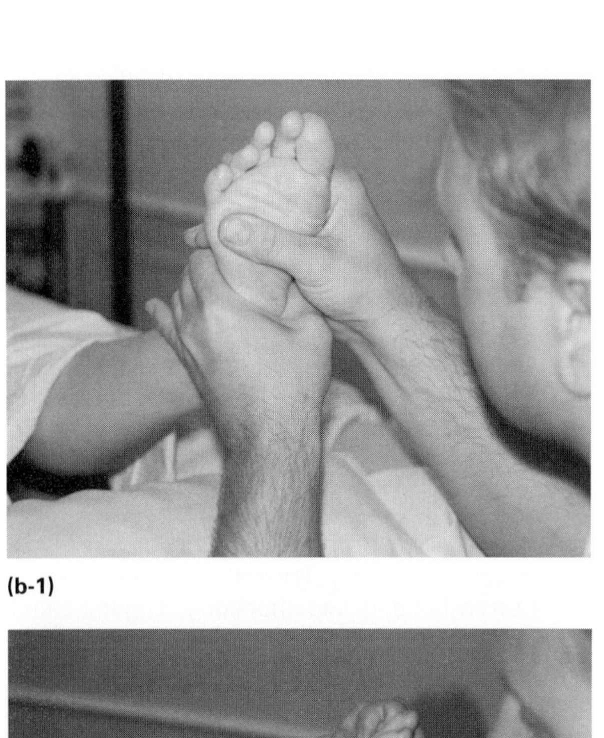

(b-1)

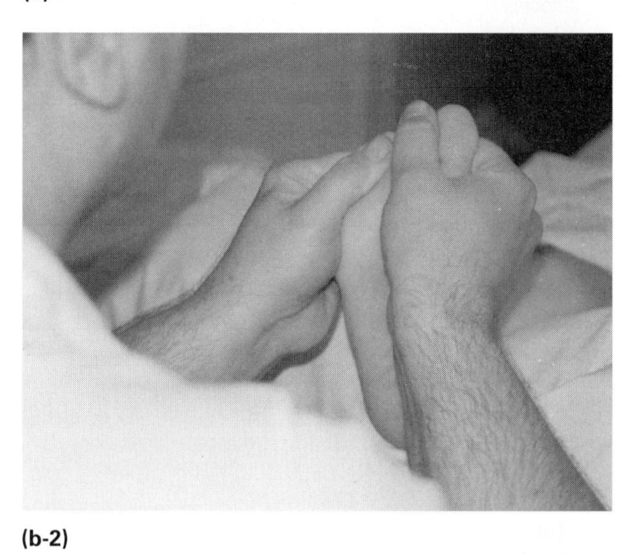

(b-2)

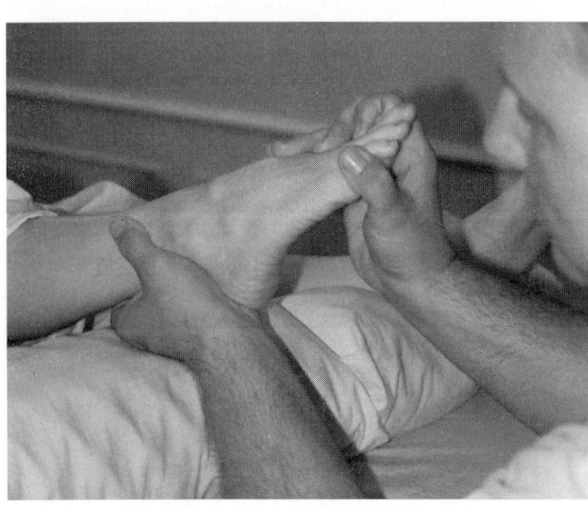

(c-1)

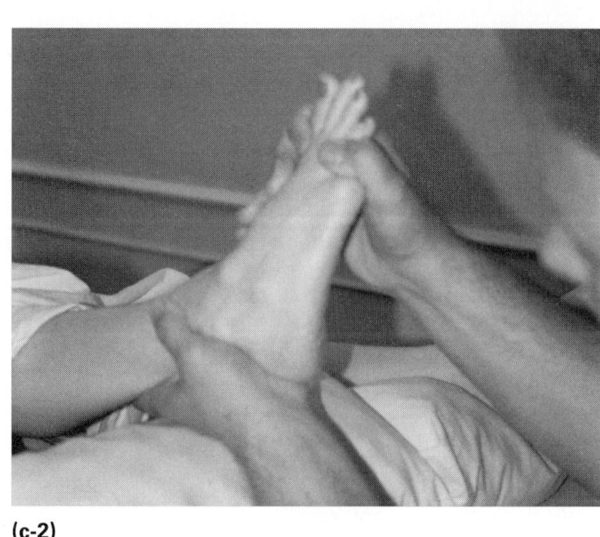

(c-2)

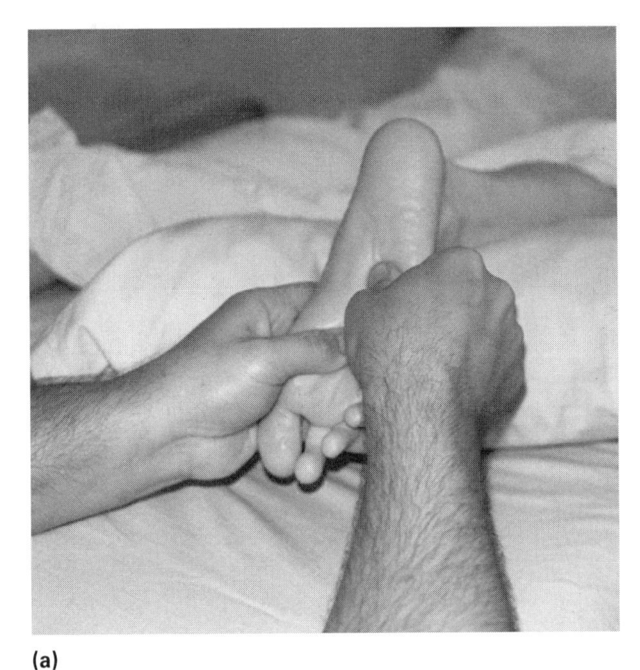

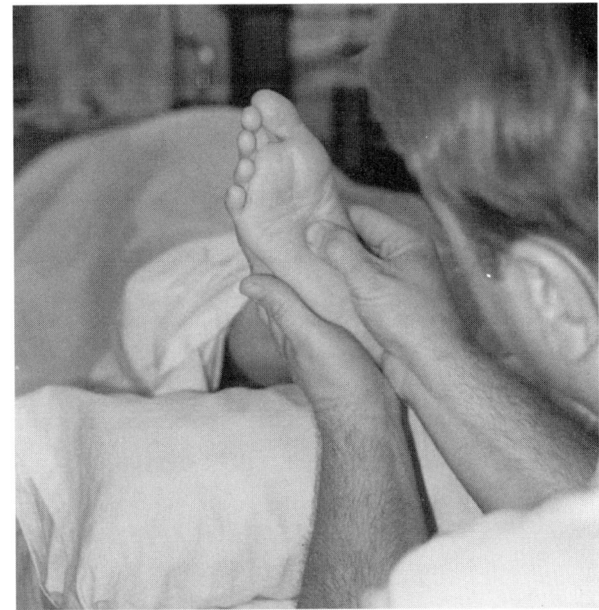

(a) (b)

Figure 18-6
(a) Using the basic holding technique; (b) using the basic thumb technique.

when using the index finger the joint should only be bent slightly, so that the inside edge of the finger can work the reflex. If the joint is flexed too far, and you use the fingertip, much of your contact with the skin is lost, and as with the thumb technique, you risk digging your fingernail into the foot during the treatment.

Another finger technique is hooking. Supporting the foot well in your holding hand, start by placing the thumb of your working hand on a reflex area (Figure 18-7b). Now hook the thumb in and back sharply to one side. To complete the sequence, you will be using the third finger technique, called reflex rotation. Start by pressing your working thumb gently onto the reflex. Now use the holding hand to rotate the upper foot around the thumb clockwise, then counterclockwise (Figure 18-7c).

Using Reflexology to Treat Individual Parts of the Body

As we have already discussed, in reflexology we use pressure or reflex points located on the hands and feet to treat individual parts of the body. Those areas which can benefit from treating the foot include the head, sinus, eyes and ears, the neck, throat, and lungs, the upper and lower abdominal areas, the spine, and the hip, knee, and leg regions. Areas of the body which can benefit from using reflexology on the hand include the diaphragm, lungs, spine, liver, hip, knee, and leg.

Using the Head, Sinus, Eye, and Ear Reflexes

When using the head and sinus reflexes, you should begin the treatment with the left foot. Start by supporting and protecting the toes with the right hand and use your left thumb to work on the reflexes. Being careful to keep your left fingers over your right, begin at the big toes, letting your thumb walk down to the base of each toe in a small caterpillar movement. When you have reached the little toe, change hands, and walk back toward the big toe again. Reverse the technique to work on the other foot.

To treat the reflex areas which correspond to the eyes and ears, begin by walking along the ridge at the base of the little toes which are formed by the metatarsal joints. With one hand, support the foot, using your thumb to pull down the fleshy skin covering the bases of the toes. Complete the sequence by using the outside edge of both thumbs to walk along the ridge in both directions.

Using the Neck, Throat, and Lung Reflexes

The reflex zone for treating the neck and throat is located at the base of the big toe. Working with this zone often not only affects the neck itself, but also the top of the spine, the tonsils, and the thyroid and parathyroid glands. Supporting the foot with one hand, use the thumb of your other hand to work around the base of the big toe from the side. Then change hands and come back in the opposite direc-

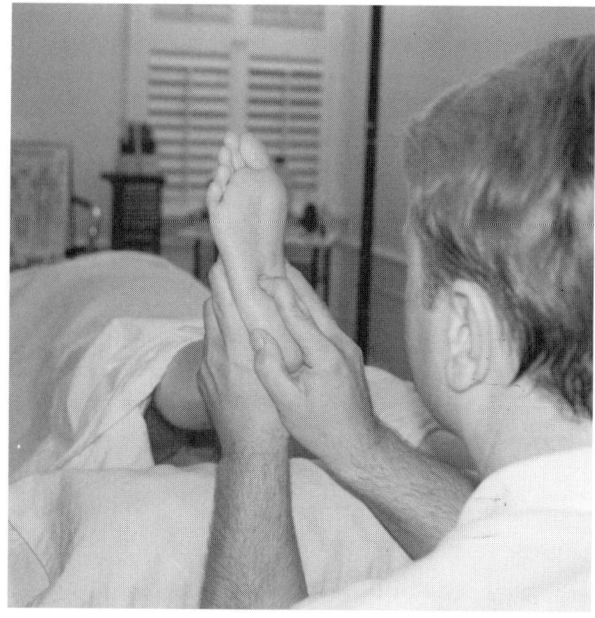

(a)

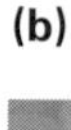

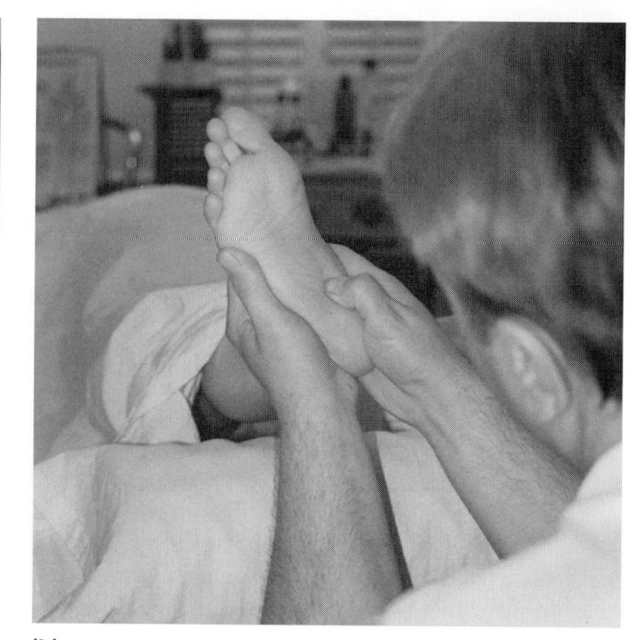

(b)

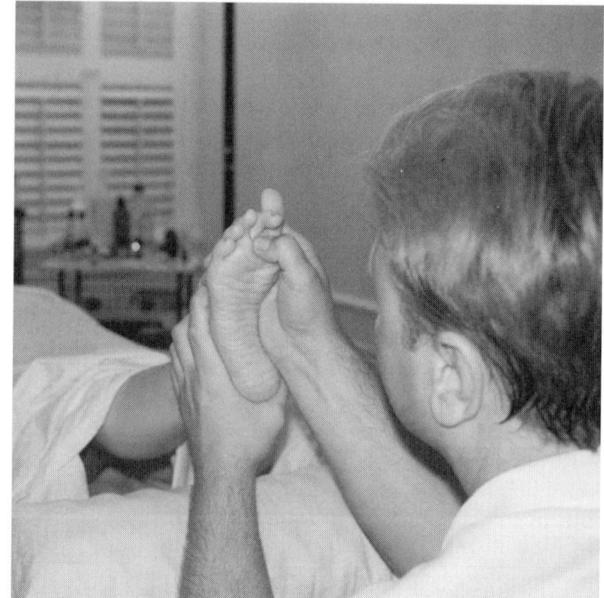

(c)

Figure 18-7
(a) Using the index finger technique; (b) using the hooking technique; (c) completing the sequence by using the reflex rotation technique.

tion, reversing which hand holds and which thumb works the reflex.

After you have worked the neck and throat reflexes, you are ready to begin to treat the lung area. This reflex area is situated between the metatarsal joints and the base of the toes on the underside of the foot, and between the metatarsal bones on the top of the foot. You should begin by first working on the lung reflex area on the underside of the foot, since this zone affects all the organs within the thoracic cavity, not just the lungs. Start by holding the toes in one hand. Then, using the medial corner of the other thumb, work up between the metatarsals to the base of the toes. Now work back in the opposite direction using the other thumb. To complete the sequence, hold the toes in one hand and use the medial, or inside, corner of your other index finger to work down between the metatarsal bones from the base of each toe. Start at the big toe and work across to the little toe. Then change hands and work back the other way. Remember, too, that your thumbs should be pushing forward on the heads of the metatarsals in order to open up the top of the foot.

Treating the Abdominal Organs

When using reflexology to treat the organs located in the abdominal cavity, the first thing you should understand is that because this area is so large, it is treated as two separate regions. The upper abdominal reflex zone is located between the waist line and the heads of the metatarsal joints (diaphragm line). Since the reflexes to organs on the right-hand side of the body are located on the right foot and vice versa, you will find that the liver reflex is located predominately on the right foot, and the stomach and pancreas reflexes can be found on the left. The kidney reflexes are located on both feet.

If you are working within the upper abdominal zone, the organ you will probably be most concerned with is the liver. To treat this area, with your holding hand on the toes, work systematically across the whole area with your thumb. Be sure you wrap the fingers of your working hand around the top of the foot to give leverage to the thumb. Once again, always make sure you alternate which hand is the working hand.

If the treatment requires you to work in the lower abdominal area, you are probably going to be most concerned with treating the ileocecal valve, appendix and ascending colon, and the sigmoid and descending colon.

Treating the Ileocecal Valve, Appendix, and Ascending Colon

To treat the ileocecal valve, appendix, and ascending colon, start by placing your left thumb on the ileocecal valve and appendix reflex. To find this reflex, walk your left thumb slowly up the inside edge of the foot until you find a tender point, just above the heel. After you have found the correct area, using the hooking technique you already learned, walk your thumb up the outside of the foot until you have reached the waist line.

Treating the Sigmoid and Descending Colon

Before you can begin to treat the sigmoid and descending colon, you must first locate their reflex areas. Start by placing your left thumb just above the heel line on the inside of the left foot. Now, move down and visualize a 45-degree angle located between the middle of the foot and top of the heel line. Then hook back and forth toward the inside of the foot a few times. Complete the sequence by changing hands and walking up the outside of the foot with the right thumb to contact the reflex to the descending colon.

Treating the Spine

The spinal reflexes are worked as one continuous movement along the inside edge of each foot, from the coccyx and sacrum area beginning at the inside edge of each heel. To work the spinal reflex, start at the inside edge of the heel and gradually walk your thumb toward the big toe. Since the skin over the reflex areas of the coccyx and sacrum are often tough, you may have to use a little more pressure than you are used to. This means you will have to wrap the fingers of your working hand around the outside of the heel bone to give greater leverage to your working thumb.

When working on the spinal reflexes, always make sure you work up the reflexes as far as you can go without ever stretching the thumb. Then move the fingers of the working hand from the outside of the heel and place them over the instep. Now, with your working hand in this position, you can continue working up the lumbar, thoracic, and cervical areas of the reflex.

Treating the Hip, Knee, and Leg

The reflex areas covering the hip, knee, and leg are what we refer to as "helper" zones, since they not only relax those individual parts of the body, but also help to eliminate congestion or tension in other areas. Their greatest benefit is provided for those patients who suffer from chronic backache.

The area covering the hip, knee, and leg reflex is quite large. It's located on the outside of the foot, extending from the fifth metatarsal to the heel, with the hip reflex surrounding the back of the ankle joint. You can treat this area either with your index finger, or with your thumb. In either case, if you are treating the entire hip, knee, and leg region, the movement involves walking across the foot in various directions. If the treatment only requires working the hip reflex, begin the sequence by first holding the foot in an upright direction with your supporting hand. You can then use your index finger to work around the ankle joint.

Using the Hand Reflexes

Many reflexologists and massage therapists agree that the main advantage of using the hand rather than the foot is simply convenience. However, the major drawback in using the hand is that it is often a less effective treatment because the reflexes are deeper, and therefore, generally more difficult to contact.

Treating the hands requires the use of your thumbs to work the palm, and your index fingers to work the grooves between the fingers on the backs of the hands. The technique for working with the thumb is the same as it is for the feet; however, the main difference is that when working with the hands, you should continually extend and flex the hand onto your thumb as it moves forward.

Understanding the Hand Reflex Chart

The hand reflex chart is used as a map which outlines the various positions of the hand reflexes corresponding to those on the feet. And, just as the hands and feet differ in size and shape, so too do their reflexes. Looking at Figure 18-8, you can see, for example, that the spine reflexes are much shorter on the hands than they are on the feet. The reflexes for the sinus also appear much larger than they do on the feet. That's because the fingers are longer than the toes. The reflexes located on the hand also seem

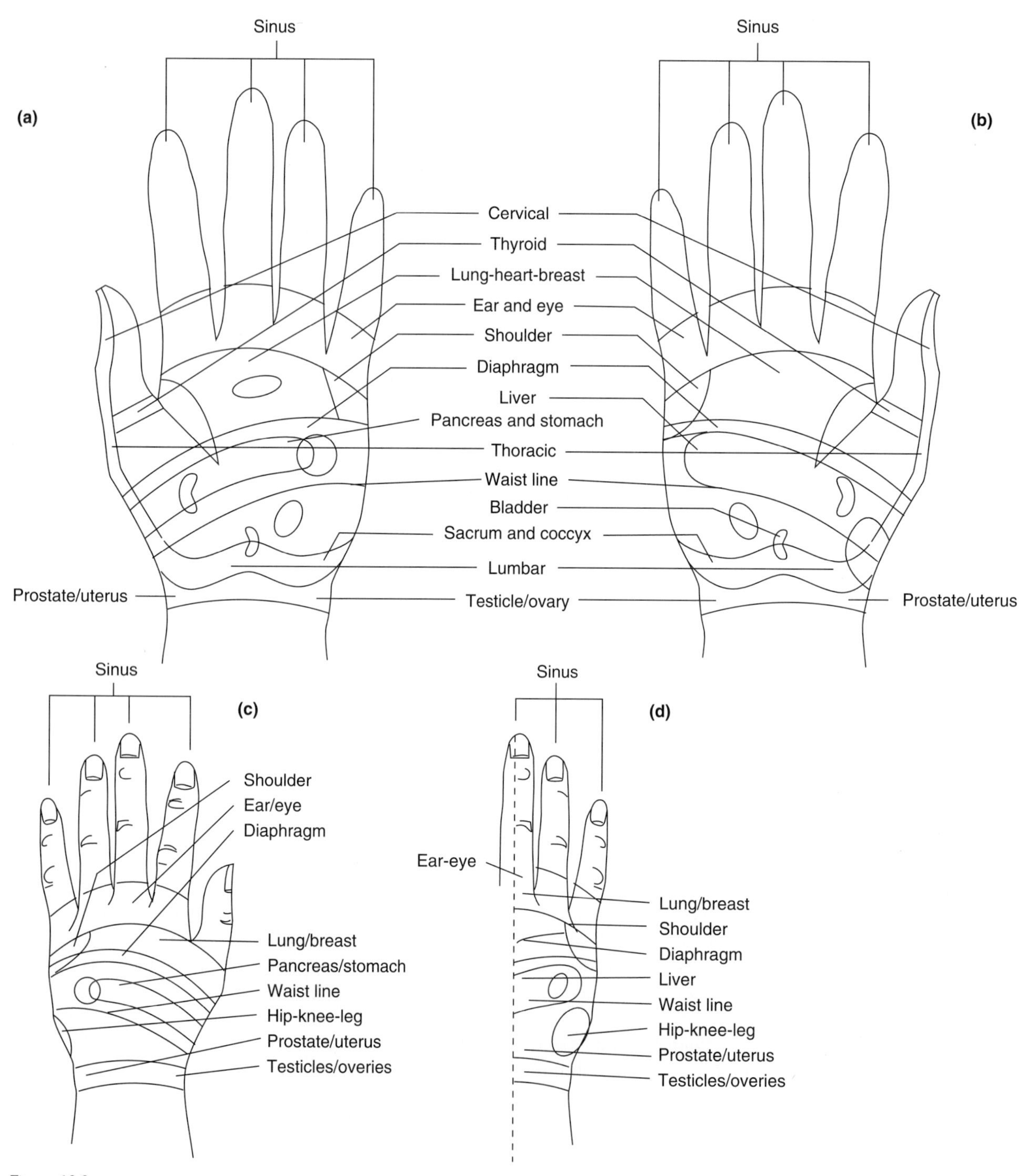

Figure 18-8
The hand reflex chart: (a) left palm up; (b) right palm up; (c) left palm down; and (d) right palm down.

much deeper than those found on the feet. This is because the hands are more exposed to the environment, and therefore, are less sensitive.

Treating the Diaphragm, Lung, and Liver

Treating the Diaphragm

The diaphragm reflex is considered the most important reflex located in the hand for relaxing the entire body. In order to find it, you must first locate the protuberances which are formed by the head of the fifth metacarpal bone, and the one which is located at the base of the thumb. The reflex can be found across both sides of the hand, just beneath those two protuberances.

Once you have determined the location of the reflex, you are ready to begin using it to treat the diaphragm. Start by holding the hand firmly in one of your hands, placing your other thumb on the middle of the diaphragm reflex. Now, gradually walk the thumb across the reflex. You can conclude the sequence by repeating it on the other hand.

Treating the Lung

The lung reflex is located just above the diaphragm line on the back and palm of each hand. It is treated by using the thumb on the palm, and the index finger on the back. Begin by holding the patient's hand in both of your hands. Now work down between the metacarpal bones with your thumb, while at the same time gently flexing and extending the fingers with your holding hand. Conclude the sequence by repeating the same movements on the back of the hand.

Treating the Liver

The area in which the liver reflex is best found is just below the diaphragm line on the right hand. To treat this area, gradually walk your thumb across the reflex, while at the same time gently extending and flexing the person's hand against it.

Treating the Spine, Hip, Knee, and Leg

Treating the Spine

The spinal reflexes differ from the others located on the hand in that they are much easier to find. To treat this area, start at the heel of the hand. Then, using the same type of caterpillar movement you used on the feet, walk your thumb along the reflex from the lower back to the cervical area.

Treating the Hip, Knee, and Leg

The reflex used to treat the hip, knee, and leg is located on the back of each hand, near the outside edge just below the waist line. To treat this area, use your index finger to gently walk over the whole area; first with one hand, and then with the other.

Summary

In this chapter, we discussed the theory and principles involved in using reflexology as a modality for treating the body. We also explained the roles of the feet and the hands in using this modality. Finally, we identified some of the most frequently used techniques and sequences used in reflexology to help treat various ailments of the body.

Review Questions

1. Briefly explain the philosophy of reflexology.
2. Briefly explain the *zone theory* used in the study of reflexology.
3. How is reflexology used to treat the foot?
4. What is the difference between *hooking* and *reflex rotation*?
5. Discuss at least one relaxation technique used in reflexology.
6. Briefly explain how reflexology is used to treat the head, sinus, eyes, and ears.
7. Briefly explain how reflexology is used to treat the neck, throat, and lungs.
8. Briefly explain how reflexology is used to treat the hips, knees, and legs.
9. Describe how the hand reflex chart is used in reflexology.
10. How is the spine treated using reflexology?

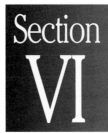

Physical Therapy Aide: Basic Concepts and Applications

19

Introduction to Physical Therapy

Performance Objectives

Upon completion of this chapter, you will be able to:

1. Briefly explain the purpose and function of physical therapy.
2. Discuss the role and function of the physical therapy aide.
3. Discuss the various modalities used in physical therapy.

Terms and Abbreviations

Active movements therapeutic movements performed by the patient, who voluntarily contracts and relaxes the muscles that control a particular movement.
Assistive movement therapeutic movement in which the patient is helped to perform the movement.
Diathermy a technique used to elevate the heat of body tissues by passing a shortwave high-frequency current through part of the body.
Hydrotherapy a process using water to treat a pathological condition.
Infrared radiation radiant heat transmitted through the air from the infrared portion of the spectrum.
Passive movements therapeutic movements performed by someone other than the patient.
Physical therapy the specialty of medicine which deals with the examination and treatment of patients with physical disabilities.
Resistive movement therapeutic movement in which the patient performs the movement against resistance.
Ultrasonic sound waves or vibrations that have a frequency above the audibility of the human ear.
Ultraviolet radiation therapy which utilizes the ultraviolet portion of the light spectrum.

Physical therapy is a medical specialty which deals with the examination and treatment of patients with physical disabilities. Often referred to as physical medicine, many health care practitioners consider this field to be both one of the newest, and yet one of the oldest branches of medicine practiced in the United States. It is one of the newest because only in the past 15 to 20 years has it been recognized as an integral part of regular medicine. It is one of the oldest because many of the physical agents used in its practice have been around for thousands of years.

Many ancient physicians knew about and employed physical agents in therapy. They even used electrotherapy in the form of shocks from electrified torpedo fish in the treatment of certain diseases. The Romans also practiced hydrotherapy and thermotherapy in their public baths. And the Greek gymnasts used massage and corrective exercises to aid them in caring for their injuries.

The modern revival of physical therapy modalities began during World War I, and was greatly accelerated both during and after World War II. Today, all branches of government, as well as private agencies, allocate millions of dollars each year for rehabilitation and physical therapy. This is through their implementation of physical therapy for injured, diseased, and disabled children, adults, and aged persons, as well as for treatment of patients suffering from conditions ranging from orthopedic, neuropsychiatric, arthritic, and pre- and postoperative diseases, to neuromuscular disorders, amputations, and injuries resulting from sports and athletic competitions.

Purpose and Function of Physical Therapy

The objectives of any good physical therapy program depend greatly on the condition for which it is being used for treatment. While many factors enter into decisions regarding the type of therapy to be employed, in general, the goal of ordering physical therapy is to increase or restore the ability of the patient's body, or any of its parts, to perform normal functional activities. Specifically, physical therapy is often used to:

- increase and maintain strength and endurance.
- increase the range of motion in joints.
- increase coordination.
- decrease pain, muscle spasm, spasticity, and swelling.
- promote healing of soft tissue lesions.
- prevent contractures and deformities.
- correct postural deviations.
- decrease gait deviations and promote independence in ambulation and transfer activities.
- teach patients and/or their families how to correctly carry out physical therapy procedures in the patient's home.

Types of Physical Therapy

Physical therapy includes using various tests and measurements of bodily functions to determine the type of treatment which may be necessary. Treatments generally range from the use of special activities and exercises to implementing specialized equipment and physical agents, such as heat, light, water, electricity, and massage.

Physical therapy may also be used to help people resume their activities of daily living (ADL). This is especially helpful for people who may have suffered some sort of disease or disability which has left them impaired by the disorder. Activities of daily living include such things as putting on and taking off clothing, walking with an artificial limb, or just standing up without pain or assistance.

The Physical Therapy Department

Most physical therapy departments or centers employ three levels of career positions. These include the physical therapist, the physical therapy assistant, and the physical therapy aide. Together, these three make up the physical therapy team. Each position has definite responsibilities, and each is responsible for working closely with the other to provide the best possible care for each patient.

The Physical Therapy Team

The Physical Therapist

The physical therapy team is headed by the physical therapist. This is a person who has completed either a four- or five-year degree program leading to a bachelor's or master's degree in physical therapy. All states require that the physical therapist be licensed at the completion of their training.

In most physical therapy departments, the physical therapist is ultimately responsible for caring for patients referred by physicians and chiropractors, to restore their bodily functions, relieve pain, and prevent disability following disease, injury, or loss of a body part. This person also reviews and evaluates the patient's condition and medical records, performs indicated tests and measurements, and evaluates findings. They use these findings to establish a patient care plan that includes setting short- and long-term goals and appropriate treatment procedures for the patient.

The Physical Therapy Assistant

A physical therapy assistant is generally trained in a community or two-year junior college and receives an associate degree upon completion of his or her coursework. Working under the supervision and direction of the physical therapist, most states require that the assistant also be licensed.

Physical therapy assistants generally are responsible for administering exercises, massage, heat, light, sound, water, electrical, and infrared treatments to patients. They may also instruct and assist the patient to learn how to improve their ability to walk, climb, and move from one location to another, and to acquire special skills which may be needed for daily living.

The Physical Therapy Aide

Under the direction of the physical therapist or the physical therapy assistant, the physical therapy aide often helps to prepare patients for treatments, transporting them to and from the physical therapy department, and removing and replacing mechanical devices such as braces, splints, and slings. Like the assistant, the aide may also be responsible for aiding the patient in therapeutic exercises, and massage, heat, light, sound, water, and electrical and infrared treatments to patients. The aide may also carry out administrative tasks, such as making appointments, acting as a receptionist, and other clerical duties assigned by the department supervisor.

Most physical therapy aides attend a one- to two-year college or vocational program; however, some health care facilities may offer their aides on-the-job training. While no certification or licensing is currently required for the aide, most facilities require their employees to seek continuing education courses in order to keep up their skills and knowledge.

Physical Therapy Modalities

Therapeutic modalities used in the care and treatment of patients with injuries, diseases, and physical disabilities are generally classified into one of eight categories. These categories include the hot and cold applications, ultrasound, hydrotherapy, paraffin bath, massage, traction, and therapeutic exercises.

Heat and Light Applications

The application of heat is one of the most commonly prescribed modalities used in physical therapy. Of the various types of applications available, those most frequently used include moist hot packs, infrared heat, diathermy, and ultraviolet radiation.

Moist Hot Packs

Because of their availability, moist hot packs are the most commonly used means of applying heat. The heating unit for moist hot packs is a small, stainless steel water tank equipped with a thermostatic control that maintains the packs at a constant temperature of 170 degrees F (Figure 19-1). The manufactured pack, a fabric envelope containing silica gel which absorbs and holds a great deal of water, has been found useful in hospitals, medical offices, and in patients' homes. After immersing the pack in the tank of hot water, it becomes a hot compress that can provide the patient with 30 minutes of intense moist heat. The degree of heat applied may be controlled by increasing or decreasing layers of toweling between the patient's skin and the hot wet pack. This type of therapy can be used up to two to three times a day, since there is less danger of burning the patient with these packs than with a hot water bottle or a heating pad, which are both commonly used by nonmedical persons.

Infrared Heat

Infrared radiation is based on the principle that heat is transmitted through the air from the infrared portion of the spectrum. Infrared radiation for physical therapy is produced primarily by using various types of lamps (Figure 19-2); however, heat can also be provided by using hot water bottles and electric heating pads. Heat lamps have a greater advantage over these, in that they require little time and attention from the health care provider, while at the same time can deliver constant heat for any desired length of time without any variation in the degree of heat being applied and without danger of burning the patient. They never come into direct contact with the part of the body being treated, so there is no weight or pressure on the part. Therefore, it is possible for the patient to remain undisturbed for prolonged periods of time. The heat which is produced by infrared lamps is also considered more effective than that produced by other sources of radiant heat, and the therapeutic effects it offers are often much more predictable.

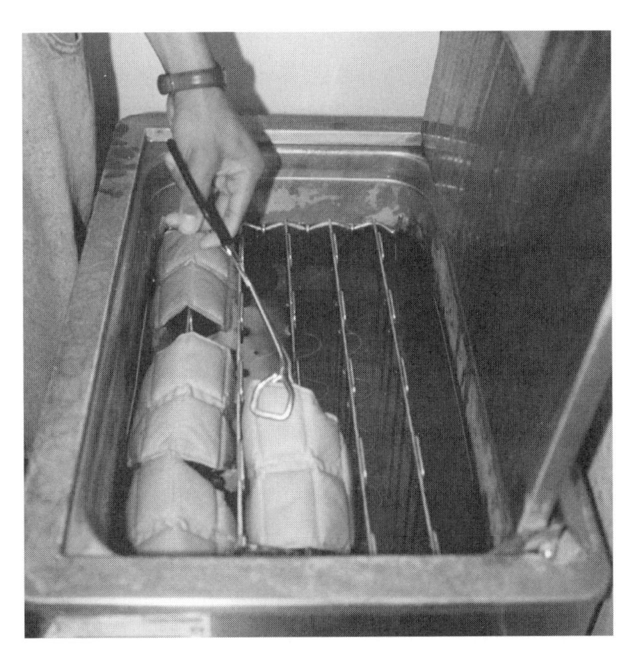

Figure 19-1
Unit used to heat moist hot packs.

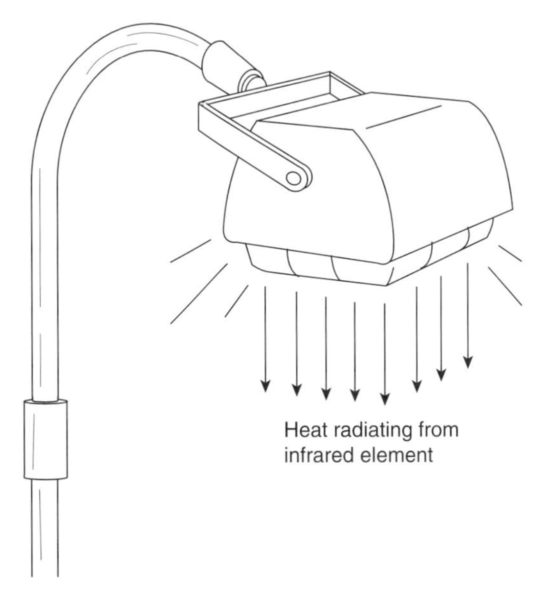

Figure 19-2
Infrared lamp.

Diathermy

Diathermy is a physical therapy technique involving the elevation of the heat found in the body's tissues. A shortwave high-frequency current is passed through part of the body, and the heat which is produced occurs as a result of resistance offered by the tissue to passage of the electrical current. The use of medical diathermy as a physical therapy modality should be a pleasant experience for the patient and should never cause pain during the time of treatment. The initial strength of the current should be adjusted according to the patient's previous experience and should then be guided by the patient's sensation of the treatment. Since the patient's sensation of heat is the principal guide for regulating the dosage of diathermy, it is extremely important that you make sure his or her sensory perception of it is normal or near normal. In acute conditions and early in the course of treatments when the degree of reaction may be uncertain to you, only a small amount of energy should be applied for about 15 minutes. Occurrence or aggravation of pain indicates that the current is too strong or has been applied for too long a period of time. Therefore, the average duration should be no longer than 20 to 30 minutes, since excessively long treatments may cause an intensive heat effect and thereby exhaust the patient.

Ultraviolet Radiation

The application of *ultraviolet radiation* is a therapeutic modality which utilizes the ultraviolet portion of the light spectrum, meaning, that portion of the spectrum which lies beyond the visible spectrum. Ultraviolet rays are of very high frequency and short length. In physical therapy, the ultraviolet radiation is provided by using a special lamp. If the intensity of the lamp is such that a minimally perceptible erythema may be obtained in 15 minutes at a distance of at least 24 inches from the reflector to the patient, the unit is classified as a therapeutic lamp.

Ultraviolet rays have a chemical action on the body. That means that they are capable of producing a latent erythema which appears within several hours after the body part has been exposed to the rays. Following intensive irradiation of the skin with the rays, the latent erythema is followed by changes in the pigmentation of the skin.

The dosage of ultraviolet radiation should be prescribed according to the desired reaction, rather than to duration of exposure. There is generally a wide variation in individual response to this therapy, with erythema of the skin being the most evident. It readily indicates a person's sensitivity to ultraviolet, and for this reason, is taken as the criterion for establishing dosage. Men are more sensitive than women, and blondes seem to be more sensitive than brunettes.

When applying ultraviolet heat, you should understand that there are five degrees of erythema which can be seen. These include the following:

- *suberythema:* there is no visible subjective skin change over a period of 24 hours after exposure.
- *minimal erythema:* there is moderate reddening of the skin within 24 hours after exposure.
- *first-degree erythema:* there is moderate reddening of the skin within 48 hours after exposure, which is followed by peeling of small patches of the skin.
- *second-degree erythema:* there is an angry reddening of the skin which may last from three days to one week, followed by peeling of large areas of skin in sheets.
- *third-degree erythema:* there is an angry reddening of the skin leading to blister formation and sloughing of the epidermis and dermis; after healing, the area becomes darkly pigmented and can remain that way from three to six months.

Cold Applications

The application of cold, including ice, is frequently used in physical therapy. This is because muscles constantly produce heat, and when they are exposed to cold, there is a need for increased production of heat, and subsequently, muscle tone is increased. Therefore, brief exposure to cold causes both an increase in the muscle's workload, as well as raises the stimulus threshold of muscle spindles, thus prolonging relaxation of the muscle.

There are many advantages, both physiological and structural, to using cold application. For example, when it is applied to a body part for a brief period of time, there appears to be no significant change in a person's blood pressure; however, an immediate constriction of the peripheral vessels of the skin does occur, which in turn drives the blood into the deeper vessels by a reflex action of the central nervous system. When it is applied to an injured part of the body, it can relieve muscle spasm and pain, reduce swelling, diminish spasticity and fatigue, decrease the risk of hemorrhage in acute trauma or muscle and ligament strain, and overall, enhance a person's ability to perform voluntary motions. A major disadvantage of cold is that it often causes some degree of discomfort, particularly in older patients who are unable to tolerate it.

When applying cold, there are some very important points which you will need to remember. These include:

- always soaking the packs in water at a temperature of 40 degrees F for at least 45 minutes.
- when treating the upper or lower extremities,

they should be treated by immersing them in a bath of ice and water at a temperature of 34 degrees F, and withdrawn within 20 to 30 seconds to avoid overexposure to the cold.

- if prescribed, you can use cold packs with alternating heat on the affected part.

Ultrasound Therapy

The term *ultrasonic* refers to sound waves which have a frequency above the audibility of the human ear. The velocity of those waves depends upon the elasticity and density of the medium through which the waves are being sent. Since the ultrasonic waves cannot pass through air, an air-free contact must be established between the applicator and the body's tissue. This is achieved by providing a coupling medium, such as mineral oil or water, between the applicator and the skin. As the sound waves travel through the tissue, part of the energy of motion is transformed into heat. This heat can penetrate to a depth of five centimeters or more. When the waves are impeded by interfaces in the tissue, such as an exit between bone and muscle, increased localized heating takes place in the region of the interface. This is often referred to as structural heating. This localized heating at interfaces produced by ultrasonic waves is not produced by any other form of heat therapy.

Physiologically, ultrasound can be very beneficial in treating such conditions as bursitis, osteoarthritis, and other musculoskeletal and arthritic disorders, such as firbrositis and rheumatoid arthritis. Through its application, heat is generated, causing the relief of edema, the increase of intracellular metabolism, and the immediate relief of pain. And patients receiving this therapy do not feel any pain or discomfort. If they do experience a sense of burning, tingling, or pain, this can be an indication that either the treatment dosage is too intense, the treatment head is not being moved fast enough or is being left in one spot too long and building up in intensity, or that the power output is too great. You can alleviate the patient's discomfort by moving the sound head away from the area of discomfort and by reducing the power setting of the generator. Remember, pain is considered the body's natural line of defense against too high dosages. Therefore, you would do well to begin with low dosages and increase them progressively in time and intensity.

Hydrotherapy

The use of water in treating diseases is an ancient practice that still has many good uses. It may be used hot, warm, cold, or in the form of ice, and all or part of the body can benefit from its usage.

Hydrotherapy takes many forms, but the most frequently used modalities include hot and cold baths, whirlpool baths, and wet compresses. There are many types of baths used in physical therapy, and substances such as oatmeal, sodium bicarbonate, sulfur, and potassium permanganate are often used to produce a therapeutic effect for the patient.

Cold Water Baths

Cold water baths are sometimes ordered because of their stimulating effect on the patient. When of short duration, they tend to increase muscle tone and energy; however, they can also produce pallor of the skin and contraction of the cutaneous fibers, causing the person to experience "goose pimples," followed by a reddening of the skin. Cold water baths can also decrease the heart rate and lengthen the period of diastole, raise the blood pressure, and increase metabolism and the amount of oxygen inspired. Cold baths of longer duration can produce stiffness, shivering, and cause the patient to experience an overall diminished functional capacity.

Warm Water Baths

Warm water baths given for short durations will tend to lessen the patient's fatigue and irritability, thus causing him or her to experience relaxation of the muscles. When given for longer periods, however, they seem to have an enervating effect. They can also stimulate the sweat glands, dilate the peripheral blood vessels, and increase the workload of the heart, causing the blood pressure to drop and the patient to gasp for air.

Whirlpool Baths

Patients suffering from acute arthritis, burns, decubitus ulcers, fractures, nerve injuries, and low back pain frequently find relief from a whirlpool bath. When such a treatment is prescribed, you must use the proper equipment. The whirlpool tub is a specially manufactured vessel of suitable size to accommodate a patient's arm or leg, and in some cases even the entire body. Water is delivered at high temperatures, usually beginning at 100 degrees F, and controlled by a thermostatic valve. It is then increased to the patient's tolerance, and mixed with air by hydrostatic pressure or by an electric mixer. The time in which a patient should be immersed in the bath is generally between 20 to 25 minutes, usually twice a day.

Wet Compresses

Wet compresses can be either hot or cold, and are often used on various parts of the body to relieve fever, swelling, and inflammation. Cold wet compresses are frequently used on the head to lessen febrile headaches, and on the throat to relieve discomfort in tonsillitis and laryngitis. Hot wet compresses are useful in inhibiting the spread of infections, and are also useful in many musculoskeletal conditions, such as lumbago, sciatica, and bursitis.

Paraffin Baths

A paraffin bath may be used to help keep a part to be treated warm and moist for a period of time, thus making the skin soft, pliable, and ready for the application of other physical therapy modalities and procedures, such as massage and manipulation. When applying the paraffin, the area to be treated must first be washed clean and dried. If the hand is to be treated, it is rapidly immersed in the melted paraffin six to eight times, until a thick coating forms. At first contact, the paraffin may feel hot to the patient; however, on reimmersion of the hand, covered with the initial layer of paraffin, the sensation of heat is decidedly lessened. After several layers have been applied, the coating of paraffin very much resembles a thick glove. The hand can either be held in the melted paraffin for a period of 20 to 30 minutes, or it can be removed, with the paraffin glove being permitted to remain in place for about 30 minutes. Once the paraffin has been removed, the hand will appear very red, moist, and soft, a condition which is quite suitable for massage or manipulation.

Massage

Massage is one of the oldest, most useful, and easily administered forms of treatment for the relief of pain and other symptoms of disease and injury. It is frequently used to increase the supply of blood to an affected part, to help in the drainage from the region of an involved joint which has been diminished by periarticular swelling, to provide muscular relaxation, and to lessen the potential for muscular atrophy. It is also helpful in the treatment of arthritis, sprains and contusions, pain caused by sacroiliac strains, and in many orthopedic conditions, including back problems.

There are five different types of massage which can be used in physical therapy: effleurage, deep stroking, petrissage, friction, and percussion.

Effleurage

Effleurage involves superficial stroking toward the body or heart, using a slow, gentle, rhythmic movement which helps to produce a reflex action. To obtain this effect, the pressure must be extremely light and each movement should be repeated in the same direction.

When giving effleurage massage, you can use one of four different types of stroking.

- *using one hand:* generally used on the extremities, back of the head, and in single massage of the neck.
- *using the thumb:* frequently used between two muscles or between a muscle and a tendon, and often to reach the interossei of the hands and feet.
- *using both hands:* frequently used upon the lower extremities on adults, on the chest and back, and when performing double massage of the neck.
- *using the tips of the fingers:* principally used around the joints.

Deep Stroking

Deep stroking massage, that is, stroking in the same direction of the natural flow of lymph and venous blood, is frequently used to aid in the emptying of veins and lymphatics and in pressing their contents in the direction of their natural flow. When using deep stroking massage, it's essential that you make sure your patient's muscles are relaxed, and that your movements are deep but not heavy.

Petrissage

Petrissage involves a process by which you use kneading, wringing, lifting, or pressing of a part to help assist in the venous and lymphatic circulation. It also helps in stretching retracted muscles and tendons, and in stretching adhesions. The strokes used in petrissage are the same as they are for deep stroking, and one or both hands may be used.

Friction

The goal of friction is to press deeply onto a part by moving your hand in a circular direction to free adherent skin, loosen scars and adhesions located deep, and aid in the absorption of local effusion. Friction is an important type of massage to use around joints of small areas, such as the hands, feet, and the face. It may also be given with the thumb, the fingertips, or with one hand.

Percussion

Percussion, which is also known as tapotement, consists of striking the part to be massaged quickly with the hand. There are four types of percussion which you can use. They include clapping with the palms of your hands, hacking with the ulnar borders of your hands, tapping with the tips of the fingers, and beating with a clenched fist.

Cervical Traction

Traction is another modality which is often employed in physical therapy when there is a need to assure a certain amount of immobilization of the spine.

It also helps in the relief of muscle spasms. When correctly applied, cervical traction straightens the spine and enlarges the intervertebral foramina to relieve compressive or irritative forces placed upon the nerve roots.

Intermittent traction is the most effective method of traction application. It relieves muscle spasm because of its massage-like effect upon the muscles and the ligamentous and capsular structures. It also reduces swelling, improves circulation in the tissues, and prevents the formation of adhesions between the dural sleeves of the nerve roots and the adjacent capsular structures.

When applying traction, you must always remember to first give the patient hot packs and massage before the traction is started. The patient is then placed in a sitting position with his or her head and neck flexed or bent slightly forward. The traction is then applied, starting with 10 pounds, and held for two seconds, followed by a rest period of three seconds. The total treatment time should be no longer than 15 minutes. As long as the patient can tolerate it, you can gradually increase the weight by two pounds at each treatment until the total weight is between 20 and 30 pounds. The usual protocol for applying cervical traction on the hospitalized patient is once a day, for no longer than 15 minutes at a time.

Therapeutic Exercise

Therapeutic exercise involves movements which are prescribed by a physician or physical therapist to help restore normal function or to maintain a state of well-being. Its application is based upon restoring, improving, or maintaining a muscle's strength, elasticity, and coordination. All therapeutic exercise programs are developed to meet a patient's individual needs, and as such, are based upon a medical evaluation of the person's disability.

Types of Movements Used in Therapeutic Exercises

There are four types of movements used in the performance of therapeutic exercises. They include *passive movements,* which are movements performed by someone other than the patient, in which no muscle action occurs and the patient exerts no effort; *active movements,* which are performed by the patient, who voluntarily contracts and relaxes the muscles that control a particular movement; *assistive movements,* in which the patient is helped to perform the movement; and *resistive movements,* in which the patient performs the movement against resistance.

Types of Therapeutic Exercises

There are several different types of therapeutic exercises which you may use to assist your patient to restore, improve, or maintain a specific muscle or group of muscles. The types most frequently employed in the physical therapy department include the following.

- *Range of motion (ROM):* movement of the joint through its full range in all the appropriate planes; may employ passive, active, or resistive movements.
- *Endurance:* exercises which use low resistance and high repetition to help increase one's endurance.
- *Relaxation:* exercises that help to promote the release of prolonged muscular contractions.
- *Postural:* exercises designed to help maintain a proper relationship between body parts.
- *Pressive resistance exercises (PRE):* exercises to help increase resistance in order to help strengthen a muscle, muscle group, or supportive structures surrounding a joint.
- *Muscle re-education:* exercises that help a muscle or muscle group to "re-learn" its normal function.
- *Coordination:* exercises to help improve precision of muscle movement.
- *Conditioning:* exercises that help to maintain and/or strengthen some or all of the body's musculature.

Using Therapeutic Exercise to Promote Wellness

There are many conditions which can be helped by the application of therapeutic exercises; however, among the most important, are the following examples.

- *Weakened abdominal muscles* With your patient in a supine position, have him or her:
  1. raise the feet, first individually, then together, with the knees extended about 10 inches above the floor.
  2. flatten the lower back against the floor, rotating the pelvis backward by contracting the abdominal muscles.
  3. with knees flexed and heels close to hips, lift the hips and hold.
  4. slowly bring the flexed knees over the chest and close to the face.
  5. alternate bending and straightening the knees as in riding a bicycle.
  6. while in the same position, bring each knee alternately to the opposite shoulder.
- *Limited movement of foot and ankle* Have the patient:
  1. rotate the foot, right foot clockwise, then left foot counterclockwise.
  2. pick up marbles with the toes.
  3. gather a towel under the foot and toes.
  4. pull up the arches; then roll the foot to the outside with the toes down.

5. rise up on the toes; then shift weight to the outside of the foot.
6. stand between two chairs with the affected foot about 12 inches in front of the other foot; rock to and fro in this position, keeping the affected foot flat on the floor.

- *Limited flexion of the knee* Have the patient:
  1. lie on the abdomen; make a complete turn of a bandage around the foot and ankle, and then grasp both ends of the bandage, attempting to flex the knee by pulling up on the bandage.
  2. from a position on the hands and knees, sit backward on the heels.
  3. standing, grasp the back of a chair with the hands; bend the knees and assume a squatting position, placing the weight of the body on the toes.
  4. bend and straighten the leg.
  5. bicycle while in a supine position.
  6. climb stairs.
- *Limited neck movement* Have the patient:
  1. move the head forward and backward.
  2. move head to the side, right, and then left.
  3. rotate the head.
  4. roll the head against towel resistance.
  5. move the head backward against hand resistance.
  6. lying on the back, with weight on the back of the head, roll from side to side.
  7. lying face down, with weight on the forehead, roll from side to side.
- *Limited shoulder movement* Have the patient:
  1. raise the arms sideward at shoulder height; then swing the arms upward and backward in a circular motion, gradually increasing the size of the circles.
  2. lie on the abdomen with the hands at back of neck and raise both elbows and the head.
  3. shrug the shoulders in upward and downward and circular motions.
- *Limited hip movement* Have the patient:
  1. stand between two chairs; then swing the affected thigh backward and forward.
  2. sit with the feet spread about 12 inches apart and roll the foot and leg inward and outward.
  3. lie on the abdomen and extend the thigh backward, keeping the knees straight.
  4. lie on the back with the knees straight; slide the legs wide apart and then return to the starting position.

Summary

In this chapter, we briefly discussed the purpose and function of physical therapy, and the role played by each member of the physical therapy team in carrying out some of the most frequently used therapeutic modalities.

Review Questions

1. Therapeutic movements that are performed by the patient alone are called:
   a. active
   b. passive
   c. resistive
2. Therapeutic movements that are performed by someone other than the patient are called:
   a. active
   b. passive
   c. resistive
3. What is the name of a technique used to elevate the heat of body tissues by passing a shortwave high-frequency current through part of the body?
4. What is the name of the medical specialty dealing with the examination and treatment of patients with physical disabilities?
5. What is the term used to refer to sound waves or vibrations that have a frequency above the audibility of the human ear?
6. Briefly explain the difference between effleurage and petrissage.
7. ______________ is the process by which people are helped to regain a satisfying life following an injury or illness that has affected their normal body functions.
8. What is the name of the process by which water is used to treat a pathological condition?
9. What is the name of a type of heat that is transmitted through air?
10. Briefly explain the five degrees of an erythema.

20

The Role of the Physical Therapy Aide

Performance Objectives

Upon completion of this chapter, you will be able to:

1. Define the role of the physical therapy aide as a member of the physical therapy team.
2. Explain the role of the physical therapy aide in assisting patients with their activities of daily living.
3. Describe the function of the physical therapy aide as it relates to positioning and transferring patients.
4. Discuss the role of the physical aide in assisting the patient to ambulate.

Terms and Abbreviations

Activities of daily living (ADL) those activities a person takes part in every day to maintain his or her body.
Ambulation the process of walking.
Dangling sitting with the feet and legs hanging freely over the edge of a bed or chair.
Prone position in which a person is lying with his or her face downward.
Prosthesis an artificial limb or body part.
Supine position in which a person is lying on their back with the face upward.

As we discussed in the previous chapter, your role as a physical therapy aide is primarily directed and supervised by the physical therapist. In most cases, however, many of your responsibilities and the clinical tasks you will be most concerned with deal with the actual hands-on techniques required to assist the patient receiving physical therapy.

It can never be assumed, just because a person has suffered an injury or has a debilitating medical problem, that he or she won't be able to function in their home or at work; therefore, many of the skills you practice will have to do with aiding the patient in learning how to get along in their daily life. Such skills as assisting and teaching a patient how to properly position or transfer him- or herself, or helping someone to learn how to walk again after he or she has suffered an injury, are examples of some of the responsibilities you must assume as a member of the physical therapy team.

Assisting the Patient with Activities of Daily Living (ADL)

The overall goal of the physical therapy department is to help the patient to achieve as much independence as possible. Attaining this goal, however, will depend greatly on the patient's disability, age, occupation, and home and work environments. In some cases, the patient may only require assistance in learning the skills involved in dressing, while in other cases, you may have to teach the patient how to move about with the help of an assistive aid, such as a wheelchair or a walker.

Evaluating the Patient's Need for ADL

The purpose of testing or evaluating the patient's need for learning *activities of daily living* is to determine his or her ability to function in everyday life.

This means learning how to function at work, at home, and during recreational times. The tests used to determine ADL include such activities as bed- and bathroom skills, dressing and undressing, gait or *ambulation* needs, and using equipment, or assistive aids, such as crutches, braces, wheelchair, or walker.

Evaluating the patient's need for ADL also includes testing for muscle strength and range of motion. This is an important part of the testing process, since any weakness or a lack of ability to move a part its normal distance could hinder the patient's ability to function.

The physical therapy team uses the evaluation process to provide information so that each member of the team can best help the patient. The therapist uses a form to record the results so that each test performed by the patient during the evaluation can be checked using symbols to indicate the response to the test being performed. In that way, if the patient appears to be having difficulty in a certain area, the physical therapy team can help solve the problem.

The individual activities which make up the ADL test include evaluation of the patient's ability to move about and transfer in and out of bed, to perform self-care, such as combing and brushing hair, brushing teeth, shaving, and putting on makeup, the ability to feed him- or herself, dressing and undressing, and activities which involve ambulating, such as walking and stair climbing. Once the ADL evaluation has been completed, the physical therapy team uses the evaluation to give it a current picture of the patient's functional ability.

Evaluating the Patient's Psychological Need for ADL

Because physical illness and disability often produce emotional and mental changes, part of the process involved in evaluating the patient's need for ADL usually includes a psychological examination. The patient's attitude toward his or her disability and recovery often determine the outcome of the entire treatment program, and these emotional and mental attitudes can have both positive and negative effects on the final outcome of the rehabilitation process. Therefore, the total evaluation process generally includes an assessment of the person's behavior and attitudes.

Evaluating a patient's psychological need for ADL involves testing in two major categories: objective and projective. Objective tests use a set of predefined standards and help the physical therapy team evaluate a person's abilities. Projective tests, which are often used to determine how a person responds to stress and anxiety, help to evaluate the patient's personality. These are done by an analysis of how a person responds to vague stimuli.

Because it is important that the patient learn new ways to perform ADL during his or her rehabilitative process, it is also important to know the patient's ability to learn. No matter how minor the injury or disease may be, the patient may need to learn verbal, motor, social, vocational, or personal adjustment skills. Therefore, part of the psychological evaluation process also includes determining the patient's readiness to learn and ability to decipher a particular problem, and how that problem is met head on. This often includes determining how the patient sees the problem, the defense mechanisms used by the patient to relieve the problem, the level of anxiety and frustration met while dealing with the problem, and the patient's acceptance and attitude toward dealing with the problem.

Alignment and Body Positioning

As an important and integral part of the physical therapy team, one of the most important areas which you should be concerned with is body alignment and positioning. One of the essential elements of comfort and good posture is good position and alignment of the various moveable parts, or segments, that make up our body. If alignment at one of these segments is not maintained, then the body will compensate in another part in its attempt to achieve a comfortable position. This in turn could lead to other physical problems. Good alignment and positioning can only be achieved when no undue stress is placed upon the body's muscles and skeleton.

Assisting the Patient for Comfort

Many of the patients you encounter in the physical therapy department are only there for short periods of time. Therefore, these patients need only to be assisted in their positioning for comfort, so that they can relax and concentrate on their treatment.

The Supine Position

In most cases, the patient who is *supine* will be most comfortable when he or she is positioned with a pillow for the head. A small towel roll also may be placed under the lower back, and one or more pillows under the knees for added comfort (Figure 20-1a). The arms should be positioned at the side.

The Prone Position

Patients who require treatment in the prone position lie with their face down and turned to the side. A pillow can also be placed under the head and abdomen if additional comfort is required (Figure 20-1b). The arms may be placed overhead or down at the patient's sides.

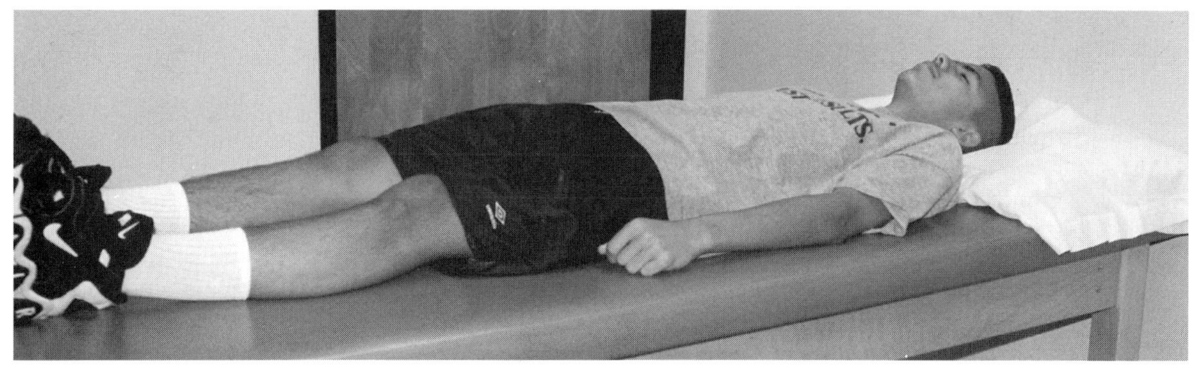

(a)

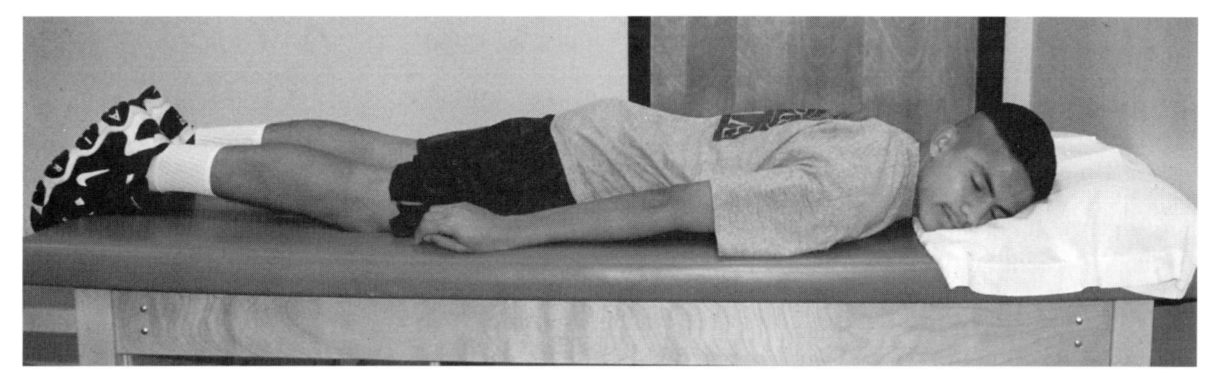

(b)

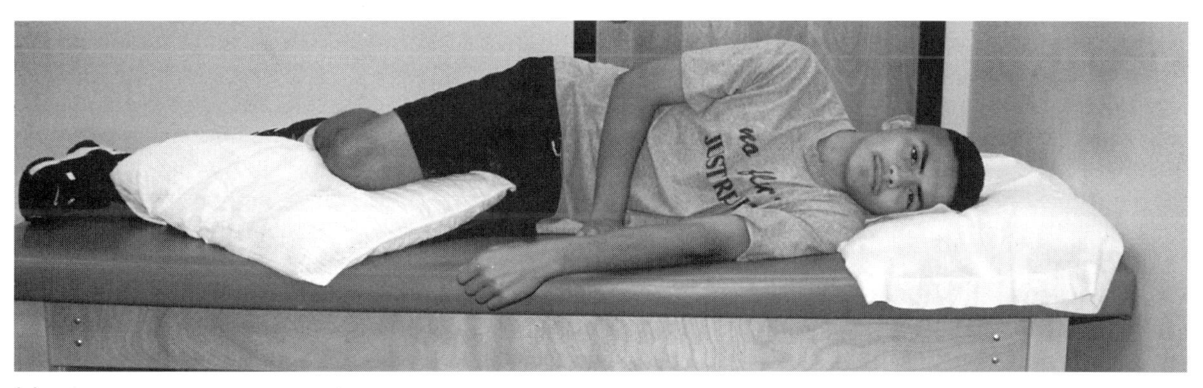

(c)

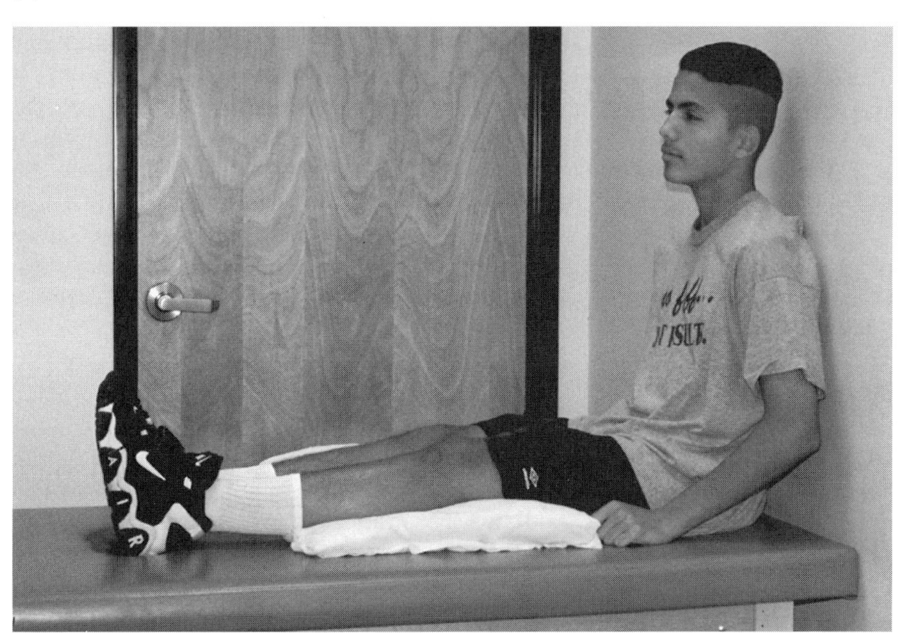

(d)

Figure 20-1
(a)The supine position;
(b) the prone position;
(c) the side-lying position;
(d) the sitting position.

The Side-lying Position

For the patient who must be positioned on his or her side, a pillow should be given for the head. Additional pillows are used to support the patient's back and trunk, so that he or she can fully relax. The weight-bearing shoulder can be positioned slightly forward for comfort, and the weight-bearing lower extremity may be bent at the knee, with a pillow placed between both knees for comfort. Support of the ankle may also be needed if it makes the patient feel more comfortable (Figure 20-1c).

The Sitting Position

If the patient is most comfortable in a sitting position, you must first assist him or her to move against the treatment table and then lean against a wall or a stack of pillows to help support that position (Figure 20-1d). This position is often used for patients who are unable to tolerate any other position.

Assisting the Confined Patient

As a physical therapy aide, some of the patients you encounter may be confined to their hospital beds for prolonged periods of time. Many patients with severe disabilities may be bedridden for days, weeks, and in some rare cases, even months at a time. These patients may find that their entire body has become stiff, and movements which previously were second nature are now difficult, and often impossible to attain without the help of another person.

For the patient confined to his or her bed for any prolonged period of time, there are many dangers. Because the blood supply can be interrupted when a bony prominence rests on the bed, the weight of the patient's body part blocks the flow of blood to the tissue under that bony area. What can result is a decubitus ulcer, or bedsore. Atelectasis, or collapse of a part or all of a lung, and muscle weakness may also occur because of the patient's inactivity.

In addition to the many physical effects which plague the bedridden patient, he or she may also suffer psychological and emotional consequences from prolonged confinement. When a person is unable to carry out his or her normal physical activity, mental attitude and spirit also tend to suffer. Therefore, it is helpful to include the person in the scheduling of daily activities, so that he or she will feel like an important member of the treatment process.

Positioning the Bed Patient

To maintain proper body alignment while the patient is confined to his or her bed, therapeutic devices are often used to provide comfort, support, and safety. These devices frequently include pillows which can be used for support, comfort, and elevation of body parts; a firm mattress to help support proper body alignment; and a bedboard in cases where the patient requires additional firm support. Adjustable hospital beds are also useful for putting the patient in different positions. The bed allows the patient to be positioned with his or her knees bent and can also be adjusted to place the person in a sitting position. Because it can be lowered and raised, the hospital bed is also useful in transferring a patient in and out of the bed, as well as preventing injury to your own back while you are working with the patient.

Patients who have sustained an injury or who suffer from an illness which requires their confinement to bed are often weak, helpless, and in some cases, even unconscious. For these patients, changing their position at least every two hours is extremely important. In some cases, the patient is able to move him- or herself alone, and may only need your help as a reminder for changing position. Other patients may require that the nursing staff or a member of the patient's family be taught when and how to position the patient. In cases where the patient is severely disabled, as a member of the physical therapy team you may be required to assist in positioning the patient in bed.

The majority of patients confined to their hospital beds because of a disability are usually most comfortable if they are positioned in a supine, side-lying, prone, or Fowler's (semi-sitting) position. To position the patient supine, you should start with his or her body in a normal anatomical position so that the body is lying flat on the back and in proper alignment. A pillow may be placed under the patient's head for comfort; however, you can use small towels rolled to help support the neck and the lower back. The hips and knees should be kept straight, and the legs supported at the sides with towel rolls. This will prevent rotation. The toes should point toward the ceiling, and a small roll should be placed under the patient's ankle to take the pressure off his or her heels. Never place anything against the bottoms of the patient's feet. The upper extremities may be positioned in a number of ways depending on the patient's disability. If possible, the arm should be abducted, or positioned away from the body, and the hand should be maintained in a functional position with the aid of a firm rolled towel.

When the bed patient requires positioning on his or her side, it's important to pay special attention to the arm and leg on the upper side of the body, since undue pull on these extremities can cause the patient additional discomfort. This can be prevented with the proper use of pillows which are placed under the arm and leg to maintain proper body alignment and elevation. The hand and elbow, as well as the knee and ankle, should not be allowed to hang down lower than the patient's shoulder or hip. Pillows may also be placed in front and behind the patient to prevent him or her from rolling forward or backward.

Assisting the patient to change his or her position so that he or she is lying prone, or with the face placed downward, often comes as a relief to the person confined to a hospital bed for long periods of time. With the patient lying face down, you can either allow the feet to hang over the mattress to prevent pressure on the toes, or you can use pillows to help elevate and support the extremities and trunk. A small pillow or rolled up towel can also be used to support the patient's head. And if necessary, you can also use a rolled up towel to help prevent the patient's shoulders from sagging into the mattress.

Assisting the patient into a Fowler's position means that you will be helping the patient to a semi-sitting position in which pillows are used under the arms and hands to prevent pulling at the patient's shoulders. A small pillow is also placed under the head for comfort. The legs are kept in good alignment with the toes pointing toward the ceiling and the knees supported in a slightly bent position.

Assisting in Transferring

Some of the patients you will work with in the physical therapy department require a wheelchair, gurney, or other assistive device to move them about. And the degree to which your help will be needed to transfer these patients from one location to another will greatly depend upon the patient's physical condition or disability. If you are required to assist the patient in moving or transferring, you must remember that no matter what the situation is, safety must always be your first and primary concern.

Whether the patient is confined to his or her bed, or is able to move about with the aid of an assistive device, prior to helping in the transfer always make sure to check all the equipment for safety. If the patient is in a bed, this means pushing the bed against the wall, and locking the wheels.

Before beginning any transfer, it's important that you first explain the procedure to the patient. This means telling him or her what you will be doing, as well as what is expected of the patient. And always use a safety belt. If one is not available, you can make one by wrapping a sheet around the patient's waist. If a person is confined to a wheelchair or gurney, you must also lock the wheels before starting the transfer. Also, make sure that the transfer surfaces are at the same height. Most hospital beds can be adjusted to the same level as the wheelchair or gurney. If the patient is being transferred to or from a wheelchair, remove the wheelchair armrest on the transfer side. Whenever possible, transfer the patient from his or her strongest side.

Another important safety measure is to make sure the patient wears shoes with nonslip soles and without heels. And never try to transfer someone who is just wearing socks, stockings, or who is barefoot.

Practicing good safety precautions also involves proper positioning on the part of the person assisting in the transfer. When helping a patient, it's always best if you stand close to prevent any possible strain to your back. This means keeping your back straight and your knees slightly flexed, and your feet about shoulder width apart, with one positioned slightly in front of the other. Creating a wide base of support will help you to balance when the patient is moving.

Helping with Assisted Transfers

While there are several types of transfers for which patients may need assistance, two that you will probably encounter most frequently include the bed to wheelchair transfer and the wheelchair to treatment transfer.

Assisting the Patient from the Bed to the Wheelchair

When assisting the patient to transfer from the bed to his or her wheelchair, you must first make sure that the head of the bed is elevated to a high Fowler's position, with both side rails in the up position. Then lower the side rail on the wheelchair side, lock the brakes on the wheelchair, and remove the wheelchair armrest on the side on which the patient is being transferred. Also make sure that the bed is the same height as the wheelchair seat. To initiate the transfer, you would:

1. Place the safety belt on the patient, and swing his or her body so that the legs are off the side of the bed.
2. Using the safety belt, move the patient's hips forward until both feet are flat on the floor.
3. After positioning yourself in front of the patient, with your knees blocking his, assist the patient to stand.
4. Once the patient has his balance, pivot him around to the wheelchair; the back of his legs should touch the seat of the chair.
5. After instructing the patient to reach back for the chair armrest, allow him to slowly sit down.
6. Replace the armrest, and raise the footrests of the chair for patient comfort.
7. To assist the patient to transfer from the wheelchair back to the bed, use the same procedure in reverse.

Assisting the Patient from the Wheelchair to the Treatment Table

When assisting the patient to transfer from the wheelchair to the treatment table (Figure 20-2), you must first ascertain the degree to which he or she is disabled, since this will determine the amount of assistance you should provide. Then, to initiate the transfer, you would:

1. Place the wheelchair close to the treatment table.
2. Using the safety belt, assist the patient to stand.
3. Pivot the patient around until his buttocks are touching the table and instruct him to sit up on the table.

Unassisted Transfers

Unassisted transfers are those in which the patient can move him- or herself without the aid of another person. These transfers include the wheelchair to car or bed transfer, the wheelchair to tub or toilet transfer, and the bed to wheelchair transfer (Figure 20-3 on p. 238). Of all of these, the most common is the bed to wheelchair transfer. To accomplish this movement, the patient first sits him- or herself up on the edge of the bed, with the wheelchair positioned close to the bed in a locked position. The patient then stands up, using the arm of the chair for support. The body is then pivoted until the backs of the patient's legs are touching the seat of the wheelchair. With both hands positioned firmly on the arms of the wheelchair, the patient completes the transfer by slowly lowering him- or herself into the chair.

Assisting the Patient Toward Independence

All of us want and need to be independent and self-sufficient. We want to be able to care for ourselves, get about, and function on our own. To provide the patient with as much independence as possible, many different types of equipment have been developed to assist the patient in walking and ambulating, and other activities of daily living.

Any piece of equipment used to assist a person toward increasing his or her independence is referred to as an assistive device. These devices can be made of plastics, leathers, metals, or wood. As a physical therapy aide, you must be able to assist your patients in learning how to use the many types of equipment available to them. Not using equipment correctly is one of the greatest problems health care providers face when we train our patients to become more independent and self-sufficient.

Choosing the Appropriate Device

When choosing the appropriate device for a patient, there are several factors which you should consider, such as the activity to be performed and the physical requirements needed to complete that activity, the psychological effects the equipment may have on the patient, the importance of the equipment in the total rehabilitation process, and the materials and design of the equipment. You should also take into account the purpose and goals for which the equipment is required. Specific purposes for using these devices include providing positioning and support for weakened body segments, encouragement of early movement and function of muscles and joints, assistance in coordination and balance, and control of spasticity. Two other functions of these devices include replacement of a lost body part and helping to increase the function of residual muscle strength and skill.

Just as important as filling the need for using these devices are the goals or objectives for which they should be used. They should help to protect the patient and his or her family from injury, help in maintaining proper body alignment, protect specific body segments from overstretching and/or overfatigue, provide independence to the patient in order to carry out his or her activities of daily living in spite of the disability, and above all, they should help the patient to build his or her self-esteem.

Types of Assistive Devices

There are many different types of assistive devices available for use by patients. The most common of these include special hospital beds, such as the circular-framed bed and the Stryker frame bed, custom-made *prostheses,* which are used to replace a body part, and as such, provide a higher degree of functional independence, and ambulatory assistive devices, such as canes and walkers (Figure 20-4 on p. 239), and crutches (Figure 20-5 on p. 240), which can be used to help the patient walk.

Helping the Patient to Ambulate

Before you can begin helping your patient to ambulate, you must first assist him or her in gait-training activities. Muscles that will be used when a patient attempts to walk must be strong. Therefore, you should encourage your patient to do strengthening exercises to their arms and legs before beginning to ambulate.

To prepare for standing, have your patient first sit up in bed. If no complaints of dizziness or nausea are reported, the patient can then be moved to the edge

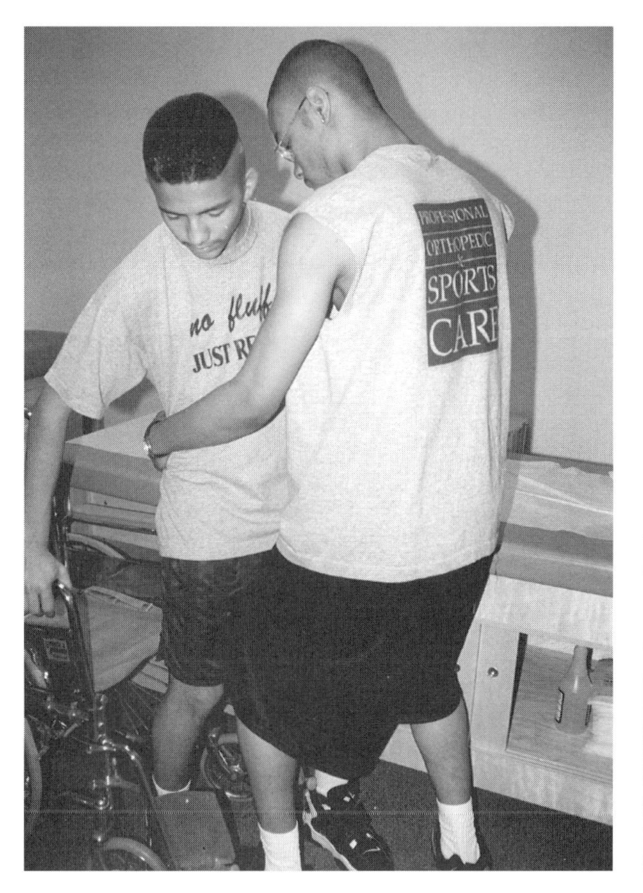

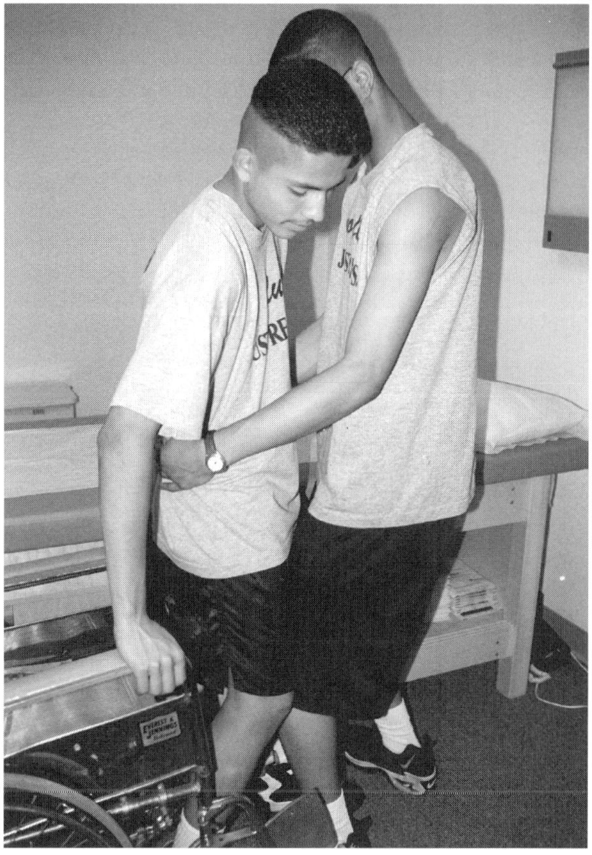

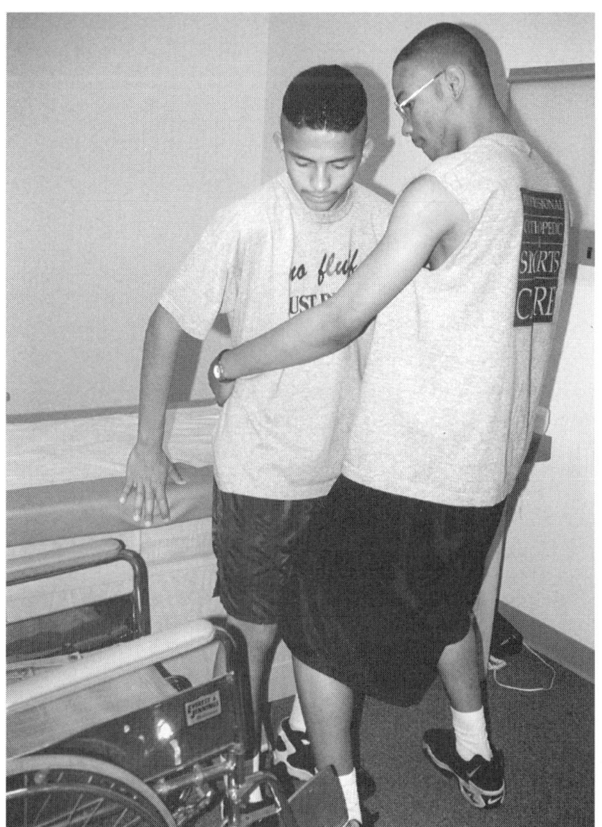

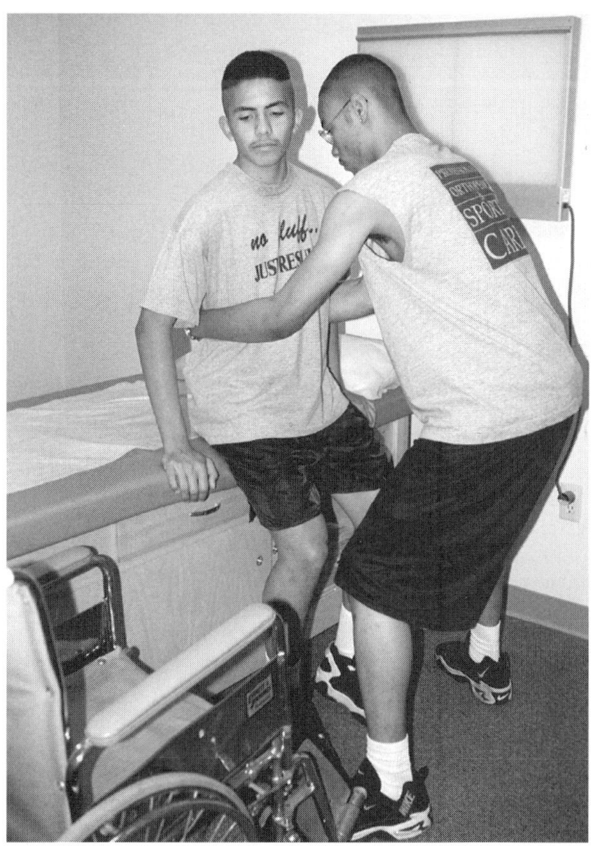

Figure 20-2
Assisting the patient to transfer from the wheelchair to the treatment table.

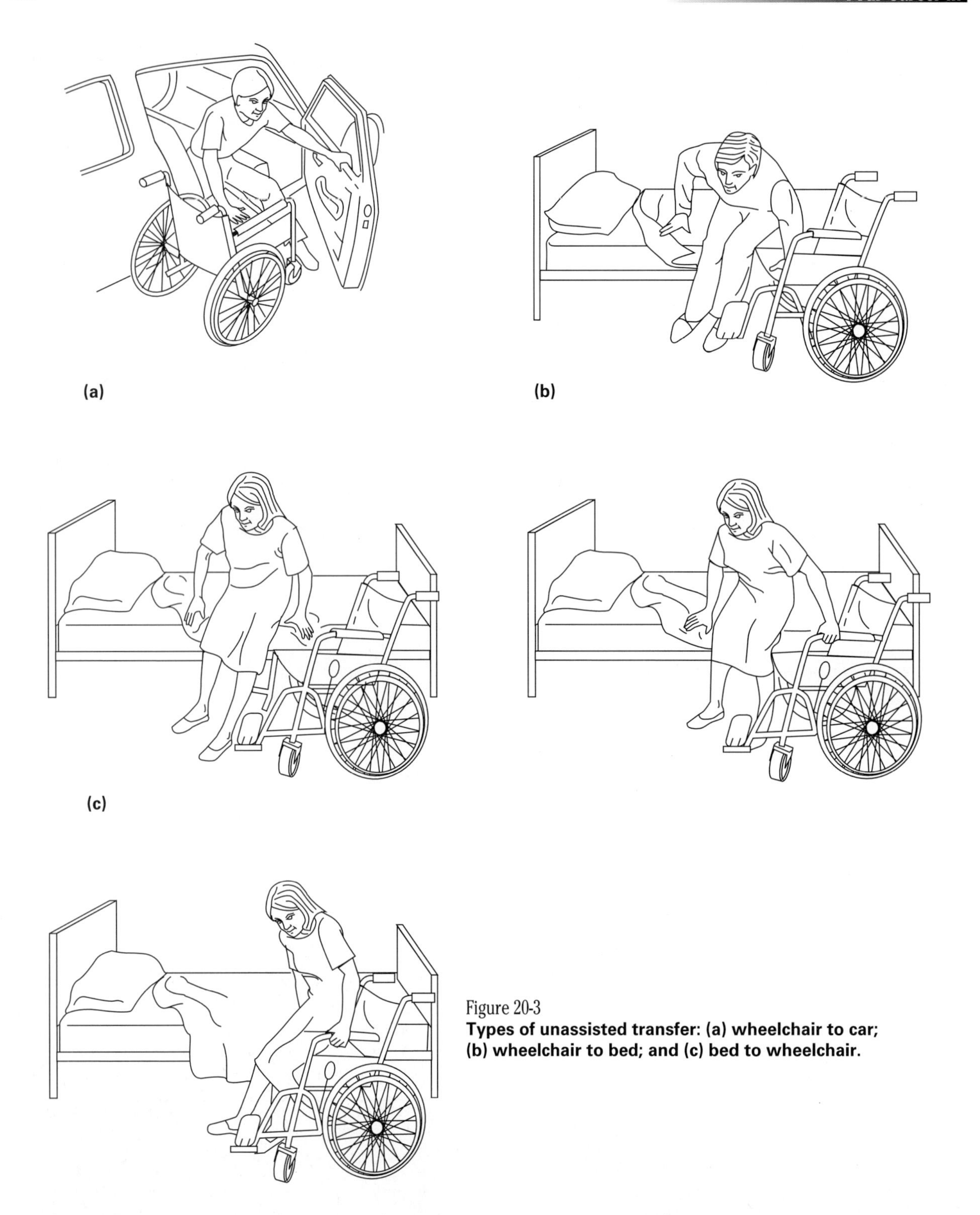

Figure 20-3
Types of unassisted transfer: (a) wheelchair to car; (b) wheelchair to bed; and (c) bed to wheelchair.

of the bed, with the legs still allowed to dangle over the edge and touch the floor. Completing this activity will help prepare the patient for standing and eventually walking. If the patient does complain of some dizziness, have him or her lie back down.

If it has been determined that your patient requires an assistive device to ambulate, show him or her the device and demonstrate how to properly use it. Also, make sure that you have a safety or walking belt close by to help provide security and support for the patient once he or she begins to ambulate.

Assisting the Patient to Use a Walker

A walker is used for support when the patient is learning to walk again. Patients who have been confined to bed for long periods of time or who have had fractures of the lower extremities can benefit from

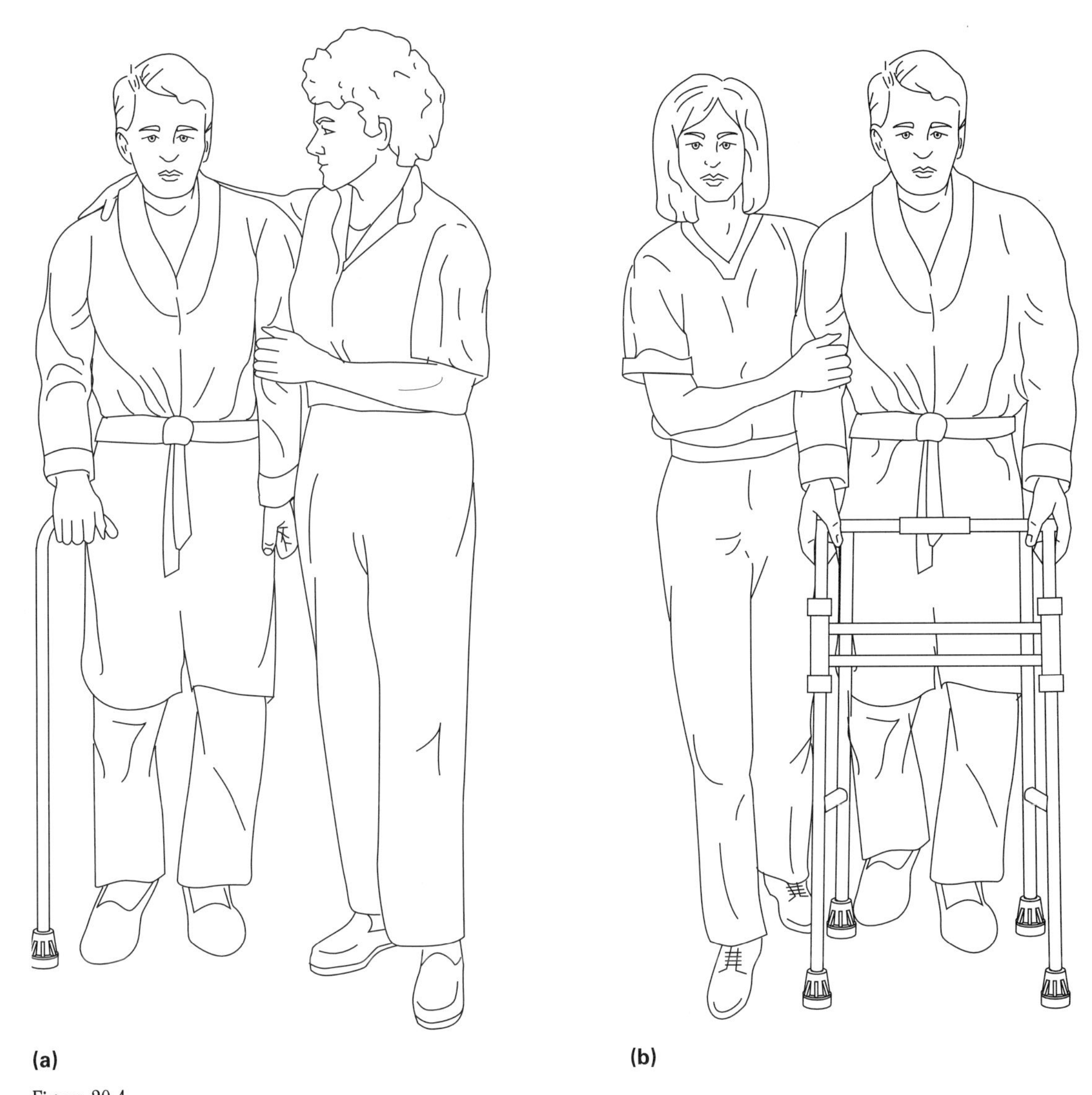

(a) (b)

Figure 20-4
(a) Assisting a patient with a cane; (b) assisting a patient with a walker.

using a walker. It can also be used to prepare a patient for using crutches. To use a walker correctly, the patient must be able to bear full weight on one foot, balance while standing, and have full use of both arms and/or hands. Most walkers can be adjusted to meet the individual needs of the patient. Your responsibility is to adjust the height of it so that when the patient rests his or her hands on the handgrips, the elbows will be bent about 30 degrees. After you have made sure that the walker correctly fits the patient's height, place it firmly on the floor in front of the patient before you allow him or her to attempt to take a step.

Assisting the Patient to Use a Cane

Canes are generally made of aluminum or wood and come in many styles and models. Frequently a patient will use the cane incorrectly by holding it on the same side as his or her weak leg. Therefore, you must instruct the patient to carry the cane on the side opposite the weak or injured leg. This will provide for a more normal walking pattern.

Assisting the Patient to Use Crutches

Crutches usually come in two types: axillary crutches, which are the most common and frequently used by persons needing short-term help, and Canadian or Lofstrand crutches, often used by people requiring permanent assistance with walking. The axillary crutches are held under the patient's axilla, or armpit, during use, while the Canadian or Lofstrand crutches have a cuff or band that fits around the forearm to keep the crutches in place.

A third type of crutch, used less frequently than the others, and usually of most benefit to patients who do not have good hand function, is called the

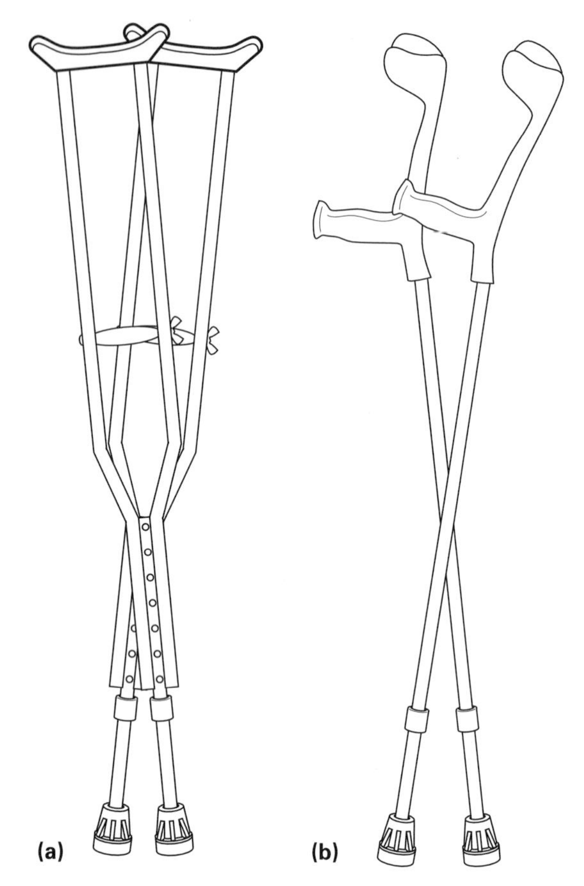

Figure 20-5
Types of crutches: (a) axillary; (b) Canadian or Lofstrand.

platform crutch. These crutches are especially helpful for people suffering from arthritis in their upper extremities.

Measuring the Crutches

It is up to the patient's physician, or in some cases the physical therapist, to prescribe the type of crutches that will be needed by a patient. To make sure that the crutches fit the patient correctly, a determination will have to be made as to the correct size. To measure patients for crutches, they should be wearing shoes even if they are being measured while they are in bed. If the patient is supine, the measurement is taken from the anterior fold of the axilla down to a point approximately six inches to the side of the heel. If the patient is standing, the measurements are taken from about two inches below the anterior fold of the axilla down to a point approximately six inches to the side of the heel. When measuring the crutches, you must also include any padding and the crutch tips. The handgrips should be adjusted to allow about 30 degrees of elbow flexion during relaxed standing, and the wrists should be slightly extended.

If the patient's shoulders are being pushed upward by the pads, or if the shoulders are resting heavily on the axillary pads, then the crutches have not been fitted properly. Two additional signs that may indicate that the crutches are not properly sized are if the crutches slip out from under the patient's arms while he or she is walking, and if the elbows are straight or bent more than 30 degrees. Crutches fit correctly only when:

- weight is on the hands with the elbows bent about 30 degrees.
- axillary pads are about two inches below the patient's armpit.
- they are out to the side and ahead of the feet in a comfortable position about six inches from the patient's toes to permit clearance of the hips.

Teaching the Patient How to Use Crutches

When teaching your patient how to properly use crutches, always make sure you use a safety belt, keeping one hand placed firmly on the belt and the other on the patient's shoulder. Then, position yourself so that you are standing behind the patient, and instruct him or her to:

- stand straight against the wall, with the crutches out to the side and ahead of the feet in a comfortable position.
- put his or her weight on the hands with the elbows slightly bent.
- shift the weight slightly forward, then advance the crutches while leaning forward on the handgrips.
- take the crutches back and return to the wall for support.

Once you have taught your patient how to assume the starting position for walking with crutches, he or she is ready to begin crutch-walking.

There are four basic types of crutch-walking gaits. The first is called a two-point gait (Figure 20-6). It is generally used for patients who can bear some weight on both of their legs. The rhythm for using the two-point gait is left crutch, right foot, right crutch, left foot. The procedure for using this gait is to have the patient:

1. stand with one crutch on each side supporting most of his or her weight.
2. advance the left crutch and the right foot.
3. advance the right crutch and the left foot.
4. repeat steps two and three.

Another crutch-walking gait, the three-point gait (Figure 20-7), is most often used for patients who are unable to bear weight on one leg. It is also quite helpful for a patient who has a cast, broken leg, or any

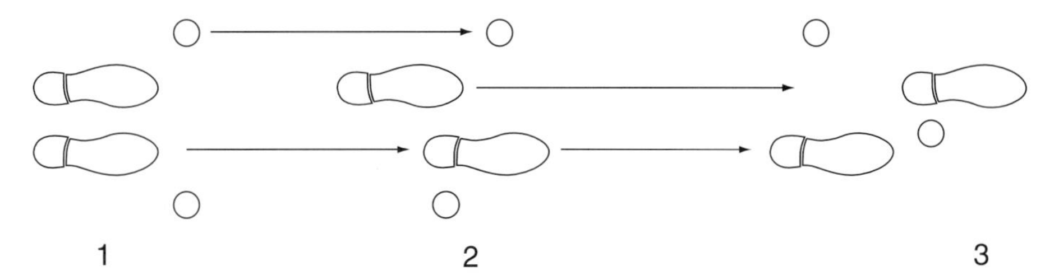

Figure 20-6
The two-point crutch gait.

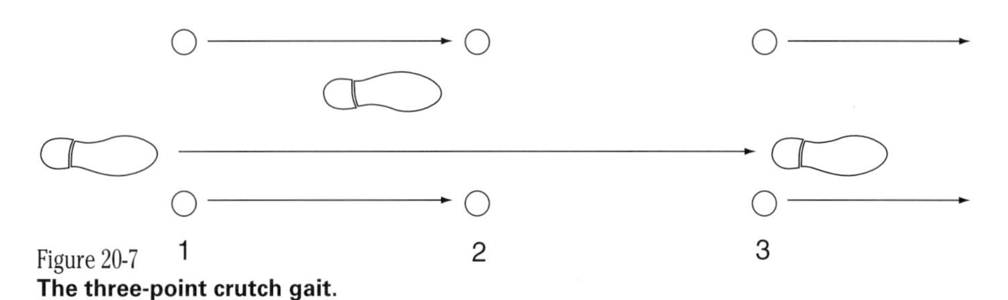

Figure 20-7
The three-point crutch gait.

other medical condition for which no weight can be put upon the leg. The rhythm for using the three-point gait is crutches, step, crutches, step. The procedure for using this gait is to have the patient:

1. stand with all of his or her weight on the stronger leg.
2. place both crutches forward at the same time.
3. take the weight on the hands, and step through the crutches, landing on the stronger foot.

A frequently used crutch-walking gait which should only be used by patients who are able to bear weight on both legs, but where one leg is weaker than the other, is the four-point gait (Figure 20-8). This gait can also be used by patients who have weakness in both legs, since it is considered to be the slowest and safest of the gaits. The rhythm for using the four-point gait is left crutch, right foot, right crutch, left foot, and repeat. The procedure for using this gait is to have the patient:

1. place the left crutch forward.
2. step forward with the right foot.
3. place the right crutch forward.
4. step forward with the left foot.

The least frequently used crutch-walking gait is the swing-through gait (Figure 20-9). It is used primarily for patients who are able to bear weight on their

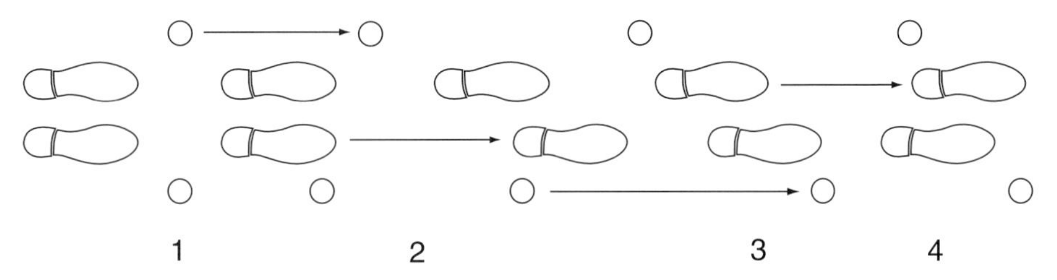

Figure 20-8
The four-point crutch gait.

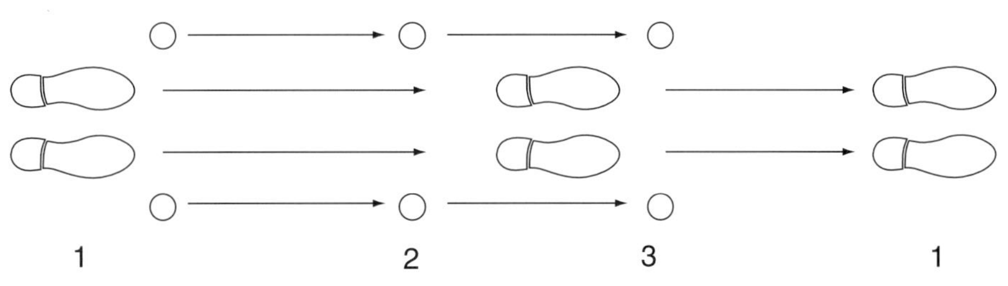

Figure 20-9
The swing-through crutch gait.

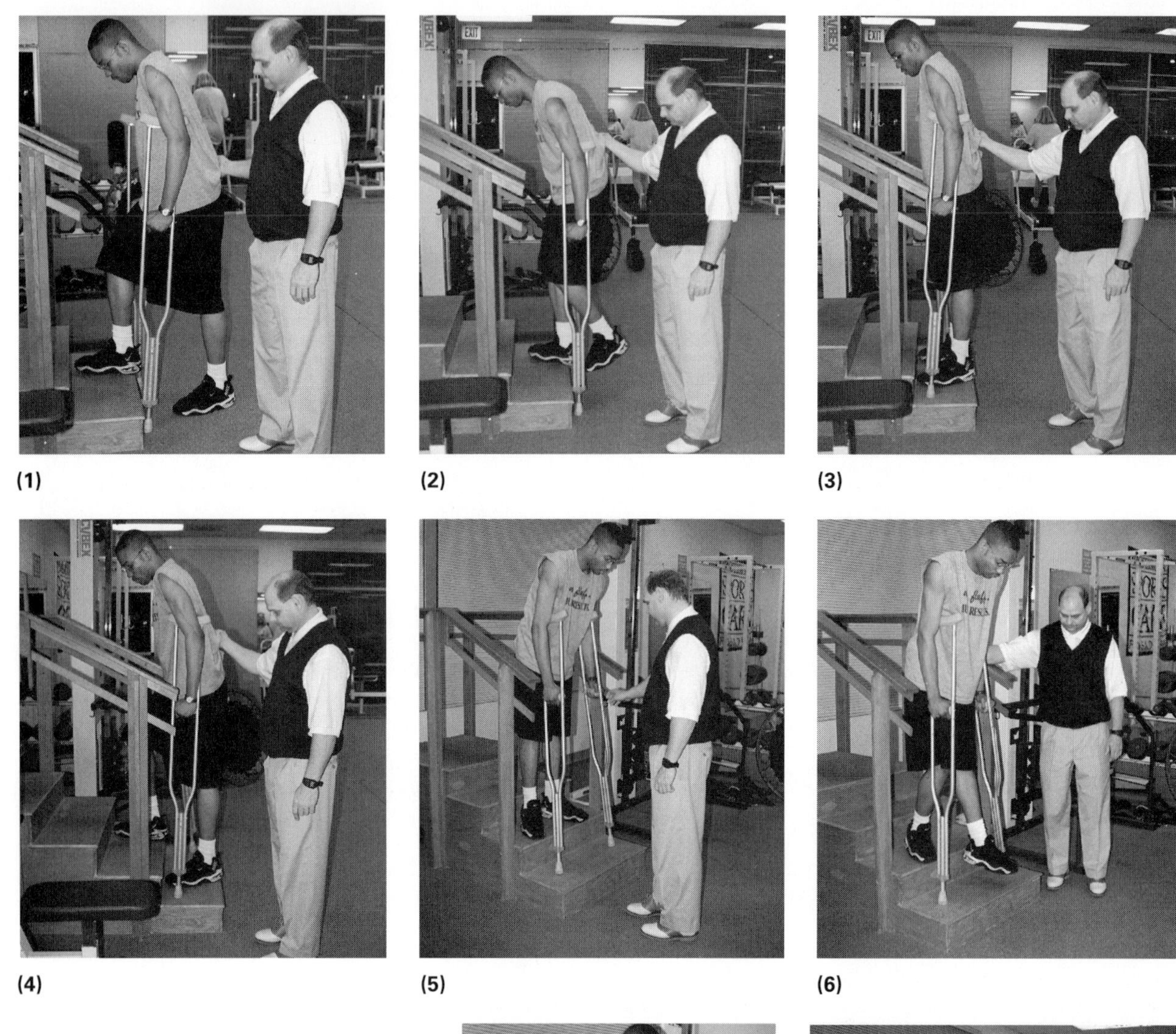

(1) (2) (3)

(4) (5) (6)

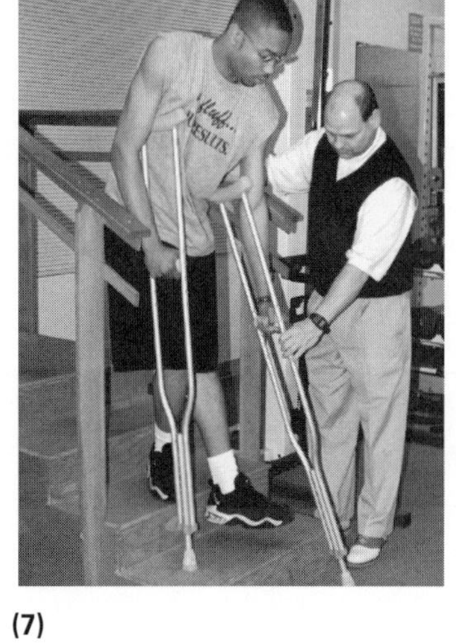

(7)

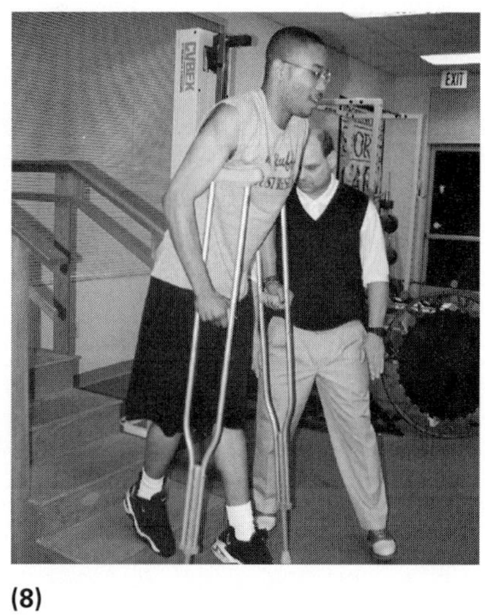

(8)

Figure 20-10
Using crutches to go up and down stairs.

extremities, but may not be able to move the extremities individually due to a debilitating medical condition such as muscular paralysis. These patients will use their arm strength and momentum to swing their legs forward and through the crutches. The rhythm for using the swing-through gait is crutches, swing, crutches, swing. The procedure for using this gait is to have the patient:

1. stand with all of his or her weight on both feet.
2. place both crutches forward at the same time.
3. swing both lower extremities through the crutches, landing on both feet.
4. repeat steps two and three.

Additional Ambulatory Movements

Patients who use crutches do not have to be confined to one place or location. With proper instruction, they can learn such movements as using a handrail to go up and down stairs (Figure 20-10) and getting in and out of chairs and automobiles.

Going Up and Down Stairs

When using crutches to go up the stairs, the patient should:

1. put one hand on the railing, and put both crutches under the other arm, holding onto the handgrips with the other hand.
2. place the strong foot on the step above.
3. push on the rail and handgrips, and bring the affected leg and crutches up to the same step.

When using crutches to go down the stairs, the patient should:

1. put one hand on the railing, and both crutches under the other arm, holding onto the handgrips with the other hand.
2. place the crutches on the step below.
3. using the stronger leg for control, slowly lower the affected leg to the step below.
4. bring down the stronger leg and the crutch.

Getting In and Out of a Chair

When using crutches, the procedure for sitting in a chair is to instruct the patient to:

1. back into the chair until he or she feels the seat on the back of the legs.
2. take the crutches out from under the arms, and hold them by the handgrips with one hand.
3. reach back with the other hand to grip the armrest.
4. slowly sit back in the chair.

When using crutches, the procedure for getting out of the chair is to instruct the patient to:

1. move to the edge of the seat.
2. hold both crutches by their handgrips with one hand.
3. place the feet under the edge of the seat.
4. put the other hand on the armrest.
5. push onto the armrest and crutch grips in order to stand.
6. reach over, take the crutch, and place it under the arm.
7. place the other crutch under the other arm.

Summary

In this chapter, we defined the role of the physical therapy aide as a member of the physical therapy team. We also explained the function of the aide in assisting patients with their activities of daily living, positioning and transferring activities, and in assisting patients to ambulate.

Review Questions

1. Give at least three examples of assistive devices which can be used to aid a person to ambulate.
2. The term ______________ refers to sitting with the feet and legs hanging freely over the edge of a bed or chair.
3. What is the difference between *prone* and *supine*?

21

Physical Therapy and Medical Disorders

Performance Objectives

Upon completion of this chapter, you will be able to:

1. Define the role of physical therapy in caring for patients with special medical conditions.
2. Discuss the role of the physical therapy aide in assisting with treatment of patients diagnosed with common musculoskeletal and neurological disorders.
3. Discuss the role of the physical therapy aide in assisting with treatment of patients diagnosed with common cardiovascular and respiratory disorders.
4. Discuss the role of the physical therapy aide in assisting the patient with an amputation.
5. Explain the role of the physical therapy aide in assisting patients with burns and common dermatologic conditions.
6. Discuss the role of the physical therapy aide in assisting patients diagnosed with common medical conditions of the eyes, ears, nose, and throat.
7. Discuss the role of the physical therapy aide in assisting patients diagnosed with common genitourinary disorders.

Terms and Abbreviations

Bursitis inflammation of the bursa.
Contracture any atrophic changes in the muscles and tendons.
Dyspnea a term used to describe painful and labored breathing.
Guillain-Barré syndrome a condition seen in patients with viral encephalitis, often characterized by the absence of fever, pain or tenderness in the muscles, motor weakness, and the deterioration of motor reflexes.
Multiple sclerosis a highly complex, chronic, and progressive neurologic disease caused by changes in the white matter of the brain and spinal cord.
Muscular dystrophy an inborn abnormality of muscle which is characterized by dysfunction and eventual deterioration.
Parkinson's disease a chronic, progressive disease of the nervous system characterized by tremor and weakness of resting muscles and a shuffling gait.
Sciatica pain in the lower back, buttocks, hips, or adjacent parts, especially the back of the thigh.

The role of the physical therapy aide in assisting patients diagnosed with various types of medical conditions is one which requires specific knowledge and understanding of some of the most basic physical therapy modalities. Much of the care prescribed by physicians often involves the introduction of physical therapy as a means of treating the patient. While most people believe that physical therapy is only useful in treating patients diagnosed with musculoskeletal conditions, many health care providers and physical therapists agree that the hands-on techniques and modalities used in physical therapy are frequently beneficial, and often essential, in meeting the needs of patients suffering from medical dysfunctions and disorders of many of our other body systems.

Treating Common Musculoskeletal Disorders

There are many physical therapy modalities that are beneficial in treating patients diagnosed with a musculoskeletal disorder. However, before a decision can be made about which type therapy can help these patients, it is extremely important that the physician perform a complete evaluation of the patient's pain, its type and location, and its severity.

The presence of a patient's pain is often considered to be a subjective decision, meaning that much of the information as to its type, location, and severity, is generally made by the patient him- or herself. Therefore, to ascertain an accurate evaluation of the pain, the doctor or physical therapist will frequently use certain factors to judge the presence, location, duration, and severity of the patient's pain and discomfort. These factors include an assessment of the following conditions.

- *pain occurring after a patient rests and then improves with movement:* this is usually a sign of osteoarthritic joints and sometimes mild sprains and strains.
- *pain occurring upon weight bearing:* this may be a sign of static deficiency or overstraining of the lower extremities.
- *pain occurring immediately after an injury:* this is often equated with the presence of a fracture or a major tear of a muscle, ligament, or tissue.
- *pain which occurs after an interval:* this usually means the presence of a minor strain or sprain.
- *pain occurring upon movement of a joint and ceasing when the joint is at rest:* this is usually a sign of an acute joint disorder or injury, or sometimes of a sprain or strain.
- *pain which radiates along the distribution of a nerve:* this usually suggests the presence of a lesion or impingement on the nerve by contracted muscles.
- *pain occurring while a person is working or after work:* this is usually an indication that the injury was sustained during the person's work time or as part of his or her occupation.

Treating Arthritis and Rheumatic Conditions

Because of the many physical therapy modalities available to the physician, he or she is sometimes at a loss in determining which to prescribe for patients suffering from arthritic or rheumatic conditions. Therefore, in most cases, the physician employs the following plan of treatment.

- *for subacutely inflamed joints:* application of moist heat or very mild infrared heat approximately 30 minutes, two to three times per day.
- *for acute stage arthritis:* no massage or exercise is prescribed during the acute stages of arthritis, except when the involved joint is moved through a full range of motion two to three times each day.
- *for subacute and chronic stages of arthritis:* in these stages, physical therapy is generally administered at least once a day in the form of heat, massage, and graded exercises; heat may be applied through moist heat, infrared lamps, warm paraffin applications, warm tub baths, or diathermy.

Assisting with the Administration of Heat Modalities

In the acute stage, heat is rarely used as a treatment for arthritic and rheumatic conditions. Therefore, during this phase of treatment, you may be called upon to assist in keeping the patient comfortable by ensuring adequate rest and using various types of splints for immobility of the affected joint(s). Medication may also be prescribed during this period. In the nonacute phase of arthritic or rheumatic conditions, however, various forms of heat are often used to provide comfort and treatment for the affected joints. These generally include the following.

- *paraffin baths:* these are particularly helpful in the treatment of hands and fingers.
- *infrared heat:* this is often considered the most convenient form of heat; treatments are usually by way of an infrared lamp, kept approximately 18 inches away from the part being treated, for a

period of 30 to 45 minutes, administered two to three times a day.

- *electric heating pad:* may be used by the patient, provided that the part being treated is wrapped in a towel to prevent burns; treatment may be two to three times a day for a period of up to 45 minutes.
- *hot tub baths:* should be taken prior to the patient beginning any form of therapeutic exercises; frequently used for treatment of hand, forearm, and feet; temperature of water should not exceed 102 degrees F, and bath should not last longer than 20 minutes.

Assisting with Administration of Massage

Massage, which is often preceded by some form of heat, is usually started soon after the acute inflammatory process in the joint has subsided. This is noted by a diminished redness, swelling, and tenderness at the affected area. The strokes which you use should be gentle, followed later by deeper stroking motions, kneading, and friction of the surrounding muscles. Superficial, or very light stroking may also be started over the affected joint. Massage should never cause the patient pain. Remember, it is usually better to give too little than too much, and unless contraindicated, every patient with nonacute rheumatoid arthritis should have this form of treatment at least 10 to 15 minutes at least twice a day.

Assisting with Range of Motion Exercises

The purpose of assisting the patient with range of motion exercises is to first strengthen the muscles that are needed to maintain good bone position within a joint; and second, to help increase joint motion. This can only be accomplished by putting a joint through its full range of motion up to the point at which a patient can tolerate the pain. An affected joint should be carried through its full range of motion at least several times a day.

All of the types of exercises can be used in the treatment of arthritis. These range from passive exercises to active exercises to active resistive. If a joint is exercised too much, however, the condition may become aggravated. If it is moved too little, motion can become limited. Therefore, to guide the patient between these two extremes, there are two points of information, or rules, which you can observe when assisting the patient with range of motion exercises. First, always remember that any exercise that produces pain during the same or the following day should be reduced in frequency or stopped altogether. Second, any exercise that is painful only at the time it is being administered, or for an hour or two afterwards, is always considered beneficial.

Range of Motion Exercises for the Hand and Wrist

The sequence for assisting the patient in performing range of motion exercises for the hand and wrist (Figure 21-1) includes the following.

- Have the patient make a fist; then instruct the patient to stretch the fingers as straight as possible. If the fingers remain bent, rest the hand, palm down, on a table. The other hand should be held firmly on top of the affected hand. The forearm of the affected arm is then raised in an effort to flatten the bent fingers. The fingers should then be spread apart.
- The patient should then touch the top of each finger to the end of the thumb, making as round a circle as possible.
- Bend the wrist forward and backward as far as possible, and move the fingers toward the thumb. Turn the wrist slowly back and forth as though turning a doorknob.

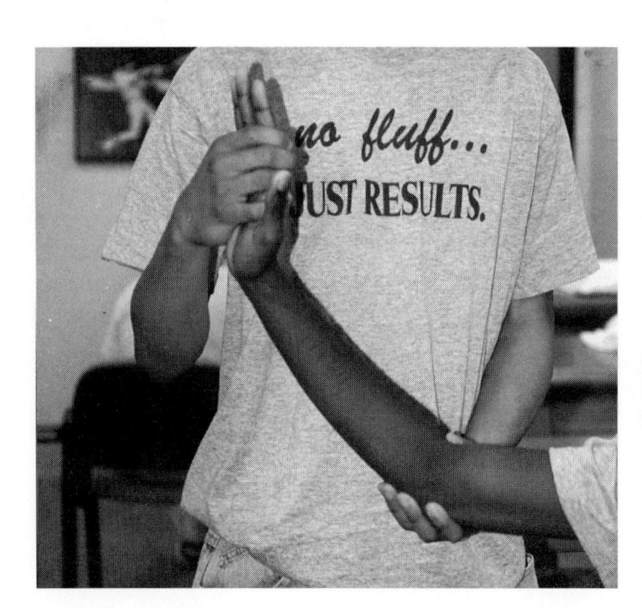

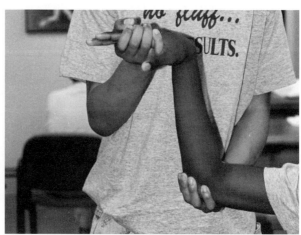

Figure 21-1
Range of motion for the hand and wrist.

Range of Motion Exercise for the Elbow

The sequence for assisting the patient to perform range of motion on the elbow (Figure 21-2) includes the following.

- Lying on the back, with the upper arm resting on the bed or table, instruct the patient to bring the fingers to the top of the shoulder.
- Then, with the palm turned upward, the hand should be brought down to the bed or table, while at the same time, straightening the elbow.

Range of Motion Exercise for the Shoulder

The sequence for assisting the patient to perform range of motion on the shoulder (Figure 21-3 on p. 248) includes the following.

- Standing with the arms resting at the sides and the palms pointed toward the body, instruct the patient to raise the arm sideways as far as possible away from the body, and then return; then raise the arm forward, upward, and as far back as it will go, and then return.
- Lying on the back with the legs straight and arms at the sides, the patient is then told to raise the arm forward, upward, and back as far as it will go; the arm is then swung out to the side and around the back to the side of the body.

Range of Motion Exercise for the Ankle

The sequence for assisting the patient to perform range of motion of the ankle (Figure 21-4 on p. 249) includes the following.

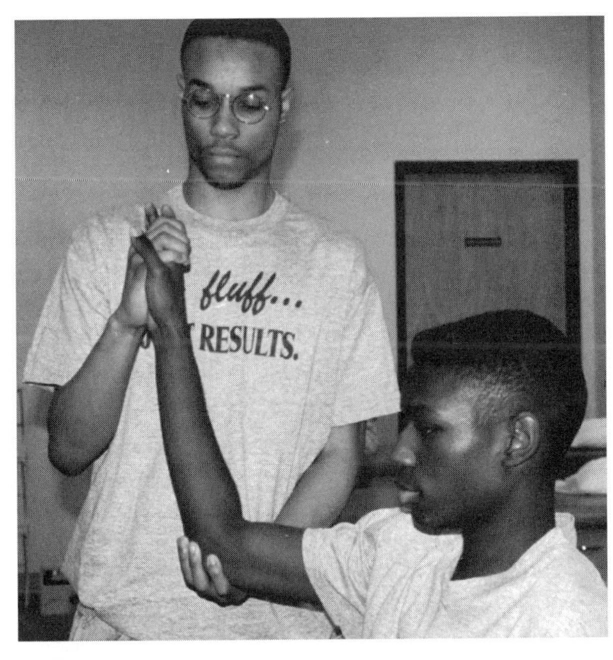

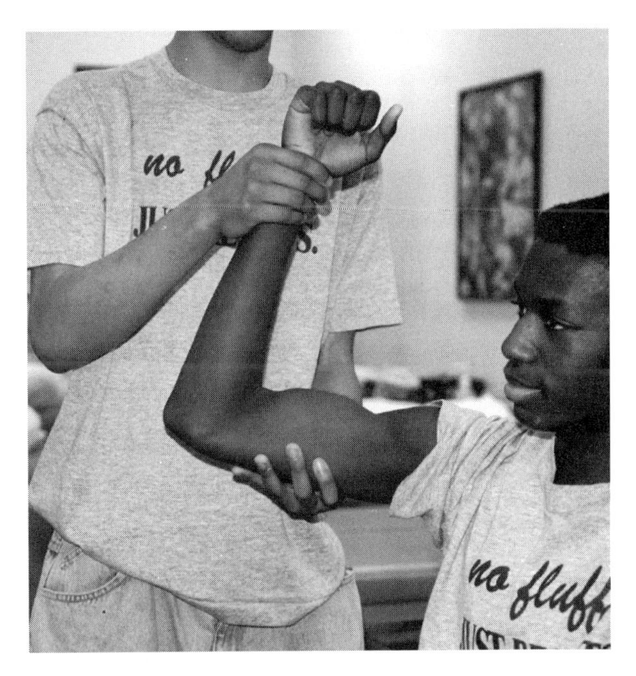

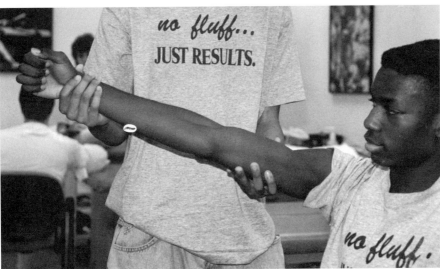

Figure 21-2
Range of motion of the elbow.

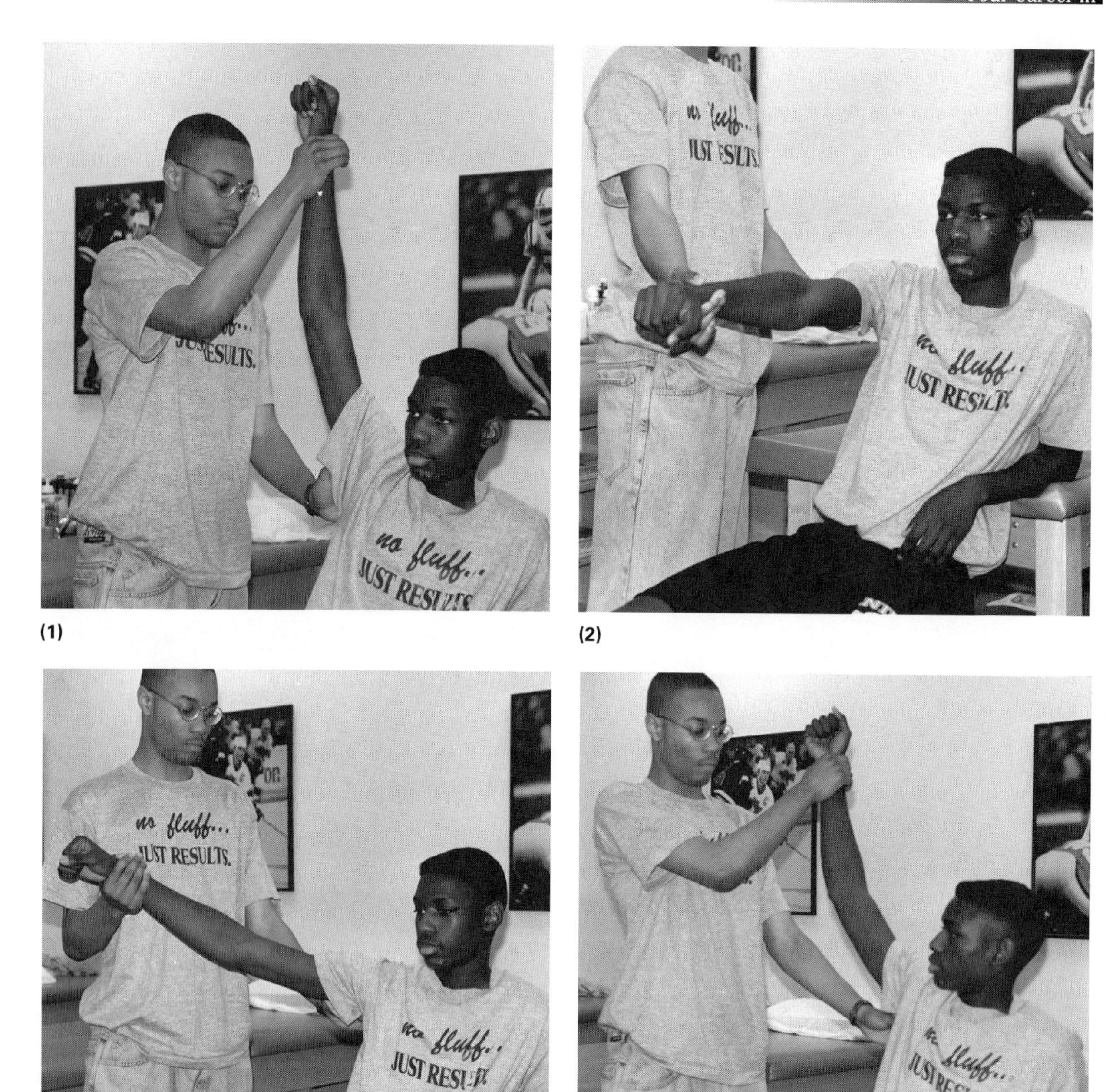

Figure 21-3
Range of motion for the shoulder.

- Have the patient bend the foot up and down slowly, and then alternately turn it in and out.
- Sitting on the edge of the bed or table, the foot should then be moved through a circular motion.

Range of Motion Exercise for the Knee

The sequence for assisting the patient to perform range of motion of the knee (Figure 21-5 on p. 250) includes the following.

- Lying on his or her back, with the leg straight, have the patient contract the muscles of the entire leg, tightening the kneecap and flattening the knee down on the surface of the bed or table.
- Then, have the patient come to a sitting position, with the legs hanging over the edge of the bed or table and above the floor. Instruct the patient to then straighten the legs and lower them again, alternating between the left and the right leg.
- Still in a sitting position, with the legs straight, the patient then raises the knee off the bed or table, sliding the foot back and thus bending and straightening the leg, alternating between the left and the right.

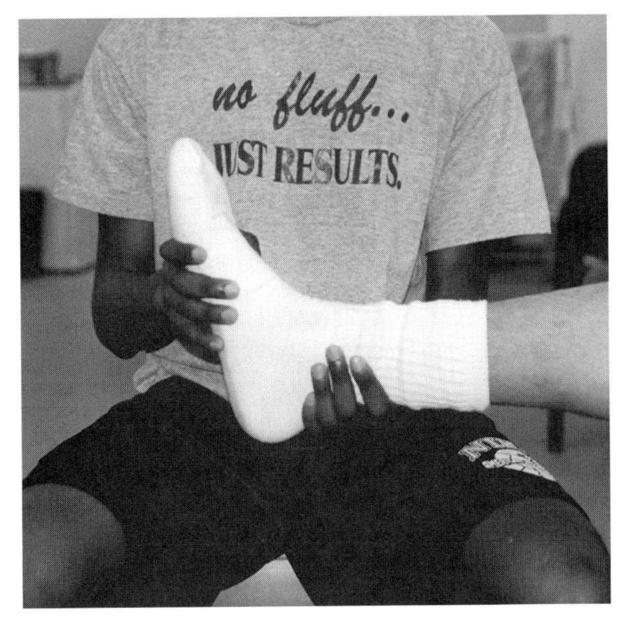

(1)

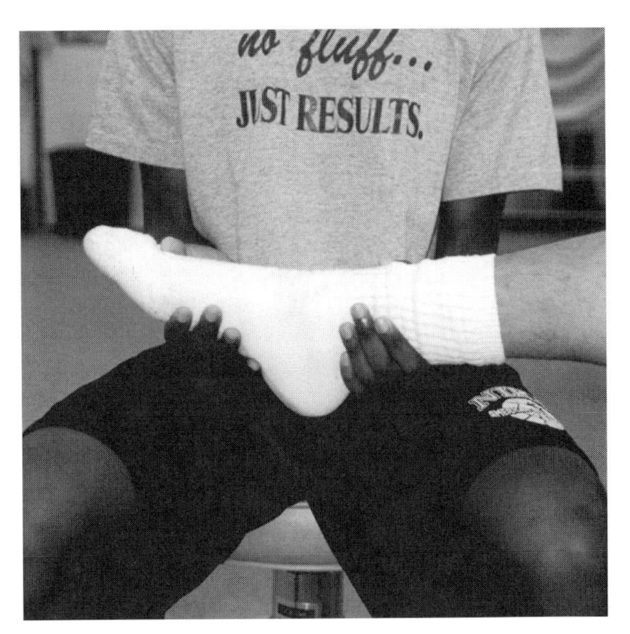

(2)

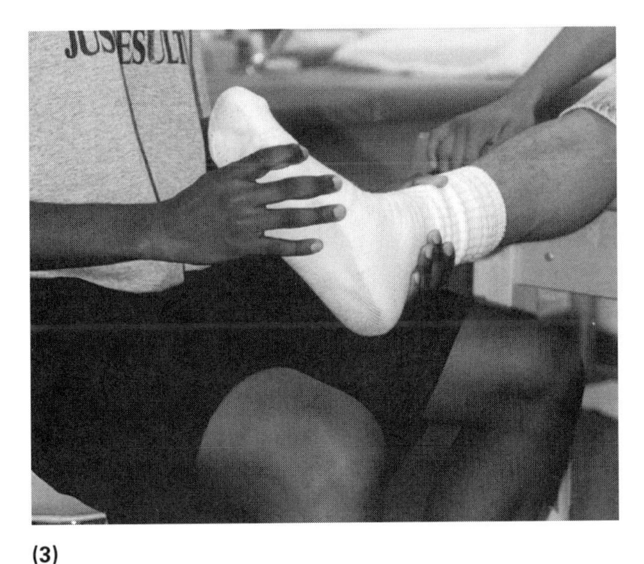

(3)

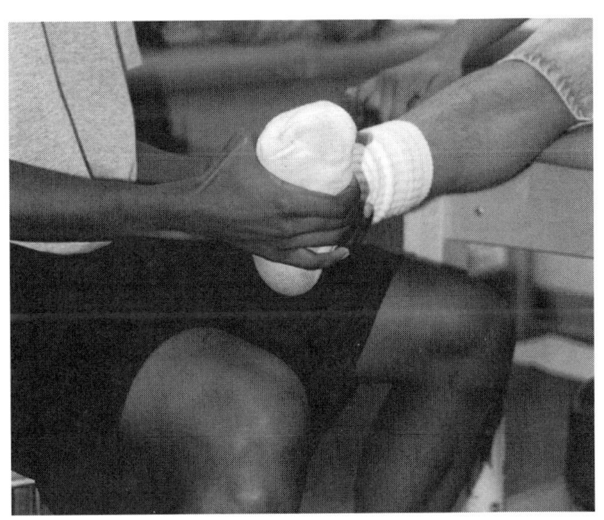

(4)

Figure 21-4
Range of motion for the ankle.

- The sequence is completed by having the patient lie on his or her back, and then "riding a bicycle."

Range of Motion Exercise for the Hip

The sequence for assisting the patient to perform range of motion of the hip (Figure 21-6 on p. 251) includes the following.

- Have the patient lie on his or her back, with the legs held straight. The legs should then be moved approximately 15 inches to the side, and then back.
- While still on the back, the patient should then raise and lower the legs slowly, with the knees first straight, and then bent.
- Then, lying face down, and with the knee kept straight, the leg is moved backward.

Treating Lower Back Pain

Unfortunately, today lower back pain is a very common condition suffered by patients of all sizes and all ages. Because of the increase of this pathology, there's a very good possibility that at some point in your career you may be required to assist in the treatment of a patient suffering from some form of lower back pain. For this reason, it's important to have an understanding of some of the differential characteristics associated with this condition. Some of the more common of these include the following.

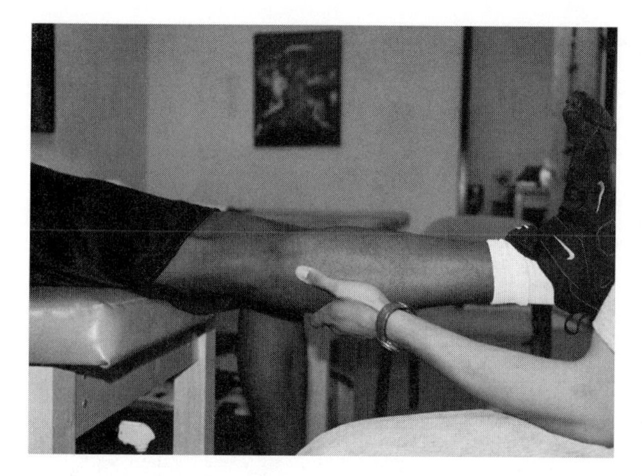

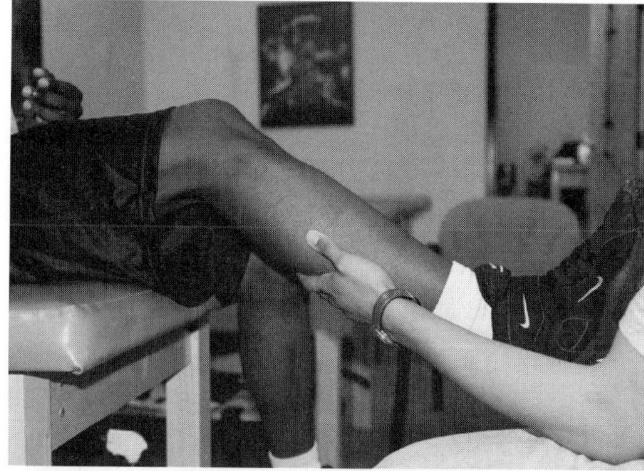

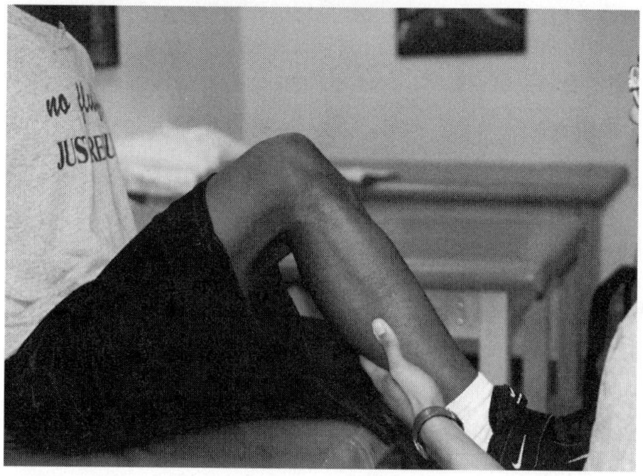

Figure 21-5
Range of motion for the knee.

- Localized or generalized lower back pain is often considered the chief symptom associated with lumbosacral and sacroiliac strain.
- Patients with a history of having been aware of something "snapping" or "slipping" in the back suggests a periosteal or ligamentous tear.
- Back pain felt upon awakening, but which rapidly seems to improve after the patient becomes involved in the day's activities, is often characteristic of mild or chronic arthritis of the spine.
- Recurring attacks of low lumbar backache with sciatica felt in the back of the leg is usually the result of a defective intervertebral disk; in most instances, the pain appears to be intensified by sneezing or coughing during periods of acute pain.
- Pain that is definitely localized, but which does not seem to radiate, often occurs when there is a fracture or abscess of the vertebrae.
- Pain that seems to disappear during the night, and then increases during the following day or evening as a backache is often associated with poor body posture.

Assisting the Patient with Back Pain

Patients suffering from back pain are often most comfortable if they sleep on a very firm mattress, lying in a supine position. Additional support to the lower back is also helpful. This may include taping, the use of a binder, or a pillow placed under the knees while the hips are flexed.

Moist hot packs administered for 20 minutes, at least three or four times a day, as well as infrared heat therapy, may also be used to treat the patient suffering from back pain. The heat should not be applied continuously, and neither should a heating pad be used all the time, or all night, since prolonged application of heat tends to increase congestion, thereby defeating its purpose.

In acute cases, massage should not be attempted, however, it may be used later as the acute stage begins to subside. Very light massage which gradually becomes deeper may be indicated; the type used will greatly depend on the degree of acuteness of the symptoms.

In some cases, you may use corrective exercises for treating back pain, but only after the acute stage has ceased and the patient has become ambulatory,

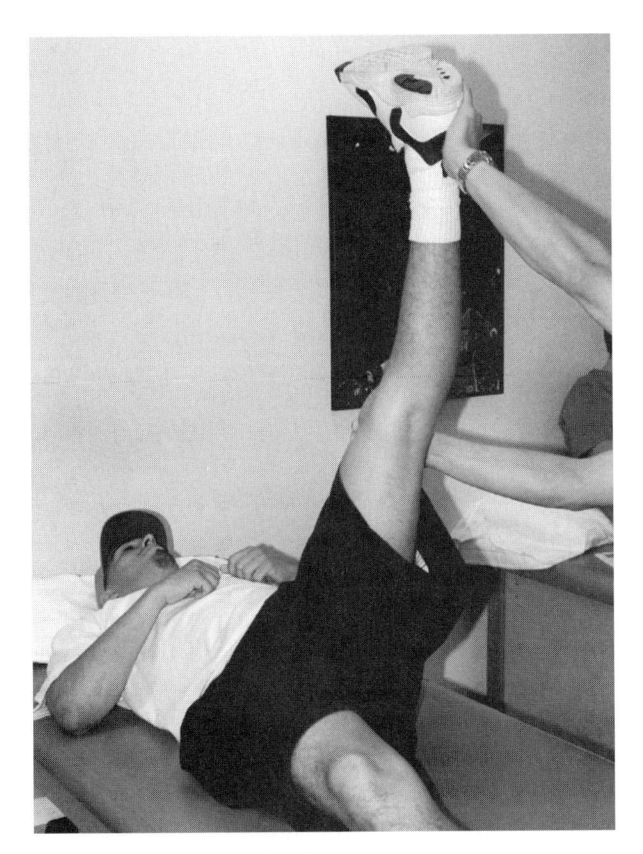

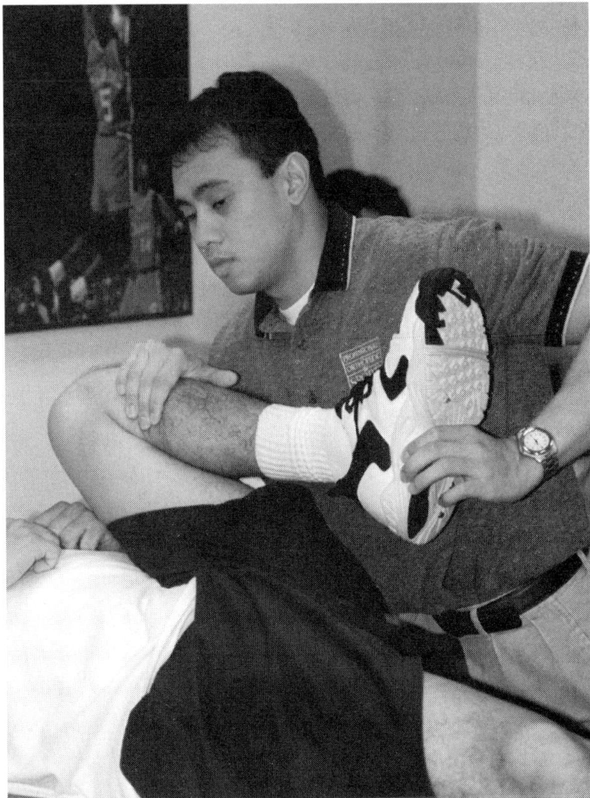

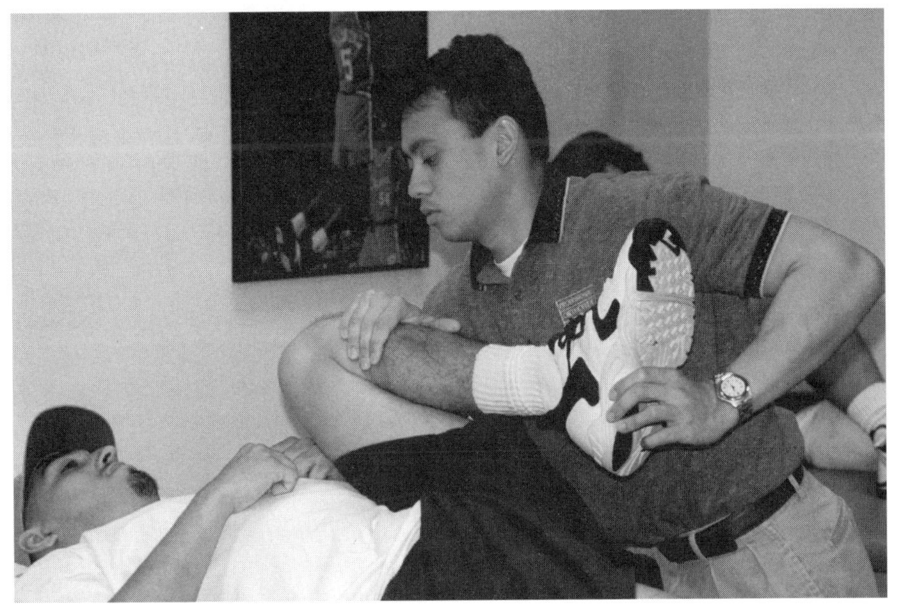

Figure 21-6
Range of motion for the hip.

or after the symptoms have become milder. Since there are many different back exercises which may be prescribed, it is often up to the physical therapist to instruct the patient in the type of exercises which would best be suited for treating a particular condition. The following exercises are designed to strengthen the stomach muscles and stretch the contracted back muscles. The patient should begin by doing each exercise at least 10 times a day and then increase by one each day until he or she is doing each exercise up to 20 times a day. Remember, too, some pain during the performance of exercises is acceptable, however, if the pain lasts for several days, the number of times the exercises should be done should be reduced.

Therapeutic Exercises for Lower Back Pain

To assist the patient in performing therapeutic exercises which will help in the treatment of lower back pain (Figure 21–7), you can instruct the patient to:

- Lie on the back with a rolled blanket or small pillow under the knees; then, with the hands held up beside the head, tilt the pelvis to flatten the lower back on the table by pulling up and in with the lower abdominal muscles; hold the back flat and breathe in and out easily, relaxing the upper abdominal muscles.
- Lie on his or her back, knees bent, with the feet placed flat on the table; with the hands up beside the head, the pelvis is tilted to flatten the lower back on the table; the legs are then straightened as much as possible with the back held flat; keeping the back flat, the knees should then return to a bent position, sliding one leg back at a time.
- Sit with the legs extended forward, placing a rolled blanket under the knees to allow slight knee bend; then pull in with the abdominal muscles, keeping the pelvis tilted back, and reach forward toward the toes, bending the lower back.
- Sit with the knees straight, and then reach forward toward the toes; then have the patient try to bend at the hip joints by tilting the pelvis forward.
- Lie on the abdomen and contract the buttocks (gluteal muscles).
- Lie on the abdomen and grasp the top of the bed with the hands; then raise one thigh, and then both thighs at the same time.
- Lie on the abdomen, grasp the side of the bed with the hands; then raise one knee and cross it over the opposite one by rotating the lower part of the back; keeping the chest and shoulders flat, the other knee is then moved in the same manner.
- Lie on the back, draw one knee up to the chest and bring it up tight with the hands; then, without allowing the knee to straighten out, return it slowly to its original position; repeat with the other knee.
- Lying on the back and drawing one knee to the chest, straighten the knee, pointing the leg upward as far as possible; flex the knee and return it to its original position; alternate with the opposite leg, repeating the cycle 8 to 10 times.

Treating Lumbosacral Strain

Strains on the back are usually caused by less severe injuries than those resulting in sprains. Therefore, the signs and symptoms are often less pronounced. However, failure on the part of the patient or the patient's doctor to recognize a strain, and then to treat it as a possible troublemaker, can often result in the patient suffering from a prolonged disability.

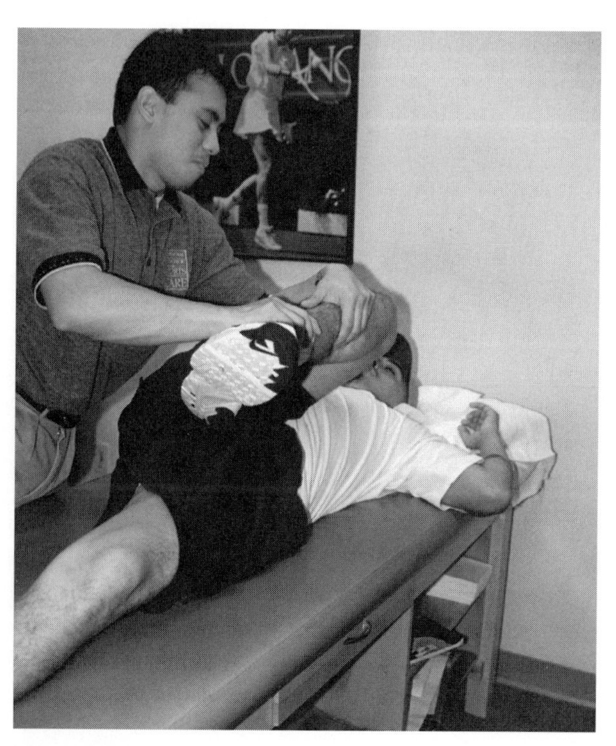

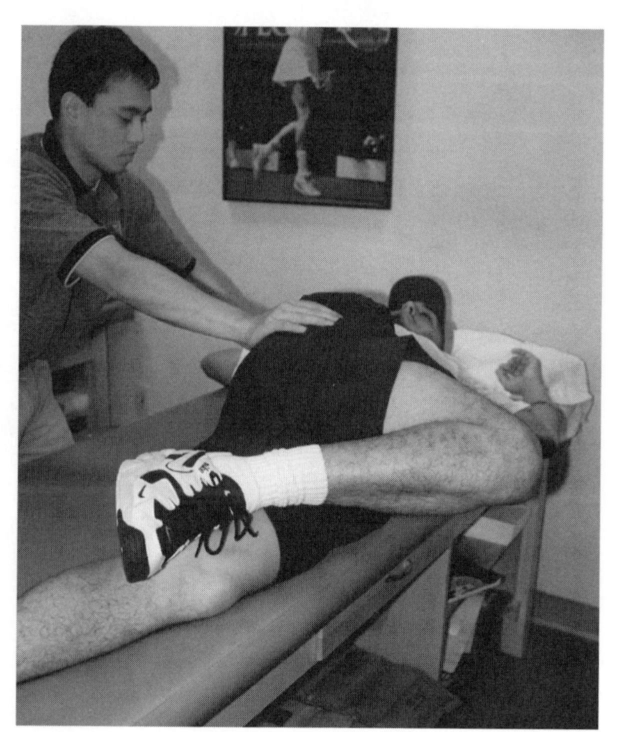

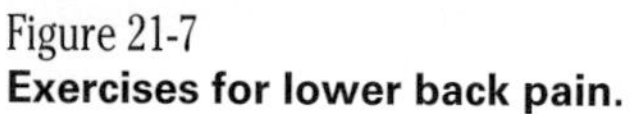

Figure 21-7
Exercises for lower back pain.

A firm binder is often applied to a patient who has suffered a lumbosacral strain. Heat, massage, and daily graduated active exercises may also be administered. Between treatments, the patient should have a hot bath daily, followed by at least 30 minutes of rest before going out of doors. If the symptoms appear to grow worse, or if they are prolonged for more than a week, it would be wise for the patient to have a few extra days of rest and receive the treatment prescribed for a back sprain.

Treating Back Sprains

Any sudden twist or fall when one is in a strained position may result in back sprain. This can be a result of slipping while straining to lift a heavy object, or not lifting the object properly. A back sprain can also be caused by suddenly having a weight thrown upon you. A back sprain can cause tearing of the ligaments and muscle attachments about the back, minute hemorrhages, ecchymoses, and often, swelling at the site of the sprain.

When a back sprain occurs, the patient often feels pain immediately, causing the person to cease his or her daily activities; however, after a few hours, the pain may subside and the person will return to these activities. Continued use of the back can aggravate the condition, and the next morning, or a day or two later, the pain can become so severe that the patient cannot even get out of bed or stand.

To provide the patient with the proper treatment, it is extremely important that the sprain be diagnosed early and the patient be placed on bed rest. Most often, these sprains are in the lower back, usually in the lumbosacral or sacroiliac area. They may not appear sufficiently serous to cause much concern, but allowing the patient to be up and about or to assume faulty posture in order to relieve his or her discomfort will only prolong the condition.

Treatment for back sprain generally starts with rest, heat, and massage during the first week, followed by daily graduated exercise to help restore function. Strapping may also be applied for two to seven days after the patient has become ambulatory, but if at all possible, it should be avoided because it makes proper massage next to impossible. If the patient does not respond to these treatments, he or she should be seen by an orthopedist. However, lack of response does not necessarily mean that physical therapy is contraindicated for sprains of the back.

Treating Bursitis

The first attack of *bursitis,* an inflammation of the bursa, can usually be relieved by the application of physical therapy. The affected part should be placed at rest, with an ice bag applied to the affected area. In some cases, infrared heat given for 30 minutes twice a day may also be administered. As the pain diminishes, careful massage and relaxed motion can also be employed. Later on, you may begin to assist the patient with active range of exercises.

Treating Cervical Disorders

There are many pathological conditions which can arise in the cervical region of the spine. Of these, the most common include whiplash injuries; arthritic changes such as those resulting from osteoarthritic, rheumatic, or traumatic origin; muscular and ligamentous strains; and cervical disk injuries caused by the compression or irritation of one or more cervical nerves at the site of a protruding disk.

The patient with an acute cervical disorder is often hospitalized, put into traction, and given such treatments as the physician prescribes. Cervical traction, which has been used for many years for the treatment of neck injuries, may be applied continuously or intermittently. When applied correctly, continuous traction assures a certain amount of immobilization of the cervical spine, straightens it, and enlarges the intervertebral opening or foramina, to relieve compressive or irritative forces upon the nerve roots, thus relieving muscle spasm. Heat in the form of hot packs is also useful in treating patients with a cervical disorder, as is massage in relieving muscle spasms. In some cases, the physician may also inject a local anesthetic or prescribe certain medications for the relief of pain.

Treating Degenerative Joint Disease (Osteoarthritis)

In caring for a patient diagnosed with degenerative joint disease, you must understand that rest is by far the most important part of the physical therapy program. Rest may be local or general, depending upon the parts of the body involved. Since overuse of affected joints is thought to bring about the symptoms and may also be a factor in producing further damage in osteoarthritis, complete bed rest may appear more rational; however, this is not really very practical for most patients, and therefore is probably not necessary. When a patient suffers an acute or severe exacerbation of the symptoms, particularly in the knees, hips, or spine, absolute bed rest for a few days may be the most rapid means of relieving the pain. Other physical therapy modalities which are frequently used in the treatment of degenerative joint disease include the application of heat, massage, and therapeutic exercise.

Treating Common Neurologic Disorders

While there are many different types of neurological disorders, the application of physical therapy can be much more beneficial to some than to others. Some of the more common disorders which can be treated with the use of therapeutic modalities include cerebral vascular accident, or stroke, Guillain-Barré syndrome, multiple sclerosis, muscular dystrophy, Parkinson's disease, and protrusion of an intervertebral disk.

Treating a Patient Who Has Suffered a Cerebral Vascular Accident

The patient who has had a cerebral vascular accident, or stroke, resulting in hemiplegia is often treated with physical therapy to prevent or correct deformity, to improve his or her motor function, and to help develop the ability to carry out the basic activities of daily living to the extent that he or she can, at least partially, take care of personal needs.

Treatment for a patient who has suffered a stroke is usually initiated as soon as possible. In most cases, it can be started within the first week following the stroke. Numerous modalities and techniques, which can be used alone or in combination, are available and helpful to the physician in the management of the hemiplegic patient. The more common of these include heat, stimulating massage, movement reeducation, therapeutic exercises, and training in the use of such assistive devices as a walker, braces, crutches, and canes.

Preventing Deformity in the Stroke Patient

There are four simple procedures which can be carried out during the acute stage following the stroke, and while the patient may still be bedridden. All of these will help prevent some of the deformities commonly seen in the hemiplegic patient. The four procedures include:

- Placing a small pillow in the axilla on the affected side to prevent adduction of that arm toward the shoulder.
- Using a footboard or applying a posterior leg splint to the affected leg to prevent toe drop and shortening of the Achilles tendon.
- Placing sandbags along the lateral surface of the affected leg to help prevent outward rotation of the leg.
- Assisting the patient to practice quadriceps range of motion exercises to help maintain and improve muscle strength needed for ambulation.

Assisting the Patient with Range of Motion Exercises

Exercise is a very important part of the treatment in hemiplegia. The type of exercise used will, of course, depend greatly on the condition of the patient's affected extremities. Various types of movement can be used, such as active and passive, assistive and resistive, as well as muscle reeducation.

When assisting the patient, it's always a good idea to start with the two of you looking in a mirror while you demonstrate an exercise, and then allowing the patient to perform the exercise before the mirror. While the patient is performing the exercise, it's important to watch closely and observe that the patient is not becoming too fatigued, out of breath, or dizzy. Also, you can allow the patient to use his or her unaffected limb to assist the affected one only when motion is impossible without assistance.

Slow passive movements of the affected extremities and your encouragement of active movements of all extremities should be started as soon as possible after the most acute stage of illness is over. Special attention should also be given to the upper extremities. The following is a list of suggestions for active exercises that will help the patient to prevent the development of contractures and deformities after a stroke.

- flexing the fingers and touching the thumb with each finger; extending and spreading the fingers; making a fist.
- flexing and extending the wrist, and then flexing the elbow, trying to touch the shoulder; extending the arm and bringing it to the side.
- using the unaffected hand to life the affected one to the head, and then to the opposite side and back.
- flexing, extending, and spreading the toes, dorsiflexing the feet, and flexing and extending the knees.
- grasping and holding objects of different sizes and shapes, then lifting them with the fingers; using a large pencil to draw large circles on a piece of paper.
- assisting the patient to attempt to walk by practicing raising and swinging the affected leg while supporting him- or herself; a walker can be used for support while doing this exercise.

Assisting the Patient with Reeducation for Walking

With proper training, many hemiplegic patients can be taught to walk again. However, the degree to which a person's normal gait can be restored greatly depends upon the amount of residual function retained by the quadriceps muscle on the affected side. If the patient is able, there are certain steps which you can initiate to help in the reeducation of a patient's ability to ambulate or walk. These steps include the following.

- getting the patient out of bed and into a standing position as soon as possible, to help prevent loss of the sense of balance and the development of muscle atrophy.
- if necessary, fitting the affected ankle with a brace to prevent plantar fixation and supination of the foot, leading to foot drop, and to give the patient confidence in weight bearing.
- using two chairs or the parallel bars for support, have the patient practice weight bearing on the involved leg.
- instructing the patient in the technique involved in the reciprocal gait, which is the normal gait for walking and which involves moving one leg and the opposite arm forward at the same time, and then the other leg and its opposite arm.
- teaching the patient to raise his or her foot from the floor by flexing the hip and knee, extending the affected leg forward at the knee, and then extending the hip until the foot touches the ground, heel first.

Assisting the Stroke Patient to Regain Arm, Hand, and General Body Control

The reestablishment of arm and hand movement for a hemiplegic patient should always begin with passive exercises to the shoulder and stretching. This helps to prevent flexion deformities at the elbow, wrist, fingers, and thumb. As soon as some voluntary movement of the arm becomes possible, the next step is to introduce functional activities which are usually assisted through the implementation of occupational therapy activities.

When assisting the patient to regain control of his or her body, it's important to understand that this always begins with teaching the patient how to move in bed so that his or her position can be changed from supine to prone and from supine to sitting. The patient must also learn how to use the unaffected leg to move or raise the paralyzed leg and how to swing both legs laterally so as to bring them over the side of the bed preparatory to standing.

The hemiplegic patient will also need instruction in how to get in and out of a wheelchair and how to propel it by using the unaffected arm and leg. Some wheelchairs are equipped with a one-arm drive mechanism which is particularly useful for patients with unilateral paralysis. Also, the patient who can learn how to walk without the aid of a cane, crutch, or brace needs to learn how to cope with different floor surfaces indoors and ground surfaces outdoors. He or she must also learn how to stand up unassisted, to sit down, to climb stairs, to step up and down a curb, and to cross a street.

Treating a Patient Diagnosed with Guillain-Barré Syndrome

Guillain-Barré syndrome is a term given to a condition often seen in patients with viral encephalitis. It is a disorder which is characterized by the absence of fever, pain or tenderness in the muscles, motor weakness, and the interruption or lack of motor reflexes.

Treatment in the acute stage of Guillain-Barré syndrome usually consists first of an evaluation of the patient's condition, followed by a utilization of passive range of motion exercises, breathing exercises, correct positioning in bed, and application of heat. In the later stages of the syndrome, rehabilitation is generally based upon an evaluation of the patient's needs and the results of tests of muscle strength. The therapeutic modalities and activities initiated at that point usually include range of motion exercises, activities to develop functional skills, reeducation of the affected muscle groups, standing and balancing, ambulation and gait training, functional activities to improve strength, dexterity, and range of motion of the upper extremities, and instruction in the performance of the activities of daily living.

Treating the Patient Diagnosed with Multiple Sclerosis

Multiple sclerosis is a highly complex, chronic, progressive, neurological disease caused by changes in the white matter of the brain and spinal cord. It is often classified as being either acute, with a sudden onset; chronic remittent, which is characterized by extensive involvement and by exacerbations and remissions that are almost complete and last over a long period of time; and chronic progressive, which are accompanied by symptoms which persist and are without periods of remission. Unfortunately, multiple sclerosis can be accompanied by many varied symptoms, and the number and degree to which the patient experiences them is usually different with each individual person.

Signs and Symptoms of Multiple Sclerosis

In most cases, the signs and symptoms of multiple sclerosis develop slowly and over a period time, although occasionally they may appear quite suddenly and be acute in nature. In most instances, there is complete recovery from the first symptoms. This period of recovery, however, is actually a remission which can vary in length from days to years. Unfortunately, when the symptoms are the result of a large lesion that causes ataxia, paraplegia, or mental deterioration, they tend to become permanent.

The most common symptoms of multiple sclerosis are diplopia, nystagmus, intention tremor, ataxia, weakness, slurred speech, and spasticity. When the cerebellus is involved, the patient often exhibits spasticity of one or both legs along with ataxia and tremor. Emotional disturbances may also accompany multiple sclerosis. When this happens, the patient may become euphoric, depressed, or emotionally unstable, and experience personality changes and loss of memory.

Sadly, the prognosis for patients diagnosed with multiple sclerosis is often unfavorable. The course of the disease varies greatly, but survival is usually estimated between 5 to 20 years. The outlook for patients with single or fewer symptoms is often more favorable than for those with a combination of symptoms, especially if the cerebellus is involved. And death is usually the result of a complication or conditions resulting from the patient's lowered resistance to infection.

Assisting in the Treatment of Multiple Sclerosis

The goal in treating patients with multiple sclerosis revolves around retraining the patient to ambulate, helping to maintain a high level of physical and mental activity, and facilitating family management of the patient in the more advanced stages of the disease. Many patients are able to continue with their work, home life, and social activities for a number of years after the onset of the disease. Therefore, your main objective in treating someone with multiple sclerosis should be to help that person to do as much as possible for him- or herself for as long as possible. The use of assistive devices will often prolong the patient's ability to do something on his or her own. And it is often more psychologically sound and beneficial for these patients to continue their regular activities within the limits imposed by their condition than for them to give up and assume the attitude of being a complete invalid.

Treating the Patient Diagnosed with Muscular Dystrophy

Muscular dystrophy is an inborn abnormality of muscle which is characterized by dysfunction and eventual deterioration. While there are numerous types of dystrophies, regardless of the type, the disease has an insidious onset, with the chief symptoms being weakness, tightness and atrophy of muscles, and absence of deep tendon reflexes.

Tightness of muscles in the upper extremities occurs primarily in the pronators of the forearm, the wrist and finger flexors, and the scapulo-humeral flexors and adductors. Tightness in the lower extremities usually occurs early and affects the gastrocnemius, coleus, and hamstring muscles, the iliotibial band, and the hip flexors. *Contractures* also occur early and are severe, usually because the muscle itself is the site of the pathological lesion. Deformities caused by these contractures are the main reason for early loss of the person's ability to walk.

Assisting in the Treatment of Muscular Dystrophy

Patients diagnosed with muscular dystrophy are encouraged to remain ambulatory for as long as possible, and exercises which help to increase flexibility of the muscles are generally started early. When indicated, the patient is also taught breathing exercises. The patient should also be encouraged to do strengthening exercises, however, it is important that he or she not exercise to the point of fatigue. Massage may also be implemented, since it often delays the development of contractures.

Braces and assistive and ambulatory devices are hardly ever used if the patient can manage without them, however, if contractures do not respond to physical therapy modalities, supportive splints or braces may be necessary and may defer the eventual need for a wheelchair.

Since the use of prolonged physical therapy may not be necessary, the patient is frequently placed on a program of home care early on in his or her treatment, and then seen by a physical therapist on a regular checkup basis. For this reason, most therapists believe that the patient should receive early and adequate instruction in procedures for carrying out their activities of daily living.

Treating the Patient Diagnosed with Parkinson's Disease

Unfortunately, for the patient diagnosed with *Parkinson's disease,* physical therapy can only offer temporary symptomatic relief and improvement. Such improvement, however, is often considered quite beneficial. Muscular rigidity can be lessened by active range of motion exercises, and under the proper supervision and encouragement of the physical therapy department, some bedridden patients may be taught to walk again, improve their posture, and ultimately, become more independent. Active exercises which are graded to the patient's tolerance can also be useful in combating atrophy. And in the event that limitation of motion occurs, causing the patient to experience pain upon movement, heat may also be used.

Treating the Patient with a Protrusion of an Intervertebral Disk

During the time in which diagnostic studies are performed to determine the possible need for surgery, the application of physical therapy is useful in most cases in which there is a suspicion of a protrusion of an intervertebral disk. Treatment usually includes complete bed rest on a firm mattress, traction to the legs or head, or sometimes both, and the use of heat and sedative massage at the painful areas. Mild diathermy of short duration and infrared heat may also be used. Frequently, symptoms of a protrusion of an intervertebral disk are relieved by these treatments within a short period of time, after which, gradual mobilization may be initiated along with the use of various exercises for muscles in the abdominal, gluteal, and lumbar regions. Patients should also be taught how to prevent further excessive back strain when stooping and sitting down, and during other bodily movements.

Treating the Patient with Sciatica

Sciatica is one of the most common neurological disorders which can be treated by physical therapy. The three types most frequently encountered include subacute and chronic sciatica associated with rheumatism and arthritis, true neuritic sciatica, and sciatica that is associated with prolapse of an intervertebral disk.

During the acute stage of this disorder, the patient is often put on bed rest, with a fracture board placed between a firm mattress and the spring. The affected leg may be partially flexed by placing a pillow under the knee and a small, firmer pillow placed under the lumbar area. Heat may also be applied to the lower gluteal region and lower back, but should be discontinued if it causes an increase in pain. Diathermy is sometimes used, but only in low intensity. Ultrasound therapy has also proved to be very beneficial.

Once the acute pain has subsided, massage and postural exercises can be used while the patient is still on bed rest. And before the patient is allowed up and able to get out of bed, he or she should be fitted with a lower back support and taught to maintain the correct posture. If one leg is shorter than the other, a heel lift may also be required.

Treating Common Cardiovascular and Respiratory Disorders

Heat is both a therapeutic modality and a powerful vasodilator which acts directly upon the blood vessels. In sufficient doses, it can increase the temperature of the blood. When it is applied to any part of the body, heat can also increase the temperature of the tissues, thus aiding in the body's metabolism.

The application of heat is often used in the treatment of many cardiovascular and respiratory disorders. Of these, those which you may encounter most frequently include peripheral vascular disorders, emphysema, asthma, and chronic bronchitis.

Treatment of Patients with Peripheral Vascular Disorders

In peripheral vascular disease, circulation of the extremities should be increased by warming the patient's trunk and thighs or opposite normal extremities. Electric heating pads and hot water bottles should never be used or applied directly to the affected extremities. Thermostatically controlled heating is the safest. Hot soaks may also be used in the treatment of such peripheral vascular disorders as gangrene and decubitus ulcers, however, the water should never be warmer than 102 to 105 degrees F. The use of cold therapy has also recently been regarded as a recommended means of safeguarding the patient against, or minimizing the result of, gangrene resulting from arterial occlusion.

In addition to heat and cold therapy, other treatments may be used for peripheral circulatory disturbances. One such modality is the introduction and use of the Buerger-Allen exercise. Consisting of three stages and lasting about 10 minutes in duration, the exercise is usually performed three to six times at each session, with the session repeated at least two to four times a day.

In the first stage of the exercise, the patient lies on his or her back, with a watch in sight, resting the legs on an inclined plane that is raised to an angle of 45 degrees. The legs are kept raised until the feet are thoroughly blanched. Usually this takes up to two minutes. In the second stage, the patient sits with his or her legs hanging over the edge of the bed or treatment table, and puts the feet and toes through a series of motions. The ankles are flexed downward, and then upward; the feet are rocked inward, and then outward; the toes are spread and then closed again. As the patient performs the movements, the feet should start becoming flushed, until eventually the entire foot to the tips of the toes are a strong pink color. This usually takes from one to three minutes. If the toes begin to look cyanotic or the patient complains of pain in them, the feet should be elevated immediately.

In the third and final stage of the exercise, the patient lies supine, with the legs horizontal, and wrapped in a woolen blanket warmed by a hot water bottle or electric heating pad for approximately five minutes. In this way, the reactionary flush achieved by the exercises in stages one and two is maintained.

Treating Respiratory Disorders

Of the many respiratory disorders treated in today's health care facilities, those which can benefit most from physical therapy include emphysema, asthma, and chronic bronchitis.

Assisting the Patient with Emphysema

Emphysema is a fairly common lung condition characterized by an abnormal enlargement of the alveolar spaces in the lungs and destructive changes in the alveolar walls, resulting in the collection of air in the interstices of the connective tissue and the intra-alveolar tissue of the lungs. These changes often cause an impairment in the most vital aspect of breathing; that is, the ability of the lungs to exchange air efficiently. Emphysema may occur at any age, and is most often seen in people who are heavy smokers.

The goal of physical therapy in the treatment of emphysema is to help the patient to breathe more efficiently without the aid of a nebulizer or other breathing apparatus. Properly executed, exercises can be used to strengthen muscles that will help more oxygen into the patient's lungs and thus reduce *dyspnea,* or painful and labored breathing. Postural drainage can also be used to help remove obstructions in the bronchial tubes.

Exercises that are helpful in the treatment of emphysema include the arm-lift breathing exercise, exercises to help increase the strength of abdominal muscles and of lateral chest muscles used in breathing, hand-clapping, and exercises to correct posture.

Arm-Lift Exercise

This exercise can be done in the standing position or when the patient is lying down. Its goal is to increase the exchange of air in the lungs. In the standing position, the patient breathes in slowly through the nose while, at the same time, raising the arms forward and upward until they are fully extended over the head. After the patient takes in as much air as is needed, the arms are slowly lowered while exhaling, using one-third more time than was used to inhale.

Exercise to Strengthen Chest Muscles

This exercise helps to strengthen not only the lateral chest muscles used in breathing, but also the abdominal and other chest muscles. With the patient lying flat on the bed or table, the knees are flexed and the feet are placed firmly on the mattress or table surface, and the trunk is raised while twisting it either to the right or to the left. The hands may be held either behind the head or raised forward to the right or left. The exercise should be repeated at least five times with the patient twisting to the right and then five more times twisting to the left.

Hand-Clapping Exercise

For the hand-clapping exercise, the patient should be standing erect. While maintaining good posture, the hands are then brought forward and clasped, with the arms thrown backward as far as they can at shoulder height. The sequence is completed by bringing the arms forward again and then repeating the entire procedure.

Assisting the Patient with Asthma

Asthma is a respiratory disorder characterized by recurrent attacks of dyspnea during which expiration is particularly labored. These attacks are often the result of a spasm of the smooth muscle of the bronchi, as well as swelling of the mucous lining causing an increase in the secretion of mucus.

In most cases of asthma, the ability to use the diaphragm in breathing and to expand the basal areas of the lungs have been compromised or lost. In addition, the chest is often tense and the neck muscles in vigorous action, making it almost impossible to practice diaphragmatic breathing. Therefore, the patient has to be taught how to relax and keep the upper thorax still, and to use the diaphragm in breathing.

Exercise to Correct Posture

In some cases, it may be necessary to correct the patient's posture before he or she can receive the maximum benefit from some of the breathing exercises. To accomplish this, the patient should stand with the shoulders erect and the chest thrust forward. Breathing is then done slowly through the nose, gradually increasing the amount of air being inhaled. The air is then expelled slowly while the chin is kept up and the correct posture maintained.

Assisting the Patient with Chronic Bronchitis

Chronic bronchitis is a respiratory condition characterized by chronic inflammation of the lining of the larger and medium-sized bronchi, usually occurring as a result of an infection. It is most common in middle-aged and older people, especially those living in industrial areas or in cold, damp climates, and those with low resistance. It may also be caused by irritations arising from some chemicals, gases, dust, and smoke.

The main goal in treating a patient with chronic bronchitis is to increase his or her ability to take in oxygen. It is also important to raise the resistance of the bronchial tree to infection. The various exercises which are used in the treatment of emphysema and asthma can also be used in treating chronic bronchitis.

Treating Common Disorders of the Eyes, Ears, Nose, and Throat

Many of the most common disorders of the eyes, ears, nose, and throat can be helped by physical therapy modalities. Although some of the treatments used may be considered by some to be old fashioned, they are both helpful and useful in the treatment of many of these conditions.

Treating Conditions Affecting the Eye

Two of the most common conditions affecting the eye for which physical therapy can be helpful in their treatment are acute conjunctivitis and chronic meibomitis. Patients who are diagnosed with acute conjunctivitis can use a cold compress applied to their eye for the first 24 hours, followed by moist or dry heat. For patients with chronic meibomitis, massaging of the lids is often very helpful.

Treating Conditions Affecting the Ear

There are two common disorders which can benefit from use of physical therapy modalities. The first is called eczema of the auricle, in which there is a scaly appearance to the outside of the ear. This is easily treated with the application of ultraviolet irradiation. Chronic otitis media, which is a chronic inflammation of the middle ear, may also be treated with ultraviolet irradiation, as well as short wave diathermy.

Treating Conditions Affecting the Nose

The most common disorder of the nose for which physical therapy can be useful is sinusitis, which is an inflammation of the nasal sinuses. Hot moist towels can be applied over the sinuses, with an infrared lamp pointed directly at the towels. Diathermy may also be used if there is drainage, however, it should only be applied at low intensity for no longer than 20 to 25 minutes, using the air-spaced technique or a special sinus applicator.

Treating Conditions Affecting the Throat

There are three conditions of the throat which can most benefit from the application of physical therapy: laryngitis, or inflammation of the larynx; pharyngitis, or inflammation of the pharynx; and tonsillitis, or inflammation of the tonsils. In the acute stage of laryngitis, heat treatments in the form of infrared irradiation or hot compresses may be helpful, as is diathermy with the electrodes placed on each side of the neck. Cold compresses are also sometimes used. Patients suffering from pharyngitis may be treated with infrared heat, diathermy, and hot compresses. Ultraviolet irradiation may also be used in the region of the inflamed pharynx. For patients diagnosed with tonsillitis, the application of hot compresses, infrared heat to the neck, and short-wave diathermy, with the electrodes placed on either side of the neck, may also be useful.

Treating Common Dermatologic Disorders

Physicians frequently use certain physical therapy modalities to treat common skin disorders before they refer their patients to a dermatologist. One such modality is ultraviolet heat, often used in the treatment of such skin disorders as acne vulgaris, alopecia areata, boils and carbuncles, eczema seborrheicum, lupus vulgaris, neurodermatitis, and psoriasis. The application of ultraviolet heat and radiation is also quite beneficial in the treatment of decubitus ulcers and in some infected wounds.

Patients suffering from an excessive buildup of scar tissue may also benefit from physical therapy. In some cases, the scarring may only involve the skin, while in other cases, it may extend into deeper tissues surrounding the joints, tendons, and nerves. Forceful manipulation of scar tissue only results in tearing and further scarring. Therefore, treatment for these patients usually involves the application of hot moist packs, ultrasonic therapy, friction-type massage, and active exercises and stretching. In severe cases, scarring may require surgical intervention.

Using Physical Therapy to Treat Burns

One of the most serious complications of burns is the development of deformities caused by the contraction of scar tissue. During the healing of burns that have destroyed the entire thickness of the skin, fibrous tissue must form to compensate for the loss caused by the burn. Once formed, this interlacing of collagen fibers undergoes a period of active contraction, and the forces exerted in this vital process are considerable. The overwhelming value of physical therapy in the treatment of burns is that it minimizes the process by which fibrosis takes place.

The degree of scarring which develops following a burn greatly depends upon the force and effectiveness of the treatment and medication, as well as the response by the patient to the healing process. In all cases, treatment should begin as soon as possible after the injury.

When using physical therapy to treat burns, the following modalities have proved most useful.

- *dry heat:* various sources can be used to help relieve pain.
- *massage:* helps stimulate the blood supply to the burned area, reduces the amount of scar tissue that develops, loosens scars and overcomes a tendency for them to retract or contract, and helps to restore function of the involved joints.
- *whirlpool bath, paraffin baths, and Hubbard tub baths:* help to increase movement and motion of the affected body parts.
- *ultraviolet irradiation:* helps to improve the patient's general condition by stimulating healing, overcoming low-grade infections, and preparing the burned area for eventual plastic surgery.
- *dry cold:* helps in overcoming traumatic and postoperative swelling.

Using Physical Therapy in the Treatment of Amputation

Following surgery, patients who have had a limb amputated are usually referred to a physician specializing in orthopedics. However, there are many physical therapy modalities which can be used before this person is ready to be fitted for his or her prosthesis.

When physical therapy is used as a treatment in caring for patients who have sustained an amputation, the main goal of the treatment is to prepare the stump for early and efficient use of a prosthesis. The modalities used for such a task generally include heat, massage, and therapeutic exercise. Whirlpool baths are considered the preferred source of heat, since they improve circulation and relieve pain which has been caused by the persistent edema and excessive buildup of periosteal connective tissue. Massage is usually administered at a later time, after it has been determined that there is no possibility of infection. Early therapeutic exercise of the remaining part of the limb results in reduction of edema and is usually good preparation for the use of an artificial limb.

Using Physical Therapy in the Treatment of Genitourinary Disorders

While there are many urinary tract infections and disorders which can be helped by the early use of physical therapy modalities, those which seem to benefit from it most include prostatic disorders, cystitis, some disorders of the kidney, and spasms occurring in the ureters. For most of these conditions, physical therapy treatments often include the use of diathermy and infrared heat.

Assisting the Patient with a Prostatic Disorder

For patients suffering from an acute inflammation of the prostate, local heating by means of diathermy, hot irrigations, or hot sitz baths are very helpful and frequently used in conjunction with medications.

Assisting the Patient with Cystitis

Patients diagnosed with an inflammation of the urinary bladder, or cystitis, often experience pain and spasms which can be greatly relieved by heat-producing methods, such as hot sitz baths, hot packs to the suprapubic area, infrared heat to both the suprapubic and perineal regions, and diathermy applied by a special electrode. While the application of physical therapy is especially helpful before the symptoms are relieved by antibiotics, it is often continued throughout the entire period of the infection.

Assisting the Patient with a Kidney Disorder

Heat applied locally to the renal area by means of warm baths, hot packs, infrared lamps, or diathermy may be a very effective measure in relieving the patient of the often dull ache and colicky pain associated with kidney disorders. Mild massage is also helpful in relieving painful muscle spasm, as is diathermy when it is used as an adjunct to other methods in the treatment of oliguria or anuria resulting from crystallization of sulfa drugs within the kidney's tubules.

Assisting the Patient Suffering from Spasms in the Ureter

When a spasm occurs in the ureter as a result of the formation of a calculus (stone) or trauma from instrumental examination of the ureter, the local application of infrared heat or diathermy is often used to help produce relaxation of the ureter.

Summary

In this chapter, we discussed the role of physical therapy aide in using various therapeutic modalities to help treat patients diagnosed with special medical conditions and disorders. In our discussion, we talked about the many types of therapeutic treatments used to care for patients diagnosed with musculoskeletal, neurological, cardiovascular, and respiratory disorders. We also discussed the usefulness of physical therapy as a modality for treating patients with amputations, burns and skin conditions, disorders of the eyes, ears, nose, and throat, and genitourinary disorders.

Review Questions

1. A neurologic condition which is highly complex, chronic, and progressive, and in which changes in the white matter of the brain and spinal cord occur is called:
   a. multiple sclerosis
   b. muscular dystrophy
   c. radiculitis
2. A neurologic condition which is caused by irritation of the spinal nerve roots, and which is manifested by pain and by alterations in perception of sensation or in muscle function is called:
   a. multiple sclerosis
   b. muscular dystrophy
   c. radiculitis
3. What is the name of the medical condition which is frequently seen in patients with viral encephalitis?
4. ____________ is a term which is used to describe painful and labored breathing.
5. What is another name for "tennis elbow"?
6. ____________ is a term used to denote a group of nonspecific illnesses characterized by pain, tenderness, and stiffness of the joints, muscles, or adjacent structures.
7. A term which refers to any condition of a joint in which trauma has been directed onto it, resulting in a disturbance in the synovial membrane, is called ____________.

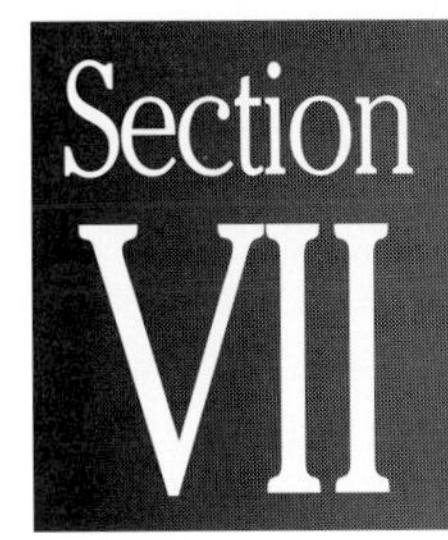

Sports Medicine Assistant: Basic Concepts and Applications

22

Recognition and Assessment of Sports Injuries

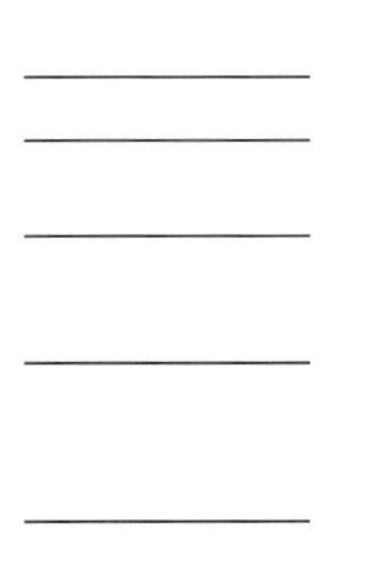

Performance Objectives

Upon completion of this chapter, you will be able to:

1. Identify the purpose of physical assessment and evaluation techniques used to determine sports injuries.
2. Discuss the relationship of fitness to recognition and assessment of sports injuries.
3. Discuss the role of a participant in preventing a sports injury.
4. Discuss injury prevention as it relates to both the young and the mature athlete.
5. Explain the functions of a spotter in sports.
6. Identify common injuries and their prevention in selected sports.
7. Briefly explain the process of wrapping, and identify when it is used to prevent injury.

Terms and Abbreviations

Atrophy a wasting away of muscular tissue.
Contusion a bruise, generally accompanied by pain, swelling, and discoloration, without breaking the skin.
Dynamometer a device used for measuring force or power.
Electrocardiogram a tracing of the heart which shows its electrical activity and which is recorded by an electrocardiograph.
Endurance the length of time that a specific activity can be sustained by a set of muscles without tiring.
Ergometer a device which resembles a bicycle, used to measure the performance of the cardiopulmonary system.
Flexibility one's ability to move his or her body parts through a full range of motion at the joints.
Shin splint pain around the anterior tibia which can be due to, or a result of, tiny tissue tears, a tibial stress fracture, or swelling of muscles which may be due to intense or prolonged exercise.
Spotter a person responsible for keeping watch for a participant during the engagement of an activity.
Strength the amount of force a muscle can exert as it contracts.
Torque a force causing a turning or twisting movement.
Torsion the condition of the body or individual body part being twisted along its long axis.
Treadmill a stress test consisting of running at different speeds and inclines to measure cardiovascular fitness.
Warm up a process or procedure used to prepare an athlete for sport or activity.

If you decide to seek a career and work in the field of sports medicine, you will soon discover that, just like the sizes and shapes of all individuals vary, so too do our physical abilities. It is for this very reason that all people who engage in any type of sports or athletic activity must first determine where their strengths and weaknesses are. This measurement is most often accomplished through the process of assessment and evaluation.

Assessment Through Physical Examination

When a person decides to begin any type of exercise program, the first step should always be to undergo a physical examination by his or her physician. Most family practice or primary care doctors can provide this to their patients. Later on, if problems do occur in connection with physical activity, the patient may need to seek out another physician whose speciality is sports medicine.

If a patient does decide to undergo a complete physical examination prior to beginning any exercise program, it is usually to determine the overall state of his or her health. Therefore, the examination is not limited to just checking for musculoskeletal problems. It also includes taking a complete medical history, both of the patient and his or her family members; measuring the patient's vital signs; examining all body parts by observing, palpating, and listening; performing blood tests and urinalysis; taking an electrocardiogram; and for women, examining the breasts and performing a pelvic exam, including a Pap smear. For those patients undergoing an examination to make sure they are able to begin an exercise program, the final portion of the assessment and evaluation process involves measuring how they rate in each of the components of fitness.

Fitness Evaluation

A fitness evaluation examination includes five components: cardiovascular and respiratory endurance, muscular strength, muscular endurance, flexibility, and body composition. Since all of these areas can be improved through a well thought out and planned exercise program, once a person's status in each area has been determined, a program can be designed which can assure that the person gets enough of the right kind of exercise.

Evaluating Cardiovascular and Respiratory Endurance

The terms cardiovascular fitness and *endurance* are frequently used when we discuss the ability of both our circulatory and respiratory systems to meet the great demands of sustained physical exercise. This is often referred to as aerobic fitness, and it is most concerned with the ability of the two systems to transport oxygen to the cells, while at the same time removing excess wastes. Cardiovascular fitness is also considered to be a very important part of our overall state of health, because of its ability to increase energy, reduce weight, and help to slow down fatigue.

When a person is being specifically evaluated for cardiovascular fitness, there are two tests which are most frequently used for the examination. They include the *treadmill* and the *ergometer.* These two stress tests are generally conducted in hospitals, clinics, health clubs and fitness centers, and sports medicine and sports physiology centers.

If a patient is scheduled for the treadmill stress test, it's very important to make sure that he or she is informed about getting a good night's sleep prior to the test. You should also make sure that the patient is told to bring running shoes and gym clothes to the examination. If the patient has not had a recent physical examination, a current weight and medical history is taken prior to beginning the test. Electrodes are attached to the patient's chest to record an *electrocardiogram* and to allow members of the staff involved in the test to monitor any appearance of cardiac abnormalities. The patient's blood pressure is also checked. If any abnormality or trouble does arise, testing should be immediately stopped.

The Treadmill Stress Test

A treadmill stress test consists of a series of at least three separate runs which become progressively more difficult. The treadmill can be programmed for different speeds and different grades of inclination, or height. If you are responsible for performing the test, the first step is to take a series of counts of the recovery heart rate at the conclusion of each run. You may then calculate the amount of oxygen being consumed by using an apparatus to collect the air being exhaled during the run. Oxygen and carbon dioxide content are determined to see just how efficiently the body is able to utilize oxygen.

The Ergometer Test

Often times, the physician or sports medicine specialist will use both the treadmill and an ergometer to evaluate the patient for the effect of exercise on his or her cardiovascular systems. The ergometer is a bicycle-like device which can be used either in conjunction with, or instead of, a treadmill to evaluate a person's cardiopulmonary fitness. Sitting on the ergometer, the patient pumps the pedals against a load that is gradually increased. Heart performance and oxygen consumption are then recorded and monitored in the same manner as with the treadmill.

Evaluating Cardiopulmonary Capacity

Both the treadmill and the ergometer tests have been designed to put stress on the cardiovascular system. Therefore, they are also capable of doing damage to people with undetected heart or lung problems, or in some cases, can even lead to a decrease in cardiopulmonary capacity. However, both of these tests are extremely valuable screening tools for identifying such potential problems or for giving a person a clean bill of health if he or she wishes to begin a sports or athletic program.

If a decrease in the person's cardiopulmonary capacity has been detected, there are two simple methods which can be used to evaluate its presence for any age group. These methods can also be used to compare levels of fitness. It's important to note, too, that neither of these tests should be used unless a person is already in some type of conditioning program and/or is under the age of 35.

The first method for evaluating cardiopulmonary capacity is by timing how long it takes a person to run/walk one and one-half miles. To do this, use an area such as an athletic track which has a mile measured and marked. You will also need to know how many laps equal one mile. The object is to see just how fast the person can cover the distance. If, for example, the distance is covered in 12 minutes while running, the person has scored well in fitness.

The second method for measuring cardiopulmonary capacity is to have the person complete a three-minute step test (Figure 22-1 on p. 268). You will need a bench or chair that is 12 inches tall. To take the test, have the person step up with one foot, and then bring the other beside it. Make sure you tell the person to straighten his or her knees and stand. Then have the person step down with the first foot, and bring the other down. This completes one cycle. The rate of stepping should be about one full set of up and down every two seconds. After stepping for at least three minutes, have the person stop, sit down, and find his or her pulse. They should wait at least one full minute, and then count their pulse for 30 seconds. A rate of 50 to 60 beats per minute indicates a high level of fitness.

Evaluating Muscle Strength and Muscle Endurance

Muscle strength and muscle endurance are extremely important for carrying out the daily tasks of everyday living. They are also important in maintaining posture and in performing sports and other athletic activities. Muscle *strength* has to do with the amount of force a muscle is able to exert as it contracts. If muscles are not used, they become weak and will eventually *atrophy,* or waste away. Muscles which are frequently tested for strength are those located in the hand. To determine the amount of grip strength of these muscles, a hand-grip manometer or *dynamometer* may be used. The person whose strength is being measured holds the instrument in his or her hand, flexes the elbow, and then squeezes the hand-grip tightly (Figure 22-2 on p. 269).

Measuring muscle *endurance* has to do with determining the length of time in which a specific activity can be sustained or repeated by a set of muscles without the person getting tired. Muscular endurance can also be measured for different body areas. Sit-ups, for example, can be used to test the person's abdominal area. They are scored by the number performed in one minute, with 35 to 40 being the best indication of the presence of a good degree of fitness. Pull-ups or a flexed-arm hang can be used to measure the person's upper body endurance. These are scored by how many can be completed; three to eight are generally considered good. The flexed-arm hang is scored by the length of time a person can hold that position. If the person cannot last at least 15 seconds, that is a pretty good indication that he or she will need more upper body endurance. Push-ups can also be used to evaluate a person's upper body strength.

Evaluating Flexibility

The ability to move our body parts through a full range of motion at their joints is called *flexibility.* It helps us to prevent muscle and joint injuries, as well as lower back pain. People who are more flexible also perform better in sports and exercise activities. Unfortunately, however, there is no single test or method to determine the flexibility of our muscles. This is because in order to achieve flexibility, all muscles and joints must be involved.

A good way to improve flexibility is to *warm up,* to stretch both before an exercise set is begun, and after the program has been completed. The person should be warned never to bounce when stretching, but rather, only to stretch to the point of tightness, but not to pain. Gradually, stretching farther and for a

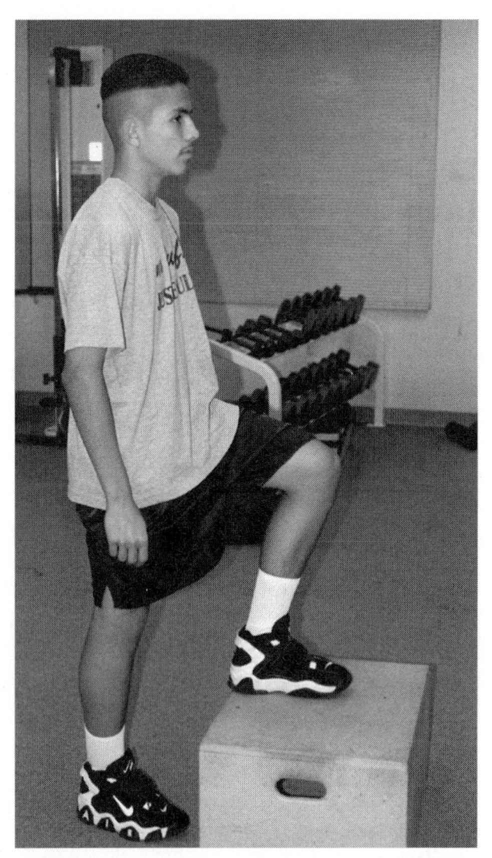

(1)

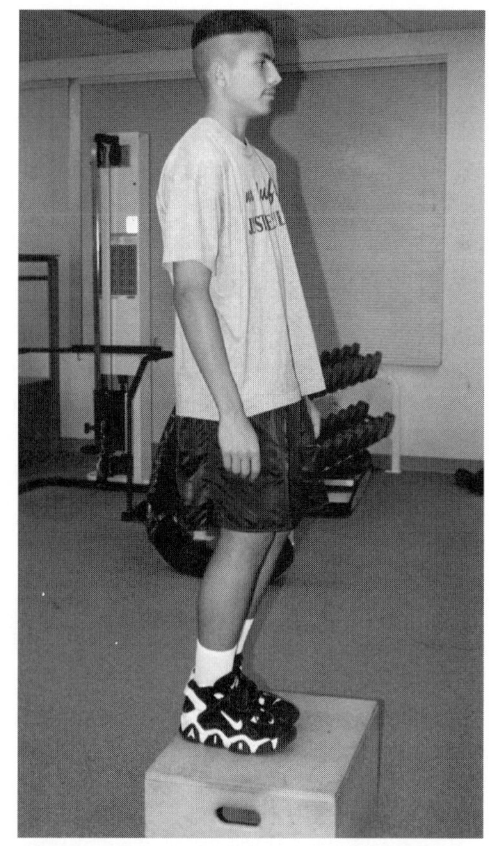

(2)

Figure 22-1
Step test.

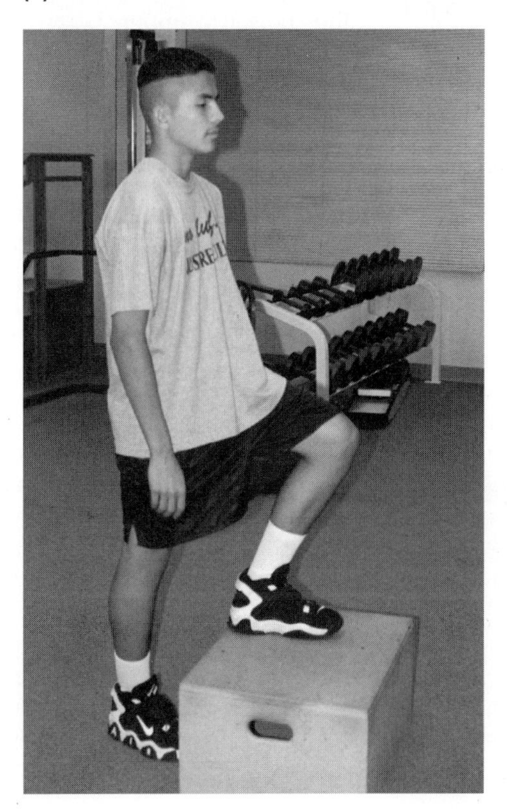

(3)

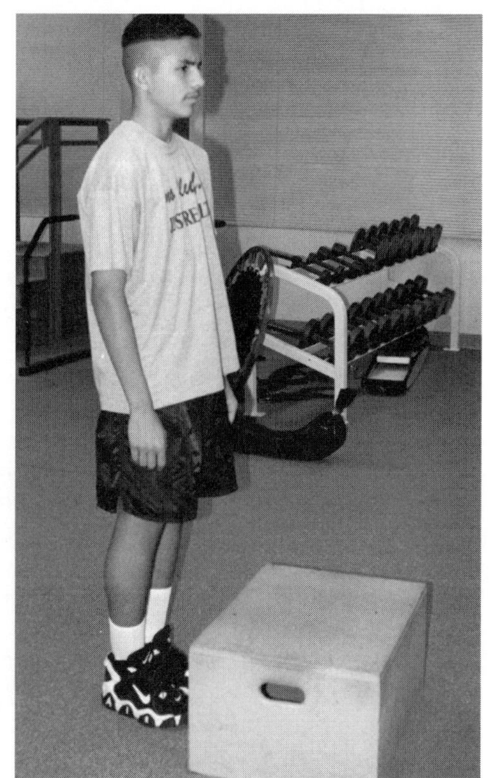

(4)

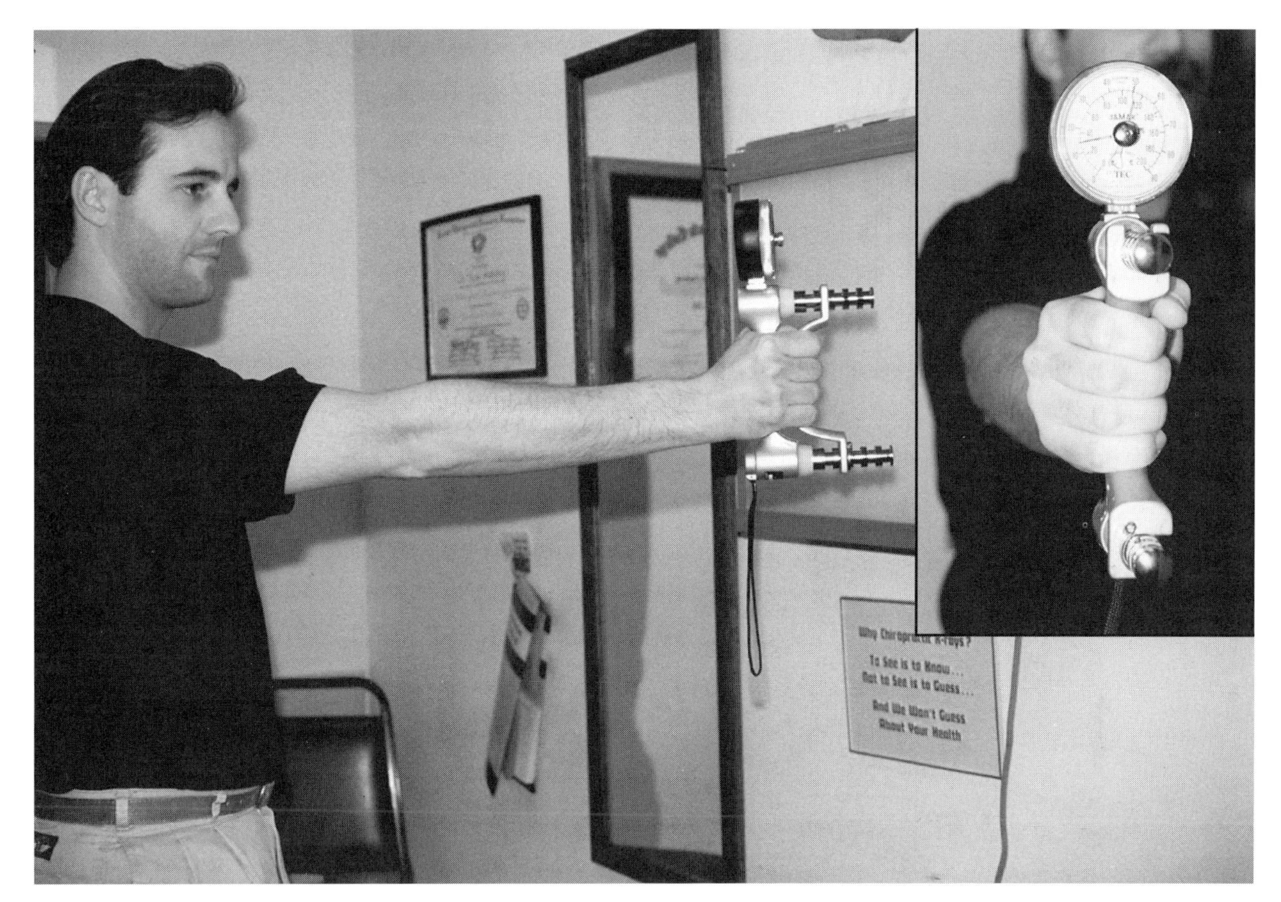

Figure 22-2
Using a dynamometer to measure grip strength.

longer time will improve the person's flexibility. Before exercise, stretching helps to warm up muscles. After exercise, it reduces tightness and thus relaxes the muscles.

Evaluating Body Composition

Body composition has to do with the proportion of body fat to muscle or fat weight as compared with lean weight. It is also the most important factor used to determine one's body weight. There are three methods which can be used to evaluate or determine one's body composition: hydrostatic weighing, the use of calipers, and the pinch test.

When the hydrostatic weighing method is used, the person must be totally immersed in a tank of water for weighing. Water displacement and other measurements are then made and used to determine the percentages of lean and fat to total body weight. This test is accurate but expensive. It is also quite time-consuming, and is generally only available in special sports medicine centers employing highly trained personnel.

Calipers is a measuring device used to determine the skin thickness from a pinched fold of skin. About half of our body fat is stored directly beneath the skin in the subcutaneous layer. From two to four sites are selected for measurement. These sites may include areas just above the triceps and biceps on the arm, the upper back just below the scapula, and at the iliac crest. Readings from the calipers are used to compute the percentages of fat to lean weight in the skin fold. This test is frequently done by a physician or fitness trainer.

The third and least accurate method for measuring a person's body composition, and thus, determining whether that person is becoming obese, is by using the pinch test. To perform this test, you will need to pinch a fold of skin on the back of the person's upper arm between the shoulder and the elbow or just below the waist on the hipbone. If the skin fold is more than one-half to one inch, this means that the person has too much adipose or fat tissue. Most physicians agree that obesity is beginning when a person is at least 20 percent or more above their normal weight for their height, body type, and age group.

Preventing Sports Injuries

Following proper methods and procedures for preventing sports and athletic injuries is just as important as properly assessing and evaluating a person for these types of activities. As a matter of fact, most members of the sports medicine community seem to agree that it is a lot easier to prevent an injury than it is to treat it. And, the probability of an injury occurring during an exercise program can be significantly decreased when the participant assumes the responsibility for his or her own safety.

Many of the responsibilities of the participant of an exercise program involve rules of basic safety and common sense. Examples of some of these rules include:

- developing the muscular strength, endurance, and flexibility which is necessary to be successful and to complete an activity.
- developing skill and accuracy with practice over a period of time, and learning skills in the order of their complexity, by first mastering fundamental skills of any activity before proceeding to more advanced skills.
- practicing good warm-up activities before starting an exercise program.
- following a skill through a completion once it has been started.
- using the principles of kinesiology to lessen injury if a fall or blow is inevitable.
- avoiding any type of horseplay or practical jokes while completing any type of exercise program individually or around others.

Preventing Sports Injuries of the Young Athlete

Whenever you are responsible for working with youngsters participating in any type of sports or athletic activity, you must give special thought to their level of maturation. This includes having an understanding of their musculoskeletal development and their overall body structure. A shorter, more compactly built teenager, for example, is far less prone to injury than a gangly uncoordinated one.

Another factor which you must take into consideration whenever you are working with young people involves comprehension of their physiological readiness to learn new skills. Since the stage of a younger person's development will vary from individual to individual, and because strength and endurance also tends to increase with age, you would be wise to begin a sports or exercise program for the younger person by first teaching them activities which use large muscles before those requiring the finer muscle skills.

A final consideration which must be given to working with young people is your knowledge of sports activities and those which should be geared to the individual rather than age group norms. Chronological age is the least accurate factor to consider.

Preventing Sport Injuries of the Mature Athlete

As we begin to age, we still need physical activities to maintain healthy bodies during our maturing years. Unfortunately, both physiological and anatomical conditions place restrictions and limitations on the types of activities we can do to prevent injury. Posture, shape, and even bone structure change with age. Flexibility starts to decrease, and joints begin to show deterioration. Strength has been shown to relate closely to age. It increases from birth to age 20 to 25 years, and then seems to level off and begins to decrease. You can see why it is so very important to make sure that a physical examination and assessment and evaluation take place before the senior or mature person attempts any exercise program.

If you choose to work with the elderly or mature participant, to ensure the selection of the appropriate exercise program you must have an understanding of kinesiology and the aging process. Activities must be done in moderation, less often, and for shorter periods of duration. Certain activities may be appropriate for one person, but contraindicated for others. Exercise must be developed on an individual basis. While jogging, for example, may still be suitable for one person, it may not be for another who is overweight or who has arthritic knees.

In addition to understanding the anatomical and physiological factors associated with working with mature athletes, there are certain factors which must be taken into account. Because of the aging process, and both the physical and emotional changes which it creates on the maturing person, you must be aware of such implications as motivation, postural improvement and maintenance, flexibility, balance, and overall aerobic fitness. All of these factors must be evaluated individually in designing program goals. While the motivation, or goals, for some participants may be overall fitness, others may desire training just to maintain activities for their everyday living. Postural changes with aging are due to joint degeneration and shortening of muscles. Therefore, exercise must encourage development of muscular strength in the shoulders, back, and abdomen to maintain correct upright alignment.

Sadly, many activities that require endurance, great muscular strength, and quick *reaction time* are often not popular with the elderly or mature athlete. Isometric exercises are also not recommended for these people, since they tend to raise blood pressure and could therefore lead to other cardiovascular problems. The mature athlete tends to enjoy more passive activities, such as walking, riding a stationary bicycle, swimming, and calisthenics, all of which help to improve posture, muscle strength, flexibility, and aerobic capacity. Aerobic capacity can also be improved through sustained activities, such as racquetball and handball, which are enjoyed by many older adults.

A nasty problem which seems to rear its ugly head with regard to the aging athlete has to do with bone porosity. As we begin to age, bone density starts to decrease due to the loss of calcium and phosphorus, thus leaving the bones brittle and prone to breakage. More porous bone also takes longer to heal once it is broken or fractured. On way to combat the onset and high incidence of this problem is to offer the mature adult endurance activities which will help to impede the onset of the porosity. You may also suggest that the person talk with his or her doctor concerning prescribing supplemental calcium.

Preventing Sports Injuries During Sports Activities

Two of the easiest ways to prevent a sports injury from occurring during an athletic or exercise activity involve the practice of the art of spotting and the use of protective equipment. A *spotter* is a person who is responsible for watching and assisting a sports participant to prevent an injury. While spotters can be used in any number of athletic competitions, they are most frequently utilized in weight lifting, gymnastics, and activities involving the trampoline. When a spotter is designated, he or she stands close enough to the participant to keep his or her forearms in a vertical position. Little weight can be absorbed when the spotter's arms are in a horizontal position. In some instances, the spotter may need to move a little closer if the athlete appears to be falling. Sometimes the spotter may also be called upon to provide a lift in order to assist with a rotation activity. To be most effective when receiving weight, the spotter should allow his or her arms and legs to bend, or "give." If the participant's motion is horizontal, the spotter may also need to take several steps to adjust his or her position (Figure 22-3 on p. 272).

While some activities require the need for a spotter, others may demand the necessity of protective equipment. Injuries such as those that happen in many team sports, like baseball, football, and basketball can be substantially reduced through the proper selection and usage of such protective equipment.

Protection Against Common Sports Injuries

There are many common injuries seen in athletic competition and sports programs. Many occur in both team sports and individual, or one-on-one, rivalry. As a matter of fact, there are certain sports which are actually characterized by specific types of injuries occurring in that particular activity. Athletic activities in which injuries seem to most frequently appear include football, basketball, baseball, bicycling, ice hockey, gymnastics, soccer, snow and water skiing, weight lifting, and running or jogging.

Football, Basketball, and Baseball Injuries

Injuries that seem to be most common to football generally include sprains, strains, bruises, scrapes, fractures, pulled muscles, and in a few cases, serious cuts. Many of these injuries are due to hard contact with another player's helmet, shoulder pad, or shoes. Others, such as spearing by one player with his head into another, for example, is a common tactic used in blocking and tackling. The impact of spearing is so devastating on a player that it can actually crush or fracture the participant's vertebrae.

Most football injuries can best be prevented by players wearing helmets and shoulder pads. Additionally, some players often use wrapping and taping to offer some extra protection from contact with other players. All protective equipment should always be kept in good condition. Players should also be instructed in fundamental tackling and blocking skills. And training programs for these athletes should emphasize muscular strength and endurance.

Injuries occurring during a basketball game are somewhat different than those seen during a football scrimmage. This is due, primarily, to the leaping under the basket and collisions with other players that take place during most basketball games.

The most frequent injuries to basketball players are those to the ankles, elbows, fingers, wrists, and head. Bruises and abrasions also occur as a result of the participants falling. The abrupt stops and starts and the frequent quick changes in direction of the players lead to ankle injuries, especially to the Achilles tendon. Fatigue also seems to play a role in decreasing the players skill and agility, thus resulting in injury.

Many of the injuries common to basketball can be prevented by providing players with the proper protective equipment. These generally include knee guards or pads, hip pads, and braces. Taping of the joints is also frequently used. Strength and endurance training of the basketball athlete should concentrate on the legs, back, arms, and shoulders. Shoes should

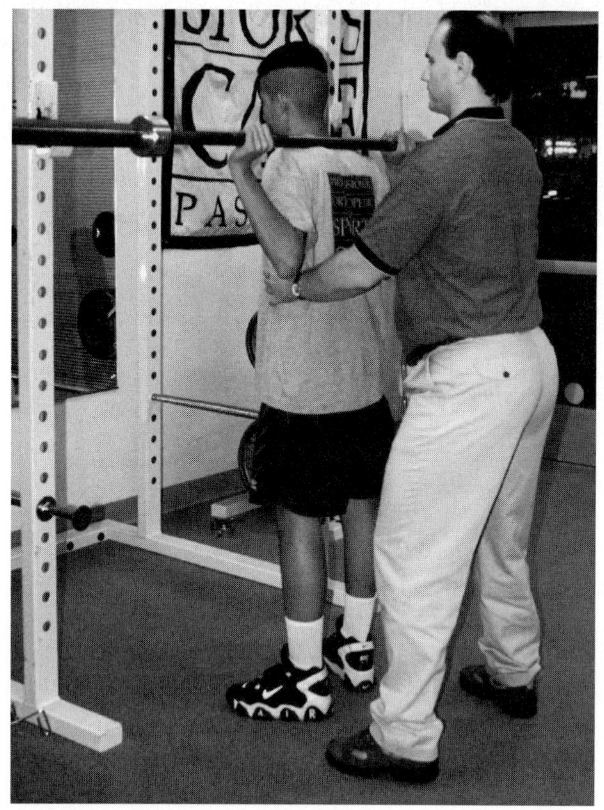

(1)

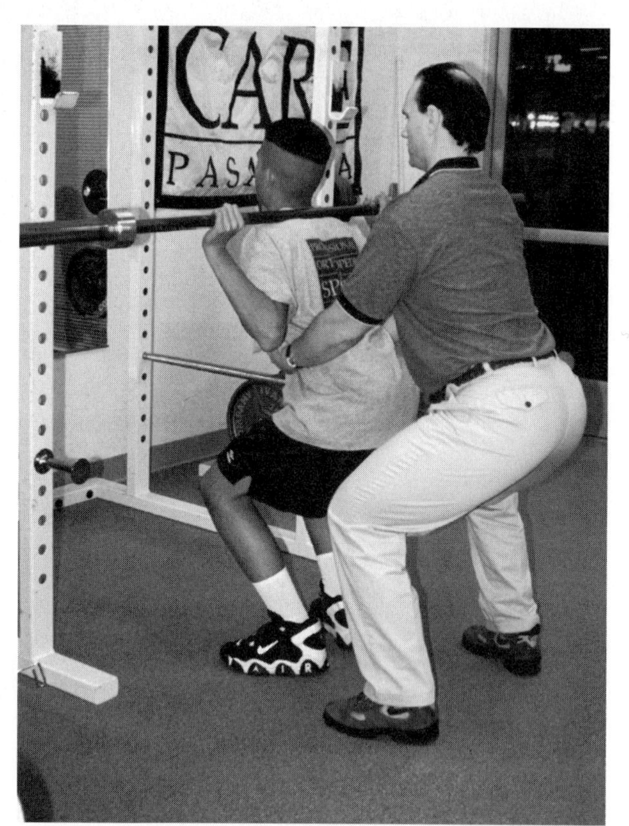

(2)

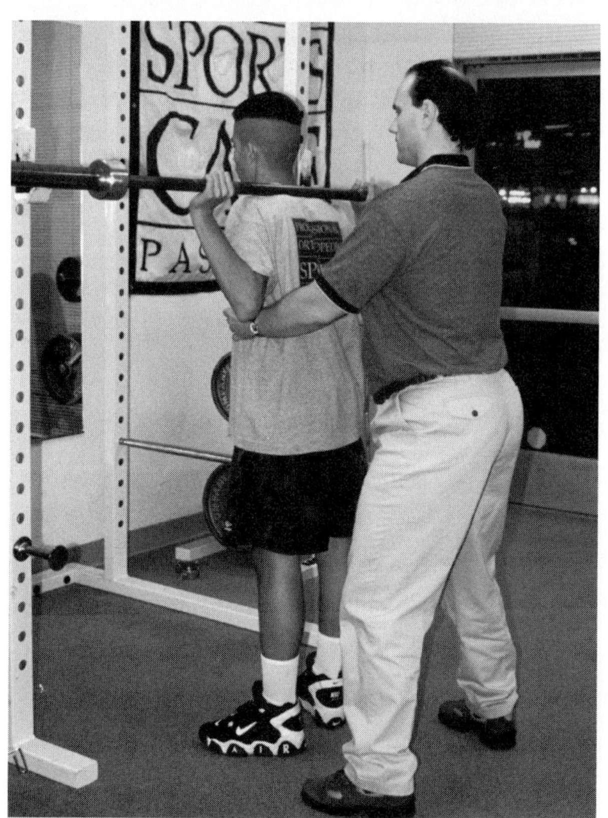

(3)

Figure 22-3
Using a spotter to prevent an injury.

also be well fitted, in good condition, and easily adaptable to quick changes in direction.

Compared to many other team sports, baseball seems to have the lowest rate of accidents. Most of the injuries that do occur during a baseball game seem to affect the players arms and legs, head, and neck. Injuries to the head and neck usually occur as a result of a blow with a ball or bat or by a collision between players. Pitching also seems to place a greater stress on the player's shoulder and arm because of the rotation and twisting motions. And many of the injuries to the arms and legs are often caused by the player sliding improperly, and by surfaces on which the slide has occurred.

Helmets are frequently used by baseball players while batting to protect their heads, and mitts and gloves are worn to lessen the impact of balls. Catchers also wear extra padding to protect themselves against the force and energy of a fast-moving ball.

Bicycling Injuries

Many of the injuries present in other sports are also seen in bicycling. These include bruises, scrapes, and fractures. Because many cycling enthusiasts travel on streets and highways, they often are in danger of being struck by moving vehicles. If this occurs, the athlete runs the risk of suffering from multiple fractures and internal injuries. The greatest concern of most cyclists is being struck or thrown from a bike, and landing on his or her head. If this occurs, brain damage is almost always certain.

The recent passage of laws in some places requiring that all cyclists wear safety helmets has helped a great deal in the prevention of many head injuries. Bicycles should also be kept in good working condition. This means that they should have reflectors, lights, and slip-resistant pedals. The brakes should also be in good working order.

Ice Hockey Injuries

Ice hockey, because of its very nature and the speed at which the game is performed, seems to have a great many more injuries than other athletic competition programs. Players may sustain injuries as a result of falls or collisions with other players or the wall, or they may be hit or struck by a hockey stick, a flying puck, or jabbed by skates.

Athletes involved in ice hockey must be adequately padded without sacrificing their speed on the ice. The position of goalie requires the greatest amount of protective padding. This includes wearing a face mask that is molded with raised ridges to distribute impact away from the goalie's face.

Gymnastics Injuries

The majority of injuries that are sustained by gymnasts result from their contact with equipment or the floor. These usually include abrasions, *contusions,* and in rare cases, fractures.

Since no protective equipment is worn by the gymnast, they must learn to check their gymnastic apparatus for safety before using it. They should also learn how to break a fall and distribute the impact over more area and time. Most gymnastic facilities use pads or mats, which can be placed on the floor to absorb the impact of falls. Spotters are also used whenever possible to assist the athlete in warding off a potential fall.

Soccer Injuries

Many of the injuries that occur in soccer are similar to those occurring in football. Eye and facial injuries seem to be the most common, mainly due to the athlete heading the ball. Injuries to the knees and ankles are also common, and, like basketball, are often due to the athlete abruptly changing his direction or from sudden stops and starts.

Except for wearing well fitted soccer shoes, the only other protection for the athlete participating in soccer comes from being involved in a well thought out and planned exercise program, in which the participant learns how to condition his body for strength, endurance, flexibility, agility, and quick reaction time.

Skiing Injuries

Many injuries can result from skiing accidents. Snow skiing accidents generally include injuries resulting from falls and collisions. The most common of these are fractures and sprains of the ankle, lower leg, and the knee. Spiral fractures of the lower leg are also common to the snow skier, often a result of boot rigidity or catching the inside edge of a ski, thereby creating *torsion.* The upper leg is rarely injured.

The best way to prevent injuries from snow skiing is to make sure that the athlete checks and adjusts all of his or her equipment before it is to be used. Unfortunately, the use of higher rigid boots has, in some cases, reduced ankle injuries, but in some instances, has made the situation worse by simply moving the injury to a higher level. Since most of the injuries that do occur to the snow skier result from falls and collisions, the best protection the athlete can take to avoid such injuries is to learn techniques for falls, that is, how to turn with the *torque* instead of away from it.

Like snow skiing, injuries sustained by water skiers most frequently result from accidents. The only difference between the two is that water skiing accidents are often more deadly, just because they occur on the water.

Most water accidents happen as a result of the skier falling into the water, colliding with an object such as another boat, dock, or pier, becoming entangled with a tow rope, or being struck by a propeller or another boat while in the water. These falls, collisions, and entanglements can cause serious injuries, unconsciousness, and in some cases, even death.

Water skiing injuries can be easily prevented by using common sense and by following boating and water safety rules. These include never attempting to ski at night, after eating, when tired, after drinking alcohol, or ingesting certain prescribed medications. Also, it is up to the boat operator to ensure the safety of his or her water skiing passengers. This means making sure that the boat is in good running order, and that operation of the boat is smooth with regard to starts, stops, and turns.

Weight Lifting Injuries

Many of the injuries caused during weight lifting involve the pulling, spraining, or tearing of muscles, tendons, and ligaments. In rare cases, a dropped heavy weight landing on a body part may also cause a body part to be fractured or crushed.

Weight lifting injuries can be prevented by teaching the athlete to use good body mechanics. This often involves learning how to lift weights as close to the line of gravity as possible and with all the body parts in alignment. In some cases, weight lifters choose to wear a wide leather belt, which helps to support the back as the weights are lifted.

Running and Jogging Injuries

The majority of injuries encountered by the runner or jogger affect the foot, ankle, lower leg, and upper leg. Running hills also seems to put undue strain on the runners lumbar spine because of excessive forward lean. This in turn leads to hamstring strains, sore feet, and pain in the Achilles tendon. *Shin splints,* which are often caused from wearing worn-out shoes, overstriding, changing running surfaces, or the increased intensity or length of training, can also be suffered by the runner. Foot pain is frequently caused by stiff shoes, improper arch support, and running on hard surfaces. Running on banked roads, muscle imbalance, or differences in leg length can also cause a tightness on the lateral side of the thigh and knee, a condition commonly known as runner's knee.

The first and most important requirement for preventing injuries associated with running or jogging is to wear a pair of well-fitting shoes. Shoes tend to break down about every 500 miles of running and therefore should be changed at least every three to four months. Runners should also learn to avoid banked roads, uneven surfaces, and running hills, since all of these tend to put additional strain on the hamstrings and feet. Finally, athletes involved in running and jogging should learn to use exercises that will keep their muscles strong and flexible. This includes completing a set of warm-up exercises prior to running or jogging.

Protecting the Joints and Bones from Injuries

Many athletes use wrappings of adhesive tape to protect against injuries to their joints and bones during competition or fitness training. These wrappings are often applied around a joint and bone to prevent injury or to halt further trauma to an area that has been previously sprained, strained, or fractured. In addition, these wrappings may also be used to restrict motion of a joint, to support bones and their surrounding tissues, to ease the stress put on tendons and ligaments, and to support muscles. Adhesive tape is used because it allows greater strength than wrappings made from cloth. To provide the greatest amount of support, the tape is applied directly to the skin. A tape adherent can also be applied to the skin, prior to the wrapping, to hold the tape in place.

Whenever preventative wrapping is used, the person responsible for wrapping the area should make sure that there is a large selection of tape widths available. Tape that is one inch wide may be used on fingers and toes, while tape that is 1½ to 3 inches wide, may be used on the athlete's arms, legs, and the torso. The backcloth for the tape may be either elastic or nonelastic. Paper tape is now available with a backing of a hypo-allergenic adhesive substance.

Before the wrapping is applied, protective padding of either tape or moleskin should be used to protect the athlete from blisters. The entire exposed area should be covered. If a blister does occur, it can be padded with cotton and then taped over, thus allowing healing to occur and the athlete to participate in his or her activities. Once you have applied the protective padding or moleskin, you are ready to begin the application of preventive wrappings.

Procedure for Preventive Wrapping of an Ankle

One of the most common locations for doing a preventive wrapping is at the ankle. To complete a protective wrapping of the ankle, you would:

- Obtain the necessary equipment; this will include elastic tape, nonelastic tape, and a pair of scissors.
- Prepare the skin with tape adherent; apply underwrap material as high as the adhesive tape will go.
- Begin at the foot, and wrap elastic tape in spirals around the foot, ankle, and up the leg to the desired height; make sure the wrapping is firm around the foot and ankle, but slightly looser up higher on the leg.
- Using the nonelastic tape, apply a series of three or four overlapping stirrups; these will begin inside the leg and extend down and across the sole and up the outside of the leg; make sure you do not cover the metatarsal bone; instead, angle the stirrups slightly forward.
- Place two or three nonelastic strips across the inner bend of the ankle; these go across, and not wrapped around; use another stirrup strip to hold down the ends of the transverse tapes.
- Wind the elastic tape around the leg in order to hold down the stirrup strips; cut the tape.

Summary

In this chapter, we discussed both the components of recognition and assessment of sports injuries, and how such injuries could be prevented. We talked about the purpose of physical assessment and evaluation techniques used to determine sports injuries, and the relationship between fitness to recognition and assessment of sports injuries. We also discussed the role of the participant in preventing his or her own injury, and the differences between injury prevention of the very young athlete and the mature or senior athlete. We explained the functions of a spotter in sports, and described some of the more common sport injuries and their prevention. Finally, we talked briefly about the process of wrapping and identified when and how preventative wrapping is used to prevent injuries.

Review Questions

1. What is a term used to define a wasting away of muscular tissue?
2. What is the name of a person who is responsible for keeping watch on a participant during the engagement of a physical activity?
3. The term ______________ refers to a process or procedure used to prepare an athlete for another sport or activity.
4. ______________ is a term used to refer to one's ability to move his or her body parts through a full range of motion at the joints.
5. A device used to measure the performance of the cardiopulmonary system is called:

   a. dynamometer
   b. ergometer
   c. caliper

6. A device used to determine the percentage of body fat is called a:

   a. dynamometer
   b. ergometer
   c. caliper

7. A device used for measuring force or power is called a:

   a. dynamometer
   b. ergometer
   c. caliper

8. An ______________ is a tracing of the heart which shows its electrical activity.
9. ______________ pertains to the length of time that a specific activity can be sustained by a set of muscles without them tiring.

23

Psychology, Rehabilitation, and Sports Medicine

Performance Objectives

Upon completion of this chapter, you will be able to:

1. Describe the relationship between applied psychology and sports medicine.
2. Briefly discuss the concept of performance, particularly as it relates to the differences between men and women.
3. Explain the role one's attitude and commitment play in achieving a positive outcome during a sports training program.
4. Discuss the relationship between stress and exercise.
5. Briefly explain the importance of achieving feedback during an exercise program.
6. Discuss the emotional implications involved in dealing with a person suffering from a sports injury.
7. Identify procedures and briefly explain types of therapies used to prepare and care for patients who have received a sports injury, including those involved in therapeutic exercise, electrotherapy, and therapeutic massage.

Terms and Abbreviations

Biofeedback a technique used to develop one's ability to control one's own autonomic nervous system.
Commitment pledging to do something.
Cryotherapy cold therapy.
Feedback the return of information to its place of origin.
Proprioception a type of internal feedback used to interpret the weight, position, and relationship of an object to the body.
Stress any tension or pressure which results from the relationship between a person and the factors in that person's environment.
Therapeutic exercise a type of exercise used to maintain or improve muscular strength, stability, and range of motion.

When we talk about psychology and its relationship to sports medicine and rehabilitation, we are actually referring to three things. The first relates to the degree of training which has been undertaken by the participant. The second deals more with the person's desire to compete in the activity. And the third deals with the modalities involved in the building up and rehabilitating of a person who may have become injured during the activity. The psychology of the training phase can easily be applied to anyone who is involved in an exercise program, as well as to competitive athletics. The second phase involves the final preparation and the anticipation and participation in a performance or contest. The third phase is available to all participants in both the exercise and competitive athletics.

Applying Psychology to Sports and Wellness

Achieving a Positive Attitude Toward Training

A positive attitude is always necessary in order to train over a period of time without becoming bored or losing interest. There are four basic steps to achieving such an attitude. These include choosing definite goals, developing a good method for measuring your progress, making sure there is plenty of variety in your program, and devising a plan for measuring your success.

The first thing the athlete or anyone participating in a planned sports program should do is to target his or her objectives or goals. To accomplish this, one should never use vague generalizations such as "losing weight," but rather, set a long-term goal with short-term goals to encourage success and accomplishments. The next step is to devise a method to measure one's own progress. This can be as simple as using a chart to show weight loss each week, or a list of how many miles you walked each day.

Another factor to consider when working toward achieving a positive attitude is to make sure there is a variety in the training program. Variety is easy to introduce in programs such as running, jogging, or walking simply by varying the routes. In activities such as calisthenics, different exercises can be used which still work the same muscle groups. Learning a new sport, especially a team sport, is also an interesting way to provide variety and lessen the chance of boredom during an activity.

In order to truly provide variety, you must be willing to change your lifestyle. This means replacing unhealthy habits with those that encourage a healthy lifestyle. For example, replace sedentary activities such as watching television with activities that help to achieve your goals in an activity program.

Finally, to really measure your success, the easiest way is to employ the basic principles of kinesiology, that is, repetition, progression, and overload. If these are applied, then the training or exercise program should provide you with clear evidence of some measure of success, such as the loss of five pounds of weight or the ability to walk four miles in 30 minutes instead of two miles in 40 minutes.

Another measure of success in a training program may be evidenced in competition. If, for example, your team wins, or you are able to beat a competitor in an individual activity, you feel your training activities have all been worthwhile.

Pledging Commitment

Commitment is a pledge, or a type of promise, to do something. There are three factors which are important in determining whether a person stays committed to an activity or sports program.

The first, and perhaps the most important factor to fostering commitment, is interest. This means selecting an activity because you enjoy doing it. Chances are, you probably won't continue a program if it becomes boring or a chore.

A second factor involved in commitment is time. It is extremely important to select a time that fits your individual schedule. This can be accomplished by first determining whether you function best in early morning or in the afternoon. Once you have determined which time is best for you, set aside that block of time, and stick to your schedule. Also, if you find that your motivation seems to be weak, do things or get involved in activities that will help you meet your commitment. This might include joining a health club, choosing a team sport, or just asking a friend to join you in your exercise program. This important factor to commitment is often referred to as companionship.

Relationship Between Stress and Exercise

It's hard to ignore the fact that *stress* is a very large part of our everyday lives. However, there is some stress that, given the right environment and opportunities, can actually be good for us and increase our performance.

The kind of stress generally seen by the physical medicine assistant often has to do with the physical stress built up by the athlete's muscles. The major concern here is that the assistant must determine whether or not the stress has been created from increased physical performance or as a result of some other internal or external factor, such as irritability, insomnia, or other physical dysfunction like gastric pain, headache, or increased blood pressure.

Any time you become aware of a stressful situation, either as a member of the health care team, caring for patients, or in your own everyday life, the most important thing you can do is to identify the problem which is causing the stress. This often means first admitting, either to yourself or to another, that you genuinely feel stress or tension. Once you have faced this fact, you can begin to start looking for solutions. The only difference here is that when you are working with a patient, your most important responsibility is to first be supportive of the patient's need to discuss his or her stress. Once you have become aware of where the stress is coming from, you will be in a much better place in helping the patient to deal with the problem or situation causing the stress.

There are many ways of dealing with stress in your life. Sometimes you can relieve stress caused by your relationships with others by simply discussing the problem with another objective person. Often these discussions can clear the air of any anger or harbored resentments you or the other person might be feeling. Rest or relaxation is another way to relieve stress. Another way is to break from your regular routine, meet new friends, or create something new. And finally, for those people involved in sports or athletic training, another excellent way of ridding yourself of stress is by taking part in physical exercise, such as walking, running, or playing a team sport. Such physical exertion generally helps a person to relieve his or her emotional stress, and at the same time, helps to provide you with a change of pace and break in your regular routine.

Performance, Feedback, and Mental Practice

Whenever we discuss the practice of physical medicine, particularly as it relates to exercise and sports, it is also important to have an understanding of how such exercise and activities are measured in terms of success and achievement. And to comprehend this concept, we must first look at the three parts which make up the "success triangle." They are performance, feedback, and mental practice.

Performance

During childhood, generally up to the age of 10 to 12 years, there seems to be few differences in athletic performance between boys and girls. And on the average, girls between the ages of 13 to 14 are often as heavy and tall as boys, or sometimes even larger and taller due to their earlier maturation. However, after puberty, major differences begin to emerge. Some of these differences may be cultural, as the girls begin to assume a more sedentary lifestyle than the boys. Other changes begin to take on physical differences. For example, strength, endurance, flexibility, and cardiovascular fitness begin to decrease, while body composition and changes in the accumulation of fat tissue begin to increase.

As we begin to mature, differences in body build and overall composition become more and more obvious. For example, in the adult male, we notice wider shoulders, broader chest, and narrower hips than in the adult female. And by the time the adult female has reached maturity, she appears shorter and lighter in weight than her male counterpart. Although the female weighs less, her percentage of body fat is usually greater by comparison. However, females who perform endurance activities, such as long distance running, tend to lose body fat and develop the same relative lean-to-fat ratio as male athletes.

In most cases, males have a tendency to have greater upper body strength. With planned weight training, however, females can develop substantial levels of strength without gains in their muscle bulk. Strength of the lower extremities is similar in both sexes when related to overall body weight. And the capacity for endurance is also quite similar or equal, when based upon lean body weight. Because of higher testosterone levels in the male, he will also have a larger overall total muscular mass.

A concern which seems to be shared by many female athletes is the effect exercise has on the female reproductive system. Many women have practically no difficulties with their menstrual cycles whether they participate in athletics or sports competition or remain sedentary. Others have menstrual difficulties. Some women athletes, during training for endurance and competitive sports, report a total absence of menstruation. According to some gynecologists, this may be a result of exceptionally low body fat deposits after intensive training. Once the rigorous training has been reduced, the regular cycle seems to return to normal. The bottom line, here, is that there is no reason to recommend or promote different exercise programs based solely on the sex of the athlete or participant.

Feedback

The term *feedback* has to do with the return of information to its place of origin, or the system that receives it. It may be either positive or negative, and may be caused by either internal or external factors.

Internal feedback deals with those mechanisms which act to increase or decrease hormone production in our body, in order to maintain homeostasis, or an equal balance within our body. *Proprioception* is a form of internal feedback that is important in the study of kinesiology and sports medicine. It originates in the nerve endings, or receptors, of the hand in relationship to the awareness of the weight, position, and relationship of objects, such as a ball or tennis racket, to the body. It also includes an awareness of different changes which are occurring in our equilibrium due to posture and movement. This internal feedback is necessary to create the body action which we desire.

External feedback, which involves our senses, such as vision and hearing, has to do with what is occurring outside our body. Distance runners, for example, use this type of feedback in order to judge their distance and timing.

One method which can be employed either by the sports medicine assistant, the trainer, or by the participant him- or herself to measure the degree of success or achievement of an activity is through *biofeedback*. This technique involves the development of a person's ability to regulate his or her own autonomic or involuntary nervous system. The person uses a monitoring device which emits a sound with a change in the person's blood pressure, heart rate, skin temperature, and brain waves, or when a muscle contracts. The patient or participant is then trained, through repetition, to set up these same conditions for causing the desired change.

Mental Practice

The third component to measuring the degree of success and achievement of one's involvement in physical activities or sports deals with the concept of mental practice. Such a practice is often used to develop higher level skills which can ultimately be applied to performance. After a person has practice in motor skills, he or she can conduct mental practice by reviewing the skill in his or her mind. Mental practice has it greatest value to those activities using fine motor skills, such as golf, gymnastics, or diving. Many athletes, before competition, are often instructed to mentally run through their expected performance.

Injuries and Sports

Despite all the precautions and safety measures that are taken during athletic training and sports activities, injuries can still occur. It is often the mental attitude of the injured athlete that can best determine how rapidly and completely he or she recovers from an injury. Each person reacts to injuries differently. Any type of injury or illness is a threat to a person's sense of security, and can often cause different degrees of disruptions or disturbances to the person's emotions.

Any injury produces emotional and mental changes in a person. At times, such changes seem to follow a characteristic pattern. Often, after the initial shock of the injury, the person may deny the seriousness of the condition. A person may think that everything is okay. Such denial is generally followed by a period of grief and depression. Once the grief and depression has passed, the person may begin to feel anger and hostility. Eventually, the person accepts his or her injury and the alterations in lifestyle or sports involvement it may have brought. While these emotional and mental changes may not be the same for everyone, it is important to remember that any changes in the person's state of mind during a time of injury are considered quite normal responses to any serious injury, illness, or disability.

A person's attitude is perhaps the single most important thing he or she can work with when it comes to determining the final outcome of the entire recovery or rehabilitative phase following a sports injury. Emotional and mental attitudes can have both positive and negative effects on the ultimate results of the rehabilitation process. The extent of the person's injury must be evaluated by trained personnel. And the total evaluation process should include the individual's attitudes, behavior, and personality.

Ultimately, whenever a person experiences a sports or athletic injury, an exercise program must be planned and goals set, as though it were any other training program. Realistic goals must be determined; that is, those that can be achieved. While there are many programs of exercise to help an injured athlete achieve his or her goals, the most important point to remember is that once the program is begun, frequent reevaluations must follow.

Rehabilitation and the Injured Athlete

In all sports and athletic activities, there is always a much greater potential for injury than in the daily activities of living. Lack of muscular strength, physical contact, imbalance, the impact of gear and athletic equipment, and being struck by propelled objects, such as a ball, can cause a wide range of injuries to the athlete. And, as we have already discussed, the majority of these injuries involve muscles, bones, and joints, and often include sprains, strains, fractures, and dislocations. Any athlete who has sustained an injury suffers from discomfort and pain. And, as we have already stated, the way the athlete accepts his or her injury often plays a key role in his or her rehabilitation.

Therapeutic Modalities of Rehabilitation

There are several modalities which can be utilized in the rehabilitation and treatment of the injured athlete. These include the use of therapeutic exercises, therapeutic and superficial heat, hydrotherapy, cryotherapy, the penetration of deep heating into the affected or injured muscles, ultraviolet therapy, electrotherapy, and massage therapy.

Therapeutic Exercises

The purpose of any *therapeutic exercise* program is to assist the injured athlete in maintaining or increasing muscle strength, developing endurance, providing for coordination and stabilization of the body, maintaining or increasing range of motion of the injured part, and developing speed in order to shorten the activity time.

If you are responsible for assisting the injured athlete with implementing a therapeutic exercise program, it's important for you to understand the three preliminary steps involved in creating such a program. The first step is to evaluate the person's present ability to take part in a program. Once this is done, you should help the person to set realistic goals. This helps the injured athlete to determine just what can be achieved within the limitations of his or her disability. Finally, after you have begun the planned program, you should set up a schedule for reevaluating the effectiveness of the program.

Most people are much more cooperative and interested in an activity when they have an understanding of why such an activity must be done. This is especially true when you are working with an injured athlete. Therefore, it's important to begin by first setting up a friendly, informal relationship. This includes making your patient feel at ease, as well as making sure that you not only give proper instructions about how a particular exercise should be done, but just as important, paying particular attention to the patient's comprehension of how he or she should complete an exercise.

One method for providing instructions to your patient is to combine a verbal explanation of the activity with an actual demonstration of the movements or actions involved in the activity. This method may involve four basic steps. The first step is to prepare the patient for the activity. Next, you must present the actual activity. The third step is to have the patient try out or perform the activity. Finally, you should provide the patient with follow-up and input regarding the performance of the activity. Once you have completed your instructions and have gone through your four-step plan of introducing the activity, you are ready to assist the patient in starting the program.

Principles of Therapeutic Exercises

Whenever you implement a therapeutic exercise program, there are some basic principles which you should know that apply to all types of exercises. These include the following.

- Always make sure that the patient is in a comfortable position.
- Always make sure that the joint which is involved or which you are working with is well supported.
- Always make sure that all movements are smooth and not jerky.
- Always make sure that the exercise program is done frequently and for short intervals.
- Always make sure you keep accurate records.
- Always make sure that the patient knows exactly why and how a particular exercise should be done.

Types of Therapeutic Exercises

There are many different categories of therapeutic exercises used in the practice of sports medicine. However, the most frequent of these include passive and active exercises, progressive resistive exercises, stretching exercises, isometric exercises, functional exercises, and exercises which involve the use of specialized equipment, such as crutch exercises, mat exercises, and parallel bar exercises.

In passive exercises, the goal of the activity is to prevent contractures from occurring. Therefore, the exercise is performed by someone other than the injured person, thus allowing the patient to remain entirely passive and relaxed. On the other hand, if the activity is to be an active exercise, the responsibility for performing the movements lies solely with the patient. In this case, you would first demonstrate the exercise in a step-by-step manner, and then allow the patient to follow your movements with a return demonstration while you observe.

Progressive resistive exercises, which are often used to help increase a person's strength, involve activities which generate repetitive contraction against some type of resistance. In these exercises, the resistance is gradually increased as the person continues to gain strength. To perform this type of activity, the person should make an active effort to move the limb or body part. Then, using some of your own body weight or some other type of weight equipment, you would provide the resistance.

Another type of exercise which helps to maintain, increase, or improve muscle strength is isometric exercise. These are accomplished by contracting a muscle without allowing joint motion to occur. This type of exercise is most common and frequently used in the treatment of arthritis and is often implemented following joint surgery.

Stretching exercises, which can either be passive or active, are often used to help a person achieve normal range of motion. Frequently, mechanical devices, such as weights, may be used to apply the stretching force.

Exercises which help or prepare a person to be able to perform within his or her limitations of a disability are called functional exercises. The most common of these are called activities of daily living, or ADL. Many of these exercises can be done in bed, on an exercise mat, in a wheelchair, or using parallel bars.

Therapeutic exercises which involve the use of mechanical or therapeutic equipment generally include mat exercises, parallel bar exercises, and crutch-walking exercises. Mat exercises are often used to teach the patient how to effectively and safely change positions, move around while sitting, balance, and move his or her affected limbs. They can also provide additional movements for stretching and strengthening the muscles. Both parallel bars and crutch-walking exercises are used to prepare the patient for walking or gait training. These types of activities help to teach the patient such things as pelvic control, how to stand up in braces and balance, how to use different steps or patterns for individual gaits, how to control a prosthetic or artificial limb, and coordination. In addition, patients who are required to use crutches also learn exercises involving turning, walking on all types of surfaces, going in and out of doors, how to properly get up from a chair or bed, and how to fall and get up from the floor without hurting him- or herself.

Therapeutic Heat Therapy

There are three basic types of heat therapy which are frequently used in the practice of sports medicine. These include therapeutic heat, which is most frequently used to relax sore muscles and to relieve pain, and often includes such items as heat lamps, hot baths, water bottles, heating pads, and hot compresses; superficial heating, often used to provide shallow penetrating heat less than 5 mm below the skin, generally with the aid of an infrared lamp; and deep heating, frequently used to provide deep heating beneath the surface of the skin.

In sports medicine, two of the most common methods used to provide deep heating therapy to the injured athlete are shortwave diathermy and ultrasound therapy. Shortwave diathermy produces high-frequency energy currents that are able to heat large areas of the body. The area which is to receive the treatment must be properly draped with one layer of toweling. The machine should then be positioned in contact with the toweling.

When using shortwave diathermy, there are two concepts which are extremely important to understand prior to placing the patient under the machine. The first is to make sure that any metal implants, jewelry, or any other metal which the patient may be wearing is not in close proximity to or near the treatment area, since metal tends to absorb the energy being emitted from the shortwave diathermy. The second is to make sure you determine the proper dosage which is to be applied and the length of time of the treatment. Dosage can easily be determined by noting the patient's sensation or sensitivity to a feeling of "gentle warmth." And, unless otherwise ordered by the patient's physician, treatment time is generally no longer than 20 minutes.

One of the most commonly used methods for applying deep heat is through the application of ultrasound therapy (Figure 23-1 on p. 282). It is a safe, easy, and relatively inexpensive type of diathermy that uses sound waves to produce mechanical vibrations within the tissues. It is frequently used to relieve pain, inflammation, and irritation in both acute and chronic conditions, such as arthritis, bursitis, myositis, and fibrositis. As the ultrasound is applied to the affected area, vibrations are able to produce both a heating and micromassage effect, as well as an increase to the permeability of the cell membrane and cell metabolism, thus increasing the circulation to the affected area. These effects are enhanced through a coupling medium or gel, which should be applied to the treatment area to provide for the penetration of the sound waves with a minimum of reflection.

To be most effective, the ultrasound should be applied either in a stationary position or with a moving technique. In the moving technique, the ultrasound head is moved in a circular or stroking motion. If the area to be treated is bony or has irregular surfaces, the ultrasound can be administered underwater. In this technique, no gel is needed, since the water acts as a conducting medium. The ultrasound head should never come into contact with the skin. Instead, hold the head approximately one-half inch from the surface of the skin while using the circular or stroking movement. This technique is especially useful when using ultrasound for treatment of the hands.

Hydrotherapy

Hydrotherapy deals with the external application of hot or warm water for the sole purpose of treating an affected area. It is a common method of treatment for many sports injuries because it has a distinct advantage over many other types of therapies in that it allows a patient to be able to move or exercise while the treatment is being administered.

One common form of hydrotherapy is the whirlpool bath (Figure 23-2 on p. 283). This is a metal tub filled with water that is agitated, with the intensity of the agitation easily adjusted by the assistant. The temperature of the water generally ranges from 98 to 115 degrees F, and treatment time is often between 20 to 30 minutes. The whirlpool bath is frequently used to treat injuries involving the extremities.

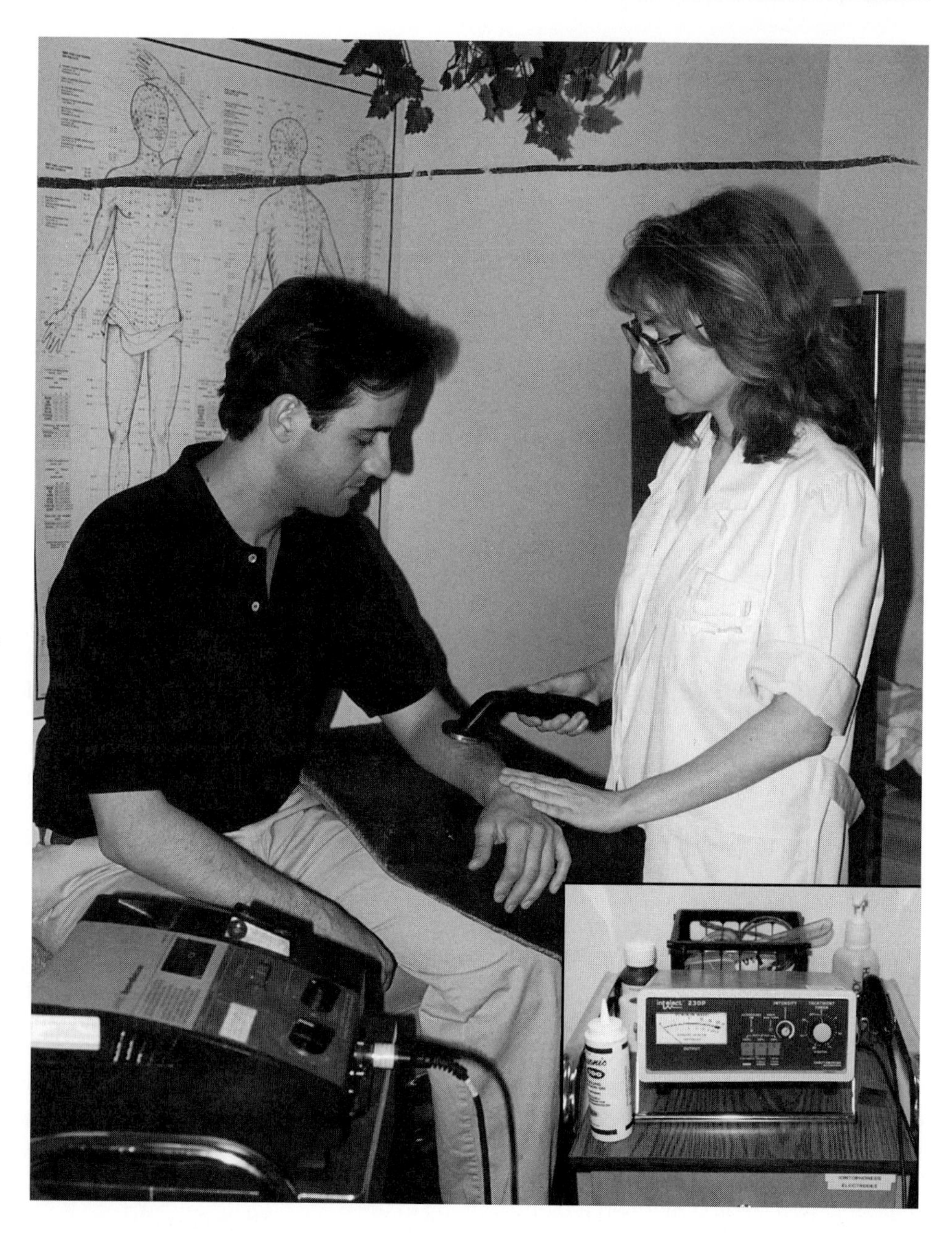

Figure 23-1
Ultrasound machine.

Another form of hydrotherapy is the use of hot packs (Figure 23–3). Hot packs come in many types and forms. They can be moist, woolen, or in the form of an hydrocollator pack. Hydrocollator packs are most commonly used in hospitals and clinics. They are kept in water-filled hydrocollator units which maintain the packs at a constant temperature of 165 degrees F. The packs are removed from the storage unit and then padded prior to use for treatment. In order to prevent burning, the packs are used with six to eight layers of padding between the pack and the patient's skin. Patients receiving hydrocollator packs should be checked at least every five minutes to make sure no burning of the skin has occurred. When using these packs, it is usually best to place them on the patient while he or she is lying face down, since lying on top of them can lead to injury and burning, and is therefore not recommended.

Two less frequently used types of hydrotherapy include a paraffin bath and the contrast bath. Contrast baths are the alternate immersion of an extremity in hot, then cold water. The bath causes the constriction and dilation of the blood vessels, thus increasing blood flow to the affected part.

A paraffin bath is a mixture of oil and wax that is heated to approximately 125 to 130 degrees F. The

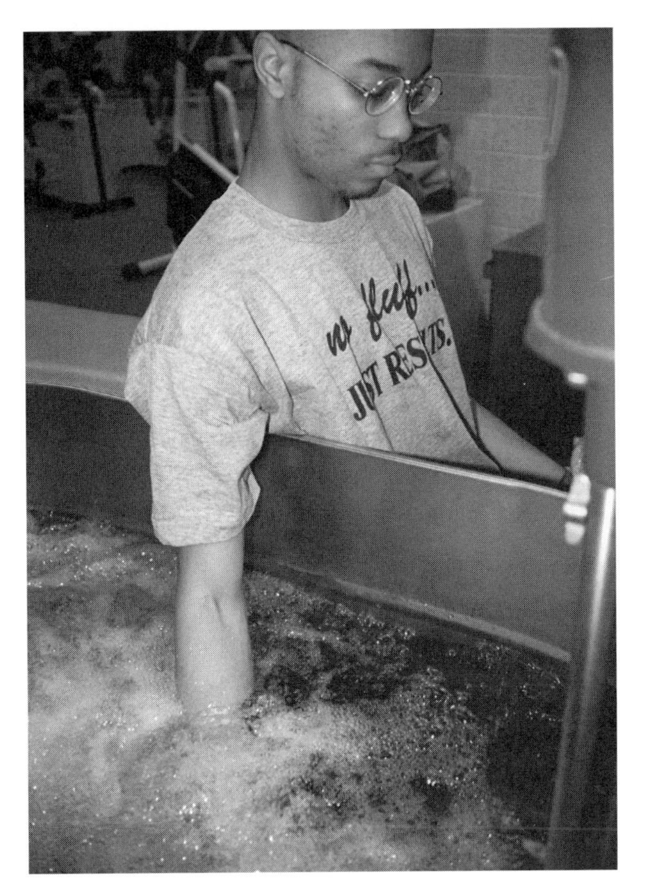

Figure 23-2
Whirlpool bath.

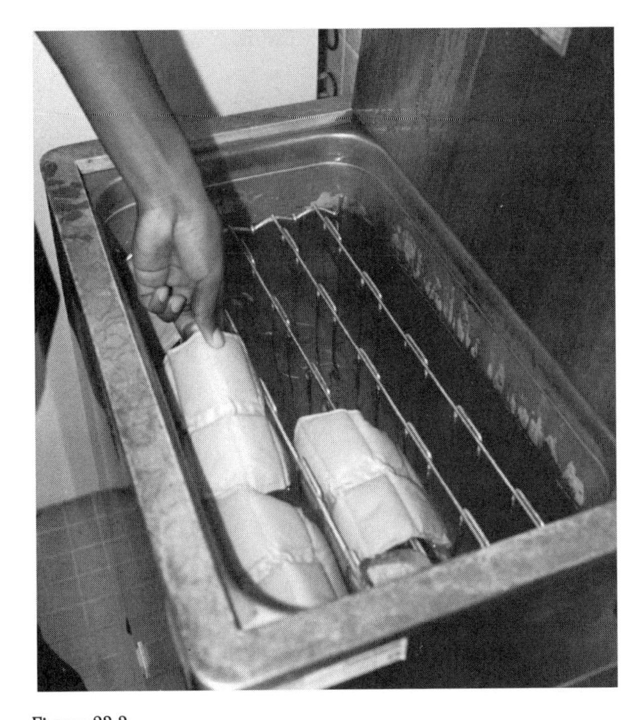

Figure 23-3
Hot packs.

oil-wax mixture allows the use of high temperatures without burning the patient's skin. This technique is generally reserved for use in treatment of the hands or feet. The part to be treated is washed, and the skin checked for any open wounds. If open areas are found, the paraffin bath cannot be used. To treat the area, the affected joint is dipped into the paraffin bath several times. The paraffin coats the joint, thereby producing warmth. The affected joint is then wrapped in plastic wrap or waxed paper and then draped with a towel to contain the heat. The entire treatment generally lasts about 20 minutes.

Cryotherapy

The purpose of *cryotherapy,* or cold therapy, is to produce vasoconstriction and a decrease in blood flow, metabolic activity, and local tissue temperature, thus, it is almost always used to reduce fever, swelling, pain, and inflammation. For most patients, the response to cold often depends upon the type and temperature of the article applied, the length of application, and the part of the body to which it is applied. Common methods of application of cold to the body include ice bags, cold water baths, cold compresses, and cold packs.

Electrotherapy

Electrotherapy deals with the use of continuous or direct electric current as treatment to an affected area. The currents are used to stimulate nerve and muscle tissue. Intensity or dosage is determined by the type of stimulation desired and the purpose for which the treatment has been ordered. Today, electrotherapy is widely used for muscle strengthening, reeducation, and pain control.

Message Therapy

Massage is one of the oldest forms of therapy known to health care providers. Therapeutic massage therapy is applied to the body by systematic stroking, using both pressure and kneading actions, and therefore, should only be provided by a trained professional.

While there are several types of massage techniques which can be used on the average healthy adult, there are only a few which should be used in the therapeutic setting. The most common of these include effleurage, petrissage, friction, and vibration and percussion. Effleurage, or stroking, can either be superficial or deep. Superficial massage is light stroking of the skin to create reflex effects. It causes dilation of the capillaries and relaxation of involuntary muscle contraction. Deep massage, on the other hand, pushes the venous blood and lymph through the vessels. When using petrissage, or a type of kneading technique, there is a gentle rolling and squeezing of the skin and underlying tissue. By lifting up and massaging the muscles, circulation is increased, and tendons and connective tissues are stretched and lengthened.

Friction is considered to be the deepest form of massage. When performed properly, you will need to use your thumb, fingers, or palm to apply deep pressure to muscles and tissues. When using this technique, movement should always be in a circular or stroking pattern following the direction of the muscle fibers.

Vibration and percussion are massage techniques often used in combination and in conjunction with positioning, to assist with the treatment of certain lung disorders. The goal of these treatments is to clear the lungs of mucus and other secretions.

In the sports or physical medicine environment, massage therapy can be used to relieve pain, to relax muscle tension, to improve circulation, and to reduce swelling. However, if you are responsible for performing any of the massage techniques previously discussed, there are some basic principles which you should understand. These include never allowing the massage to cause the patient pain, placing the person in a comfortable position, providing support to the affected part during the treatment, only using slow, rhythmical strokes in the same direction, using maximum hand contact to the skin, and never using too much or too little lotion.

Summary

In this chapter, we discussed the roles which applied psychology and rehabilitation play in sports medicine, and their relationship to one another. We discussed the concepts of performance, attitude, commitment, and the relationship between stress and exercise. We also talked about how we achieve feedback during an exercise program. Finally, we discussed sports injuries, and identified the many types of therapies used to prepare and care for patients who have received an injury during a sports or exercise program.

Review Questions

1. ______________ is a technique used to develop one's ability to control his or her own autonomic nervous system.
2. What is the name of a technique used by sports medicine professionals when the hands tap the body during massage?
3. The systematic stroking of the body using pressure and different types of kneading actions is called:
   a. feedback
   b. massage
   c. diathermy
4. What does the term *commitment* mean?
5. What does the term *cryotherapy* mean?
6. What does the term *proprioception* mean?
7. ______________ ______________ refers to a type of exercise used to maintain or improve muscular strength, stability, and range of motion.
8. ______________ is a term used to identify the return of information to its place of origin.
9. What is the term used to describe any tension or pressure resulting from the relationship between a person and the factors in that person's environment?

24

Nutrition and Sports Medicine

Performance Objectives

Upon completion of this chapter, you will be able to:

1. Briefly explain the importance of maintaining body weight.
2. Discuss the appropriate ways in which one can properly gain, lose, or maintain an ideal body weight.
3. Identify and briefly discuss the four food groups.
4. Identify the role nutrients and water play in nutrition, and briefly discuss the function of each.
5. Identify special diets and briefly discuss their relationship to maintaining balanced nutrition.
6. Discuss the impact of eating disorders on the human body.

Terms and Abbreviations

Additive any substance which has been added to food to enhance flavor, taste, or texture, or to preserve it.
Calorie a unit of heat.
Carbohydrate food source that supplies energy for the body.
Diet any food or liquid regularly consumed.
Empty calorie a calorie which only provides energy, and therefore, few actual nutrients.
Enriched food food which has had vitamins and minerals added to it.
Fat a major class of energy-rich food.
Glycogen a starch found in the liver, muscles, and other tissues in animals.
Mineral any chemical from the earth which has been found in foods.
Nutrient any food which supplies the body with a necessary element.
Nutritional supplement any vitamin and/or mineral which has been added to a food.
Obesity an abnormal amount of fat on the body.
Protein an essential constituent of all living cells.
Recommended Daily Allowance (RDA) U.S. government recommendations concerning the appropriate intake of nutrients.
Vitamin a nutrient which is needed for normal body growth, development, and maintenance.

Most young people who are involved in sports, athletic competition, or fitness training are concerned with achieving or maintaining their ideal body weight. It is vital because it not only affects our overall state of health, but also, the speed, strength, and endurance which is necessary and often required to achieve a positive outcome in any athletic or fitness training program.

How do we know if we are at our correct body weight? How many times have you asked yourself if you are too thin? Of if you should go on a diet because you weigh too much? Body size and shape varies due to individual bone size and musculature. Weight itself does not verify or validate fitness. If three people weigh exactly the same, one may be considered fit and the other two grossly out of shape.

In fact, an athlete, such as a football player, with an outward appearance of well-developed muscles may look like he is overweight, when, in fact, he is actually maintaining his ideal body weight.

Energy, Diet, and Body Weight

People engaged in sports and fitness training are often concerned with their energy level. Energy is required for all movement and mental activities. Even sleeping or resting requires some outlay or release of energy.

The amount of energy used in the performance of an activity is determined by one's body size, the amount of work being performed, and the speed at which that work is completed. All energy is measured in units of heat, called *calories.* If your diet is poor in foods which produce energy, your body will burn energy which it has stored. The best source of maintained energy is a well-balanced diet and a planned exercise program.

Planning and Maintaining a Proper Diet

The foods we eat, or fail to eat, affect not only our weight and energy levels, but also our overall appearance, disposition, and productivity. Since advertisers make it difficult to choose a proper diet by surrounding us with a variety of different things to eat, it is a lot easier to determine one's ideal weight by consulting a standard weight chart (Table 24-1 and Table 24-2 on p. 288). Once you have determined what your correct weight should be, you can decide whether to gain or lose weight and select a diet which best meets your individual needs.

When planning a diet, the first and most important step is to determine the correct number of calories required each day, which can be safely consumed by the body without causing a weight gain. Approximately 15 calories are required to maintain one pound of weight. So, for example, if a person weighed 120 pounds, and she wanted to maintain that weight, she would need about 1,800 calories a day to stay at that weight. If you want to determine the number of calories it takes to maintain your own ideal weight, after consulting the weight chart, multiply the number shown as the ideal weight for your age group, by 15. That will give you the number of calories necessary to maintain that weight. If your actual weight is above or below your ideal weight, you should begin to look for ways to change the amount or types of foods you are consuming.

Loosing Excess Weight

Each pound of fat has approximately 3,500 calories. To lose one pound each week, you would have to eat at least 500 fewer calories each day. Subtract this amount from the maintenance amount. Using our example of the 120 pound athlete, she would be able to consume a daily total of 1,300 calories and still lose at least one pound per week. Remember, to lose weight, you must first decrease the number of calories you consume in food and increase the number of calories you spend in exercise. Exercise also helps us to decrease our appetite.

Increasing Weight

If you are at least 15 percent below the ideal weight for your age, height, and body size, you are considered underweight. When this occurs, you must increase the number of calories consumed. The easiest way to accomplish this is to eat between-meal snacks, and at the same time increase your intake of foods which are high in complex carbohydrates. Exercise is also helpful when trying to increase one's weight, since it adds firm muscle tissue and not flab.

Eating Well and Staying Healthy

Eating well and making wise food choices is not difficult, in principle. All that is needed is to eat a selection of foods that supply the appropriate amounts of the essential nutrients and energy. Yet to master the principle and put it into practice may be extremely difficult for some. The physical medicine or sports medicine assistant can help clients and patients make appropriate food selections for good health. In this role, you can help your patients or clients by guiding them in a direction in which they can become more knowledgeable about nutrition, thus providing them with a meal pattern they can understand and follow.

There are four steps you can follow to assist the patient or client in beginning his or her journey to eating well and staying healthy. The first step is to become more knowledgeable about nutrition. Next, you can go beyond this by obtaining readings and keeping up with articles written about nutrition by professionals in the field. Being a role model and practicing healthy eating habits is the third step to assisting your patient or client. This shows a commitment to good, sound nutrition. And finally, finding a local resource in nutrition, such as a registered dietician, capable of giving sensible responses to your questions is another step you can take in helping the patient or client toward achieving good health by eating well.

Table 24-1
Height-Weight-Age Table for School-Age Girls

Ht. (in.)	6 yr	7 yr	8 yr	10 yr	11 yr	12 yr	13 yr	14 yr	15 yr	16 yr	18 yr	Ht. (in.)
38	33											38
39	34											39
40	36	36										40
41	37	37										41
42	39	39										42
43	41	41	41									43
44	42	42	42									44
45	45	45	45									45
46	47	47	48									46
47	50	50	50	50								47
48	52	52	52	53								48
49	54	54	55	56	56							49
50	56	56	57	59	61	62						50
51		59	60	61	63	65						51
52		63	64	64	65	67						52
53		66	67	68	68	69	71					53
54			69	70	71	71	73					54
55			72	74	74	75	77	78				55
56				78	78	79	81	83				56
57				82	82	82	84	88	92			57
58				84	86	86	88	93	96			58
59				87	90	90	92	96	100	103		59
60				91	95	95	97	101	105	108	111	60
61					99	100	101	105	108	112	116	61
62					104	105	106	109	113	115	118	62
63						110	110	112	116	117	120	63
64						114	115	117	119	120	123	64
65						118	120	121	122	123	126	65
66							124	124	124	128	130	66
67							128	130	131	133	135	67
68							131	133	135	136	138	68
69								135	137	138	142	69
70								136	138	140	144	70
71								138	140	142	145	71

Nutrients and Food Groups

There are six groups of *nutrients* which the body requires, all of which are found in most foods. These include *proteins,* which help to build and repair body tissues, *carbohydrates,* which provide energy for the body, *fats,* which are a necessary part of every cell because they protect internal organs and carry fat-soluble vitamins, *vitamins* and *minerals,* which regulate body processes, and water, which is the most important of all nutrients, because of its necessity in the many chemical reactions in the body. In fact, about 60 percent of the body is made up of water.

Energy Nutrients

Energy nutrients, which are made up of carbohydrates, proteins, and fats, contain calories and energy which can be used in several ways. They help to create heat; they help in the building of body structures;

Table 24-2
Height-Weight-Age Table for School-Age Boys

Ht. (in.)	6 yr	7 yr	8 yr	9 yr	10 yr	12 yr	13 yr	14 yr	16 yr	18 yr	19 yr	Ht. (in.)
38	34											38
39	35											39
40	36											40
41	38	38										41
42	39	39	39									42
43	41	41	41									43
44	44	44	44									44
45	46	46	46	46								45
46	48	48	48	48								46
47	50	50	50	50	50							47
48	52	53	53	53	53							48
49	55	55	55	55	55							49
50	57	58	58	58	58	58						50
51		61	61	61	61	61						51
52		63	64	64	64	64	64					52
53		66	67	67	67	68	68					53
54			70	70	70	71	71	72				54
55			72	72	78	74	74	74				55
56			75	76	77	77	78	78				56
57				79	80	81	82	83				57
58				83	84	85	85	86				58
59					87	89	89	90	90			59
60					91	92	93	94	96			60
61						96	97	99	103			61
62						101	102	103	107	116		62
63						106	107	108	113	123	127	63
64						109	111	113	117	126	130	64
65						114	117	118	122	131	134	65
66							119	122	128	136	139	66
67							124	128	134	139	142	67
68								134	137	143	147	68
69								137	143	149	152	69
70								143	145	151	155	70
71								148	151	154	159	71
72									155	158	163	72
73									160	164	167	73
74									164	170	171	74

they assist in the movement of body parts; and they can be stored as body fat. The energy values of these nutrients are:

1 gram of carbohydrate = 4 calories
1 gram of protein = 4 calories
1 gram of fat = 9 calories

Practically all foods contain a mixture of carbohydrates, fats, and proteins, although they are sometimes classified by the predominate nutrient. A protein-rich food, like beef, for example, actually contains a lot of fat as well as protein. A carbohydrate-rich food, such as corn, also contains fats and protein. Thus, it is incorrect to say we are eating a protein when we are eating meat. We are actually eating a protein-rich food that also contains other nutrients, such as fat. Only a few foods are exceptions to this rule, the most common being sugar, which is almost a pure carbohydrate, and oil, which is almost a pure fat.

Essential Nutrients

The human body is so unique that it can actually make certain nutrients from other nutrients. For example, it can convert some amino acids into carbohydrates, if need be. It can manufacture one of the vitamins, niacin, from a certain amino acid. There are, however, certain compounds absolutely indispensable to bodily functions that our body cannot make for itself. These are called essential nutrients. In this context, essential means the nutrient is needed in the diet because the body cannot make it for itself. There are about 40 different nutrients we must be concerned about. It may be a relief to discover that diet planning can be reduced to a few simple principles to ensure that we take in all the nutrients in the appropriate amounts without having to count and weigh each one. The use of a food group plan makes it possible to design a diet that meets all the nutrient needs.

Food Planning and the Basic Four Food Groups

The four food groups make up the most widely used eating plan. This plan is simple and has great flexibility. You might remember being taught about the basic four food groups back in elementary school, and in fact, those groups still remain the best model to teach nutrition principles. This plan specifies that a certain quantity of food must be consumed from each group. For the adult, the number of servings recommended is two, two, four, and four (Table 24-3 on p. 290). Most selections of food based on this plan will supply 100 percent of the recommended amounts of all nutrients for men and all except iron for women. Women miss getting the full daily recommended amount of iron by only 10 percent.

You can use the four food groups plan to teach others how to make wise food choices, to plan menus for nutritious meals, to grocery shop, and to assess a diet to determine if it's nutritionally sound. By advising your patients or clients to follow the three easy principles below, you can help others to make better food choices using the four food groups.

- Eat foods from all four food groups every day.
- Include a variety of foods.
- Practice moderation.

There are many foods which do not fit into any of the four food groups. For example, butter, margarine, cream, salad dressing, mayonnaise, jelly, coffee, and alcohol do not fit into any group. Therefore, these items are grouped together into the "others" category. Although some of them do contribute nutrients, either they are not foods or their nutrient content is not significant enough to characterize them as a food. Many years ago health professionals labeled these "other" foods as *empty calories,* meaning that they contained more calories than nutrients. Today, however, most nutritionists use the concept of nutrient density. This is a measure of nutrients per calorie. A nutrient-dense food provides more nutrients at a low-calorie cost. Therefore, a non-nutrient-dense food is one that contains more calories and/or fat and fewer nutrients, such as cookies, potato chips, cake, and soda pop.

At first, the four food group plan may appear quite rigid, but it can be used with great flexibility once its intent is fully understood. For example, you can suggest to your patient that yogurt be substituted for milk because it supplies protein, calcium, and riboflavin in about the same amounts. Dried beans and peas, as well as nuts, are alternatives for meats. The plan can even be adapted to casseroles and other mixed dishes and to different national and cultural cuisines. It can also be used for people who exercise or train regularly. Eating more servings from the groups that provide carbohydrates (fruit and vegetable group and grain group) will help athletes and active individuals meet their requirements for energy foods.

Teaching the four food groups not only helps people learn the number of servings required from each group, but also helps them realize which foods will provide the leading nutrients. For example, people who want to know food sources of vitamin C need only review the four food groups chart to see which foods will provide that nutrient. The four food groups method of diet planning is a simple and an educational means of assuring an adequate, well-balanced diet for most patients and clients.

Meeting Nutritional Needs

The United States government publishes recommendations concerning the appropriate intake of nutrients for the people of this country. These are called *Recommended Daily Allowances* or *RDA,* and are shown in Table 24-4 (on p. 291). The RDAs are used in food labeling to express the nutrients of the RDA in percentages.

Unfortunately, the use of RDAs has been very much misunderstood. To put them into perspective, you should understand that the RDA is published by the government, but the study group that recom-

Table 24-3
The Four Food Groups

I. Milk Group	Key nutrients provided include calcium, protein, and riboflavin.
Servings:	2 servings daily for adults 3 servings daily for children 4 servings daily for teenagers
One serving equals:	1 cup milk 1 cup yogurt 1 ounce cheese 1/2 cup cottage cheese 1/2 cup ice cream
II. Meat Group	Key nutrients provided include protein, niacin, iron, and thiamine.
Servings:	2 servings daily for all ages
One serving equals:	1 egg 2 tablespoons peanut butter 2 to 3 ounces lean meat, fish, or poultry 1/4 cup nuts, seeds 1/2 cup peas, beans
III. Fruit and Vegetable Group	Key nutrients provided include vitamins A and C.
Servings:	4 servings for all ages 8 servings for athletes involved in heavy training
One serving equals:	1 medium apple, banana, or orange 1/4 cup dried fruit 1/2 cup juice 1/2 cup vegetable, fruit 1/4 cantaloupe 1/2 grapefruit
IV. Grain Group	Key nutrients provided include carbohydrates, iron, niacin, and thiamine.
Servings:	4 servings for all ages 8 servings for athletes involved in heavy training
One serving equals:	1 ounce ready-to-eat cereal 1 1/2 corn tortillas 1/2 flour tortilla 1 slice bread 1/2 English muffin 1/2 cup pasta, rice, cooked cereal

mends them is composed of nutritionists and other scientists. Also, you should understand that RDAs are only recommendations, not requirements, and certainly not minimum requirements. They include a margin of safety that is so substantial that two-thirds of the RDA is often deemed adequate, except for calorie intake. Here, it's important to note that RDAs recommend a range within which most of a healthy person's intake of nutrients probably should fall. Individuals' needs differ. While two-thirds of the RDA may be adequate for the general population, it may not be adequate for some. A physician who can provide a complete blood chemistry test should therefore be the person responsible for making the final assessment as to the individual's nutritional needs. And finally, remember, the RDAs are for healthy people only, and the presence of any medical problem may alter a person's nutritional needs.

With the understanding that RDAs are approximate, flexible, and generous, they can be used as a yardstick to measure the adequacy of diets in whole populations. It must be understood that as a member of the sports or physical medicine team, your role is not to assess a person's diet using the RDA. This should be left to the person's doctor and/or a registered dietician. You can, however, make dietary suggestions by using the four food groups approach, suggesting variety and moderation.

Table 24-4
Vitamins Recommended Daily Allowances

Vitamin	Source	Adult RDA
Fat-Soluble		
A	Liver, fortified milk, margarine, butter, egg yolk, leafy green and yellow vegetables, dried apricots, cantaloupe, peaches	800–1,000 I.U.*
D	Fortified milk, egg yolk, fish, and sunlight (absorbed through the skin)	400 I.U.
E	Vegetable oils, wheat germ and whole grains, nuts	30 I.U.
K	Leafy green vegetables, cabbage and cauliflower, tomatoes, wheat bran, milk (adults also produce vitamin K in their intestines)	70–80 mcg**
Water-Soluble		
C	Citrus fruits, tomatoes, strawberries, melons, potatoes, broccoli, green peppers	50–60 mg***
B_1 (thiamine)	Pork, organ meats, legumes, whole-grain and enriched cereals and breads, wheat germ	1.0–1.5 mg
B_2 (riboflavin)	Organ meats, milk and dairy products, whole-grain and enriched cereals and breads, eggs, fish, leafy green vegetables	1.2–1.8 mg
niacin	Fish, liver, meat, poultry, eggs, peanuts, grains, legumes	13–19 mg
B_6 (pyridoxine)	Meat, cereal bran, wheat germ, egg yolk, legumes	1.6–2.0 mg
B_{12}	Liver, kidney, meat, fish, milk, cheese	3.0 mcg
folic acid (folacin)	Green vegetables, organ meats, lean beef, eggs, fish, dry beans, lentils, asparagus, yeast	180–200 mcg
pantothenic acid	Whole-grain cereals, organ meats, eggs, vegetables (found in most plant and vegetable foods)	2.0 mcg
biotin	Liver, egg yolk, peanuts, yeast, milk, legumes, bananas, cereal	100–200 mcg

*International Units
**micrograms
***milligrams

Vitamin and Mineral Supplements

Because there seems to be a lot of concern and confusion in most consumer's mind's over what makes up a nutritionally balanced diet, and since most people don't really understand the RDA, many Americans turn to supplemental vitamins and minerals as a type of nutritional insurance plan. The question that arises here is should most people be taking a supplement? Generally, no. People who take a simple one-a-day type of vitamin or mineral supplement that does not exceed the nutrient levels of the RDA is probably not doing any harm. Most of us do not need to take the supplement, however, this type of one-a-day supplement does little harm even to the pocketbook. The consumer or patient who limits food selection and calories may have a difficult time getting the recommended levels of nutrients. In this case, a multiple one-a-day could be recommended. Of greater concern to most physicians and nutritionists is the supplement taker who has a whole medicine cabinet full of supplements. These individuals take a handful of supplements for breakfast, perhaps several tablespoons of nutritional yeast and assorted pills containing trace minerals, powdered protein, and herbs. These people are asking the pills and supplements to play a role that is better delegated to food. Takers of self-prescribed supplements need a warning about the risks of overdosing. Concern should be expressed if individuals are taking high doses of fat-soluble vitamins, such as A, D, E, and K. These particular vitamins are stored within the body, and toxic levels have been found in people who take megadoses of these nutrients.

Water-soluble vitamins, such as the B complex and C are not stored within the body, and therefore any excesses are excreted in the urine. It was once thought that a toxic level of water-soluble vitamins was impossible. But recent research shows that if a person continues to ingest megadoses of water-soluble vitamins, those vitamins, too, can reach toxic levels.

Vitamin toxicity usually affects the nervous system. Both vitamins A and B6 are known to produce adverse neurologic reactions, such as nerve transmission, when ingested in megadoses rather than the recommended nutritional doses. The symptoms of vitamin or mineral toxicity are vague at best; diarrhea, vomiting, skin rashes, and overall lethargy, generally accompanied by a sense of "just not feeling well." Because these symptoms could easily describe any disease or illness, if you are working with someone who experiences or expresses these signs, it is best not to make recommendations about vitamin toxicity, but rather to suggest that the person seek professional medical advice about the symptoms. Encourage the person to take his or her supplements to the doctor and/or dietician for proper assessment.

Calcium Supplementation

Many people can meet the recommendations of the RDA by making wise food selections from the four food groups. However, for women, one of the nutrients most often lacking is calcium.

The need for calcium is greater during adolescence than in either childhood or adulthood. Approximately 45 percent of an adult's skeletal mass is formed during the pubertal growth spurt. The RDA for calcium for females 11 to 24 years of age is 1,200 mg. If calcium intake is inadequate during peak adolescent growth, it may predispose some individuals to osteoporosis in later life. Consumption of low-fat dairy products which are rich in calcium should therefore be encouraged.

There are many ways to incorporate calcium foods into the diet to meet the daily requirement of 1,200 mg. For example, two glasses of skim milk and two ounces of low-fat mozzarella cheese contain the recommended dietary allowance for young women. A combination of skim milk, low-fat cottage cheese, and frozen yogurt is also appropriate. Calcium can also be incorporated into the diet through a number of other ways, such as:

- preparing canned soup with skim milk instead of water.
- adding grated low-fat cheese to salads, tacos, and pasta dishes.
- drinking hot chocolate made with skim milk.
- adding nonfat dry milk to soups, stews, casseroles, and even cookie recipes.

Since it has also been reported that decreased physical activity has an effect on reducing the efficiency of calcium utilization and may also contribute to bone loss, it would be wise to encourage women to take part in a lifelong exercise program in addition to consuming calcium-rich foods.

Iron Supplementation

Like calcium, iron also plays a key role in many of the chemical reactions continuously taking place in our body. It is present in all of the cells of the body, plays a vital role in the transport and activation of oxygen, and is present in several pathways that create energy. Various studies have found the diets of women to be low in iron. One of the problems with dieting and limiting calories is that a woman may not be able to meet her iron requirements while trying to cut calories and lose weight. Because women face a potentially greater chance of lacking iron because of low caloric intakes and increased iron loss through menstruation, it has been suggested that they consider routine use of iron supplements, particularly during periods of heavy physical activities or exercise training.

Iron supplementation in nonanemic women has not been shown to be useful, and may be potentially harmful. Clearly, there is some hazard from prolonged administration of large doses of iron to persons who are not iron-deficient. The hazard of serious iron overdose resulting from megadoses of iron could expose them needlessly to hemosiderosis, a disorder of iron metabolism in which large deposits of iron are made in the liver. Therefore, it is important that routine screening for early detection of iron depletion be undergone by women who may be predisposed to iron deficiency or anemia.

Meeting Nutritional and Dietary Guidelines

During the mid 1960s, a select committee on nutrition and human needs was formed to study the nutritional status of the United States population. For about 17 years, the committee held hearings on malnutrition, hunger, obesity, nutrition, and heart disease. Reaching the conclusion that there appeared to be many connections, the committee published their document entitled *Dietary Goals for the United States,* which emphasized sugar, fat, cholesterol, and salt as items to avoid. In the three years that followed, critics of the committee's findings continued to react violently to the goals. Bowing to these criticisms, the committee eventually published a revised edition that suggested weight reduction, if necessary, and avoiding the overuse of alcohol. The committee disbanded in the late 1970s, and in 1986, the Department of Health and Human Services, working jointly with the Department of Agriculture, published the *Dietary Guidelines for Americans.* This document, while varying somewhat from the original goals, emphasizes that all Americans:

- Eat a wide variety of foods.
- Maintain their ideal body weight.
- Avoid too much fat, saturated fat, and cholesterol.
- Eat adequate amounts of starches and fiber.
- Avoid too much sugar and sodium.
- Consume alcohol only in moderation, if at all.

There have been many different reactions to the goals and guidelines, however, most health care professionals seem to agree that some of the guidelines are desirable, especially the ones which emphasize reducing fat, saturated fat, and cholesterol.

Nutrition and Exercise

While people who exercise seem to be much more aware of nutrition than those who do not take part in any exercise program, they still do not always know how to apply that knowledge, or in some cases, even fall prey to the myths and fallacies that surround nutrition. Such lack of knowledge is most often related to the function and roles played by water, carbohydrates, proteins, vitamins, and minerals.

Water Consumption and Hydration

Water, to the athlete, is by far the most important nutrient. For optimal performance, fluids must be replaced before, during, and after exercise. Most people rely on thirst as an indicator of how much water is lost. Unfortunately, however, thirst is not an accurate indicator of fluid loss. Therefore, water losses can and must be monitored by one of two methods. The first method involves the patient or client weighing him- or herself before and after an exercise workout. For each pound of body weight lost, two cups of fluid must be consumed. In the second method, the participant checks the color of his or her urine. If the urine is a dark gold color, there is an indication that the person is dehydrated. A pale yellow or no color means that this person is headed toward a state of hydration.

Rules for Fluid Replacement During Prolonged Exercise

In order to ward off the potential for dehydration during prolonged exercise, you can encourage the patient or client to follow two rules:

- Encourage the consumption of at least three to six ounces of cold fluids every 10 to 15 minutes during a workout, since cold fluids empty from the stomach most quickly.
- Encourage the consumption of sports drinks if the exercise or workout lasts longer than 90 minutes of continual work, since after this prolonged period of time, muscle glycogen has been depleted and the body needs a source of carbohydrates; if the workout is less than 90 minutes, then water is the best source of fluid replacement.

Carbohydrate Consumption

Another area of confusion to the exercising population has to do with how much carbohydrate food should be consumed. Most people have absolutely no idea how many calories they need, let alone the percentage of carbohydrates from the total calories they consume. Generic advice such as "eat 50 to 70 percent carbohydrates" means little to most people. Grams of carbohydrate mean more and are easier to calculate than percents. The best way you can help your patient or client is to provide them with a list of common foods in grams of carbohydrates. Recommend that they consume between 400 to 500 grams of carbohydrates daily for optimal *glycogen* storage. The list can also serve to show them which foods contain a high proportion of carbohydrates and should therefore be included in their daily diet.

Carbohydrate Loading

Muscle glycogen depletion is a well-recognized limitation to endurance exercise that exceeds 90 minutes. Athletes using glycogen supercompetitive techniques, or "carbohydrate loading," can nearly double their muscle glycogen stores. Obviously, the greater the preexercise glycogen content, the greater the endurance potential.

Since there are many adverse reactions which can occur when the body doubles its consumption of carbohydrates, this type of regime is generally reserved for those athletes involved in athletic competition. And before such a drastic method is undertaken, its usefulness for the participant should be assessed by a physician or nutritionist. Once it has been approved, six days before the competition, the athlete exercises hard, that is, at least 70 to 75 percent of aerobic capacity, for at least 90 minutes. This is followed by a consumption of a normal diet providing at least 50 percent carbohydrates. On the second and third days, training is decreased to 40 minutes at 70 to 75 percent of aerobic capacity and again the athlete consumes a normal diet. On the next two days, the athlete consumes a high carbohydrate diet providing at least 70 percent carbohydrate (about 550 gm, or 10 gm/kg), and reduces training to 20 minutes at 70 to 75 percent of aerobic capacity. On the last day, the athlete rests while maintaining the high carbohydrate diet. This regimen results in muscle glycogen storage equal to those provided by a classic diet low in carbohydrates.

Protein Consumption

As recently as 1987, research has shown us that protein may play a much greater role in providing energy for exercise than previously thought. However, protein intakes of most exercising individuals are adequate, if not excessive. When assessing protein intakes for your patients or clients, guidelines should be used. Generally, for adolescents, 1.0 gm protein/kg of body weight is used. For adults involved in very heavy weight training, that is, at least one hour or longer, or those involved in endurance training, the recommendation is 1.5 gm protein/kg of body weight. This added quantity is still easily attained in the average diet, and no protein or amino acid supplements should be encouraged. Potential problems with excessive protein or amino acid intakes include excessive weight gain, dehydration, and excessive loss of urinary calcium. High protein intakes may also impose a heavy burden on the liver and kidney to secrete excess nitrogen.

Vitamin and Mineral Consumption

All of us are bombarded with information about what to eat, what not to eat, and what supplement we should or should not be taking. What's most interesting is that when we look at the food records from people who exercise on a regular basis, we quickly see that these people seem to get more than enough of what is required for their vitamin and mineral intake from the food they eat. For the most part, athletes who use supplements have adequate diets; those with less adequate diets, generally due to calorie restriction or dieting, do not use supplements.

When working with people who augment their food consumption with vitamin and mineral supplements, always remember that consideration should be given to the individual's nutrient deficiencies, toxic levels, and unnecessary supplementation. Deficiencies of vitamins and minerals can be damaging to work performance and growth in young adolescents because of their role in releasing energy from food. However, this does not mean that adding additional vitamins or minerals to their diet will further improve a person's performance if that person is already well nourished. Actually, many sports nutritionists seem to agree that when a person consumes less than 70 percent of the RDA in his or her diet, some diet modification may be indicated, and perhaps, even a multiple one-a-day supplement should even be added.

Food Additives

Food *additives* are substances that can be combined with a food product to enhance its flavor or add color to it. Most additives, which generally include preservatives to prevent spoilage and stabilizers, emulsifiers, and thickeners to change the product in some way, are often added to the product. It's important that all consumers be aware of these additives, since some may not show up on labels.

When vitamins and/or minerals are added to enhance the nutritional value of a product, such foods are said to be *enriched,* as in the case of enriched bread. And as we have already discussed, vitamins and minerals may also be added to food. In this case, they are referred to as *nutritional supplements.*

Diets and Nutrition

Recommendations and diversity as to the proportions of different nutrients in our diets vary with the individual person or the specific group publishing such recommendations. However, according to most nutritionists and physicians specializing in the field of sports and physical medicine, in order to meet the RDA, a good, well-balanced *diet* should contain at least 58 to 60 percent carbohydrates, 20 to 30 percent fats, and 12 to 20 percent proteins. The best way to ensure the proper intake of these nutrients is to make sure you eat a well-balanced diet. A normal, balanced diet will, according to the experts, supply you with all the needed nutrients.

People involved in sports medicine need to be aware of various types of diets which are often used or advocated for training or weight loss. These include the process of loading or packing carbohydrates, as well as specific dietary programs, such as those which are high in protein and low in carbohydrates, or those very low in calories, or very high in carbohydrates.

Dispelling Dietary and Nutritional Myths

Unfortunately, there are many myths associated with dieting and nutrition, particularly as they relate to sports medicine. The most common of these include the following.

- *Large amounts of protein increases strength and size.* This is untrue. In fact, there is no evidence to show that consuming excess amounts of protein will increase one's muscle strength or size.
- *Consuming foods high in sugar content, such as candy bars, soft drinks, or honey, before competing in an athletic activity will provide a quick burst of energy.* This is actually a very dangerous myth. Since these foods have a high sugar content, eating them before competition can cause an increase in the production of insulin and can cause the sugar in the blood to be removed too quickly. Low blood sugar can result, thereby causing the person to feel fatigued and weak.

- *Drinking water before and during exercise causes an upset stomach and cramps.* Since water is the most important nutrient to someone who is exercising, restricting it during exercise periods, especially in hot weather, can cause severe dehydration and thus limit one's performance.
- *Muscle cramps are caused by consuming inadequate amounts of salt.* Cramps happen when excess water loss has occurred through perspiration. Therefore, water should be consumed before, during, and after exercise to prevent dehydration. Ingesting salt tablets can actually aggravate existing dehydration by drawing water out of the body tissues and into the stomach.
- *Crash diets are the quickest, most effective way to lose weight.* While large amounts of weight can be lost by following a crash diet, the weight lost is muscle mass, glycogen stores, and water, not excess body fat. As a result, a person's endurance is impaired. Additional problems associated with crash diets include electrolyte imbalances, calcium and iron deficiencies, and other vitamin and mineral losses.
- *Special supplements such as brewer's yeast, ginseng, and ascorbic acid can be used to improve an athlete's performance.* This is absolutely untrue. In fact, there is no scientific evidence to show these compounds contribute anything to one's athletic performance. In fact, some of these supplements may even be harmful.

Eating Disorders and Nutrition

According to most experts in the field of nutrition, one of the most common health problems in the United States is *obesity,* or an abnormal amount of fat on the body. Although metabolic disturbances can cause obesity, this problem is often the result of a larger calorie intake than calorie expenditure, or in other words, overeating. Persons who are overweight seem to tire more easily, may have frequent backaches, are more susceptible to some diseases, and generally have more difficulty doing physical work. Those who are underweight tend to be more irritable and restless, and have less physical agility and endurance.

Some people, usually teenagers, and often females, deny themselves food because they have an obsessive fear of obesity. Each views his or her body as overweight although, in reality, the body may be gaunt from starvation. These individuals may have a psychological problem dealing with accepting themselves as they are or an irrational fear of growing up. Such a disorder is referred to as anorexia nervosa.

Another eating disorder seen especially in young women is called bulimia. A person with this condition stuffs themselves with large amounts of food and then forces regurgitation, fasts, or uses laxatives. This pattern of abnormal behavior is called binging and purging. A person with bulimia generally appears normal in her appearance, thereby often making diagnosing of this problem quite difficult.

Sadly, in addition to the psychological and emotional disturbances associated with eating disorders, these abnormalities often lead to other physical problems affecting many of the body's systems. There may be upsets in the digestive system, dental problems, and hormonal imbalances throughout the body. The reproductive system in the female may become so involved that the breasts do not develop and menstrual cycles are disturbed or stop altogether. Muscle tissues may become injured when no fat remains for energy. And in severe cases, death may even result. Treatment for these disorders must include both dietary reeducation and psychological counselling to learn how to deal with the underlying causes.

Summary

In this chapter, we discussed the relationship between nutrition and sports medicine. We briefly explained the importance of maintaining one's body weight, as well as ways in which one can properly gain, loose, or maintain an ideal body weight. We also talked about food planning and the four food groups, the role nutrients and water play in nutrition, and special diets and supplements required to maintain balanced nutrition. We identified some of the most common myths about dieting and nutrition. Finally, we concluded our discussion by identifying some of the most common eating disorders affecting the general population, and their affect on the human body.

Review Questions

1. An ______________ is any substance which has been added to food to enhance its flavor, taste, or texture, or to preserve it.
2. ______________ pertains to an abnormal amount of fat on the body.
3. What is the name given to any starch found in the liver, muscles, and other tissues in animals?
4. A ______________ is any food which supplies the body with its necessary elements.
5. Briefly explain what an *empty calorie* is.
6. Briefly explain what a *nutritional supplement* is.
7. A ______________ is defined as a unit of heat.
8. ______________ are nutrients which are needed for normal body growth, development, and maintenance.
9. ______________ refers to any chemical from the earth which has been found in foods.
10. A ______________ refers to any food or liquid which is regularly consumed.

25

Care and Treatment of Sports Injuries

Performance Objectives

Upon completion of this chapter, you will be able to:

1. Briefly explain how sports injuries can be prevented.
2. Discuss sports injuries according to how they are classified.
3. Identify common sports injuries of the upper body, back, and lower extremities.
4. Identify some of the more common medical emergencies encountered in sports medicine and briefly explain the role of the sports medicine assistant in providing basic first aid procedures for such emergencies.

Terms and Abbreviations

Bandage material that is applied as a dressing or is used to hold a dressing in place.
Bones the structural scaffolding of the body and which are joined to other bones through synovial joints.
Bursa fluid sac which prevents friction between two moving surfaces within the body.
Compression the process of pressing down to reduce volume, as in chest compression.
Dressing material which is applied directly to a wound.
First aid the immediate and temporary care provided to a victim of a sudden illness or accident.
Immobilize the process by which movement is made impossible.
Level of consciousness (LOC) one's ability to respond to his or her surroundings and stimuli.
Ligament structure which limits any abnormal movement of bones.
Muscles structures which are attached to bones through tendons, thus allowing for muscle pull to be concentrated through a small space.
Shock the depressed state of all vital body functions.
Sling a bandage which is triangular in shape, used to support the weight of the arm.
Splint device which can be used to protect and immobilize a body part; generally used to immobilize an extremity.
Swathe a bandage which can be used to immobilize the arm by binding it around the chest and the arm.
Synovial joint joint that is lubricated with synovial fluid and contained with a capsule to allow for movement.
Trauma an injury or wound.

Anyone who has attended a sports event has seen athletes injured during participation. In some cases, the injuries are less serious, and the athlete is allowed to return to the sport immediately. Other injuries may be more serious, even life-threatening, and require that the player be removed from the field for evaluation and treatment. It is for this reason that most competitive sports events and training facilities require physicians or sports emergency medical personnel, such as sports medicine assistants and trainers, to be present whenever people are involved in any form of sporting or athletic activity. If you are called upon to provide basic first aid to the injured athlete, such treatment is often the result of a serious injury or emergency situation.

Injury Prevention

In most cases, sports injuries can be prevented by adhering to sensible practices and using common sense. This often includes proper training and learning the right techniques involved in the sport or activity, as well as making sure the athlete wears the proper clothing and footwear. Possibly the most fundamental and important axiom the athlete needs to follow is that one needs to be fit to play sports rather than using sports as a means of getting fit.

Training and Technique

Each and every one of us, from the athlete who walks 10 miles without becoming short of breath to the weekend hiker who thinks nothing of doing 30 miles in one day, has a baseline fitness. An improvement in performance and fitness is only going to occur if the training load is modified, either by training harder, longer, or more often. However, it's important that you understand that whatever route the athlete chooses as his or her form of exercise or athletic competition, any increase of more than 10 percent of that activity in a given week is an open invitation to an overuse injury.

An easy way to prevent overuse injuries is for the athlete to learn and follow proper techniques early on in his or her career. Such a person is much less likely to become injured. There is, however, no substitute for experience, but this knowledge can only be acquired and learned slowly over a period of time and through practice.

Choosing the Right Attire

Although fashions follow particular sports, there is often a good reason for wearing special types of clothing. Sports played in the summer, for example, usually require any increase of the core body temperature to be minimized. This can be achieved with light, loose-fitting clothing which also allows circulation of air, reflection of the sun's rays, and absorption of sweat. However, specific areas of the body may need warmth maintenance, such as the hamstrings in sprinters, who often wear long cycling shorts. Dark colors retain heat and are more suitable for winter wear, though participants in long-distance stamina events need to anticipate extremes of temperature, and should therefore be prepared. If in doubt, it is always easier for the athlete to shed the clothing during competition than to put it on.

Protective Clothing

Out of necessity, many contact sports require the participants to protect themselves against injury. Some of the items used may appear to be little more than fashion accessories, and any protective clothing must be effective enough, yet the player or athlete should not be lulled into a false sense of security by ignoring dangerous situations. Such situations can often become worse if the clothing fails in its primary task. It is also important that the protective clothing worn by one athlete not injure another participant.

Much of the clothing worn by athletes is used to protect the person from injuries to vital organs and parts of the body which are more apt to be injured during a particular sport. These protective articles include helmets and eye protectors, padding, genital protectors, and socks and footwear appropriate for the activity.

Preventing Injury Through Warm-Up Activities

Although many people involved in sports warm up, it is often in a somewhat haphazard fashion. The first part of any warm-up should be stretching of all the relevant muscle groups. A stretch should consist of the person slowly moving a limb into a position which is just uncomfortable, but never painful. It should also be held for no longer than 30 seconds before slowly returning to the original unstretched stance. There should never be any rocking, a process which will trigger stretch reflexes within the muscle and thus could lead to a tear. Having stretched all the relevant muscle groups, the athlete should then commence gentle jogging and exercising to increase his or her metabolism and raise the heart rate. Finally, a few strides at submaximal speed should leave the person some 5 or 10 minutes to adjust clothing, visit the restroom, and mentally prepare for the activity.

Warm-Up Exercises for the Neck, Shoulders, and Upper Extremities

While there are many warm-up exercises that the athlete can practice to prevent an injury to the neck, shoulders, or upper extremities, some of the more common include neck stretches, above-the-head shoulder stretching, bent arm shoulder stretches, "windmill" and shoulder shrugs, triceps stretch, and arm circling.

Neck Warm-Up Exercises

Neck stretches (Figure 25-1). To perform the neck stretches, the participant should be directed to:

1. Stand up straight, lift the head, and look upwards.
2. Slowly bring the head forward until the chin is resting lightly on the chest.
3. Raise the head, turning it slowly to one side, and then hold that position for at least five seconds.
4. Roll the head around to the other side, keeping the chin down, and hold position for five seconds.
5. Repeat the exercise five times.

Shoulders and Arms Warm-Up Exercises

Above-the-head shoulder stretch (Figure 25-2 on p. 300). To perform the above-the-head shoulder stretches, the participant should be directed to:

1. Stand to the side, facing the patient.
2. Clasp the shoulder joint with one hand; use the other hand to grasp the wrist.
3. Gently raise the arm above the head and hold for at least five seconds.
4. Repeat the exercise five times.

Bent arm shoulder stretch (Figure 25-3 on p. 300). To perform the bent arm shoulder stretch, the participant should be directed to:

1. Bend his or her right arm back over the head and right shoulder.
2. Hold the elbow with the left hand and then gently pull it toward the left shoulder.
3. Repeat the exercise on the other side.

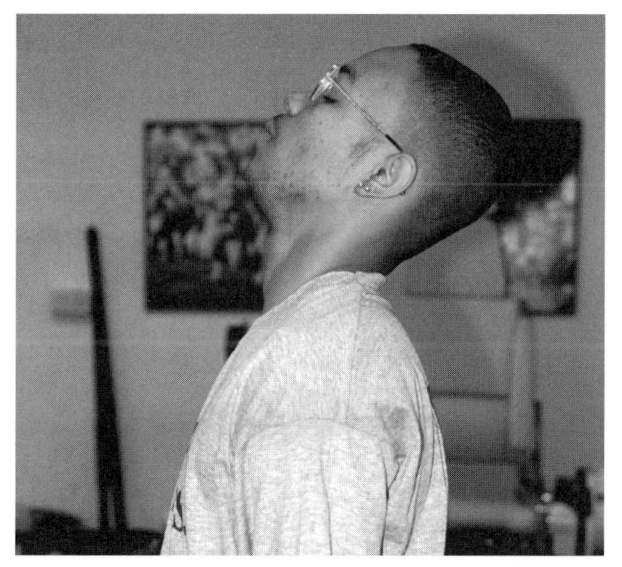

(1)

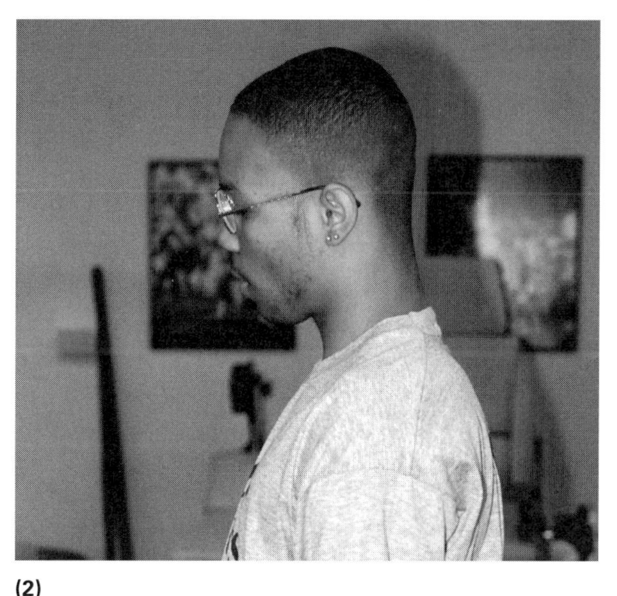

(2)

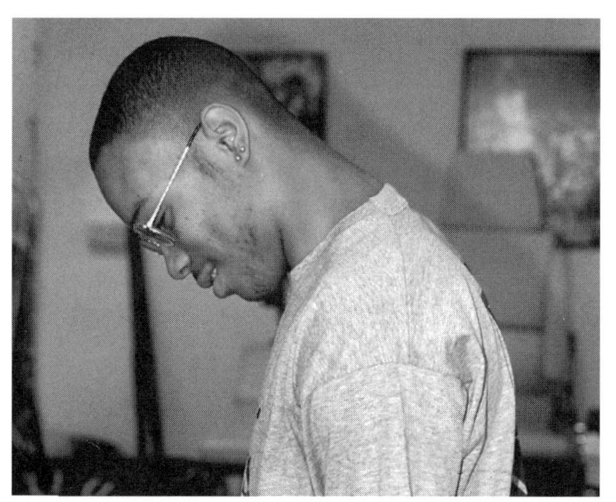

(3)

Figure 25-1
Neck stretches.

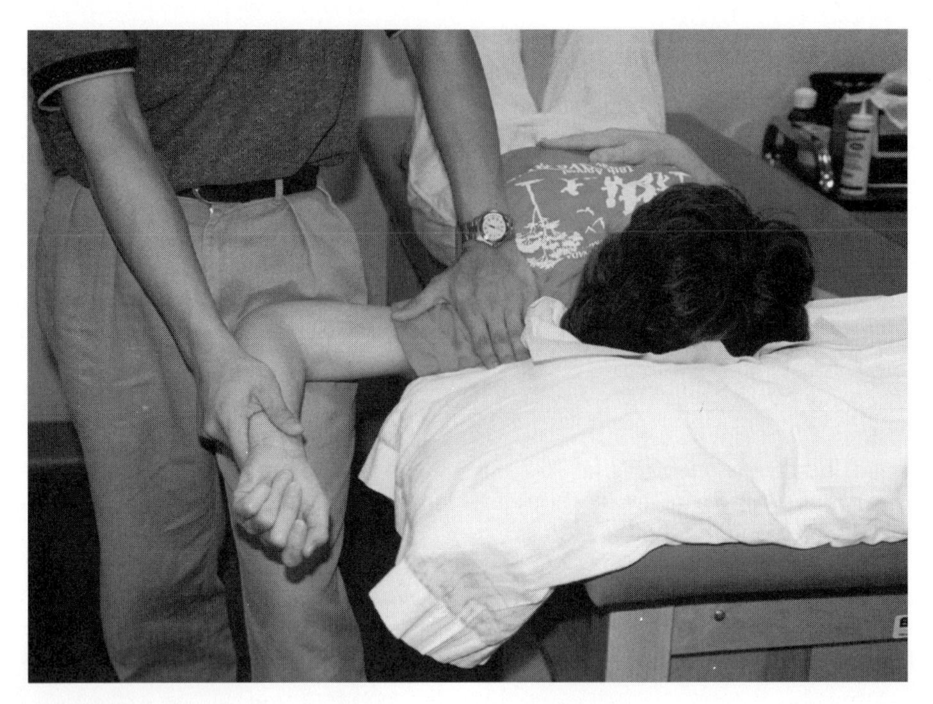

Figure 25-2
Above-the-head shoulder stretch.

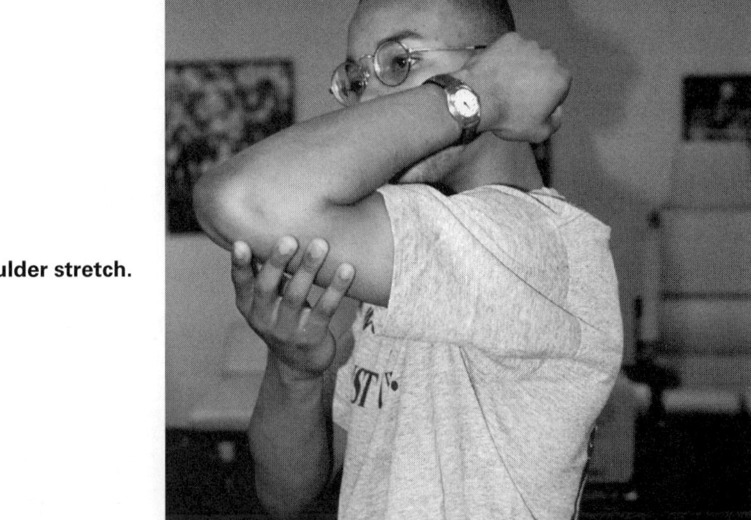

Figure 25-3
Bent arm shoulder stretch.

The windmill (Figure 25-4). To perform the windmill, the participant should be directed to:

1. Stand up straight with both arms hanging at his or her sides.
2. Swing the right arm forwards and up and around behind in a circle.
3. Repeat the exercise with the right arm five times.
4. Repeat the exercise with the left arm five times.
5. If the participant wishes, he or she may repeat the entire exercise again with both arms.

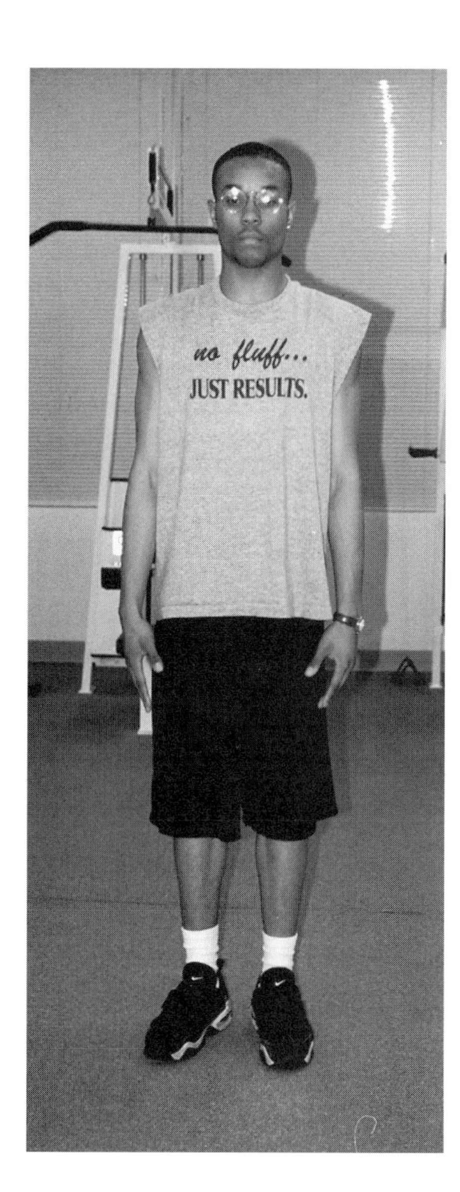

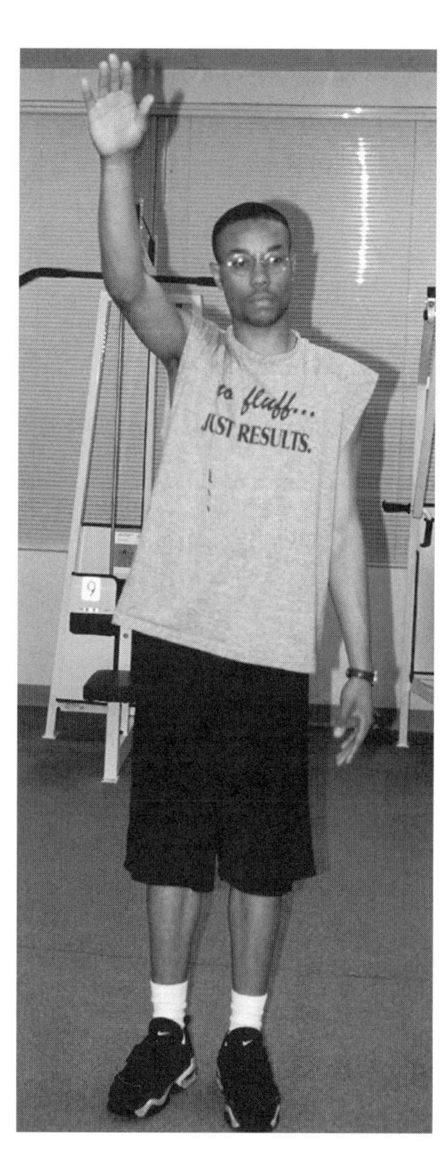

Figure 25-4
The windmill.

Shoulder shrugs (Figure 25-5). To perform the shoulder shrugs exercise, the participant should be directed to:

1. Stand up straight with his or her hands resting on the hips.
2. Shrug the shoulders, rotating them slowly backwards 10 times.
3. Then reverse and shrug them in a forwards rotation 10 times.

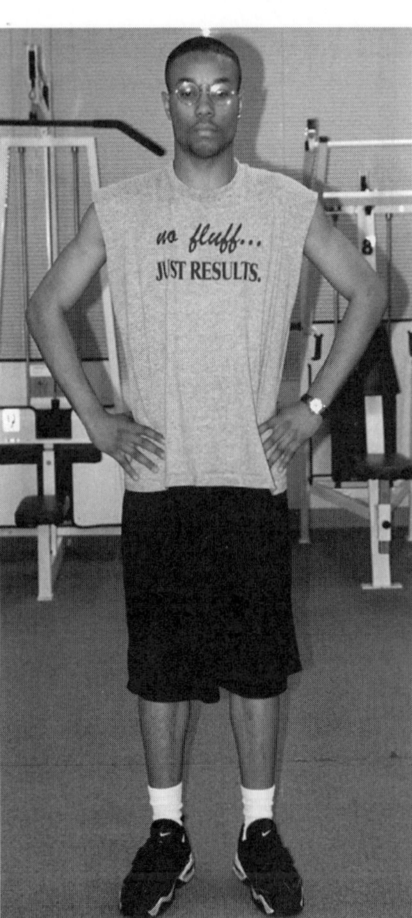

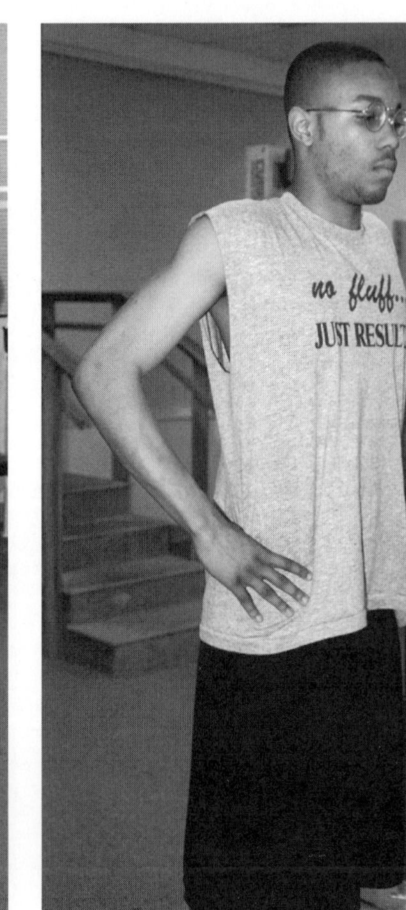

Figure 25-5
Shoulder shrugs.

Triceps stretch (Figure 25-6). To perform the triceps stretch exercise, the participant should be directed to:

1. Stand up straight and raise his or her right arm with the fingertips resting on the right shoulder.
2. With the left hand, push against the right elbow.
3. While pushing against the right elbow, try to lower the fingers down the back.
4. Hold for a count of eight and then repeat on the other side.

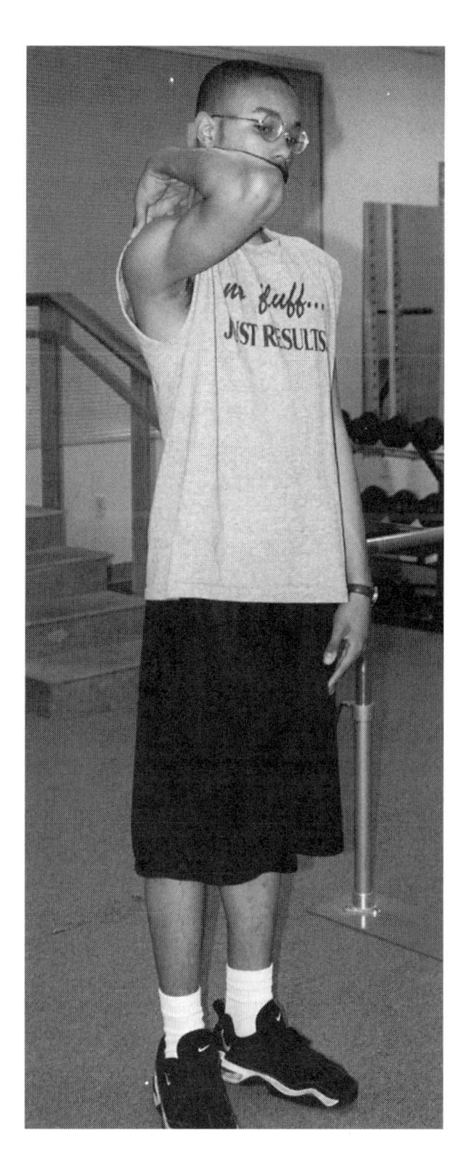

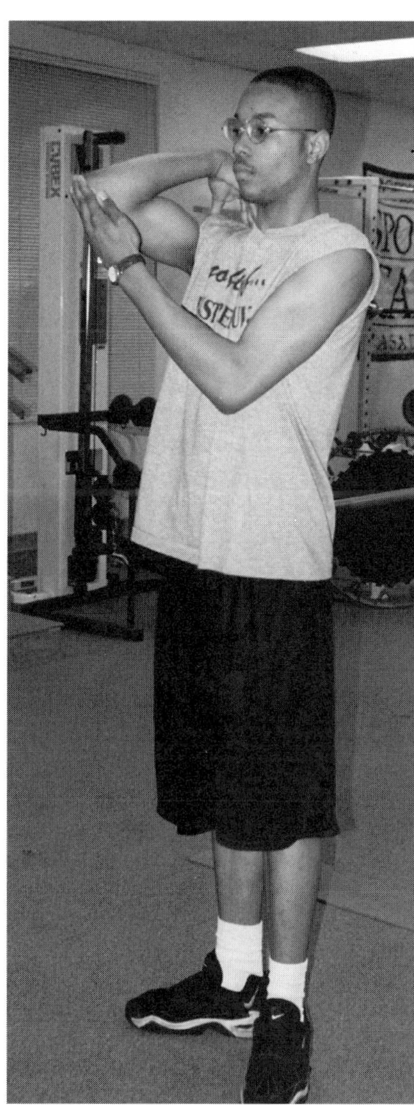

Figure 25-6
Triceps stretch.

Arm circling (Figure 25-7). To perform the arm circling exercise, the participant should be directed to:

1. Stand up straight with his or her feet shoulder width apart.
2. Stretch the arms out to the sides at shoulder level and then circle them forwards 10 times.
3. Repeat 10 times in a backwards motion.
4. Make the circles as large as possible.

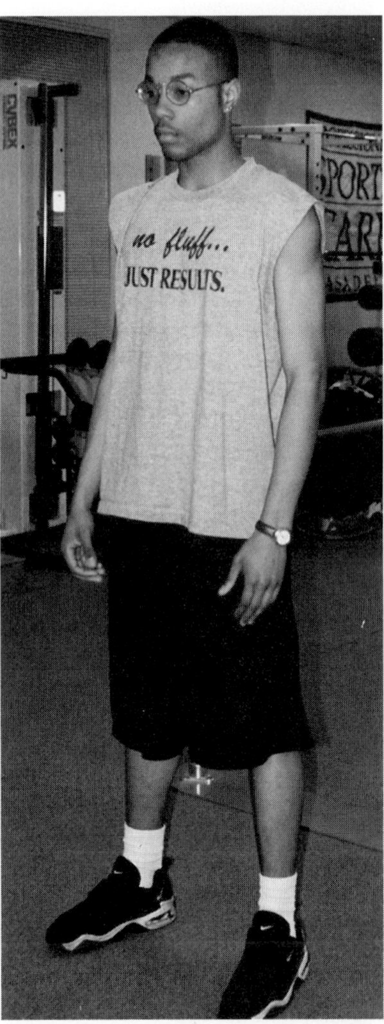

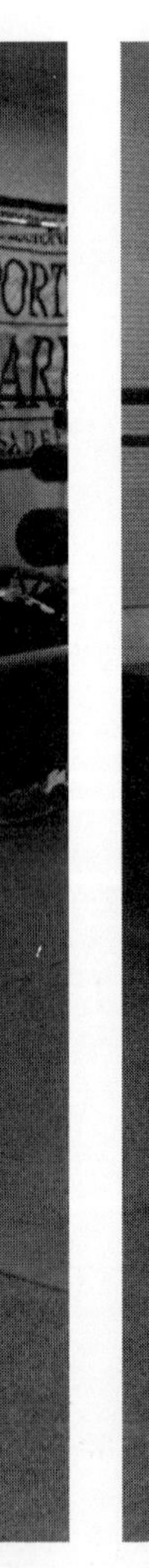
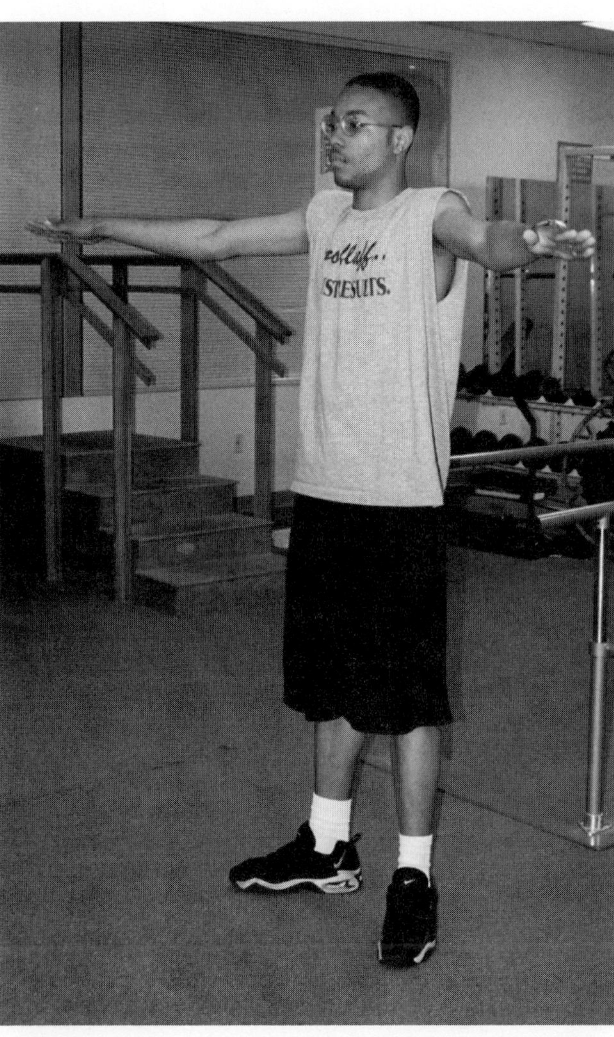

Figure 25-7
Arm circling.

Warm-Up Exercises for the Trunk and Chest, Hip and Groin, and the Lower Extremities

Like the neck, shoulder, and upper extremities, there are many different warm-up activities which can be used by the athlete to prepare him or her for various sports and athletic events. However, for our purposes, we will identify the most common of these, which include the following: torso stretch, trunk rotations, side bends, chest flings, upper and lower back stretches, lumbar stretch, side stretch, knee flex, ski stretch, hip rotations, groin stretch, adductors stretch, gluteal stretch, hamstring stretch and "hurdler's" hamstring stretch, quadriceps stretch, and calf stretch.

Trunk and Chest Warm-Up Exercises

Torso stretch (Figure 25-8). To perform the torso stretch, the participant should be directed to:

1. Stand with the feet shoulder width apart and slowly rotate the body from the waist only.
2. Stretch forwards and then around to the right side, backwards, and then around to the left.
3. Repeat the stretch in the opposite direction.

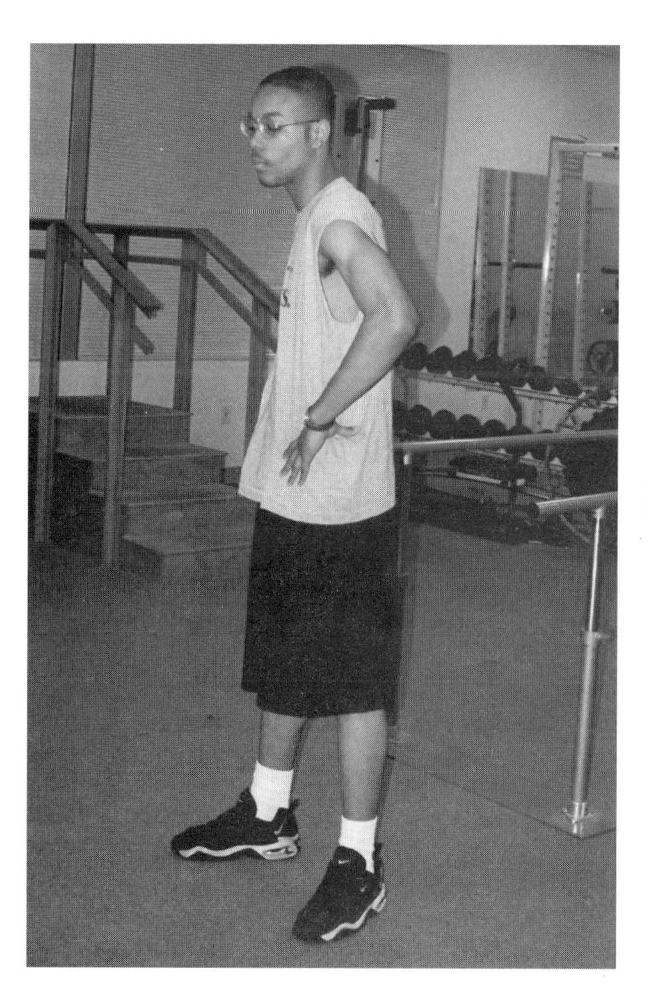

Figure 25-8
Torso stretch.

Trunk rotations (Figure 25-9). To perform the trunk rotations, the participant should be directed to:

1. Stand with the feet shoulder width apart and knees slightly bent.
2. With fingers interlocked behind the head, bend from the waist and touch the right knee with the right elbow.
3. Rotate the trunk to the left to touch the left knee and back to the starting position.

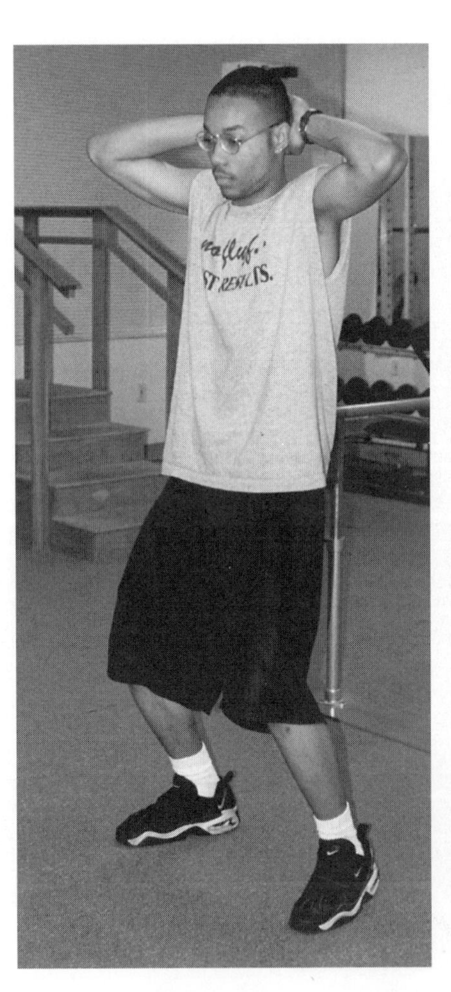
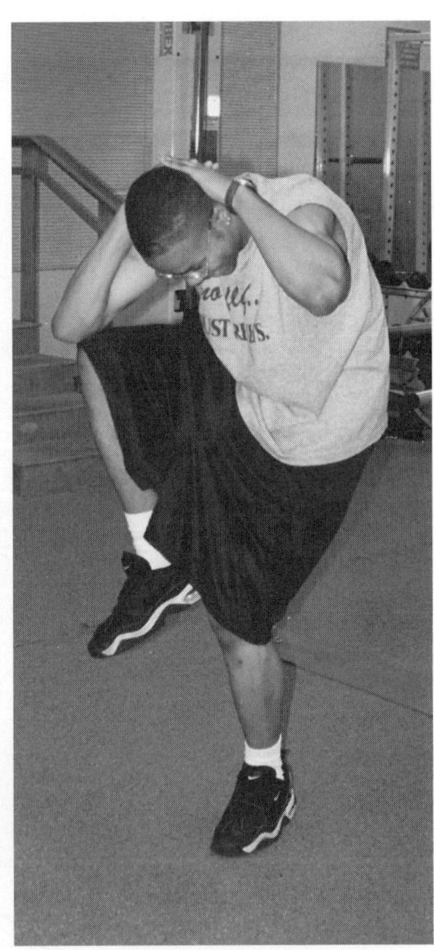

Figure 25-9
Trunk rotation.

Side bends (Figure 25-10). To perform the side bends, the participant should be directed to:

1. Stand up straight with the hands by the sides and the knees slightly bent.
2. Slowly raise one arm high above the head, easing the other arm down the leg.
3. Pull the arm over the head as far as it will go while pushing down on the thigh.
4. Return to the starting position and repeat on the other side.
5. Do three repetitions on each side.

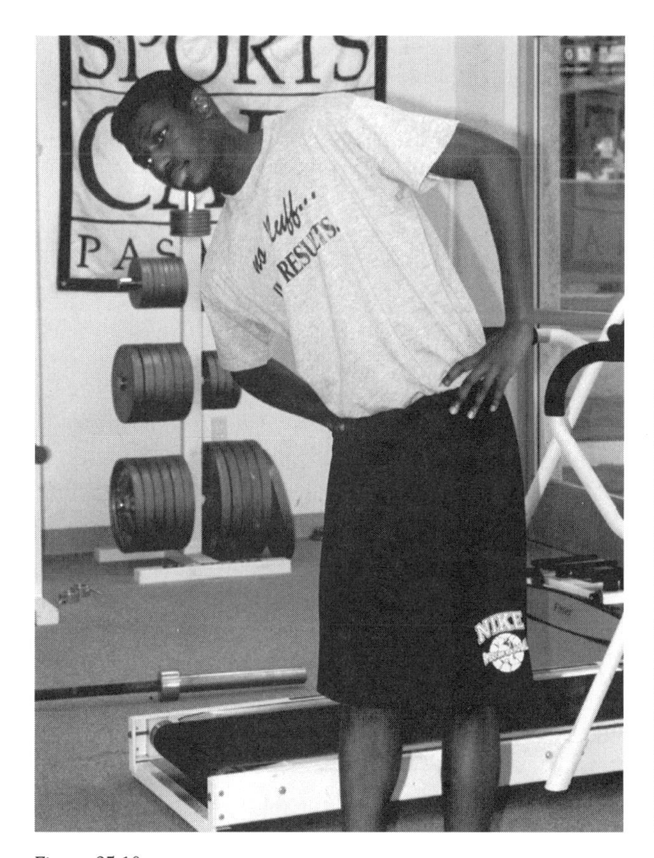

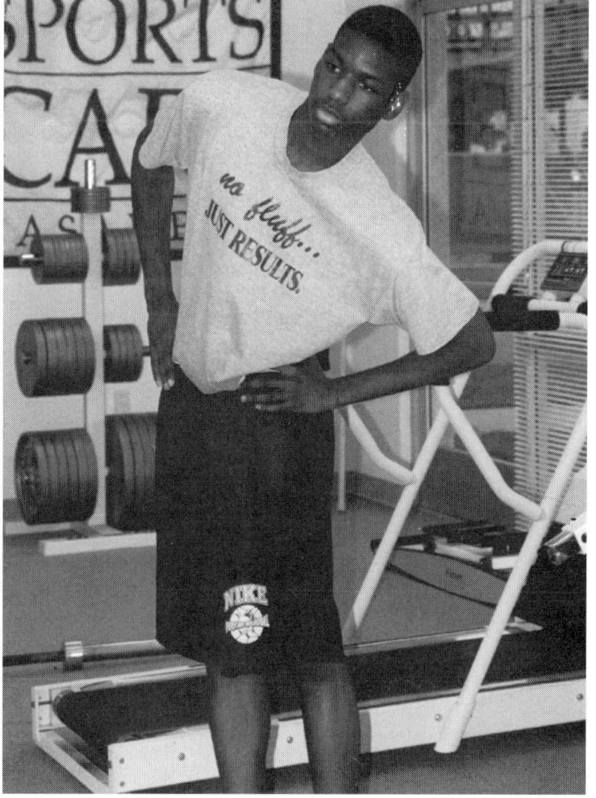

Figure 25-10
Side bends.

Chest flings (Figure 25-11). To perform the chest flings, the participant should be directed to:

1. Stand up straight with the feet shoulder width apart, elbows bent at shoulder height, and fingertips touching.
2. Fling arms out gently backwards at shoulder height and then return to the original position.
3. Repeat 10 times.

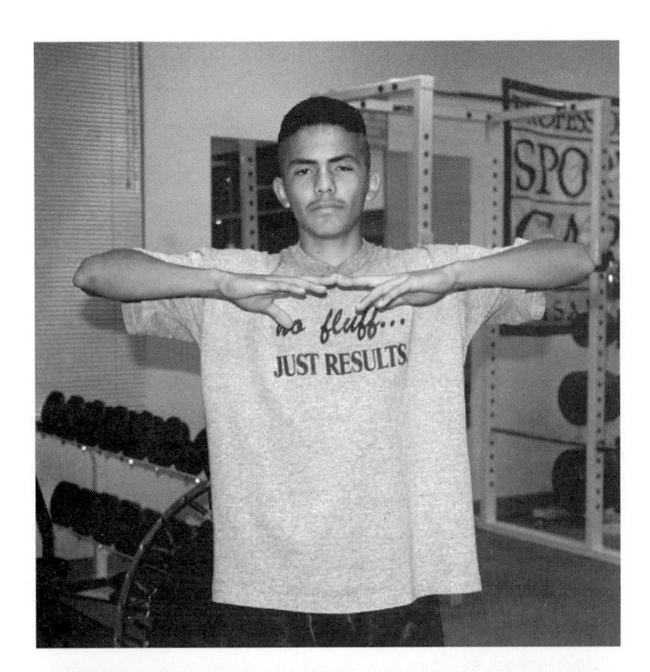

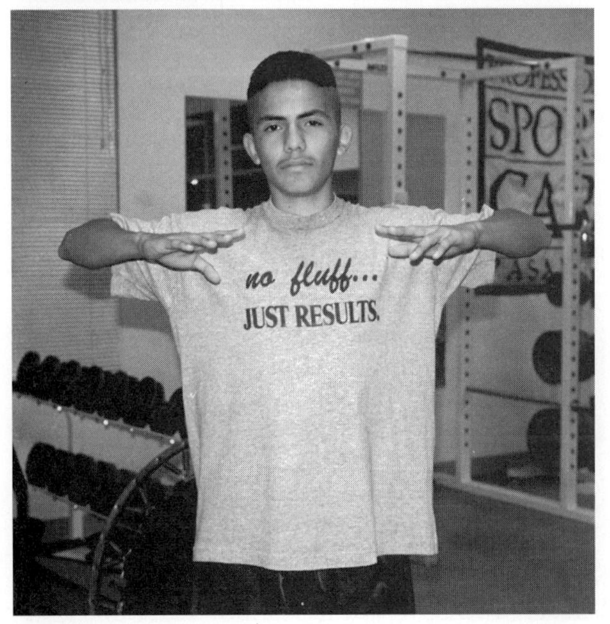

Figure 25-11
Variations of chest flings.

Upper back stretch (Figure 25-12). To perform the upper back stretch, the participant should be directed to:

1. Stand to the side with both arms extended out.
2. Place your right hand on the patient's right hip and your left hand on the patient's right shoulder.
3. Ask the patient to bend the right leg while extending the left leg.
4. Gently roll the patient to the left and hold for five seconds.
5. Repeat five times and change to opposite side.

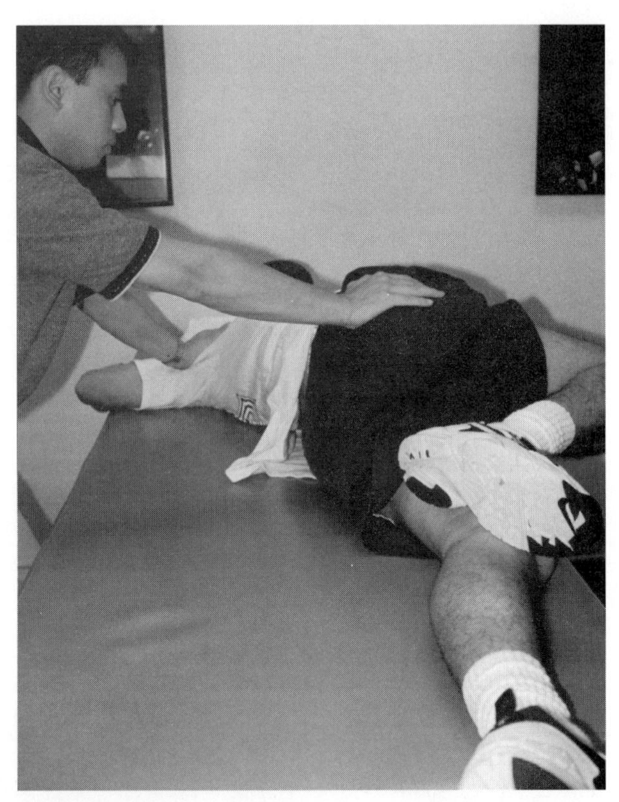

Figure 25-12
Upper back stretch.

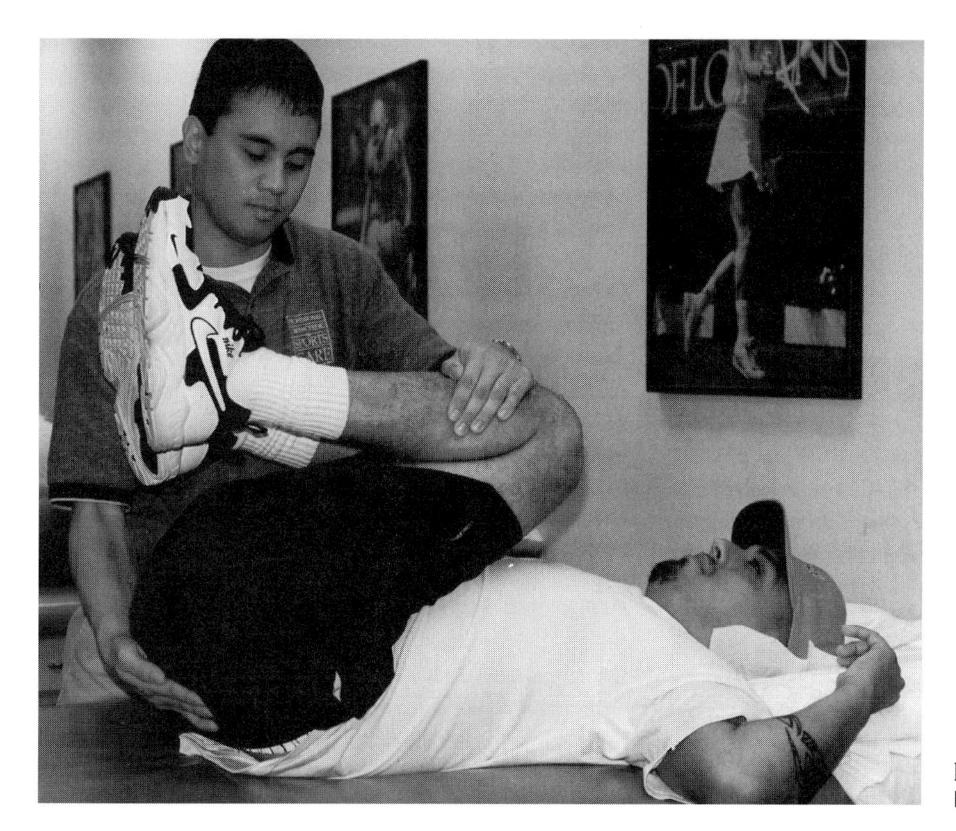

Figure 25-13
Lower back stretch.

Lower back stretch (Figure 25-13). To perform the lower back stretch, the participant should be directed to:

1. Have participant lie on his or her back with knees bent and feet pulled up.
2. Stand to the side with your right hand placed on the left buttock and your left hand placed just below the left knee.
3. Gently rock the left leg toward the right side of the body.
4. Hold for a count of five and release, letting the body go back to its original position.
5. Repeat the exercise five times for each side.

Lumbar stretch (Figure 25-14). To perform the lumbar stretch, the participant should be directed to:

1. Lie on the ground.
2. Raise the upper body by supporting the weight with the hands, palms flat on the ground.
3. Keeping the arms straight, gently stretch upwards, raising the head and chin.
4. Repeat three times.

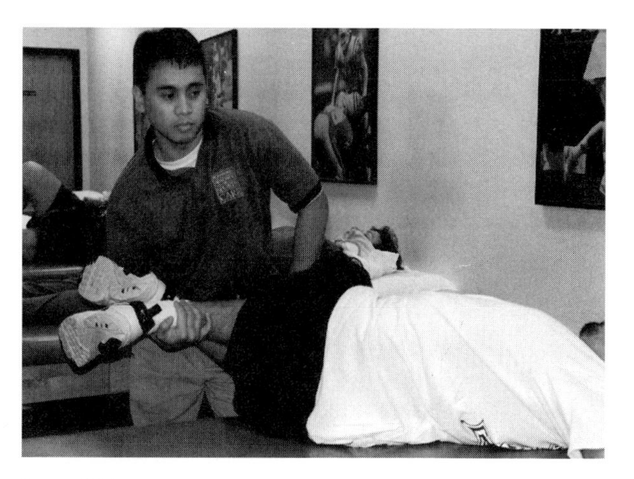

Figure 25-14
Lumbar stretch.

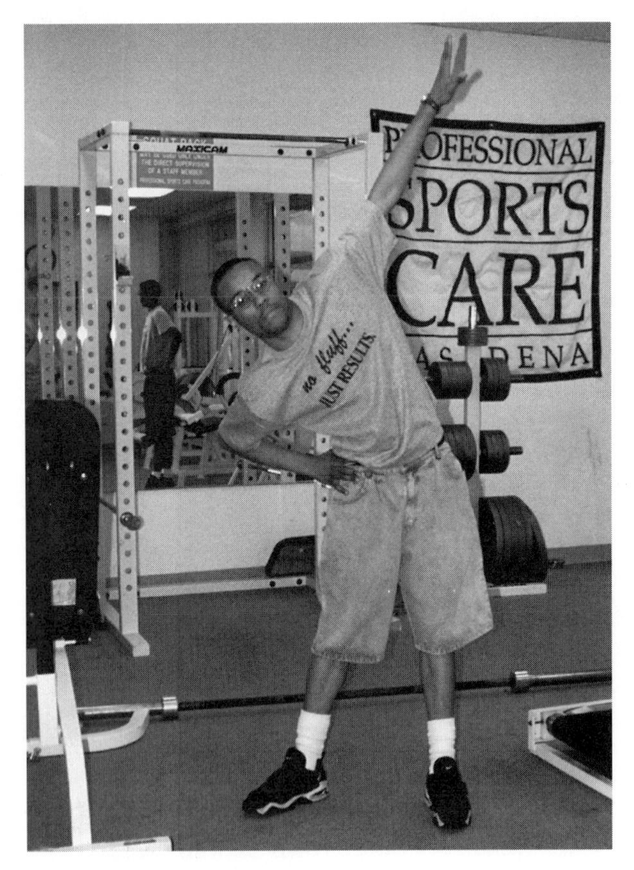

Figure 25-15
Side stretch.

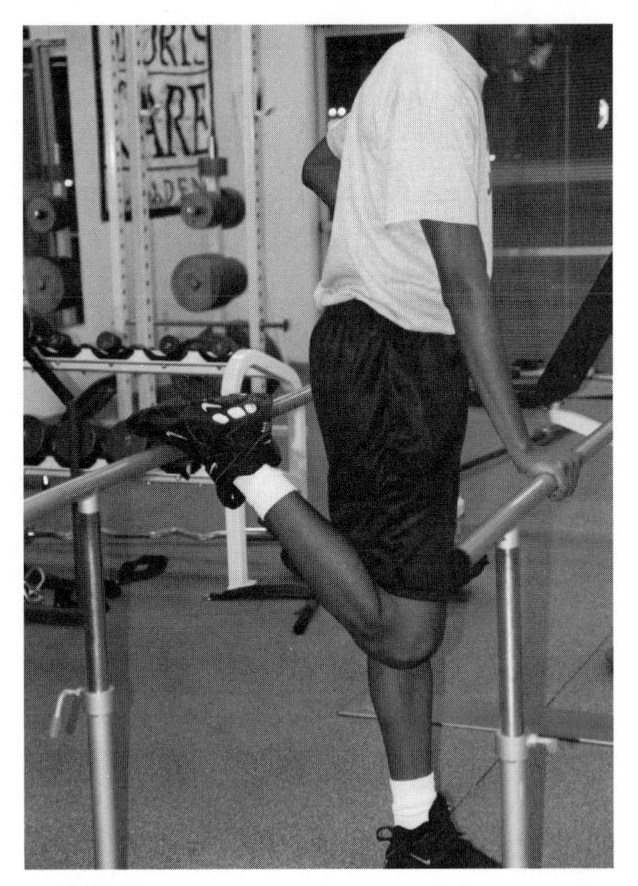
Figure 25-16
Knee flex.

Side stretch (Figure 25-15). To perform the side stretch, the participant should be directed to:

1. Stand beside a chair or table and raise the leg until it is at right angles to the supporting leg and resting on the chair.
2. Hold for the count of five and then lower and repeat with the other leg.

Hip, Groin, and Lower Extremities Warm-Up Exercises

Knee flex (Figure 25-16). To perform the knee flex, the participant should be directed to:

1. Raise one leg and place the foot on a chair, making sure that the supporting leg is straight.
2. Hold the stretch for a count of 10, then lower and repeat with the other leg.

Ski stretch (Figure 25-17). To perform the ski stretch, the participant should be directed to:

1. Stand with one foot forwards and one foot behind in a lunge position.
2. Slowly lower the body, bending the front leg until the weight is resting on the hands.
3. Keep the back leg straight with the heel off the floor.
4. Hold for a count of 10 and then change legs.

Hip rotations (Figure 25-18). To perform the hip rotations, the participant should be directed to:

1. Have participant lie on his or her back with left hip turned to the right.
2. Place your right hand on the left shoulder, and your left hand on the left hip.
3. Gently twist at the waist and rock the left hip forward.
4. Hold for a count of five seconds and repeat the sequence five times for each leg.

Groin stretch (Figure 25-19). To perform the groin stretch, the participant should be directed to:

1. Have participant stand up straight and place one leg about one stride in front of the other.
2. With right hand resting lightly on the right thigh, bend the back leg, transferring the weight onto it.
3. Keep the back leg bent, while stretching the front leg straight, and hold for a count of five.
4. Repeat five times with each leg.

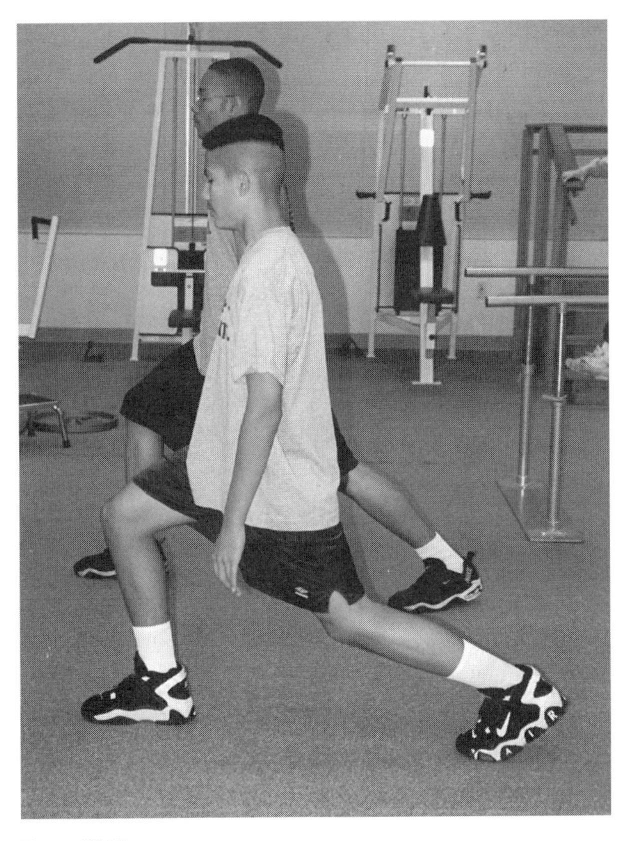

Figure 25-17
Ski stretch.

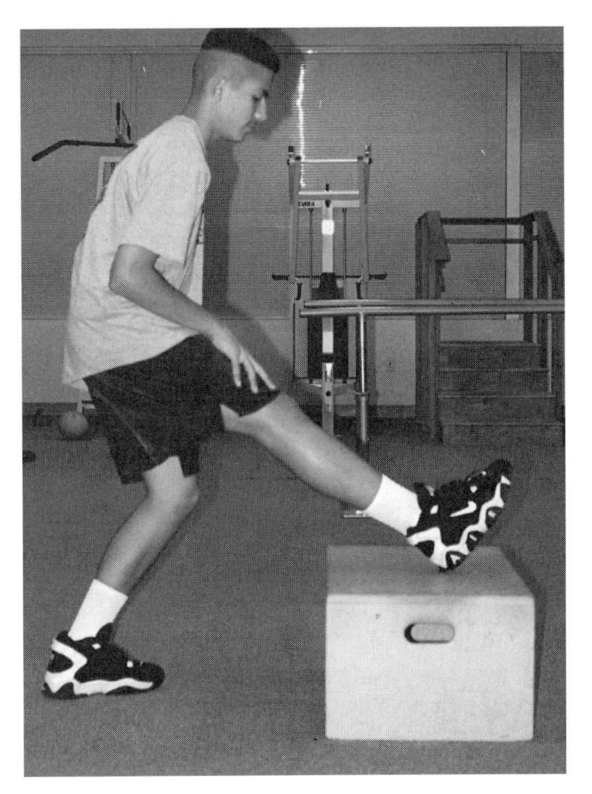

Figure 25-19
Groin stretch.

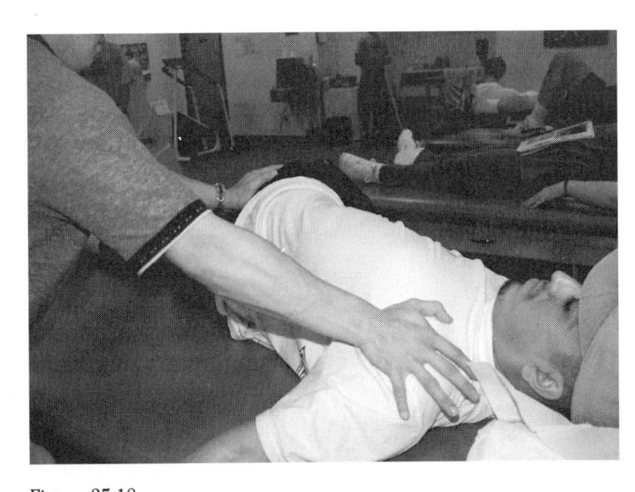

Figure 25-18
Hip rotations.

Adductors stretch (Figure 25-20 on p. 312). To perform the adductors stretch, the participant should be directed to:

1. Sit on the ground with the soles of the feet pressed together.
2. Clasp both feet with the hands.
3. Leaning forward from the hips, gently try to lower the knees toward the floor.

Gluteal stretch (Figure 25-21 on p. 312). To perform the gluteal stretch, the participant should be directed to:

1. Stand up straight, raise the right leg, and interlock the hands under the raised knee.
2. Hold for a count of 10.
3. Lower the leg and then repeat on the other side.
4. Do three repetitions on each side.

Hamstring stretch (Figure 25-22 on p. 312). To perform the hamstring stretch, the participant should be directed to:

1. Sit on the floor with the legs wide open.
2. Grab the right thigh with both hands.
3. Without bending the knees, slide the hands down the right leg as far as it feels comfortable.
4. Change legs, and repeat three times on each side.

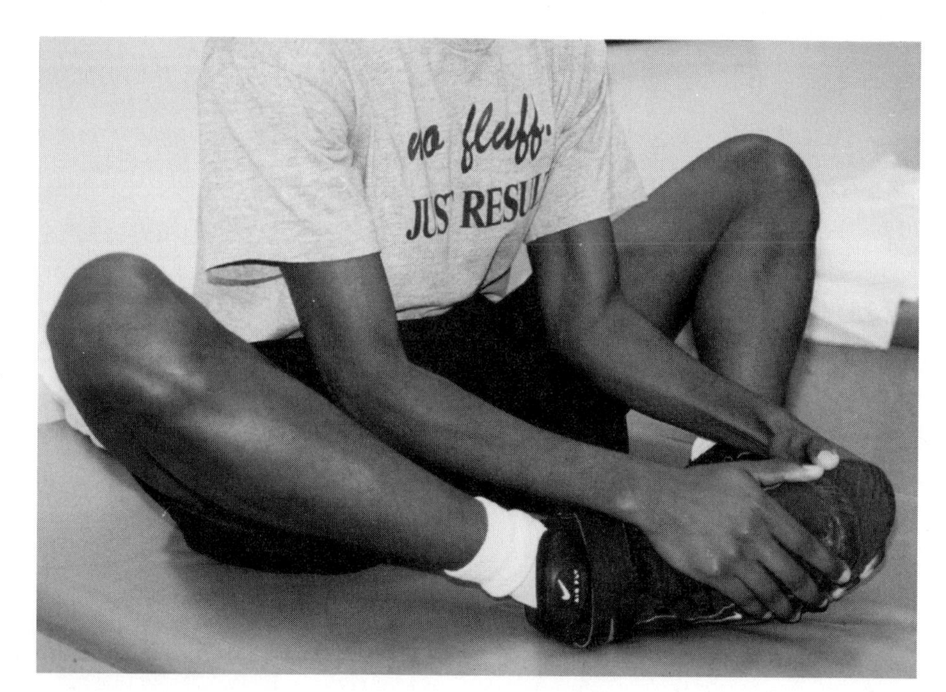

Figure 25-20
Adductors stretch.

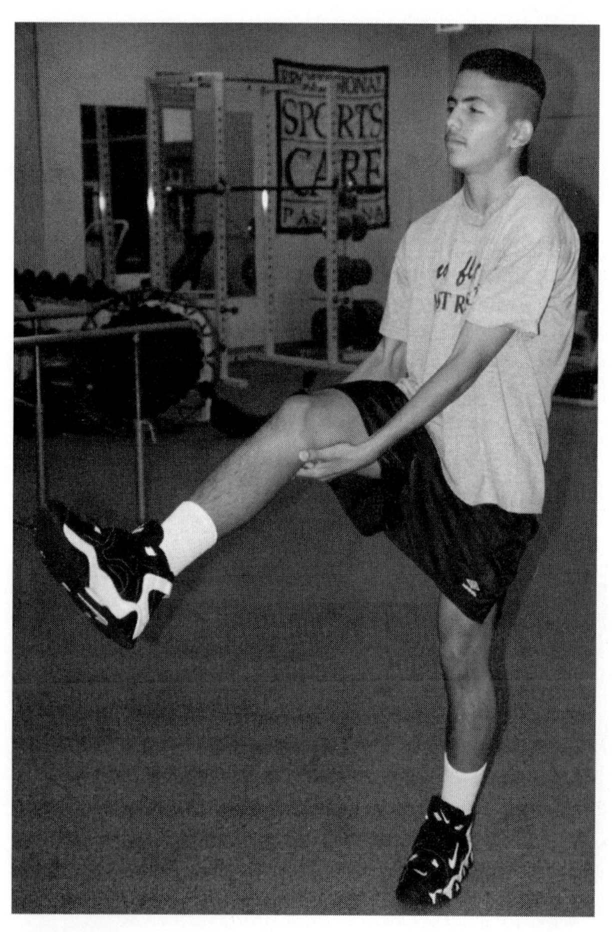

Figure 25-21
Gluteal stretch.

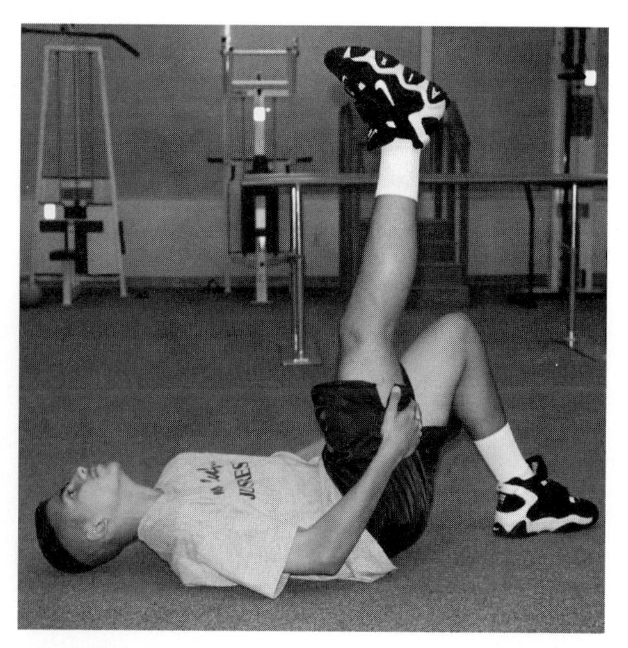

Figure 25-22
Hamstring stretch.

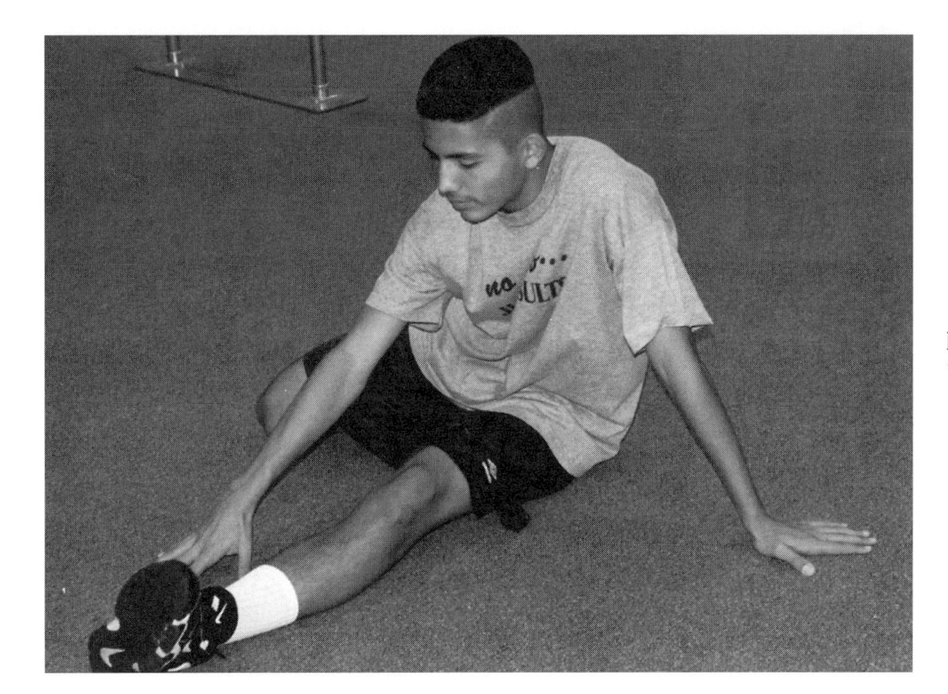

Figure 25-23
"Hurdler's" hamstring stretch.

"Hurdler's" hamstring stretch (Figure 25-23). To perform the "hurdler's" hamstring stretch, the participant should be directed to:

1. Sit down with one leg stretched out in front and the other leg bent at the knee at 90 degrees to the body.
2. Slowly lean forward from the hips, sliding the hands down the outstretched leg as far as feels comfortable.
3. Repeat on the other side.

Quadriceps stretch (Figure 25-24). To perform the quadriceps stretch, the participant should be directed to:

1. Stand up holding onto a bar or chair back with the feet shoulder width apart.
2. Raise the right knee and grasp the right ankle in the right hand.
3. Take the leg back until the heel is close to the buttock, being sure to keep the knees together.
4. Hold for a count of 10 and repeat with the other leg.

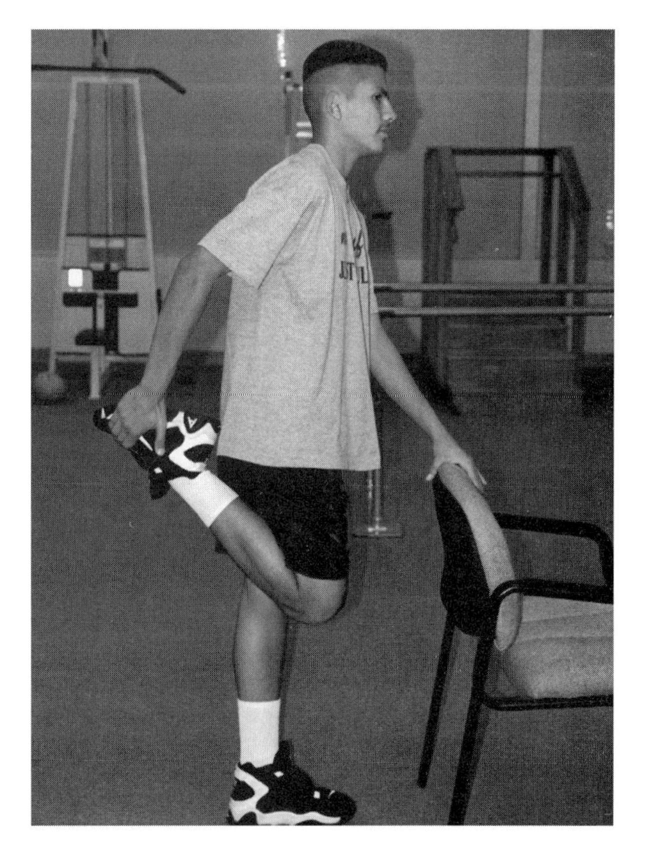

Figure 25-24
Quadriceps stretch.

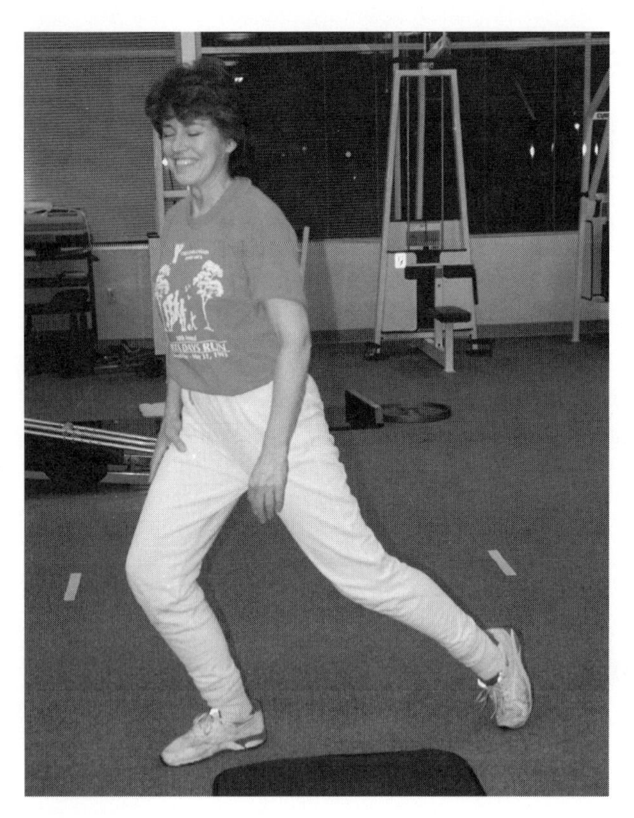

Figure 25-25
Calf stretch.

Calf stretch (Figure 25-25). To perform the calf stretch, the participant should be directed to:

1. Stand up straight facing a wall with the knee nearest the wall bent, and the other slightly behind.
2. Place the right hand on the right thigh and slowly lean forward, keeping the right foot flat on the ground, and the left heel slightly raised.
3. Gently "lunge" forward, hold for five seconds and return to upright position.
4. After completing five repetitions, change to left side and repeat.

Classification of Sports Injuries

Sports injuries, or *traumas*, may be classified in a variety of different ways. While many of the injuries occurring to the participant may be sport-dependent, the majority of them are simply classified according to those which happen as a direct result of an external force, those which are due to overuse, and those which happen as a result of an internal force.

Many of the injuries which occur both externally and internally show up as either a macro- or microscopic tear with some disruption of the surrounding blood vessels and other soft tissues. The greater the amount of bleeding, the longer the injury is likely to take to heal, so any steps you can take to minimize this are welcome. An easy way of remembering this is to use the mnemonic RICE: **R**est; **I**ce; **C**ompression; **E**levation.

Treatment of Injuries Using the RICE Method

Ice should be wrapped in a soft damp cloth and applied to the injury for no more than 15 minutes at a time, though in some cases this can be repeated every hour. *Compression* acts as a counterpressure to blood which may be leaking from the damaged vessels, but should not be so tight as to restrict arterial blood flow. Elevation helps to reduce the pressure within the leaking blood vessels when the injured limb is higher than the heart.

If you have any suspicion whatsoever that a bone may be broken or fractured, especially when that bone is used for weight bearing, then you should refer or transfer the patient to a hospital for an X-ray and further treatment. If an ambulance is not available, and the injury is one which has occurred to the lower extremity, both lower limbs should be splinted together using a piece of wood with soft padding between hard surfaces. The patient should then be lifted carefully in and out of the vehicle being used for the transfer.

Injuries resulting from bones being bruised are far more common than fractures. The pain felt by the patient is generally the result of separation of the periosteum which covers the bone and bleeding between the layers. This bruise, or hematoma, often cannot escape and takes a long time to be reabsorbed. Most people have an irregular bony surface along the front of their shins, often caused by childhood trauma to the periosteum.

Stress Fractures

A stress fracture is very much like a crack in a china cup. The bone is technically broken, but it is being held together by surface tension and surrounding tissues. This type of fracture generally results from repetitive movement and is often characterized by an increase in pain the more the movement is repeated. Diagnosis is not always simple and may require X-rays and bone scans. If an athlete ignores the symptom of increasing pain, he or she is liable to end up with a complete fracture. Treatment of stress fractures rarely necessitates the use of immobilization and casting the injured limb, however, avoiding the exercise that provokes the pain should be closely adhered to. Stress fractures in short bones generally take three to four weeks to heal, while those which occur in long bones often take as long as six to eight weeks.

Muscle Tears

Muscle tears, or ruptures, may be either complete or partial. A complete rupture of a muscle may cause profuse bleeding and look horrific, leaving two bumps and a gap between the torn ends. Amazingly, this rarely causes the athlete to suffer much disability, since other muscles take over the lost function. Surgical repair of a complete tear of a muscle is generally not required, although sensible retraining of other muscles is.

When a muscle undergoes a partial rupture, it generally involves part of the muscle bundle sheath. This causes the potential for blood to escape from the site of the injury, so although there may be much visible evidence of bruising, the effects are minimized and healing often occurs within a couple of weeks if the RICE method is followed.

When there is an intramuscular tear, the waste blood and tissue fluid cannot escape, sometimes causing the formation of an intramuscular hematoma. This is often accompanied by pain, tenderness, and limitation of movement at the affected side. If this occurs, treatment generally requires the use of the RICE method, however, after 48 hours, regulated and increased activity and movement is vital to prevent stiffening and scarring within the muscle. Physical therapy is also very helpful for partial tearing of muscles.

Injuries Involving Tendons

Tendons, which are composed of bundles of collagen fibers, are structures that join muscle to bone. Because they are surrounded by soft tissue, most of the injuries involving tendons are due either to overuse or as a result of sudden stretching.

One of the most common injuries involving a tendon is a complete or partial rupture of the Achilles tendon. In a complete rupture, the injury can happen so suddenly and noisily that the victim may imagine that he or she has been shot. The Achilles tendon and biceps are most commonly affected and naturally there is no function following the injury. Bleeding may also occur between the split ends, causing a clot to form. If this injury occurs to the nonathlete, treatment usually involves the application of a cast, which allows Achilles tendon immobilization, and thus, time to heal. For the sports participant, however, who is anxious to regain better function after the injury has healed, treatment often involves surgical repair of the tendon.

Upper Body Injuries

So far as the health care professional is concerned, all head and neck injuries are considered serious until they are proved otherwise. While some injuries occur more or less deliberately in contact sports, others are accidental and may range from a simple bleeding laceration to death from brain damage. Intermediate states may include concussion with amnesia or coma. Apart from a surface laceration, the safest and best course with any head injury is immediate referral to the emergency department of the nearest hospital. Here a full assessment can take place, with X-rays and scans ordered if the injury necessitates them. This is even more pressing if the patient appears vague or disoriented.

Neck and Spinal Injuries

Many sport activities, such as falling off a horse, taking part in a football scrimmage, or even diving into shallow water, can produce a spinal injury. The injured player may be conscious or unconscious. First aid to the unconscious head or neck injured player requires immediate action to maintain an airway, making sure the victim is able to breathe, and that circulation is being maintained, so that the heart and lungs can pump blood throughout the body. If these are satisfactory, the player should not be moved until a specialist is at hand to prevent possible worsening from the injury.

Eye Injuries

Eye injuries are not uncommon in athletic events. However, since it is usually inappropriate to attempt to treat them at the site where the injury occurred, the victim should be referred to a specialist in a hospital, so that the injury can be properly assessed and treatment undertaken.

Upper Extremity and Shoulder Injuries

Although muscles within the upper extremities can be injured and often require treatment with RICE and rehabilitation in the usual way, it is the joints that most often cause serious problems. This is because of their variable designs. A principal shoulder joint, for example, is inherently unstable, for although the bony components permit a wide range of movement, this mechanism also permits many injuries. The structure of the joint is maintained by four major muscles and several other minor ones, producing the rotator cuff. If an injury occurs to the rotator cuff, the tendons may be torn or even ruptured. Such an injury may be sudden or forceful, or may be a result of constant repetitive movements. In either case, many of the injuries of the rotator cuff are accompanied by swelling and inflammation.

If the upper arm is forced out of its socket by a fall or wrenching action, it commonly dislocates in a forward direction. When this occurs, pain is usually present and the patient is unable to move his or her arm outward.

If the injury involves the upper arm or shoulder, it is generally observed as being asymmetrical with the other shoulder. Since it is possible to sustain a fracture of the humerus at the same time, it is also important not to attempt to reduce the dislocation at the time of the injury, or to send the player back on the field after you have assessed the situation. Rather, the patient should be referred to a facility where the injury can be assessed and if necessary, X-rays taken.

Two injuries which are common to the shoulder include a painful arc and a frozen shoulder. A frozen arc injury is caused by an overuse of the shoulder muscles that can result in pain as the upper arm is moved outwards in the range above and below the horizontal. Because the person finds it extremely painful and avoids movement, there is further limit to the range. Early treatment using physical therapy, massage, and sometimes steroid injection will minimize the disability and prevent chronic pain affecting the person, which in some cases can last for many months, or even years.

The term "frozen shoulder" is used to describe a condition in which the shoulder is literally frozen after some form of overuse. Initially, it is best to let the shoulder rest, but an initial dose of anti-inflammatory drugs, ice, and mobilization under the guidance of a physical therapist should limit the time to full recovery. In many cases, however, this may take a long time in spite of all the therapies that medicine has to offer.

Another injury which can affect the shoulder and upper arm, particularly the biceps muscle, is called biceps tendinitis. This is an inflammatory and extremely painful condition which occurs when the long head of the biceps passes through a groove in the humerus, or upper arm bone. Testing for this injury can be performed by opposing elbow bending, which will cause pain. If physical therapy and anti-inflammatory drugs fail to settle the condition, an injection of cortisone may be successful.

Elbow Injuries

While there are several injuries which can affect the elbow, for the sports-minded person, the most common of these include tennis elbow, golfer's elbow, thrower's elbow, and tenosynovitis of the forearm.

Tennis elbow, or what is also referred to as lateral epicondylitis, is commonly caused by sports involving the overuse of the wrist. It is a very painful condition, with the greater degree of pain being felt on the outside of the elbow. Despite its name, it is more frequently seen in sports involving the whole arm rather than in those involved in tennis. The overuse produces pain at the origin of the muscles that extend the wrist at the lower outer end of the humerus. The overstretching causes pain, inflammation, and classic discomfort when engaging in typical activities like opening doors or pouring from a coffee pot. Because it is an inflammation, implementation of the RICE method is generally the first line of treatment for tennis elbow, however, it may not prevent it from returning.

The injury which is equivalent to tennis elbow, but differs in that it affects the muscles originating from the inner side of the elbow, is called golfer's elbow. It is less common than tennis elbow and is frequently associated with golfers using poor technique and hitting divots. The same practical treatments used in tennis elbow also apply, except that to stretch the damaged muscles, the wrist should be pulled backwards, though the best advice may well be to take a lesson from a professional golfer!

Thrower's elbow is a condition which particularly affects athletes who have to extend their elbow, such as javelin throwers, to its fullest extent. This imposes stress on the inner side of the elbow where a ligament can be partially torn away and if allowed to continue unchecked may very well finish the thrower's career because of his or her inability to fully extend the elbow. A combination of good coaching, reduced training, physical therapy, and a steroid injection often alleviates the condition, though in many cases treatment may be unavailing.

A common injury often affecting the upper arm is tenosynovitis. Although the condition presents in various ways, this painful injury of the muscles of the forearm usually causes a great deal of swelling and discomfort when moving the wrist or fingers. It is often caused by overuse of these muscles, especially where there are rapid, repeated wrist movements, such as in gymnastics. Examination produces pain if contraction of the muscles is resisted, and there is often a crackling sensation felt as these muscles are moved. Treatment by anti-inflammatory drugs, execution of the RICE method, and cessation of the provoking action may relieve the condition. Injection of steroids can also produce a rapid reduction of symptoms. Since poor technique may have a bearing on the cause of the original injury, good coaching can also help to prevent further recurrences of tenosynovitis.

Wrist and Hand Injuries

Injuries which are most common to the wrist and hand include de Quervain's disease, fractures of the wrist and hand, Mallet finger, and sprains to the individual digits.

De Quervain's disease is caused by an overuse of the tendons responsible for pulling the thumbs outwards. It produces pain and swelling over the outer side of the wrist, and is commonly found in people who continuously use rapid movements of the thumb. If application of the RICE method fails to relieve the problem, a steroid injection to the inflamed sheath of the tendon will usually effect a complete cure.

A fracture of the wrist is often caused as a result of a fall onto the hand or wrist. An X-ray is almost always required to confirm the diagnosis, and treatment generally involves immobilization of the injured part for a period of four to six weeks.

Fractures of the hands are generally quite obvious because of their noted deformity immediately following the injury. If the injury athlete can be dissuaded from playing the sport, treatment may simply be a case of taping two fingers together. A medical assessment should be sought at all times, however, to exclude permanent deformity.

A less common injury to the hands, that if left untreated can lead to a rupture of the tendon used to straighten the end of the finger, thus limiting the person's ability to fully extend it, is called Mallet finger. Treatment of Mallet's finger is quick and simple. The injured player must wear a splint for six weeks to enable the ruptured tendon to rejoin the bone before active mobilization is encouraged.

Probably the most common injury to the hands and wrists are sprains. These injuries often occur when a thumb and finger are wrenched backwards, thus causing a strain of the *synovial joint* capsule. The pain is so great following a sprain that many injured players believe they have sustained a fracture. Once an X-ray has been taken and a fracture has been excluded, treatment consists of active immobilization when it is safe to do so.

Common Sports Injuries Affecting the Back

Backache is universal and is no more common in the athlete than the nonathlete, though it may be associated with many sports. Where excessive and uncontrolled twisting, lifting, and contact are concerned, low back pain may be the result.

Posture and Back Pain

The person who frequently slouches often develops a backache whether or not he or she plays in a sport, and any athlete with nonspecific, yet recurrent backache should seek proper medical and physical therapy advice. By learning to stand and sit properly, possibly with a lumbar and thigh support, and education in the correct and incorrect methods of lifting, most backaches can be greatly alleviated, if not completely eliminated.

Common Injuries of the Back

As a sports medicine assistant, some of the more common injuries and conditions affecting the back you may encounter include a slipped disc, sciatica and sacroiliac pain, groin pain, hernia, hip disease, osteitis pubis, and trochanteric bursa.

A sudden backache is as likely the result of a ligament tear or muscle spasm as a slipped disc, in which the inner gelatinous core of the flattened disc between the vertebral bones seeps out to cause pressure on a nerve root emerging from the spinal canal. And, any time a sudden backache does occur, especially if it happens during a sporting event or a physical activity, it must be assumed to be the result of a slipped disc until proved otherwise. The action must be stopped and the sufferer made to lie down in a comfortable position.

If the backache or slipped disc is accompanied by severe pain radiating down the leg, this pain is referred to as sciatica. This is a key symptom of a severe back injury, and as such, requires immediate assessment by a physician. If a slipped disc is ruled out, treatment usually involves bedrest and anti-inflammatory drugs to relieve the pain. On the other hand, if the injury is diagnosed as a slipped disc, and a regimen of bedrest, immobilization, and physical therapy has not relieved the condition, additional medical intervention such as traction, manipulation, or even surgery may be necessary.

In some cases, the back pain suffered by an athlete may occur in the joints which attach the spine to the pelvis. These are called the sacroiliac joints, because they are located on each side of the sacral bone. Each is about four inches in length and is capable of a small degree of movement. It is not clear whether the pain occurs in the ligaments which hold it together, or within the joint itself, but pain may often be felt in the buttock or the top of the back of the thigh. Where disease (ankylosing spondylitis) is not involved, sacroiliac pain is often the result of poor hip and lower back flexibility, thus the pain from this area can frequently be eliminated if hip flexion and lumbar extension exercises are used.

A common complaint of many athletes, though its cause is generally not related to activity itself, is groin pain. The pain is often caused by an infection which may have originated in the lower extremity. The result is a swelling of the lymph nodes located in the groin area. Complete cessation of the pain is almost always achieved, as long as treatment with antibiotics begins early. However, if the pain persists, the underlying cause may be a weakness in the lower abdominal wall. This weakness is called a hernia. In obvious cases, the hernia allows part of the abdominal organs to balloon through a narrow opening, thus causing the groin swelling, a condition that is worsened by coughing. In severe cases, the only treatment is immediate surgical intervention to repair the hernia.

Many older athletes experience groin pain which radiates or is referred from the hip or pubis. If the pain seems to be coming from the hip, assessment and X-rays of the condition, followed by physical therapy and bedrest, is generally indicated. If, on the other hand, the condition is not relieved by conservative methods, it may be a result of the development of severe arthritis, in which case a hip replacement operation may be necessary.

A condition which causes severe pain in the center of the groin, and which is often due to an instability at the meeting of the two pubic bones, is called osteitis pubis. This is common in athletes who play football or where the pelvis has been tilted, such as when the legs are unequal in length, a not unusual circumstance. With prolonged rest, the condition may settle, but all too often, even with steroid injections and physical therapy, the player is left disabled.

If an athlete experiences extreme pain over the outside of the hip joint, it may be due to an inflammation of the *bursa* that overlies it. This condition, frequently caused by overuse or trauma, is called trochanteric bursa. In some cases, the pain may become especially severe, particularly if the athlete tries to force the straightened leg outwards, against resistance.

Common Sports Injuries Affecting the Lower Extremities

Many of the injuries affecting the athlete's lower extremities involve the quadricep muscles, the knee, the shin and calf area, and the ankle. The most common of these include quadricep and hamstring tears, arthritis, tearing of the meniscus, chondromalacia and ligament strains of the patellae, rupturing of the Achilles tendon, and ankle sprains.

Injuries of the Upper Leg and Knee

There are three main groups of muscles responsible for moving the upper leg: the quadriceps in front; the hamstrings posteriorly; and the abductors on the inside of the thigh, which produce inward movement. Injuries most frequently affecting these muscles include tears and strains, arthritis, and chondromalacia.

A common injury of one of the muscles of the upper leg, usually accompanied by sudden pain when sprinting or kicking a heavy ball and often produces local tenderness when touched, are quadriceps muscle tears. An easy way of testing for this is by having the patient straighten his or her opposing knee. When a gap can be felt between the two halves, indicating a complete tear, with swelling on each side, the RICE method should be used before muscle training and strengthening. If it is a partial tear, physical therapy can be used along with the RICE method. In either case, it is likely that the injury will take two to three weeks to repair itself.

Hamstring tears often affect athletes involved in sprinting and jogging. They usually occur while the person is in the act of sprinting, and the sufferer experiences pain between the lower buttock and the knee. Stretching the muscle when bending forward with the knee straight will produce discomfort. If the tear is central, the athlete will suffer considerable pain with little bruising to show for it; however, if the tear occurs in the periphery of the muscle group, there will be visible bleeding and discoloration with much less pain. Treatment must be the RICE method, followed by gentle and graduated stretching.

A part of the athlete's lower extremity often affected by injury is the knee. In its most basic anatomy, the knee is simply the junction of two sticks set one upon the other, held in place by collateral ligaments at the sides, which allow motion to and fro. Ligaments pass through the center of the joint, crossing each other to prevent the lower leg bone, the tibia, from moving backwards and forwards. The joint is surrounded on all sides by half moon pads called cartilages or menisci, which provide the knee with its ability to rotate and move. The most common knee injuries suffered by athletes include arthritis, tearing of the meniscus, and ligament strains.

Arthritis of the knee is an inflammatory condition often suffered by the older athlete, a result of many years of wearing out and tearing of the joint. It is generally accompanied by swelling and pain within the knee joint itself, and is often relieved by rest, warmth, anti-inflammatory medications, physical therapy, and cortisone injections. In some cases, however, while conservative treatment may help to alleviate the symptoms and inhibit the wearing out process, invariably the athlete may be faced with a knee replacement.

Any type of sudden or twisting movement of the knee can lead to the tearing of the cartilage surrounding the knee. Commonly referred to as a torn meniscus, it may cause locking of the knee or increased pain as the knee is slowly fully extended. Diagnosis is generally through a procedure called arthroscopy, which involves making a small cut into the side of the knee through which a fiber-optic scope is passed, enabling the surgeon to visualize the interior of this or any other joint. By further insertion of small instruments, dead or damaged tissue may be removed. Following the procedure, the knee must be fully mobilized before any sport is attempted.

Another common injury to the knee, generally caused by pressure exerted on the outside or the inside of it while attempting to force it laterally, and which is accompanied by pain and swelling at the site of the injury, is a strained ligament. The pressure stresses either the medial or lateral collateral ligaments, which allow the knee's hinge movement forwards and backwards. Since the ligaments are vital for the knee's stability, they must be allowed to heal properly. Therefore, implementing the RICE method to heal the ligament and muscles is extremely important. Straight leg training exercises may also be used to assist in the healing process and stabilize the knee. Once the training exercises have been started, the strength of the knee should be regularly tested by a physician or physical therapist to ascertain full and complete rehabilitation from the injury.

A condition which results in the kneecap failing to move smoothly in the groove at the bottom of the upper leg bone, where it acts as a pulley allowing the knee to be straightened, is chondromalacia patellae. Since this injury also involves the mechanisms of the quadriceps, treatment generally includes straight leg exercises and physical therapy. In severe cases, where the injury is so painful that it inhibits the athlete's ability to walk, the patient may elect surgery, however, the results of the operation are not particularly encouraging. Therefore, concentration on straight knee exercises will usually cure the problem if they are done on a regular basis.

Injuries of the Lower Leg

Injuries involving the lower leg generally affect the calf, shin, and ankle. The most common of these include calf strains, ruptured Achilles tendon, and sprained ankle.

A calf strain is often caused by a sudden awkward and uncontrolled movement of the ankle causing the heel to drop. It is frequently accompanied by sudden pain, especially noticeable when the athlete attempts to stand on his or her toes or to stretch forward with the heels to the ground. Treatment should be started, using the RICE method, for at least 48 hours before gentle stretching commences. Over the course of three or four weeks, this must be increased until calf movements are painless and as full as in the other ankle, and before strengthening begins.

The Achilles tendon is a structure which joins the calf muscle to the heel bone. Because of its very poor blood supply, it may be easily injured in any number of ways. The most common of these is a rupture. Generally, when a rupture of the Achilles tendon occurs, the athlete hears a very noticeable "snap." The person is unable to stand on his or her tiptoes, and there is immediate swelling and discomfort, a result of the palpable gap between the split ends of the tendon. Treatment is required if the athlete is to walk, let alone compete again, and surgery is often the method of choice, though some surgeons prefer to put the ankle in a cast and allow it to heal while it is immobilized. Full Achilles mobilization must be completed before any attempt at resuming sports or athletic competition can be contemplated.

One of the most common, and probably the most poorly treated of all injuries to the lower extremities is a sprained ankle. While it can occur throughout one's life, it seems to be more common in athletes who slip or play on an uneven surface. The majority of injuries involve inversion, so that the three ligaments joining the fibula to the talus, the bone enclosed by the mortice, become wrenched and one or more may totally or partially rupture. This causes considerable pain, especially when the foot is moved inwards, and there may be visible bruising to the outside of the foot. It may be impossible to differentiate this injury from a fracture unless an X-ray is performed.

At first, the treatment for a sprained ankle involves the implementation of the RICE method, avoidance of weight bearing in severe cases, and the use of crutches before gentle mobilization is attempted after 48 hours. The more severe cases may require wrapping of the ankle with an elastic bandage, however, the benefits of this must be weighed against the consequent disuse of the ankle muscles, which are required to provide stability and strength during the recovery process. Initially the patient should aim to increase the range of movement, always comparing the injured ankle with the uninjured. Once mobility has been obtained, the athlete should walk about in bare feet alternately on heels and toes, then the insides and outsides of the feet. Strength can be regained by standing on a lower stair and performing calf-strengthening and step-climbing exercises.

Emergencies and Basic First Aid

If you have ever attended a sports event, chances are you have seen an athlete injured during participation. Some injuries are less serious, and the athlete can return to the sport immediately, while others appear more serious, even life-threatening, causing the player to be removed from the field for evaluation and treatment. It is for this reason that physicians, emergency personnel, and sports medicine assistants are usually in attendance at professional sporting events and high school meets and college competitions.

While at times you may be required to perform life-saving measures such as CPR on an injured athlete, in this section we will concentrate on the assessment measures and basic hands-on skills required for administering basic first aid to those less serious sport injuries which you are more apt to encounter during your day-to-day activities as a sports medicine assistant.

Some types of injuries seem to prevail in sports. These include those we have already discussed, such as sprains, strains, muscle tears, and fractures. During the summer months, heatstroke and heat exhaustion must also be taken into consideration; drowning and lacerations from propellers and tow ropes are also associated with water sports. Heart attacks can occur to older athletes at any time on the jogging track or at a health club. Unexpected medical emergencies can occur in any one of many sport locations—tennis courts, golf courses, and ski slopes. Therefore, as a member of the sports medicine team, it's important that you understand basic first aid as it relates to athletics.

First aid is the immediate and temporary care provided to a victim of a sudden illness or accident, and should never be considered a substitute for standard medical diagnosis and care. It is important that you can identify an emergency situation that may require first aid and know the indicated procedures that may be necessary for that situation.

Performing a Patient Assessment

One of the first things you have to do in an emergency is determine the needs of the injured. To complete this process, you should:

- Check the scene to be sure it is safe to approach the victim; this also means protecting yourself—you will not be able to aid the victim if you become injured.
- Attempt to rouse the victim by talking or touching; if there is no response, check the victim's airway to make sure he or she is breathing.
- Check the circulation for pulse or heart beat; if the heart has stopped, you must begin cardiopulmonary resuscitation (CPR) and call out for help.
- Check the victim for severe bleeding, and control the bleeding if necessary.

All of these things should be done immediately to evaluate the seriousness of the emergency. Then, if it is established that the victim is breathing, that the heart is beating, and that there is no immediate danger of death from loss of blood, other actions must be taken. This involves calling for help and, when a helper appears, dispatching that person to notify the proper authority. The helper must be able to convey the proper information regarding the location of the accident, what has happened, how many people may be involved, what type of help is needed, and what aid has already been provided.

When an emergency situation is encountered, in addition to checking the victim for breathing, circulation, and bleeding, you must also check for *level of consciousness,* or *LOC.* This is the ability of a person to respond to his or her surroundings and stimuli. There are five levels of consciousness.

1. *Alert:* awareness of one's surroundings and responds appropriately if asked name, date, or location.
2. *Restless:* showing hyperresponsiveness to one's surroundings and stimuli.
3. *Confused:* being disoriented to one's surroundings, and oftentimes having difficulty remembering.
4. *Stuporous:* responds poorly to one's surroundings but is able to respond to stimuli such as pain.
5. *Comatose:* showing no response to stimuli, including pain; unconscious.

A person's level of consciousness is determined by the victim's responses or lack of responses. Most accident victims requiring CPR are comatose when they are found, while the majority of victims of exercise or sports injuries are alert and able to explain how the injury occurred.

Surveying the Victim's Injuries

Assessing the victim for injuries involves a primary survey, followed by a secondary systematic survey of the entire body, beginning at the head and continuing toward the feet. The primary survey commences by you looking for the cause and results of a trauma. Then you may proceed with the secondary survey by:

- checking the head, neck, and face for bruises or wounds, noting the temperature of the victim's forehead with your hand.
- looking for drainage or blood from the nose or ears.
- looking for fractures, bruises, or wounds on the shoulders, collarbone, arms, and hands.
- checking the victim's ribs and back by gently touching them with your hands.
- avoiding any movement of the victim or touching of an injury.
- noting any distention or wounds in the abdominal area, and gently pressing the sides and top of the pelvis to check for tenderness.
- examining the victim's legs and feet for any wounds, bruises, and edema.

Administering Basic First Aid for Wounds

Some of the more frequent emergencies encountered during a sporting event include wounds, bone and joint injuries, and eye injuries.

If an athlete has suffered a wound injury, the first thing you must determine is what type of wound has been sustained.

There are four basic types of wounds: abrasions, lacerations, incisional, and puncture. The two most common wounds are abrasions and lacerations. An abrasion occurs when the skin is scraped against a hard surface, such as pavement or artificial turf in a football stadium. This usually tears tissue away from the body. A laceration is a wound in which the skin is torn, leaving a jagged edge. An incisional wound is the result of a cut, generally leaving smooth edges. And a puncture wound is a result of the skin being pierced, producing a hole or opening at the wound site.

No matter what type of wound has been sustained, the first step in performing basic first aid is to make sure you control any bleeding. This can be accomplished by placing direct pressure over the wound until the bleeding stops. As long as there is no evidence of a fracture, continue to apply pressure while you elevate the injured limb. A pressure bandage may be used. Once the bleeding has ceased, apply a wrapping or *bandage* firmly around the affected area to hold the pressure dressing in place and maintain compression.

If bleeding does continue, apply pressure where the artery passes over bone, that is, over the pressure point (Figure 25-26). For a major trauma, such as uncontrolled bleeding or accidental amputation of a limb, you may have to apply a tourniquet to control the bleeding. A tourniquet is a wide strip of material placed just above the bleeding wound. The band should be tightened enough to stop or slow down the surface bleeding without stopping the flow of blood in the deep circulation. You must understand that it is extremely dangerous to apply a tourniquet to a wound, therefore, this measure should only be used as a last resort if all else fails. Application of a tourniquet completely stops the flow of blood to an extremity. Tissue deprived of the blood supply quickly dies. Thus, there is a real danger of losing a limb if a tourniquet is used. Also, once a tourniquet has been applied, you must never remove or cover it. Instead, put a notation, such as the letter T or TK, on the victim's forehead indicating the time in which the tourniquet was applied. The tourniquet will be removed when the victim is seen for treatment in the emergency room or health care facility.

In addition to the application of a tourniquet, some wounds may require that the affected limb be *splinted* to immobilize it, thus preventing the possibility of further injury. A well-stocked sports medicine facility will contain several types of splints for emergency situations. The application of an air splint is appropriate to stop bleeding when no fracture is present. Once the splint has been applied, the victim should be taken to a medical facility as soon as possible.

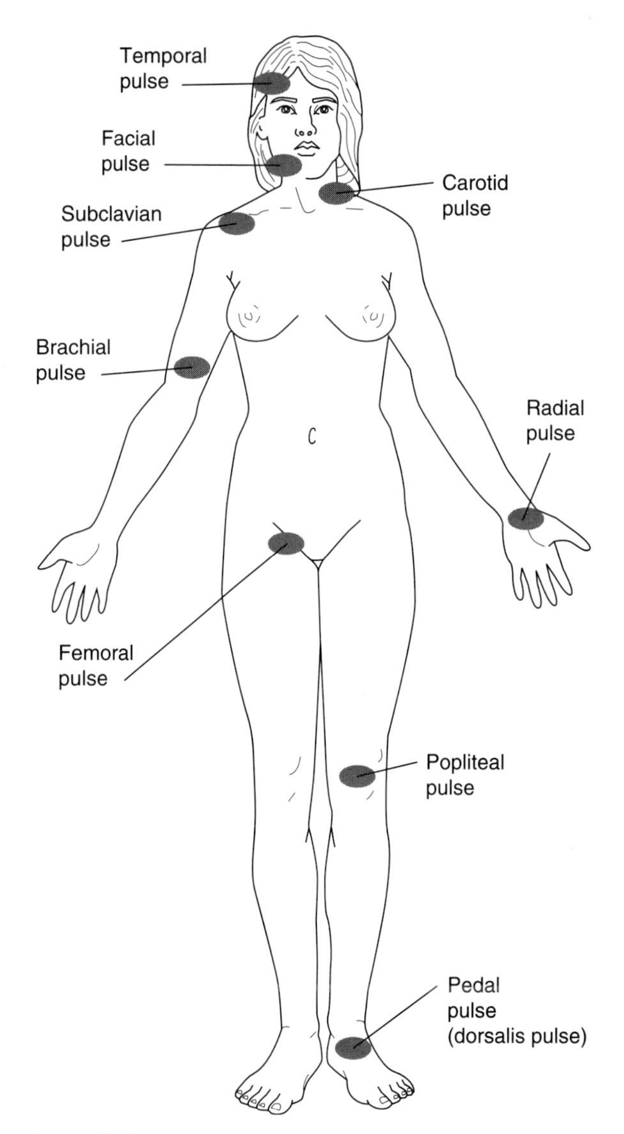

Figure 25-26
Pressure point sites.

Administering Basic First Aid for Bone and Joint Injuries

As we have already stated, another type of emergency frequently seen in sports and athletic events, is bone and joint injuries.

One of the most common types of bone injuries is a fracture. A fracture means that the bone has been broken. There are five types of fractures. In a simple fracture, the bone is broken, but there is no external wound. An open fracture means that the bone is broken, with an open wound. The wound may result from external causes or from tissue damage from the broken ends of the bone. In young children, a bone often breaks on one side only, and some of the bone fibers are not injured. This is because the bones of young children are more pliable than adults, and have not yet fully developed. This type of break is called a greenstick fracture. Another type of fracture is a comminuted fracture. This occurs when the bone has splintered into pieces, often due to the force of a blow or porosity of the bone. A spiral fracture occurs when a limb has been twisted, thus causing the bone to break diagonally downward. This type of break often occurs to the legs of a skier, as a result of a twisting fall.

One of the most common injuries to an athlete's joint is a dislocation, when a bone end has been displaced from a joint. An example of this is the lateral displacement of a player's patella, or knee, as a result of being tackled during a football scrimmage. If tissue is torn at the joint, it is called a sprain.

The basic first aid treatment for any bone and joint injury is to prevent motion of the injured part and of the adjacent joints. This is usually done by

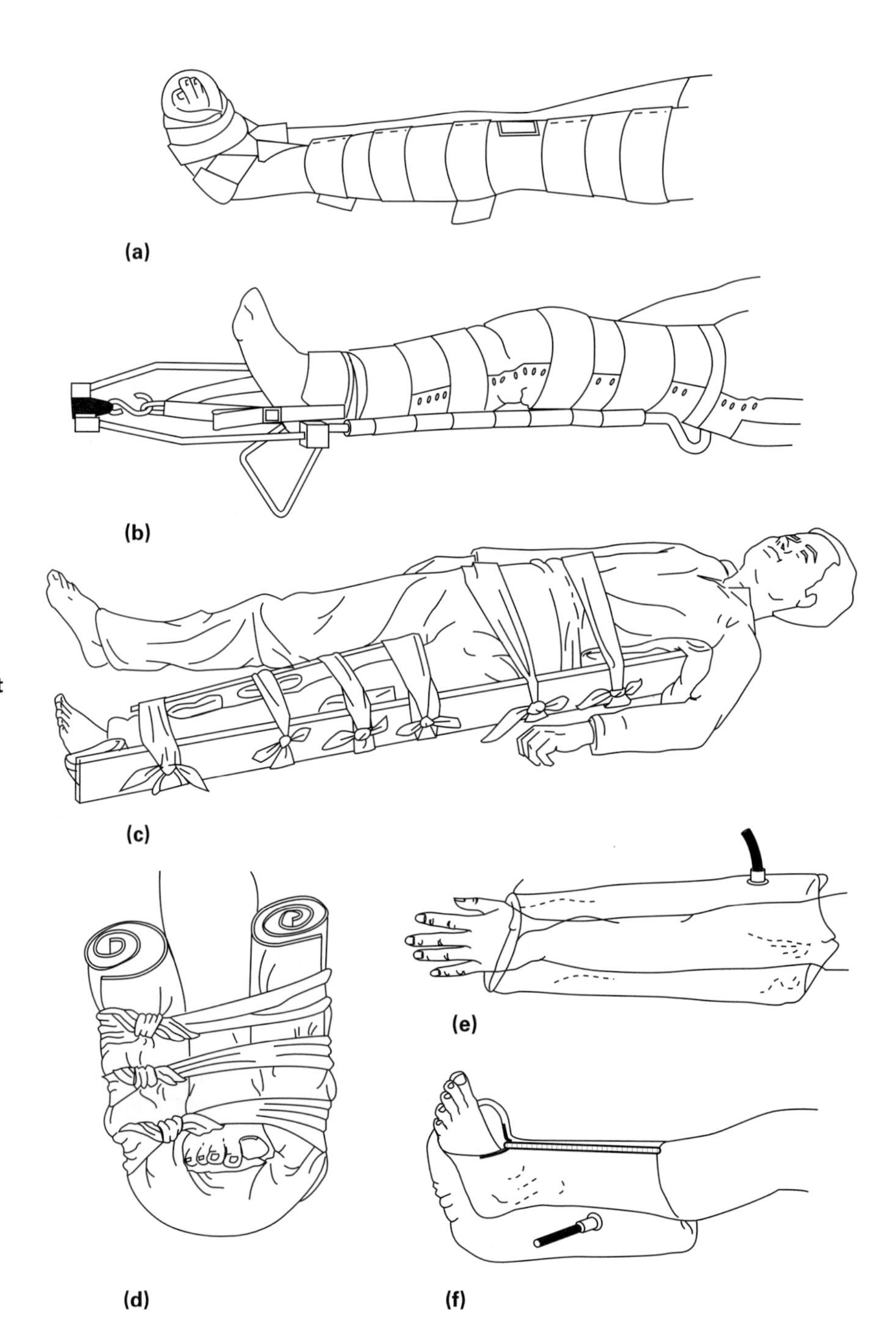

Figure 25-27
Types of splints: (a) Leg splint for fracture of leg; (b) long-board splint for hip fracture; (c) using slats of wood to splint fractured leg; (d) using rolled towel to splint ankle fracture; (e) inflatable splint for lower arm fracture; and (f) inflatable splint for ankle fracture.

splinting the affected limb. The material used as a splint may be wood, shaped metal, plastic, or an inflatable plastic splint (Figure 25-27). Whatever the material, the purpose is to support and protect the injured part. In an emergency, almost any firm object can be used as a splint: a magazine, folded newspapers, or pieces of cardboard may all be used as improvised splints. The splint is placed under or alongside the injured part and secured by tying it with a bandage. When a leg has been injured, it may also be splinted by tying it to the other uninjured leg.

If an athlete has suffered an injury of his hand or arm, a *sling* is often used to support the affected limb. This is a triangular bandage which is positioned so that the injured part is supported. The bandage is tied around the person's neck with the knot to the side of the neck, so that the hand is kept higher than the elbow. In cases where it may be necessary to completely immobilize an injured upper limb, a *swathe* may be used to bind the injured arm to the person's body.

Whenever you suspect a fracture or injury of the back or neck area, you must be particularly careful not to move the victim, since any type of movement can cause or lead to potential or additional damage to the spinal cord. Instead, try to immobilize the victim, and wait for emergency help to arrive. If there is no emergency help immediately available, and the victim must be moved, he or she should be log-rolled or lifted as one unit onto a firm support and then secured to prevent movement prior to transport. If at all possible, if you do suspect a back or neck injury, use a backboard splint and a collar (Figure 25-28) to transport or move the victim.

Administering Basic First Aid for Eye Injuries

Objects in the eye must sometimes be treated as emergencies. When treating a victim's eyes, always find out if the person is wearing contact lenses before beginning treatment. The first thing to do is to flush the eye thoroughly with water to wash the foreign body out. If you can see the object on the inside of either eyelid, you may remove it carefully by using a clean cloth or tissue. In washing the eye, make sure you let the water run from the nose side of the eye to the side of the face. This will avoid the possibility of contaminating the other eye.

Trauma to an eye which results in bleeding into the inside of the eyeball or fracture of the bones form-

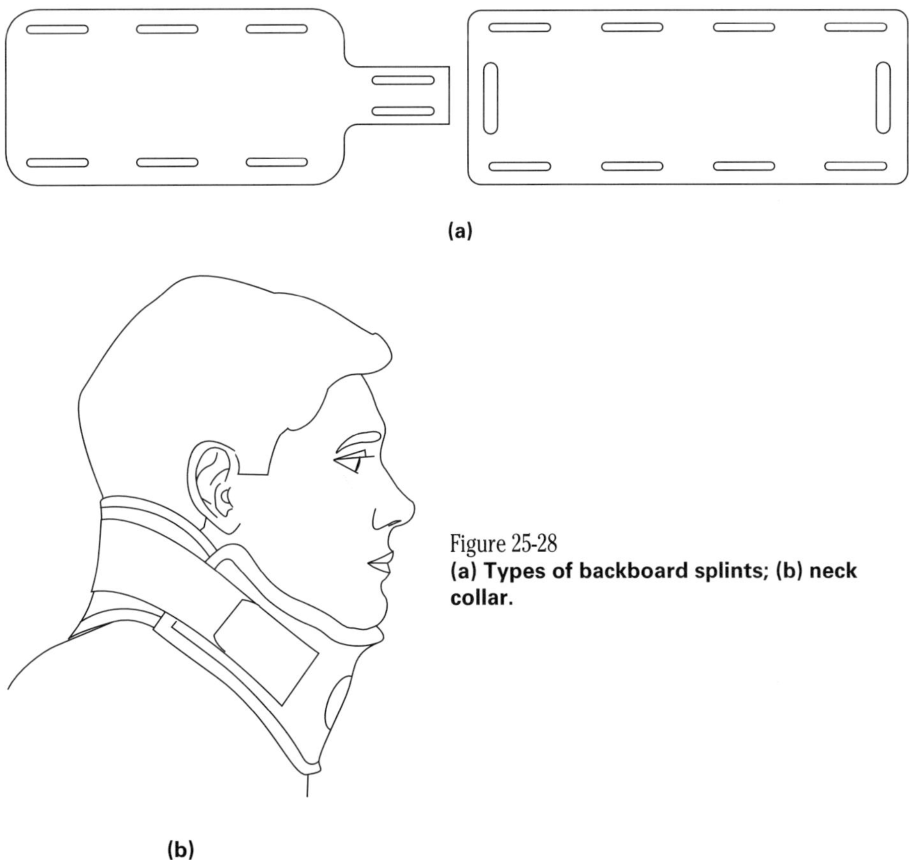

Figure 25-28
(a) Types of backboard splints; (b) neck collar.

ing the orbit are potential injuries suffered by athletes who are required to wear head gear for their events. With either of these injuries, the injured eye should be protected with some type of shield, and a bandage or patch placed over the eye to minimize movement of both eyes. This person must then be assisted to a health care facility for further treatment.

Administering Basic First Aid for Shock

Injury-related or traumatic shock is another emergency that may require the immediate administration of first aid treatment. *Shock* means a depressed state of vital body functions. It may result from severe injuries, poisoning, or some illnesses. The person in shock appears pale and cyanotic and feels weak. The skin is moist and clammy, and the pulse is rapid and shallow. The pupils may be dilated, and the eyes may appear to stare. The person may also lose consciousness. If shock is not immediately treated, body temperature falls, and the person may die.

The first aid treatment for shock is to keep the victim lying down. This helps to maintain a good blood supply to the head. The person should be covered to prevent any loss of body heat, and the feet and lower part of the body should be elevated about six inches unless they are fractured or unless shock accompanies heart attack, severe lung disease, or a head injury. If you suspect a person to be suffering from shock, do not allow the person to have anything to eat or drink. You should also seek medical help as soon as possible.

Summary

In this chapter, we discussed some of the more common injuries sustained by the athlete, and the role of the sports medicine assistant in providing care and treatment for those injuries. We also explained how sports injuries are classified. We talked about common sports injuries affecting the athlete's upper and lower extremities and the back. Finally, we identified some of the more common medical emergencies encountered in sports medicine, and briefly explained the role of the sports medicine assistant in providing basic first aid procedures for such emergencies.

Review Questions

1. What is the general term to describe any injury or wound?
2. The term ______________ pertains to the grating sound heard or felt when the ends of broken bones are rubbed together.
3. Briefly explain what is meant by *level of consciousness.*
4. A ______________ refers to a device which can be used to protect and immobilize a body part.
5. A ______________ is a type of bandage which can be used to immobilize the arm by bounding it around the chest and the arm.
6. Briefly explain what occurs as a result of a compression injury.
7. Briefly explain what occurs during shock.
8. ______________ are structures which are attached to bones through tendons which allow for movement through a small space.
9. What is the name of the fluid sacs that prevent friction between two moving surfaces within the body?

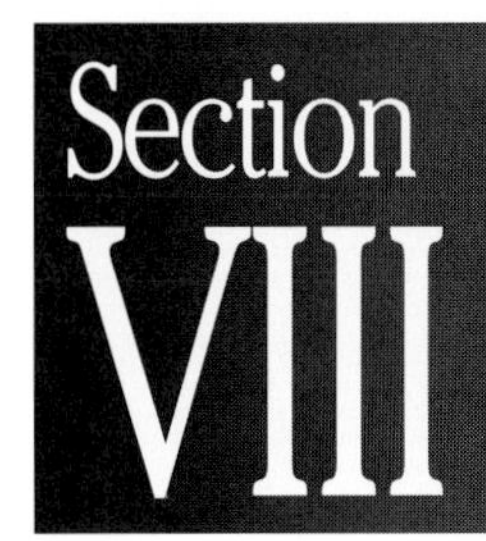

Personal Fitness Trainer: Basic Concepts and Applications

26

Introduction to Physical Training

Performance Objectives

Upon completion of this chapter, you will be able to:

1. Discuss the importance of health screening and evaluation as it relates to beginning a physical training program.
2. Identify common medical disorders and conditions which may affect exercise.
3. Briefly explain the effects of medications on the body's heart rate and one's response to physical exercise.
4. Define the parameters for referring a client to a physician for medical clearance prior to beginning a physical training program.

Terms and Abbreviations

Angina chest pain or discomfort, often described as "pressure or tightness," and usually experienced by a person when blood supply is limited, causing an increased demand for oxygen to the heart.

Atherosclerosis a process whereby fatty deposits of cholesterol and calcium accumulate on the walls of the arteries, causing them to harden, thicken, and lose their elasticity.

CAD abbreviation for coronary artery disease, which occurs when the buildup of cholesterol and calcium affects the arteries that supply the heart.

Today, more than ever before, caring for our bodies and meeting both the physical and emotional needs of our existence have become so important that some members of our society have even become obsessed with how they look, feel, and act. While some people have crossed the line between taking care of themselves and becoming obsessed with how they look, others, like those of you who may be interested in working in sports medicine or physical training, have come to the realization that good health can only be achieved through good living. And part of that good living must involve some type of exposure to a physical activity or training exercise program.

Purpose of a Physical Exercise Program

The purpose of any good exercise program is to improve the quality of one's life. However, while most of us may believe that we have the skills and knowledge to set up and implement a good program, the fact is that the average person has very little knowledge or understanding of the techniques and concepts involved in creating a physical training or exercise program based upon a healthy and medically safe foundation.

If the goal of the program is to establish a base for ensuring the quality of good life, then it stands to reason that any medical condition which might aggravate such a program would be counterproductive to meeting this goal. Therefore, to set up the most effective exercise program part of your responsibility as a personal trainer is first to evaluate your client's medical condition and individual goals. One means of doing so is to first screen your clients for any potential or pre-existing medical problems.

Performing the Physical Screening

The client's medical history is very important, but it has definite limitations because it defines only the conditions that the client is aware of and remembers to report. A client may be completely unaware of a significant risk factor. Thus, the purpose of the physical evaluation is to identify these unknown conditions and to further delineate a known condition. The physical screening is also important to establish an initial baseline and in discovering specific areas that may need work. Finally, it communicates to your clients that you are interested in them and in designing a program which is unique to them alone.

The two most important aspects of the physical screening are blood pressure and heart rate. As we discussed earlier in this text, normal blood pressure in our society has been defined as 120/80. Many factors, such as obesity, heart disease, and stress can raise blood pressure. Exercise, which can raise one's blood pressure, can also be used to correct and lower it. However, exercise in a person with uncontrolled high blood pressure can be dangerous and should be postponed until the condition is properly treated. Blood pressure greater than 140/90 in an adult is considered high and needs the attention of the client's doctor.

The normal heart rate in an adult is usually between 60 to 100 beats per minute and is regular in rhythm. Well-trained endurance athletes have developed an efficient cardiovascular system and often have a heart rate in the low 40s. If your client's resting heart rate is greater than 100, or less than 60, or if his or her heart rate is irregular, medical clearance is generally recommended before starting any exercise program.

The next part of a client's physical screening process deals with observation. Observations should actually begin the very first time you meet your client. At that time, you should notice whether the person is short of breath even at rest. How is the person's posture? Does he or she walk with a limp? Remember, part of your responsibility as a trainer is being aware of any physical characteristics or limitations that may influence the design of the person's exercise program.

The final two parts of the screening process have to do with determining the client's flexibility and strength. Fitness is defined by flexibility, strength, and endurance; however, most people neglect flexibility training. As a trainer, your job is to help your clients develop total fitness while at the same time reducing the risk for injury. Good flexibility is of prime importance to a client's overall success, and loss of it is often associated with reduced performance of the muscle, increased incidence of injuries, strained muscles and overuse injuries from altered biomechanics, and reduced circulation leading to longer tissue healing. The purpose of the flexibility evaluation is to identify areas of restriction that are at risk for injury. This information can be used to alert you to areas which may need more concentrated stretching as well as to modifications which may be necessary because of your client's poor flexibility.

Testing a person's strength is also important in establishing a baseline and in determining muscular imbalances which would have negative impact on a person's performance. For example, weak rotator cuff muscles of the shoulder could offset the muscular balance and biomechanics of the shoulder. While this may not normally be a problem, during increased exercise the imbalance predisposes your client to shoulder injury.

Medical Disorders Affecting Exercise

Unfortunately, there are always some risks involved in starting an exercise program. However, identifying these risks is the first step to preventing them. Injuries that occur in sports or from prolonged exercise generally come from aggravating an existing medical condition which may or may not be known by the client, and from precipitating a new condition. And the primary body systems usually injured with exercise are the cardiovascular and musculoskeletal systems. Therefore, having a client complete the health history form (Figure 26-1) is usually the best insurance you can take as a personal trainer to obtain needed information related to these areas.

Cardiovascular Disorders

Of the many cardiovascular disorders which can affect the outcome of exercise, the two which are most harmful are *atherosclerosis* and *coronary artery disease* (*CAD*). In atherosclerosis, there is a buildup of fatty deposits of cholesterol and calcium which accumulate on the walls of the arteries, eventually causing them to harden, thicken, and lose their elasticity. When this process affects the arteries that supply the heart, it is called coronary artery disease. As with

Patient's name ______________________________

Address ______________________________ Phone ______________

______________________________ Msg. phone ______________

Marital status: ( )S ( )M ( )D ( )Sep ( )W Sex: ( )M ( )F Age: ____

No. of children __________ Occupation ______________

Referred by: __________

Family history: Father ________ Sister(s) ________

Mother ________ Brother(s) ________

Cancer ______ Arthritis ______ Mental illness ______

Heart disease ______ Epilepsy ______ Gout ______

Diabetes ______ Nephritis ______ Goiter ______

Obesity ______ TB ______ Other ______

Past history: Mumps _____ Measles ______ Chickenpox _____ Diptheria _____

Thyroid _____ Pneumonia _____ STD(s) ________ Other _______

Women only: Onset of menstruation __________ Duration __________ Pain __________

No. of live births _____ No. of miscarriages _____ No. of abortions _____

Medications: ______________ Allergies: ______________

______________ ______________

______________ ______________

Hospitalization(s): ______________________________

Operation(s): ______________________________

Habits: Coffee/Cola/Tea (number cups or glasses per day): __________

Smoking: Cigarette (packs/day): ___ Cigar (no. per day): ___ Pipe (hours per day): ___

Exercise (type & frequency per week): ______________________

____

Stress (high, medium, low): ______________________

Recreational drugs: ______________________

Other lifestyle/factors influencing health: ______________________

Hobbies/Interests: ______________________

Occupational exposure: ______________________

Seat belts: ______________________

Alcohol (frequently, moderately, never): ______________________

Present complaints: ______________________________

____

____

Figure 26-1

The health history form.

other muscles, the heart contracts when we exercise. The increased contraction of the heart muscle is made possible by an increased supply of oxygenated blood which provides the body with its needed nutrients. The greater the exercise load, the larger the demand is for the blood and oxygen to make its way to the heart muscle. If the vessels that supply the heart with this blood are narrowed from atherosclerosis and cannot stretch, the blood supply diminishes and the demand for increased oxygen by the heart cannot be met. In some cases, this can result in a type of chest pain called *angina,* while in other cases the supply of blood to the heart can become so limited that the ensuing outcome can lead to a heart attack, or myocardial infarction.

Risk Factors in Cardiovascular Disease

Sadly, many people who experience coronary artery disease or atherosclerosis have no known symptoms and are usually unaware of their potential for a heart attack. However, long-term studies of these diseases have helped cardiologists and researchers identify several factors which seem to correlate with a person's increased risk for cardiovascular disease. Of these factors, the most significant include elevated total cholesterol greater than 240 mg/dl, cigarette smoking, a history of diabetes mellitus or hypertension in which the systolic blood pressure is greater than 160 mmHg or diastolic blood pressure is higher than 90 mmHg, and a history of coronary or other atherosclerotic disease in parents or sibling prior to reaching the age of 55.

The greater number of risk factors a person has, the greater his or her chance is of either having or developing coronary artery disease. Therefore, the goal of any exercise program should be to minimize these risk factors as much as possible. Any client with two or more of these risk factors should be referred to a physician before you begin a fitness evaluation or the client starts a vigorous exercise program. In addition, the American College of Sports Medicine recommends that males over the age of 40 and females over the age of 50 have a complete medical evaluation including a maximal exercise test prior to beginning any vigorous exercise program. The client's doctor and his or her personal trainer can then work together to set up the ideal program.

Metabolic Disorders

There are many metabolic diseases whose presence can affect or interfere with our body's metabolism. Two of the more common of these are diabetes mellitus and thyroid disorders. In diabetes mellitus, the body is unable to metabolize blood glucose properly. All of the cells in the body require sugar, or glucose, to function. Insulin, which is a hormone produced in the pancreas, helps the blood glucose move into the cells.

There are two types of diabetes mellitus. In the first type, called Type I, the person becomes insulin-dependent, meaning that he or she may require injections of insulin for cellular survival. In Type II diabetes, the person can produce insulin, but not in sufficient quantities to regulate the cellular need for glucose. Type II diabetes is usually linked to obesity and is often treated with proper diet and exercise. However, persons diagnosed with this form of diabetes often progress to the point in their disease where they may require either oral medication or insulin to control their glucose.

For the diabetic, taking part in a good exercise program must be part of one's lifestyle. Along with a specific diet and medication, it is often considered the mainstay of treatment. However, it is also important for the diabetic client to take care of him- or herself. This means taking the appropriate steps to meet the varying demands for glucose and insulin during exercise. If the need for glucose to cells is not properly met, the imbalance can lead to dizziness, coma, or even death. To avoid such complications, the person needs to thoroughly understand the effects of diet, exercise, and medication on their blood sugar.

The other type of metabolic disorder which can frequently interfere with one's ability to exercise has to do with a dysfunctional thyroid gland. The thyroid is a very small gland located in the neck which secretes a hormone that regulates the rate of metabolism, including the heart rate. Clients diagnosed with hyperthyroidism have an increased level of this hormone and, as such, also have a higher metabolic rate. Persons with hypothyroidism have a reduced level of the hormone and thus may require medication to increase their metabolism to normal. Because exercise also increases the metabolism, it could be dangerous in a person with uncontrolled thyroid disease. Therefore, if you have a client who has been diagnosed with either diabetes or thyroid disease, you must require that person to seek the approval of their physician prior to initiating any exercise or physical training program.

Musculoskeletal Disorders

As we have already discussed in previous chapters, the musculoskeletal system consists of many muscles, bones, tendons, and ligaments that function to support and move our body. This system is also the most commonly injured during exercise. In addition to the pain and discouragement of an injury to this system, there are many other factors which both you and the client must contend with. Changes or modifications in an exercise program may become necessary to accommodate an injury. Motivation is also a big factor to contend with in these situations. Furthermore, as a personal trainer, you may be legally liable for a client's injury. Therefore, it is extremely important that you be cognizant of any potential hazards before they happen. Most minor sprains and strains are easily managed, but a persistent problem or a more serious injury often requires a referral to a physician, followed by appropriate treatment. Medical referral is not only for a client's protection, but for yours as well.

The musculoskeletal evaluation is crucial to identifying both old injuries and possible risk factors for new ones. The most common type of injury sustained by people participating in aerobic activities is the overuse injury. These types of injuries are usually the result of poor training techniques, poor use of body mechanics, or sometimes both. Essentially, the injury is caused by exercise which is too much, too soon, or too fast for a particular tissue involved in the activity to adapt. The result is repetitive stress upon the tissue without enough time for recovery, thus overwhelming the body's ability to heal itself. During repetitive activity, our body is in a dynamic balance between breaking down and repairing of tissue. The overuse mechanism tips the balance toward the breaking down side. Two examples of overuse injuries are swimmer's shoulder (pain in the shoulder) and runner's knee (pain in the knee). To avoid aggravating the existing injury and to allow for proper healing, part of your responsibility as a trainer is to help your clients with overuse injuries by modifying their exercise program.

Two other common musculoskeletal injuries are sprains, involving ligaments, and strains, involving muscles or their tendons. In these conditions, there is a partial or complete tearing of the respective tissue. Again, like the overuse injuries, sprains and strains must be identified before starting any exercise program so as not to worsen the condition. A client with an injury more severe than a simple sprain or strain must have a doctor's approval before beginning their program. If specific weakness of the muscle or looseness of the joint exists, medical referral is also indicated.

Another common condition which can affect a client's back is straining or spraining of the lumbar or lower back area. For this person, designing a good exercise program which will not aggravate the area is extremely important. Insisting that your client also use proper biomechanics, practice good posture, and use the appropriate technique during their exercise program are all essential to good back care, especially when a person has a history of back pain.

As a personal trainer, you may encounter some clients with a history of arthritis, which is a general term used to describe any inflammation of a joint. These clients often experience pain, stiffness, swelling, or limitation of motion at the involved joint. While there are many different forms of arthritis, the most common is osteoarthritis, in which there is a wearing away and tearing around the joint area. The client may also suffer from an arthritic or degenerative back, hip, or knee. While these conditions are frequently aggravated by high impact activities such as running or jumping, they often respond favorably to the lower impact movements, such as those used in cycling, stair climbing, and nonweight bearing activities like swimming. Knowing that your client has an arthritic condition, and being able to identify which joints are affected, will enable you to tailor an appropriate workout program. If you have any doubts as to what exercise would be appropriate for your arthritic client, you should seek out advice and assistance from your client's physician.

Evaluating the Client's Need for Medications

Another important area which must be addressed in evaluating a client's ability to take part in a physical training or exercise program is their use or need for medications or drugs. These substances alter the body's biochemistry and, as such, may alter a client's ability to perform or respond to exercise. Therefore, if you have any doubt about the client's use or need of such substances, you should discuss them with the client's physician.

In designing and supervising a client's exercise program, it is important for you to realize that many over-the-counter medications, prescriptions, or illicit drugs affect the heart's response to exercise. Medications may be referred to by the manufacturer's brand name or by the scientific generic name. There are hundreds of thousands of different drugs on the market, so to gain an understanding of the specific effect of an individual drug, you should look at the general category under which it is grouped. The drugs in each group have similar properties, and each group is thought to have a similar effect on the average person, although there may be individual variations.

Table 26-1 identifies medications that can affect a person's response to exercise. The particular response is dose-dependent, meaning, the larger the dose, the greater the response. The effect also depends on when the medication is ingested; as a medication is metabolized, its effects start to diminish. If you have any questions concerning a client's use of medications, it is usually advisable to discuss them with a physician.

Table 26-1
Effects of Medications on Heart Rate and Blood Pressure

Medication	Resting Heart Rate	Exercise Heart Rate	Blood Pressure
Beta-adrenergic Blocking Agents	lowered	lowered	lowered
Calcium-channel Blockers	elevated lowered maintained	elevated lowered maintained	lowered
Diuretics	maintained	maintained	lowered
Antihypertensives	elevated lowered maintained	elevated lowered maintained	lowered
Antihistamines	maintained	maintained	maintained
Decongestants	elevated maintained	elevated maintained	elevated
Antidepressants	elevated maintained	maintained	maintained lowered
Tranquilizers	maintained lowered	maintained	maintained lowered
Bronchodilators	elevated maintained	elevated maintained	elevated maintained
Amphetamines	elevated maintained	elevated maintained	elevated
Caffeine	elevated maintained	maintained	elevated maintained
Alcohol and Nicotine	elevated maintained	elevated maintained	elevated maintained lowered

Meeting the Needs of the Client

One of the most important items when obtaining your client's medical and health history is to identify his or her exercise goals and the level of commitment he or she is willing to work toward to meet those goals. You must determine if the client's primary objective is to lose weight or build muscle. Is the client engaging in the training program to look or feel good, or is the client simply there because his or her doctor recommended it to reduce the possibility of future cardiovascular or musculoskeletal problems? Obtaining answers to these questions will help you to set up the best type of program for your client.

Determining a client's level of commitment toward his or her exercise program means ascertaining what the client is willing to do to achieve his or her ultimate goal. Does the client want to start the program now, or wait until another time? Is the client already in an exercise program but lacks motivation to keep up the program? Is the client willing to commit to a predefined schedule to complete his or her program? And are the goals which the client has set realistic in view of his or her degree of commitment? Frank consideration of these questions will provide both yourself and your client with a clear understanding of the best program, as well as reduce any misunderstandings either of you may have in the future.

It's very important that the client's goals coincide with your own. For example, if you notice that your client has underdeveloped arms and could benefit from an upper extremity strengthening program, but the client indicates that he does not want strong arms, you should not force your own objectives onto him. Instead, you should acknowledge the client's goals and motivate him toward achieving these goals.

Summary

In this chapter, we discussed the importance of exercise as a vital component of health. As part of our discussion, we defined the goal of a good exercise program, stating that overall, it should improve the quality of one's life without aggravating or precipitating an injury or illness. We also talked about performing a medical screening and obtaining a health history, and identified some of the most common medical disorders and types of medications which could inhibit a person's benefit from physical exercise.

Review Questions

1. ______________ is defined as a type of chest pain or discomfort described as pressure or tightness, and usually experienced by a person when blood supply is limited.
2. What does the abbreviation *CAD* mean?
3. Briefly explain what occurs during *atherosclerosis.*
4. Briefly explain the purpose of performing a physical screening.
5. Identify at least three medical disorders which can be affected by exercise.
6. Briefly explain the difference between *Type I* and *Type II* diabetes mellitis.
7. What does the term *swimmer's pain* mean?
8. Briefly explain why it is important to evaluate a client's need for medications before beginning any exercise or fitness training program.
9. What effects do antihistamines have on the heart rate and blood pressure?
10. What effects do calcium-channel blockers have on the heart rate and blood pressure?

27

Testing and Evaluation for Physical Training

Performance Objectives

Upon completion of this chapter, you will be able to:

1. Define the purpose of testing and evaluation for physical training.
2. Identify the differences between required evaluation and optional evaluation of a client interested in a physical training program.
3. Discuss the components involved in cardiovascular testing and evaluation.
4. Explain the process and techniques involved in body composition testing and evaluation.
5. Explain the process and techniques involved in flexibility, muscular strength, and endurance testing and evaluation.
6. Discuss the process involved in follow-up consultation and testing.

Terms and Abbreviations

Auscultation the procedure of using a stethoscope to listen to a body process or structure.

Body composition the quality or makeup of total body mass.

Flexibility the range of motion of any given joint.

Muscular endurance the ability to exert a submaximal force either repeatedly or statically over a set period of time.

Muscular strength the greatest amount of force that a muscle can produce in one single maximal effort.

Palpation the process by which one uses their fingertips to feel a structure.

Rockport Fitness Walking Test a routinely used test to assess cardiovascular fitness.

Because of its ability to provide both the trainer and the client with valuable and necessary information, testing and evaluation of a client's capacity to benefit from a personal fitness or exercise program is often considered the most important step in the training process.

The purpose of testing and evaluating your client prior to designing his or her exercise program is to provide you with important information to assess your client's current level of fitness and his or her ability to benefit from such a program. It also helps to identify specific areas of health or injury risks which may need possible referral to appropriate health care professionals. Finally, performing early testing and evaluation will assist you in developing an individual exercise program for your client. It does so by providing you with a keen sense of insight and understanding as to what motivates your client to achieve his or her goals in completing the exercise program.

While the specific tests administered during the early assessment phase may vary among your clients, sound fitness testing should assess heart function, blood vessels, lungs, and muscles. Most comprehensive testing and evaluation programs involve measuring the client's cardiovascular efficiency, muscular strength and endurance, muscle and joint flexibility, and body composition.

Measuring Cardiovascular Efficiency

While not all clients need or require comprehensive exercise testing, some form of early cardiovascular measurement is usually required. Determining a person's cardiovascular risk can be ascertained by ensuring the client's completion of the health history form (see Figure 26-1 p. 329) and an exercise history and attitude questionnaire (Figure 27-1 on p. 336). In addition to filling out these forms, it is also important to measure the client's blood pressure and heart rate.

Determining a Resting Heart Rate and a Resting Pulse Rate

The resting heart rate is usually measured by placing your fingertips directly onto a pulse site, or by listening through a stethoscope (Figure 27-2 on p. 337). To obtain the most accurate resting heart rate, you should encourage your client to measure it just prior to getting out of bed in the morning.

To determine a person's resting pulse rate per minute, the pulse is usually taken for one full minute, or for 30 seconds and then multiplied by two. The most accurate way of measuring it is by placing your index and middle fingers over the radial artery, and then palpating it by applying light pressure (Figure 27–3 on p. 337).

Determining Exercise Pulse Rate

Measuring a client's exercise pulse rate is most accurately determined by *palpating* it from the larger carotid artery located just to the side of the larynx (Figure 27-4 on p. 337). It's important to remember that you should never use heavy pressure when palpating the carotid arteries. This is because they contain baroreceptors that sense increases in pressure and respond by slowing the heart rate. An exercise pulse should be taken for at least 10 seconds, counting the first pulse beat as zero at the start of the 10-second period. If you are measuring it by *auscultation,* place the bell of the stethoscope on the third intercostal space to the left of the sternum.

Interpreting Heart Rate

A person's resting heart rate can vary widely for both the endurance-trained athlete and the nonconditioned client. Therefore, interpreting one's resting heart rate as it relates to his or her cardiovascular fitness is difficult at best. A normal resting heart rate varies from as low as 40 beats per minute to as high as 100 beats per minute, with the average being 70 to 72 for men and 72 to 75 for women. People who practice endurance training exercises usually have a lower resting heart rate. This is due to the increased amount of blood their heart pumps during each beat.

Measuring Cardiorespiratory Endurance

The assessment of cardiorespiratory endurance can be made either by direct measurement of oxygen consumption during a person's maximum graded exercise test, or indirectly by estimating the person's oxygen consumption from the heart rate response to a progressive increase in submaximal workloads. Of the two, the direct measurement of maximal oxygen consumption is by far the most accurate method; however, it does require specialized equipment in addition to a maximal aerobic challenge. Depending on your client's age and cardiovascular risk, this method is often limited to either clinical or research facilities and, as such, is usually performed in the presence of a physician well trained in advanced cardiac life support.

The Submaximal Exercise Test

Before you begin to administer the submaximal exercise test, it's important that you observe specific safety precautions and obtain the appropriate written consent from your client. While the submaximal aerobic exercise test carries a relatively low risk of cardiovascular and other medical complications, as a trainer, it's essential that you follow the accepted standards of procedure in the assessment of cardiovascular and other medical risks before testing or training a client. According to guidelines established by the American College of Sports Medicine (ACSM), before administering the test to any client, a cardiovascular risk assessment should be given and reviewed. The ACSM recommends that anyone over the age of 35 with one or more major risk factors, and everyone over the age of 45 should undergo a physician-supervised maximal graded exercise test prior to taking any test or beginning any physical training program. The cardiovascular risk assessment given to the client before testing should include questions related to all the major risk factors recognized by the ACSM.

After you have determined that your client can undergo the submaximal exercise test and have obtained the appropriate written consent, you are ready to begin the testing. You should understand, however, that the submaximal exercise test only provides

Name ______________________ Hm. phone ______________
Address ______________________ Wk. phone ______________
______________________ Age ______________
Doctor's name ______________________ Phone ______________
Address ____

EXERCISE HISTORY

1. Do you find yourself starting an exercise program, but then are unable to stick with it?
   YES _____ NO _____
2. How much time are you willing to devote to a regular exercise program?
   minutes/day _____ days/week _____
3. Are you currently involved in a regular endurance exercise program?
   YES _____ NO _____
4. How would you rate the amount of exertion you put out during an exercise program? (circle one)
   (1) light (2) fairly light (3) somewhat hard (4) hard
5. How long have you been involved in a regular exercise program?
   _____ months _____ years
6. Are you able to exercise during your work day?
   YES _____ NO _____
7. Would an exercise program interfere with your job?
   YES _____ NO _____
8. Do you think an exercise program would benefit your job?
   YES _____ NO _____
9. Have you been involved in any other exercise, sport, or recreation program in the last:
   6 months _____ 2 years _____
10. What types of exercises most interest you? (please check)

Jogging ________	Walking ________	Strength training ________
Cycling ________	Aerobic ________	Swimming ________
Tennis ________	Dance ________	Stationary bike ________
Rowing ________	Stretching ________	Racquetball ________

11. If you would like to start a regular exercise program to lose weight, by how much would you change what your current weight is?
    (–) ________ lbs.
12. How would you rank your goals in undertaking an exercise program?

Extremely Important				Somewhat Important				Not Important at All	
1	2	3	4	5	6	7	8	9	10

____ a. Improve cardiovascular fitness
____ b. Lose body fat
____ c. Improve performance
____ d. Improve flexibility
____ e. Increase strength
____ f. Increase energy level
____ g. Improve moods and ability to cope better with stressful situations
____ h. Enjoyment and overall feeling better about self
____ i. Reshape or tone body
____ j. Other

Figure 27-1
Exercise history and attitude questionnaire.

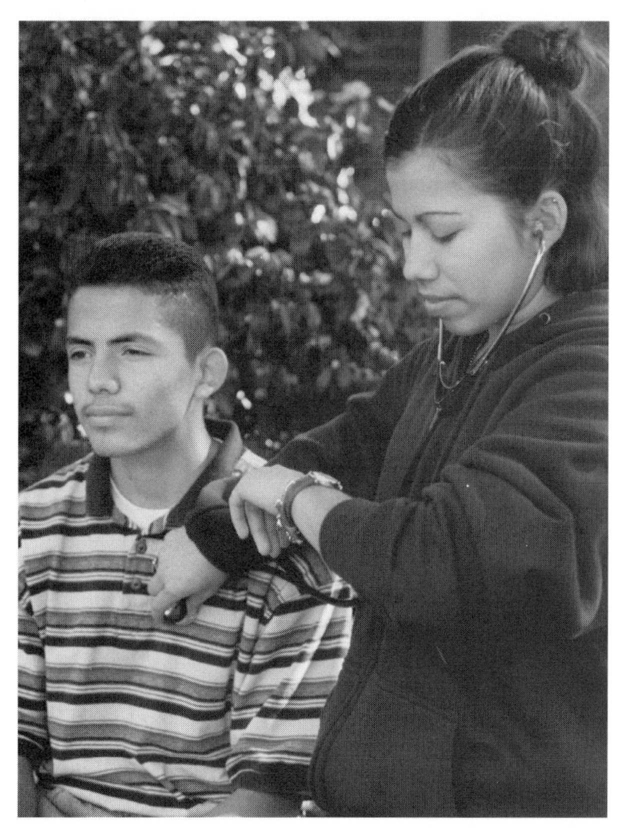

Figure 27-2
Placement of stethoscope to measure resting heart rate.

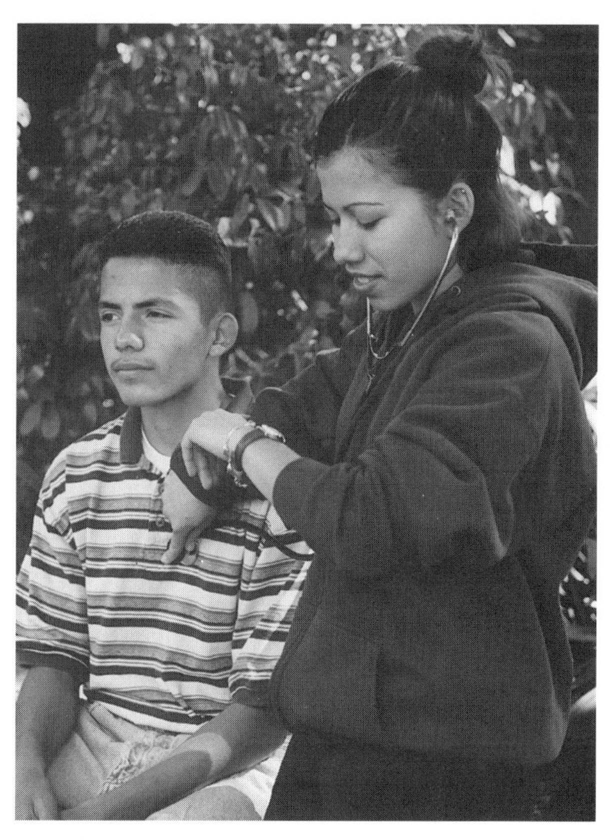

Figure 27-3
Measuring resting pulse.

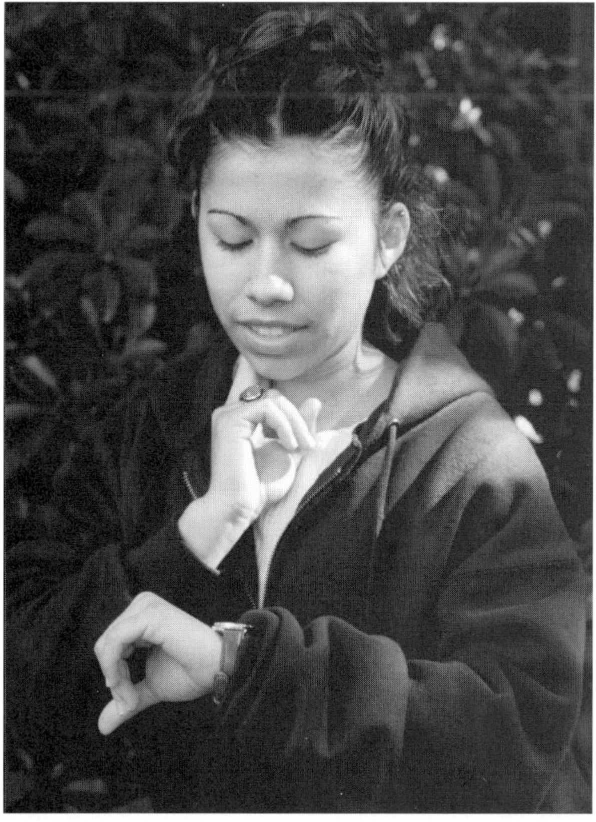

(a) **(b)**

Figure 27-4
(a) Measuring exercise pulse rate at the carotid artery; (b) measuring exercise pulse rate by auscultation.

a reasonably accurate prediction of maximum work capacity and estimation of maximal oxygen consumption. Therefore, the maximal work capacity and maximal oxygen consumption can be estimated from the rate at which the heart rate increases with progressively increasing workloads.

The limitation of the submaximal estimation method lies in the prediction of the maximal heart rate which uses a formula of

estimated maximal heart rate = 220 – age.

This is usually accurate within plus or minus 15 beats per minute. Estimations of maximal work capacity and maximal oxygen consumption are both based upon the prediction of maximal heart rate. Therefore, if a person's maximal heart rate is over- or underpredicted, so too is the maximal work capacity and maximal oxygen consumption. While there may be some error in the estimation of maximal oxygen consumption, the heart rates collected at the submaximal workloads appear to be very accurate and reproducible. Thus, it is the comparison of the heart rates at equivalent workloads during follow-up testing that will provide you with a relative change in a person's aerobic fitness. If the heart rates are accurate and used to estimate maximal oxygen consumption, a change in oxygen consumption will be valid as a measurement showing relative change in the person's aerobic fitness.

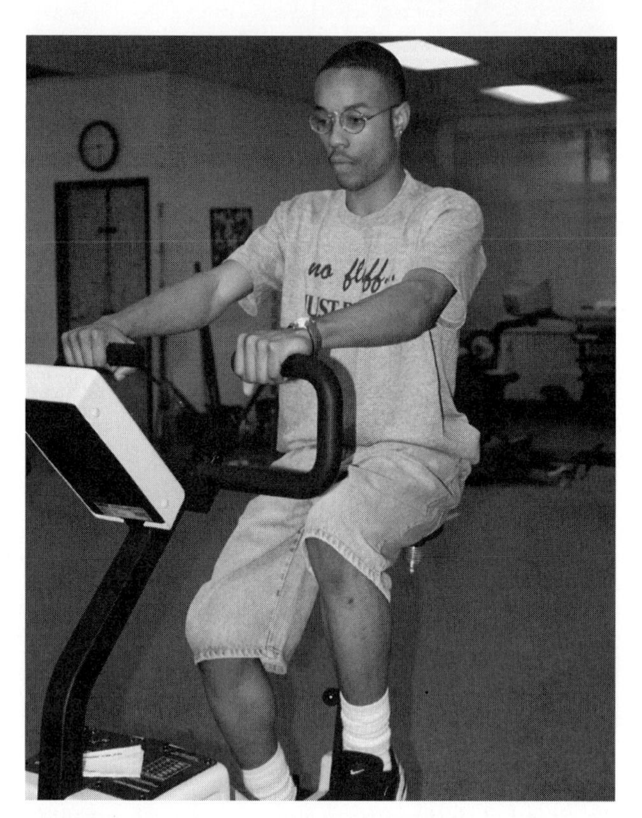

Figure 27-5
Position of client on bicycle ergometer for submaximal testing.

The Submaximal Bicycle Test

The submaximal bicycle test was developed to evaluate a person's physical working capacity, while at the same time estimating the amount of maximal oxygen uptake. Its purpose is to establish a relationship between the heart rate and the workload. To maintain the validity of the test, the two heart rates used in the estimation of maximal exercise capacity must be greater than 110 beats per minute and less than 85 percent of age-predicted maximal heart rate.

The test uses a bicycle ergometer (Figure 27-5). It should be accurate, easily calibrated, and have a range of 1–2,100 kilogram-meters per minute. It is used in place of a treadmill because it is less expensive, requires little space, is easily transported, makes it easier to measure one's heart rate, and requires little or no training or practice, because its external work is known. In addition to the ergometer, to administer this test you will also need a metronome set at 50 or 100 beats per minute to maintain the correct rhythm of the test, a timer to measure the test's duration, a stopwatch or heart-rate monitor to time the heart rate, a stethoscope to count the heart rate, and testing forms to record the data.

To administer the test, the client begins by setting the bicycle at 150 kg per minute and then progresses according to his or her heart rate response at the first workload. The metronome should be set to either 100 beats per minute or 50 beats per minute to maintain a constant pedal rate throughout the test. Before beginning, you should make sure that the seat of the bicycle is properly adjusted so that the client's leg is straight when the heel is in contact with the pedal on the down stroke or lowest point of rotation, and/or the knee is slightly bent when the ball of the foot is placed on the pedal at the same low point of rotation. Record the seat position on the data sheet so that it can be used for retesting. Once the test has begun, you should also check the bicycle's calibration to make sure that the belt tension has been released and the flywheel is stationary.

The Submaximal Step Test

Another test used to measure cardiorespiratory endurance is the three-minute step test. The procedure used in this test involves the delivery of a measured aerobic stimulus which is controlled by stepping to a standardized cadence. This test is much easier to administer than the bicycle ergometer test because it requires less equipment, is less costly, and can be used to test large numbers of people at the same time. However, the major disadvantage of using this test is that it is relatively inaccurate when compared to the bicycle test and, as such, tends to lack the appropriate data which may be necessary for comparing it to retesting data.

Before administering the test, it's usually helpful to the client if you demonstrate it first. Instruct your client to face the bench, and remind him or her that the stepping will be for three minutes, after which he or she will be told to be seated to count the pulse rate for one full minute. Once you have explained the test, begin by first setting a metronome to 96 beats per minute. The client should then be instructed to start stepping to a four-beat cycle; up, up, down, down (see Figure 22-1 on p. 268). While it makes little difference which foot the client begins stepping with, it is important that both feet come into contact with the top of the bench on the up portion of the cycle, and both feet come into contact with the floor during the down portion. The lead foot may change during the test.

During the test, you should check the client's stepping rhythm, announcing when one minute, two minutes, and two minutes and 30 seconds have elapsed. To further aid your client, you can also provide verbal cues by clapping your hands or saying "up, up, down, down" in cadence with the metronome. At the conclusion of the three-minute period, with your client seated, immediately begin counting their heart rate for one full minute.

Cardiorespiratory Fitness Treadmill Testing

An effective way to determine a person's cardiorespiratory fitness, and which can be administered either in a private home or in a health club, is to have your client walk one mile on a level treadmill at a fixed rate. After stretching, but before beginning the timed mile, have your client warm up on the treadmill, and then establish an exact pace that can be held for one mile. Once the pace has been established, the client should be able to walk for the time necessary to complete the mile at the fixed rate. At the completion of the mile, immediately take and record your client's pulse rate for 10 seconds. This should be followed by having the client cool down by walking slowly for at least five minutes.

Measuring Body Composition

People carrying around excess body fat are often susceptible to such health risks as heart disease, diabetes, hypertension, and arthritis. They also tend to have a greater risk of injury, while at the same time their level of endurance and ability to perform basic exercises may be largely reduced. The most common reason adults begin an exercise program is that they want to lose weight. And to do that, the first step is to determine what their accurate and ideal body weight should be. This is done by assessing the person's body composition. Once the body's composition has been assessed, a sound exercise program can be developed.

Body composition refers to the quality or makeup of one's total body mass. Total body mass can be divided into lean body mass and fat mass. Lean body mass is composed of bone, muscle, and organs; and fat mass is composed of adipose tissue. The assessment of body composition determines the relative percentages of lean body mass and fat mass.

There are three methods which can be used to determine a person's body composition. The first, and often considered the standard method, is called hydrostatic weighing, or weighing a person while he or she is underwater. The test involves suspending the client, seated in a chair attached to a scale, in a tank of water. Body density is then calculated from the relationship between normal body weight to that of underwater weight. From body density, the percentage of body fat is calculated. Although accurate, a properly administered hydrostatic weighing is often impractical because of the expense, time, and equipment which is involved.

A more popular method of determining a person's body composition is by measuring bioelectrical impedance. It is based on the principle that the conductivity of an electrical impulse is greater through lean tissue than through fatty or adipose tissue. Assuming the client has remained well-hydrated and has not exercised for at least six hours or consumed any alcohol for at least 24 hours, pairs of electrodes, through which an imperceptible electrical current is passed, are carefully placed on the client's hand and foot. Then, an analyzer, which consists of an ohmmeter and a computer, measures the body's resistance to electrical flow in ohms, and from that computes the body density and percentage of body fat. Using this method to assess a person's body composition has proved to be both fast and easy, however, it can be costly, with the analyzers ranging from $300 to $5000, depending on the design and data reporting capabilities.

Measuring skinfolds is the most common and relatively inexpensive way to determine body composition. The results are both valid and reliable, as long as the measurements are taken properly. The method, which is based upon the principle that approximately 50 percent of our total body fat is located under the skin, involves measuring the thickness of the skinfolds at standardized sites. These measurements are calculated, summed, and then applied to one of many equations available. Calculations are often simplified through the use of a table or nomogram. And calipers specifically designed for skinfold measurement, which range in cost from $20 to $300, is the only piece of equipment needed for this method of body fat assessment.

The procedure for assessing your client's body composition using the skinfold measurement method is as follows:

1. Identify the anatomical location of the skinfold using only the right side of the body.
2. Grasp the skinfold firmly with your thumb and index finger of your left hand. Then, holding the calipers perpendicular to the site, place their pads approximately one-quarter inch from your thumb and forefinger.
3. Read the dial to the nearest 0.5 millimeter for approximately one to two seconds after the trigger has been released.
4. Take a minimum of at least two measurements at each site, waiting at least 15 seconds between measurements; this will allow the fat to return to its normal thickness.

Location of Skinfolds

When assessing your client's body composition using the skinfold measurement method, it's important that you understand and be able to recognize the various locations where you can place the calipers (Figure 27-6). For men, the sites include the chest, abdomen, and thigh, and for women, the sites that can be used include the triceps, suprailium, and the thigh.

Measuring Flexibility

The term *flexibility* is used to describe the range of motion of any given joint, and it is frequently associated with muscular flexibility, which is the extent to which range of motion is limited by muscles and tendons surrounding the joint. Flexibility is also greatly influenced by the amount of freedom permitted by the ligaments which connect the bones that make up a given joint.

When we refer to flexibility, we are usually referring to a condition which affects both our health and our fitness. However, unlike cardiorespiratory assessment or body composition measurement, there is no single flexibility test that will provide us with a prediction of a person's range of motion of the joints of their body. Each joint must be assessed individually with a specifically designed test. Figure 27-7 (on p. 342) gives some examples of a few of the more commonly tested joints.

Measuring Muscle Strength and Endurance

Muscular strength is the greatest amount of force that a muscle can produce in a single effort. *Muscular endurance* is the ability to exert a submaximal force either repeatedly or statically over a period of time. Both are equally important for optimal health and athletic performance.

While muscular strength can be assessed independently of muscular endurance to some degree, the determination of one's muscular endurance can also measure one's strength. It's important that you pay particular attention to and give careful consideration of your client's health and fitness before you choose a specific muscular strength test. The lower-weight higher-repetition muscular endurance tests are more appropriate for less fit persons and those with more health-related exercise strength goals, especially if they have been previously inactive. Two common endurance tests that are both reliable and easy to administer are the one-minute timed sit-up test and the push-up test (Figure 27-8a, b[on p. 343], and c [on p. 344]). Another endurance test is the bench-press test (Figure 27-9 on p. 344). It's an absolute test of muscular endurance, meaning that the weight used is standardized, and therefore, results do not vary as a function of body weight.

Procedure for Completing the Sit-Up Test

The procedure for assisting your client to complete the timed sit-up test includes the following:

1. Instruct your client to lie face up with the knees bent at right angles and the heels about 18 inches from the buttocks; the fingers should be placed next to the ears.
2. Inform your client not to pull on the neck or head and to make sure the buttocks are kept on the mat; this will help to avoid any possibility of neck injury or discomfort.
3. Hold your client's ankles firmly so that the feet are kept in contact with the floor; then count the number of sit-ups performed for one full minute. A complete sit-up is defined as each time the person's shoulders touch the floor.

Procedure for Completing Push-Up Test

The purpose of performing a timed push-up test is to assess your client's endurance and strength of his or her triceps, anterior deltoids, and pectoralis major. The push-up position is different for men than for women. Men use the push-up position with only the hands and

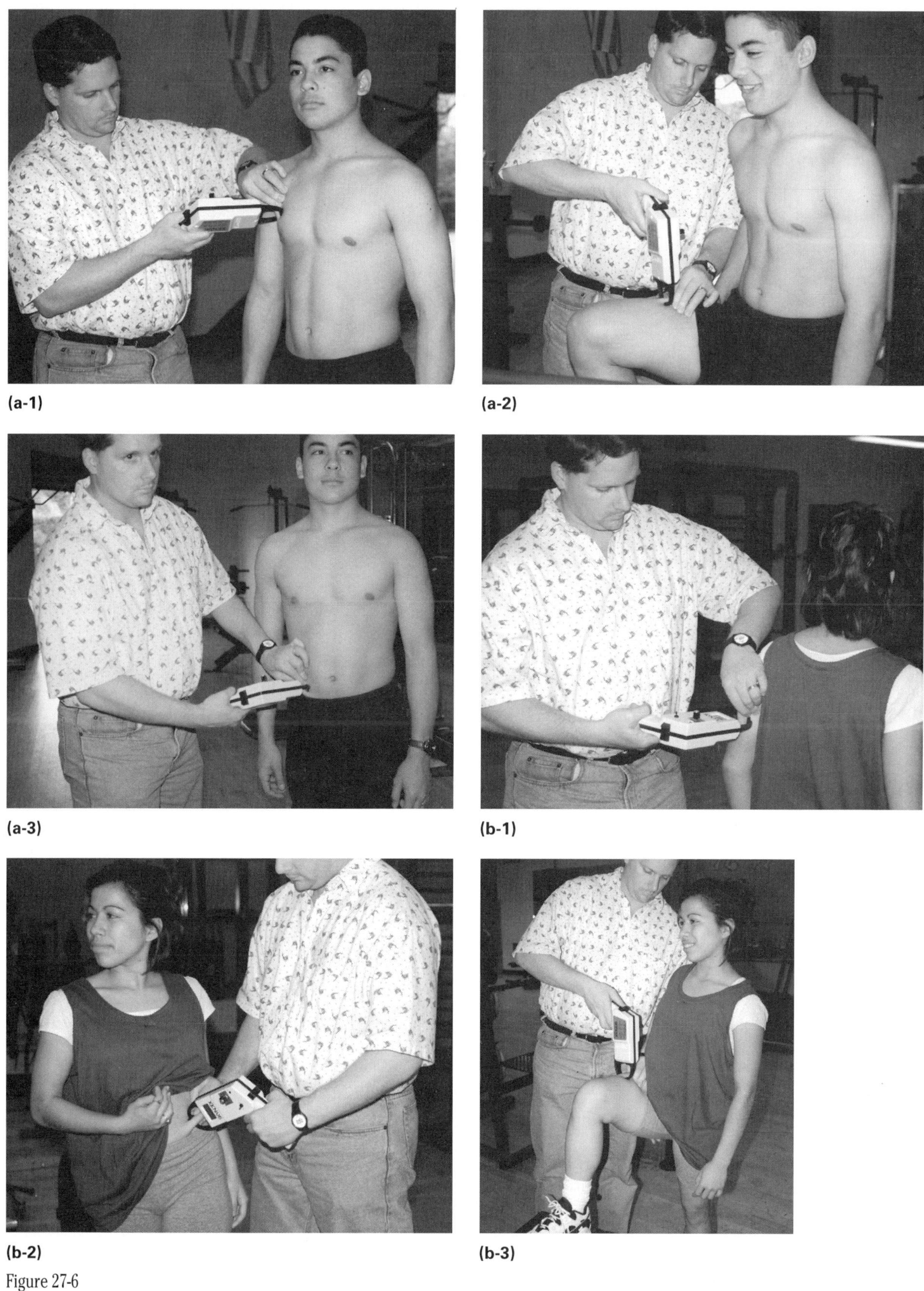

Figure 27-6
(a) Skinfold sites for men; (b) skinfold sites for women.

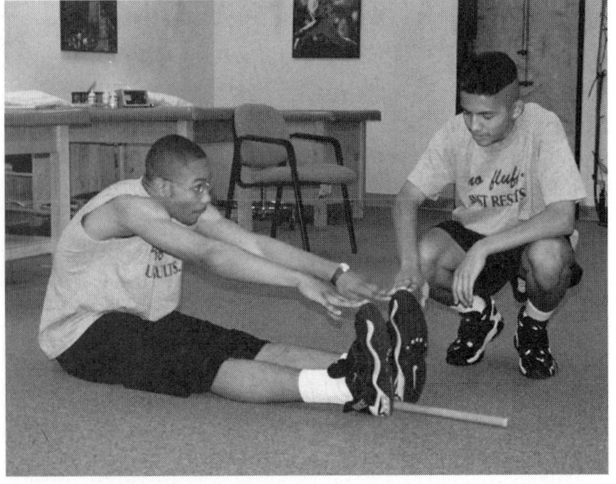

(a-1)

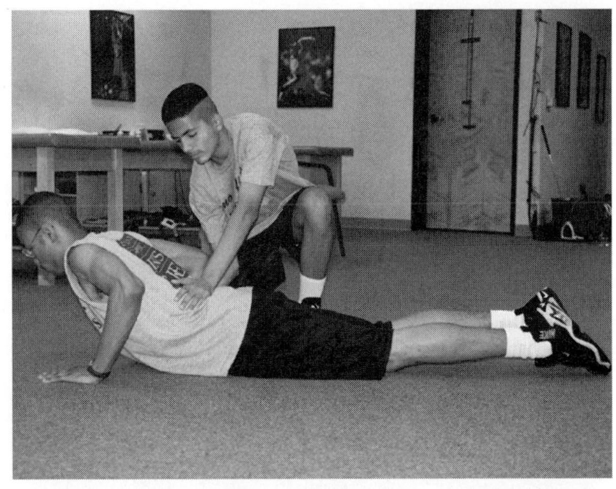

(a-2)

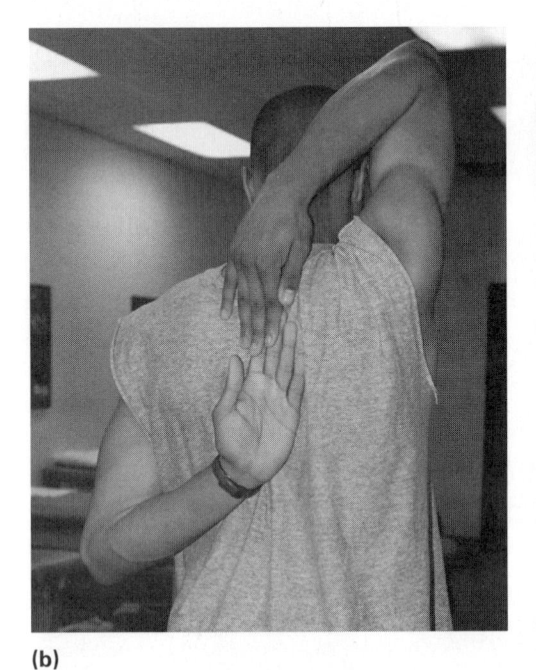

(b)

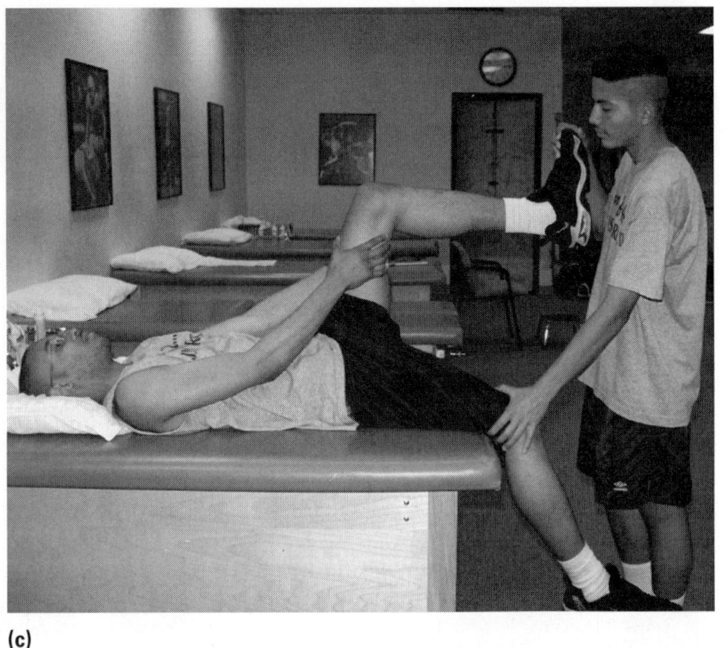

(c)

Figure 27-7
(a) Sit-and-reach flexibility test for trunk flexion; (b) assessing flexibility of the shoulder; (c) assessing flexibility of the hip.

toes in contact with the floor, while women use the bent-knee position. To assist your client in completing the timed push-up test, you should:

1. Instruct your client to assume an appropriate up position, with the body rigid and the hands about shoulder-width apart. Make sure that the client remains rigid throughout the motion, and that the chest comes within three inches of the floor.
2. Place your fist beneath the client's chest. This will serve as a guide for the client.
3. Score the test by adding up the total number of push-ups which have been performed to the point of exhaustion.

Procedure for Completing Bench-Press Test

The bench-press test using standardized weight is an excellent method for testing the endurance and strength of your client's chest and shoulders. However, the disadvantage of using this test is that it uses a fixed weight which can often be a drawback for

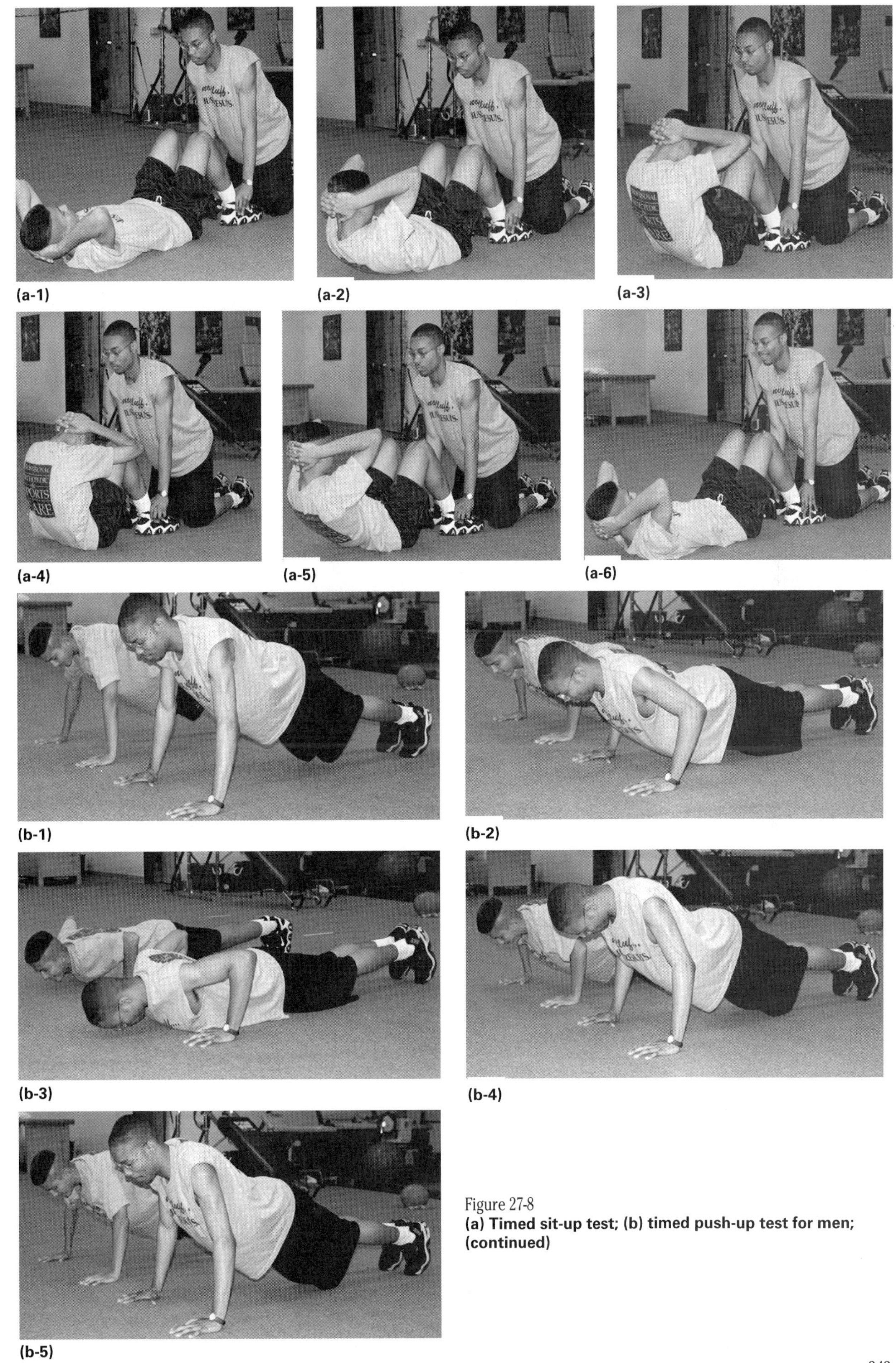

Figure 27-8
(a) Timed sit-up test; (b) timed push-up test for men; (continued)

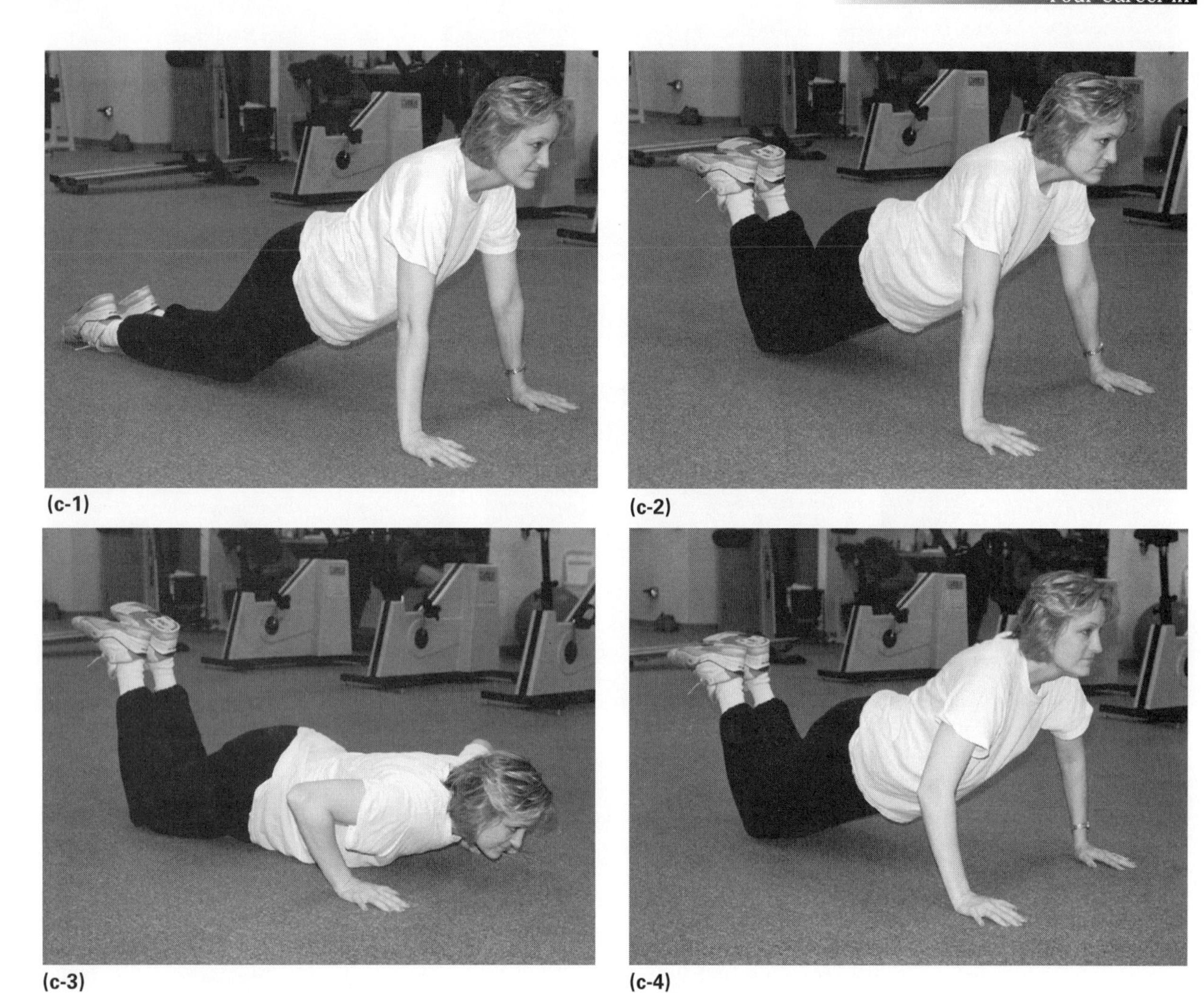

Figure 27-8 (continued)
(c) timed push-up test for women.

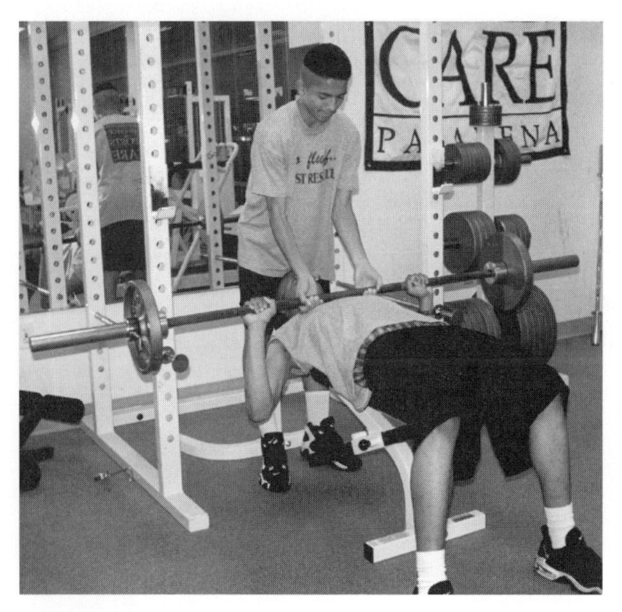

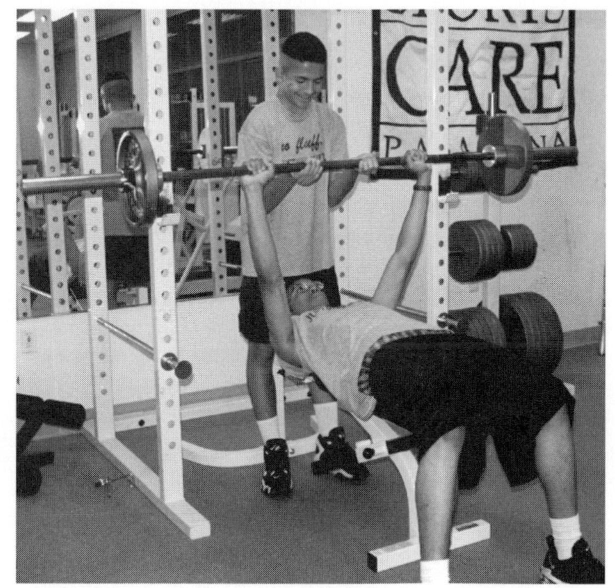

Figure 27-9
The bench-press test.

your client. To assist your client in completing the bench-press test, you should:

1. Make sure you use the appropriate weight barbell; for men, you should use an 80-pound barbell; for women, use a 35-pound barbell.
2. Instruct a spotter to be present during the test. If no one is available, do not allow your client to perform the test.
3. Set a metronome to 60 beats per minute.
4. Instruct the spotter to hand the weight to your client in the down position, that is, with the elbows flexed and the hands shoulder-width apart.
5. Before allowing your client to begin, he or she should be informed that an up or down movement should be in time to a 60-beats-per-minute rhythm; this would equal 30 lifts per minute.
6. Count each repetition when the client's elbows are fully extended. After each extension, the bar should be lowered to touch the chest.
7. You should terminate the test when your client is unable to come to a full extension or when he or she falls behind the 60 beats per minute rhythm.

Providing the Client with Follow-Up Data and Results

Following testing and evaluation, it's important to provide your client with their results. Ideally, this should involve a consultation regarding data you obtained from the testing and evaluation exercises, as well as information pertaining to any future testing or training sessions. You should inform your client that the frequency in which follow-up testing occurs greatly depends upon the quality and quantity of the exercise training, as well as the design of the testing and training program being offered. While many people begin to feel the positive effects of exercise and physical training in a relatively short period of time, for others, measurable changes can often take as long as four to twelve weeks. For that reason, the first follow-up session with your client should not be scheduled until he or she has reached at least the four-week point.

Summary

In this chapter, we discussed the importance of testing and evaluation as a foundation for a well-designed exercise and fitness training program. We determined that a valid testing and evaluation program should include ways in which to assess a person's cardiorespiratory efficiency, muscular strength and endurance, flexibility, and body composition.

Review Questions

1. What does the term *auscultation* mean?
2. What does the term *palpation* mean?
3. Briefly explain the difference between muscular endurance and muscular strength.
4. When is blood pressure considered abnormally high?
5. What is the name of a test which is routinely done to assess cardiovascular fitness?
6. ____________ ____________ refers to the quality or makeup of total body mass.
7. Why is it important to obtain a client's exercise history and attitude questionnaire before initiating any exercise or fitness training program?
8. Briefly explain how to determine a resting heart rate and a resting pulse rate.

28

Fitness Program Design and Implementation

Performance Objectives

Upon completion of this chapter, you will be able to:

1. Identify and discuss factors which must be considered when designing a fitness or exercise training program.
2. Discuss the signs of overtraining or overexercising.
3. Design a fitness workout program which can provide a client with the appropriate techniques and information necessary to maintain his or her lifestyle.

Terms and Abbreviations

Lean body mass fat-free weight.

Personal trainer an exercise professional who works with a variety of clients with different goals, likes, and dislikes in designing fitness or exercise programs which specifically meet the individual needs and lifestyle of each client.

As we discussed earlier in this text, your goal as a personal fitness or exercise trainer is to help your client develop an individualized program designed to meet his or her specific lifestyle. In order to do this, you must be able to take all the knowledge and hands-on techniques which you have learned in your own training, and apply them to meeting the needs of your client. As a personal trainer, you must have the ability to work with many different clients, each with their own unique set of goals, and each with his or her reasons for undertaking an exercise program. Therefore, it would be almost impossible for you to design one or even several exercise programs and then expect them to meet the individual needs of each and every one of your clients.

Every one of us, assuming that we are healthy and free of disease, is capable of achieving some level of competency in an exercise or fitness program. As a trainer, your responsibility is to assess your client's current state of fitness through a system of screening and evaluation, identifying measurable and realistic goals, and ultimately, developing a training program that is capable of aiding the person's accomplishment of those goals.

Designing an Individualized Program

When designing an individualized training or exercise program as a *personal trainer,* it's important for you to consider the basic physiological or biological components of fitness. As we discussed in Chapter 27, these components include cardiovascular endurance, muscular strength and endurance, flexibility, and body composition. Since each of your clients comes to you with varying degrees of these components, your task will be to design a program that addresses the client's greatest needs, while at the same time remaining aware of other areas.

Another important factor which you should be

concerned with when designing an individualized training program is that each and every one of your clients comes to you with their own reasons or goals for taking part in an exercise program. However, part of the conflict which the client often faces is that his or her reasons may not be in sync with his or her needs. When this occurs, part of your responsibility is to educate your client to help him or her understand the importance of adding appropriate exercises or deleting others.

Factors Involved in Designing the Program

In designing a good program of exercise, as we have previously noted, there are four areas which we must take into consideration: cardiovascular fitness and endurance, muscular strength and endurance, flexibility, and body composition.

Cardiovascular Fitness and Endurance

Cardiovascular fitness involves assisting your client with exercises that help increase the functional capacity of a person's heart, lungs, and blood vessels, so that oxygenated blood can be transported throughout the body. These exercises are also capable of offering us additional benefits, such as aiding in weight control and control of blood pressure.

When designing a program that meets the requirements necessary for cardiovascular endurance, the most important factors to consider are the mode, intensity, duration, and frequency of the activity. When considering the depth or intensity of cardiovascular activities, you should not overlook the principles of overload and specificity. The exercises should be aerobic; to qualify as aerobic exercises, they must involve continuous, rhythmical, and sustained movements using large muscle groups. These types of activities often include brisk walking, swimming, stair climbing, cycling, and various recreational activities which can be performed continuously with few or no periods of rest.

After you have completed designing a program of exercises which meets the standards of the cardiovascular component, you must also teach your client how to monitor his or her performance of its intensity. Remember, it's often quite difficult for a client just beginning a program to gauge the amount of intensity correctly. Therefore, you should talk to your client about using individualized exercise target heart rate zones, and subjective ratings of the amount of action or exercise which may be needed to complete the program in a safe and efficient manner.

Muscle Strength and Endurance

In addition to meeting the needs of your client's cardiovascular system, the program which you design for him or her must also take the musculoskeletal system into consideration. Sufficient maintenance of a person's muscular tone and strength will assist him or her with meeting such goals as reducing one's risk of musculoskeletal injuries, weight reduction, improvement in physique and posture, and achieving greater endurance in both daily and athletic activities.

Meeting the musculoskeletal component of a good exercise program involves understanding seven important principles. These include always making sure that safety is of primary concern; training each body segment independently by working it against a resistance capable of overloading the muscles; planning an exercise so that it can be performed throughout its full range of motion; ensuring that the speed in which your client performs an exercise is slow and controlled; creating an exercise program that is well balanced between agonistic and antagonistic muscle groups; preventing injuries by training those muscle groups requiring special attention because of daily misuse, athletic pursuits, and muscular imbalances; and also, providing at least one day of rest between workouts of the same muscle groups. And, just as in designing exercises which help in cardiovascular endurance, when you develop a musculoskeletal program, you must also consider the variables of intensity and the number of repetitions and sets.

Finally, when designing a good musculoskeletal training program, you should also take into account how many muscle groups will need to be exercised and the length of time required for each session exercising these groups. To determine this, you will first have to decide which type of training method you should use to help overload each muscle group. The three methods include free weights, weight machines, and body-weight, or calisthenic, exercises.

Ultimately, the training program should consider not only your client's initial workouts, but also the potential progression of the routine as he or she begins to achieve intermediate goals. Progression takes many forms, from adding exercises to a program, to increasing the amount of resistance and altering repetitions, sets, frequencies, and durations of specific activities. Regardless of the method you choose to use, it's both essential and critical that you always address the need for change and variety in a client's program.

Flexibility

Adequate muscular flexibility is extremely important in both preventing injuries and in maintaining one's range of motion. Unfortunately, however, it is often overlooked or underemphasized when designing a good and well-balanced fitness or exercise program. When considering one's overall level of fitness, most people generally think of flexibility in the same way they think of muscular strength or cardiovascular endurance. Also, since flexibility is unique to each individual joint, it cannot easily be improved or maintained by simply performing one or two quick stretches. As a fitness trainer, it's essential that you include flexibility training as part of your client's program so that you can create a balance between muscle groups that might be otherwise overused during physical training sessions or subject to chronic tightness due to a person's daily activity or inactivity. And it's also important to consider not only the muscles and subsequent joints being exercised, but your client's limitations and goals as well. A good flexibility program should include all major muscle groups.

When incorporating flexibility into your client's program, there are some basic principles which you should understand. First of all, it's important to understand that all muscles and tendons seem to stretch better when they have been properly warmed up. To ensure this, the best way is to have your client stretch after five to ten minutes of light aerobic warm-up and/or at the completion of the training session. Next, always make sure you isolate each muscle or muscle group. Remember, your client should not be allowed to stretch in a manner that will put unnecessary or undue strain on his or her ligaments or joints. A third principle is that you should always recommend slow, passive, static stretching. Static stretching involves a slow, gradual, and controlled elongation of the muscles. Ballistic or dynamic stretching is hardly ever recommended, since it incorporates an action which uses higher force and shorter duration. Another point to remember is that when your client performs a static stretch, it should only be to the degree in which he or she feels tension in the muscle, not pain. That means that the stretch must be held no more than 15 to 30 seconds. Finally, when performing flexibility stretches, the client should be instructed to do no more than three to five repetitions of each stretch.

Body Composition

Because one of the most common goals of a good exercise program is weight reduction, body composition is usually considered the final component of a well-balanced and health-related program. As we discussed earlier in the text, body composition is composed of both *lean body mass* and body fat. If your client's primary goal is to lose weight, you should design a program that will generate a negative caloric balance so that he or she is expending more calories than are being consumed. Since aerobic exercises often burn the most calories, usually between 300 to 500 calories per activity session, you should recommend that your client engage in these types of activities up to five times a week. For all intents and purposes, to lose one pound of body fat, he or she must have a negative caloric balance of at least 3,500 calories. Taking part in aerobic exercise for the recommended time will have the greatest impact on helping your client to lose the weight he or she desires.

Most physicians agree that exercise must be an important part of any good weight-loss program to maintain lean tissue. The strengthening component of the workout will also increase lean tissue that may have been lost during sedentary activity, dieting, injury, or immobilization. Not only does exercise increase the amount of lean tissue a person may have lost living a sedentary lifestyle or going up and down the dieting scale, but it also improves a person's muscle tone and appearance. And if your client likes the way he or she looks after losing body fat, there may be more incentive to keep up his or her newly acquired health habits to maintain that new and healthier looking appearance.

Signs of Client Overtraining

Just as important in designing a well-balanced fitness or exercise program is your responsibility in assessing your client's progress and being aware of the potential for signs and symptoms of overtraining. While you may find that some of your clients seem challenged to work hard at their program, others, in their quest to achieve their goals more quickly, may be overzealous and drive their body too hard. Therefore, it's important that you be attentive to this potential problem and communicate with your client about any noticed signs of discomfort or overtraining.

While many people believe the "no pain, no gain" theory of exercise, following such a hypothesis can often lead a person to symptoms of overtraining and injuries. As such, part of your responsibility is to educate your clients about the most sensible approach to exercise. This includes informing the person about the importance of obtaining proper rest and in working a program that is appropriate in its intensity, duration, and frequency. It also involves being aware of your client's susceptibility to such irregularities as insomnia, irritability, loss of appetite, fatigue, depression, and elevated pulse and blood pressure.

Designing a Workout Program

Each of your clients should expect an exercise or training program that is tailored specifically to meet his or her individual needs. This can only be done by obtaining data and information from your client's health screening and fitness evaluation. From this information, your task is to choose an appropriate beginning workload or exercise program that is consistent with your client's health and level of fitness.

When designing the program, it's also important to consider the type of equipment and facility options which may or may not be available to your client. Moreover, you must be able to recognize your own limitations. This means never attempting to show a client how to complete an exercise or use a specific type of equipment unless you are fully skilled with it yourself. Likewise, since clients often view their trainer as a role model, you must use caution to ensure that your clients do not try to do too much too soon in an effort to be just like their trainer. Rather, you should encourage your clients to work at their own levels, always emphasizing the fact that every person has his or her own set of exercise goals and abilities. Also, never assume that your client knows what to do. Remember, it's your responsibility to teach the client, spot the client, and do whatever it takes to ensure his or her safety. That means always designing a program that will not put your client at undue risk.

In addition to creating a program or workout session that is safe and effective, you should also have a specific goal for each of the exercises designed in your client's program. They should be varied to keep both yourself and your client interested in the training, and creative, using different options and combinations. Listed below are some examples of routines that are both safe and creative, and which you can use to accomplish your client's goals.

Routine #1

- **15-Minute Warm-Up:** These can include aerobic activities such as walking and cycling. During the 15 minutes, your client can spend either the entire time on one piece of equipment, or use several, or engage in a combination of both.
- **35-Minute Strength Training:** The client can use either manual or weight resistance to train first the upper body, then the lower. This can be reversed at the next session.
- **10-Minute Cool-Down:** Have your client perform some gentle cycling or walking, followed by stretching of the exercised muscle groups.

Routine #2

- **30-Minute Aerobic Training:** This includes having the client gradually warm up, focusing on one or more aerobic activities. Examples might include instructing the client to first work the upper and lower body by cycling for 10 minutes, and then jog on a treadmill for 30 minutes.
- **20-Minute Strength Training:** Have your client perform a variety of body-weight exercises, such as push-ups and floor exercises.
- **10-Minute Flexibility Training:** Have your client complete the workout by stretching all the major muscle groups, or the specific muscle groups that were emphasized in the work-out.

Routine #3

- **10-Minute Warm-Up:** Have the client work on cardiovascular equipment, followed by a brief stretching period prior to starting the next phase of the workout.
- **40-Minute Circuit Training:** Have the client progress from one weight machine to the next, performing 15 to 20 repetitions at each station and then quickly moving on to the next station. Then have your client alternate between strength-training stations and cardiovascular stations.
- **10-Minute Cool-Down:** Have your client do gentle walking or cycling followed by flexibility exercises.

Summary

In this chapter, we discussed the role of the fitness trainer in providing his or her clients with a program that is both well balanced and which meets the specific needs and lifestyle of the individual person. We did this by identifying and then discussing the factors involved in designing a fitness or exercise training program. We also explained how to look for signs and symptoms of client overtraining and overexercising. Finally, we completed our discussion by looking at some examples of fitness programs designed to provide a client with the appropriate techniques and information necessary to maintain his or her lifestyle.

Review Questions

1. What is meant by *lean body mass*?
2. Why is it important to design an individualized exercise program for a client?
3. Briefly explain the factors involved in designing an exercise or fitness training program.
4. What is involved in meeting the musculoskeletal component of a good exercise program?
5. Why is it important to know a client's body composition when designing an exercise or fitness training program?
6. Give at least one example of a sign that the client may be overtraining.
7. Give an example of a routine exercise program which covers aerobic training.
8. Give an example of a routine exercise program which covers strength training.
9. Why is it important to provide the client with a warm-up exercise and a cool-down exercise?

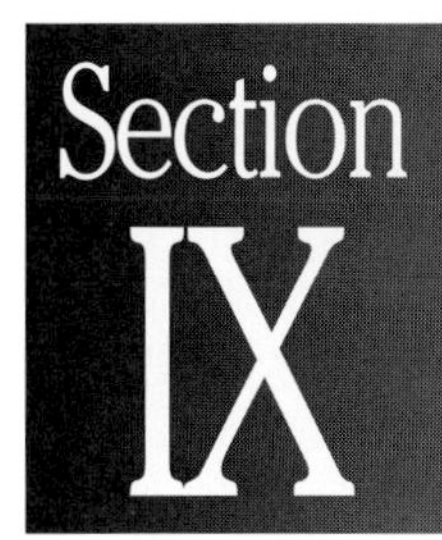

Administrative Skills in Physical Medicine: Basic Concepts and Applications

29

Administrative Management and Office Maintenance

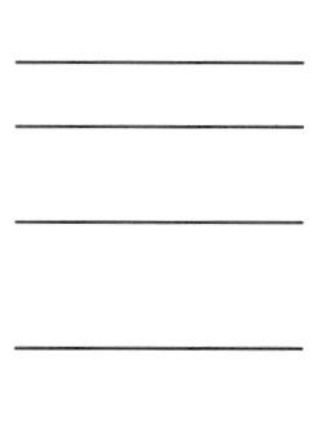

Performance Objectives

Upon completion of this chapter, you will be able to:

1. Discuss factors which influence the effectiveness of an administrative medical office environment.
2. Describe the purpose of maintaining all areas within a health care facility or medical office.
3. Explain why it is important to follow an equipment maintenance program.
4. Discuss the purpose and function of a supply and inventory ordering system.
5. Identify responsibilities of the physical medicine worker as they relate to drugs and their storage in a department or health care facility.
6. Discuss the purpose and function of a department office procedure manual.

Terms and Abbreviations

Inventory a list of all supplies and equipment on hand in an individual department or health care facility, usually updated either on a monthly or annual basis.

Office procedure manual a written guide kept in an individual department, a private medical office, or a health care facility which provides information related to all office procedures and routines.

PDR abbreviation for *Physician's Desk Reference,* a guide to pharmaceutical drugs.

Preventative maintenance a maintenance contract which can be purchased for specific equipment, in which a service person comes to the department or facility on a regular basis to check the equipment; if necessary, make minor adjustments; and repair the equipment as needed.

Whether you are employed in an individual department within a health care facility or by a private medical doctor, chiropractor, or a specialty physical therapy or rehabilitation center, you should understand that care for the physical environment in which you work is the responsibility of all members of the staff. A facility that is lit adequately and maintains a temperature which is comfortable and pleasant to all members of the staff and the patients is a healthy and enjoyable place to work.

As you progress through your career in physical medicine, you may be given the opportunity to manage a department, or even a private practice. If you can show your supervisor that you possess both the leadership qualities required of a supervisor, and the commitment to not only perform your job, but just as important, increase the productivity of both your work and your employer, you may find yourself in a very exciting and rewarding management position.

Physical Maintenance of the Health Care Environment

Maintenance of both a healthy and a comfortable environment is a task often delegated to the administrative medical worker; however, in most individual departments within a hospital or clinic it also becomes the responsibility of all health care team members. As a member of this team, it's important for you to be sensitive not only to the basic housekeeping duties of the facility, but to other factors that influence both the staff and the patients in their quest to feel comfortable in the facility.

When dealing with the physical maintenance of a health care facility, there are four areas which you must be concerned with. These include lighting, sound, temperature, and flooring.

All health care facilities require excellent lighting to perform the daily tasks required of the facility. The best lighting is uniform, as in the case of most medical facilities, which utilize fluorescent lights. If you are working for a private physician or chiropractor, you may want to maintain the reception area by using separate lamps strategically placed throughout the area. If you are using separate lamps, you must also remember to place them at reading level, where the light will not shine into the eyes of the reader or other patients waiting to see the doctor.

In planning an effective maintenance program for your department or office, you will also need to ensure for the privacy of all patients coming into the facility. This means maintaining a facility in which there is adequate soundproofing of walls to prevent confidences between patients and medical staff from being overheard. If you find that talking and conversations can be heard through the walls or between treatment or examination rooms, you will need to be sensitive to it, and let your supervisor or the doctor know as soon as possible.

Another aspect of patient comfort in an individual department or a private health care facility has to do with the proper maintenance of the facility's temperature. For most facilities, 70 degrees F seems to be the optimum temperature for the patient reception area. If your facility or department treats a number of senior citizens, you may want to recommend that the office be kept a little warmer. It's also important to maintain the correct flow of air throughout the facility. Air should be kept circulating, either by an air conditioning system or by open windows. You must, however, be careful not to allow drafts to enter the facility, as patients don't tolerate drafts well and may become quite uncomfortable.

The last area dealing with the physical maintenance of your facility is ensuring the adequacy of your facility's flooring. In most cases, carpeting is used to cover the floor in a reception room and office area. In treatment and examination rooms, however, washable flooring is used for hygienic purposes. In areas which are not covered by carpeting, it is important to make sure that floors are not slippery, which could cause either patients or staff to slip and fall. Additionally, it is never a good idea to use rugs in the treatment or exam rooms, especially if they are not tacked down, since they can easily move, increasing the possibility of trips or falls.

Cleaning and Maintenance

As a professional health care provider, your duties will not include responsibility for the heavy-duty cleaning of your facility; however, you may be responsible for performing basic cleaning tasks which involve the maintenance and "top cleaning" of reception and administrative areas, the clinical areas, such as the lab, examination, and treatment rooms, the restrooms, and storage areas. These tasks may involve picking up toys and magazines in the reception area and performing minor housekeeping duties that keep the reception area clean, tidy, pleasant, and free from odors.

If your job also includes basic maintenance and cleaning of other administrative and clinical areas, you will need to consult with your supervisor as to what is required. You may be responsible for the reception desk, the telephone, various business machines, and record storage areas. If this is indeed the case, you should use great care to make sure that steps are taken to keep desks neat and items are not moved out of their original place. All records should be kept out of sight of patients to assure complete privacy. Remember, an organized and well-maintained office gives both your patients and your co-workers the immediate impression that you are in control and that your facility runs in an efficient and effective manner.

Maintaining the Clinical Areas

Maintaining the clinical areas of a department or a private health care facility generally involves the basic cleaning and organization of treatment and examination rooms, medical and physical therapy equipment rooms, the laboratory, restrooms, and storage areas. There is nothing more upsetting and utterly devastating to a patient who may already be anxious than being ushered into a treatment or examination room that is disorganized or dirty. This means taking responsibility for seeing to the appropriate cleaning and removal of specimens of prior patients before new ones enter the room, providing areas which are spotless and free of clutter, such as soiled linen, towels, and tissues, and making sure that all examining tables have clean, fresh paper or linen on them before the patient enters the room.

One of the best and perhaps easiest ways to ensure the proper maintenance of your facility is to perform periodic checks of the facility's physical appearance and cleanliness. These periodic services generally include replacing light bulbs, cleaning out refrigerators, reorganizing cabinets and drawers, and watering plants. Most health care facilities have a specific plan for assigning such infrequent and basic tasks. Your responsibility will be to make sure that you are clear on what is assigned to you, and follow through when such duties are assigned.

Maintenance and Care of Equipment

If you are working in an individual department of a health care facility or are employed by a small private medical office, you may be responsible for monitoring the *preventative maintenance* agreements for equipment used by your facility. These agreements are usually kept in individual files, along with instructions for equipment maintenance, as well as operating instructions and invoices for repairs which might be necessary.

Another aspect of maintaining and caring for equipment has to do with keeping control over supplies used in the facility. Most facilities have a variety of supplies that need to be counted, or inventoried, on a monthly or annual basis. An *inventory* is a listing of all equipment and supplies found in the facility, and contains valuable information which may be needed for preparing income taxes and other information which might be necessary regarding equipment which has been stolen or damaged as a result of a fire, earthquake, or water damage.

The time at which an inventory is taken will depend upon the needs of your individual facility. In most cases, all capital purchases, such as furniture, medical equipment and instruments, laboratory equipment, office machines, and large decor items such as wall paintings, are inventoried on an annual basis. Other smaller, less costly items, may be inventoried more frequently.

All inventory systems generally include a method of ordering supplies. If you are responsible for completing the inventory, chances are that you will also be responsible for ordering supplies. Most of these supplies are itemized into three categories: office supplies, which include stationery, accounting supplies, desk items, and appointment materials; medical supplies, which include such disposable items as gowns, drapes, towels, lubricants, tongue blades, syringes and needles, bandages, and in some cases, medications; and general supplies, which usually consist of such items as soap and towels for the restrooms, tissues, cleaning supplies, and coffee for the employees.

It's important to keep separate forms for each individual category of supplies. Each form should provide you with information and space for diminishing supplies, so that you will know when it's time to reorder. Oftentimes, salespeople, or "detail" men or women, will come by your department or office, which will make your ordering a great deal easier. Mail-order houses are also available which allow you to make orders over the telephone.

Maintenance and Storage of Drugs and Medications

Depending upon your position and employer, in some rare instances you may be responsible for the proper maintenance and storage of drugs and medications used in your facility. This is often the case in situations where the physical medicine worker is employed by a clinic or a private medical office. If you are responsible for maintaining the storage of drugs and medications, you should start by keeping an accurate inventory of what is on hand, making sure that all drugs are accounted for, and that supplies do not run out. This may mean that you may also be in charge of contacting a pharmacy or drug salesperson to place an order.

Some smaller medical offices keep a low inventory of drugs and medications and generally rely on free samples provided to them by drug companies. Other offices, such as those not as accessible to the drug supplier may keep larger inventories. Drug and medication supplies in hospitals are often kept in a locked drug cart or storage area within the nursing station.

In many cases, different drug companies may provide your facility with their own ordering system. Their salespeople, who are often referred to as "pharmaceutical representatives" or "detail representatives," can be given access to the drug storage area and stock the drugs themselves. If your department or facility does not allow this practice, you may be responsible for restocking and checking the expiration dates to make sure that your facility is not giving out expired medications. If a patient has a drug reaction and notices that the drug has expired, there is great potential for a lawsuit.

Depending upon your job duties and responsibilities, you may also be responsible for organizing the drug storage area. All drugs can be organized by their name in an alphabetical system. They can also be organized according to the system listed in the index to the *PDR,* or *Physician's Desk Reference.* Categories in the *PDR* include analgesics, antiemetics, cardiogenics, antibiotics, and so on.

No matter where you work, accidents do happen, and the storage and usage of drugs and medications in the health care facility is no exception. If, for example, during storage a drug's label is accidently removed, the drug and its package should be immediately discarded. Most can either be poured down a drain or flushed down the toilet. They should never be left in the trash where unauthorized people can easily take them. Of course, when drugs are discarded, you must always keep a careful record as to their disposal.

Maintaining the Office Procedure Manual

All health care facilities, individual departments, and private medical and chiropractic offices, keep *procedure manuals* which provide important information regarding everything from office tasks to in-depth instructions for performing various clinical treatments and procedures. An office manual must be kept up to date, and doing so is often the responsibility of the office or department manager. In addition to providing information regarding how specific procedures are performed, manuals often contain job descriptions to help guide each staff member in performing specific tasks. A well-designed manual makes clear to all employees what exactly is expected of them. It is also a valuable document for training new employees and can provide assistance to a substitute employee.

Updating of all office and procedure manuals, including job descriptions, is mandatory in our rapidly changing health care environments. If you are responsible for maintaining these manuals, you should ask each staff member to assist you by updating his or her assignment listings. Remember, that suggestions from the entire staff can be used to create the most current manual possible.

Summary

In this chapter, we discussed the factors which most effectively influence the efficiency of the administrative medical office environment, noting that maintenance of the facility is the key to efficiency of a smooth-running facility. We also talked about how such maintenance is performed, including how to maintain the physical and hygenic appearance of the facility, how to maintain a running inventory and ordering system for supplies and equipment, and how to properly store and order drugs and medications. Finally, we discussed the importance of the office procedure manual, noting that such manuals must be kept updated as to job descriptions, employee tasks, and instructions pertaining to specific procedures and treatments, on a regular, ongoing basis.

Review Questions

1. What does the abbreviation *PDR* mean?
2. Briefly explain the concept of preventative maintenance.
3. A ______________ is a list of all supplies and equipment on hand in an individual department or health care facility, and which is usually updated either on a monthly or annual basis.
4. Briefly explain the maintenance and storage of drugs and medications in a department or private medical office.
5. What is the purpose of an office procedure manual?
6. Who is generally responsible for maintaining the office procedure manual?

30

Billing and Banking Procedures

Performance Objectives

Upon completion of this chapter, you will be able to:

1. Discuss the purpose of banking procedures used in the health care environment.
2. Describe and be able to demonstrate basic bookkeeping and billing principles and procedures used in the health care environment.
3. Identify the basic duties of the health care provider responsible for billing and banking procedures in the health care facility.

Terms and Abbreviations

A/C abbreviation for accounts payable, a term for amounts which are owed to a creditor for regular business operating expenses.

A/R abbreviation for accounts receivable, a term for claims which arise from services rendered.

Assignment of benefits an agreement by which a patient agrees to assign all insurance benefits to another party, usually a medical care provider.

ATM abbreviation for automated teller machine, a machine installed on the outside of a bank or other facility, allowing for deposits and withdrawals 24 hours a day.

Bank statement a periodic list of transactions of a checking or savings account.

Bill a statement of fees owed by a patient for services rendered.

Bookkeeping the analysis and recording of business transactions which are necessary to report the financial condition of a business at a later date.

Check an order for a bank to pay against an existing checking account.

Checking account an account against which checks can be written, often with no interest being paid.

Computerized system a type of bookkeeping system utilizing a batch-type service or telephone linked shared service.

Cycle billing a billing procedure in which itemized statements are sent to patients according to an alphabetical breakdown.

Daily record a record of daily business transactions; also called a daybook or a daysheet.

Deposit slip a form used to itemize deposits made to a bank.

Disbursement record the chronological listing of monthly and yearly business expenses.

Double-entry system a type of bookkeeping system that involves the maintenance of equality of both debits and credits.

Endorsement the process of signing one's name or the name of a business on the back of a check, indicating that all rights in the check are transferred to another party.

General ledger a record containing all financial statement accounts.

ICD-9-CM Codes abbreviation for *International Classification of Diseases, 9th Edition, Clinical Modification,* which is a coding system for classifying diseases and diagnoses.

Medicare a government health insurance program which provides coverage for people over the age of 65, and others with specific disabilities.

Pegboard system a type of bookkeeping system used in most health care facilities, which uses a lightweight board with pegs and forms layered one on top of the other.

Petty cash a small amount of cash kept in a health care facility, which should only be available for small office expenses.

Service charge a charge authorized by a banking institution used for the purpose of maintaining accounts and processing transactions.

Single-entry system a type of simple bookkeeping system which uses a daily record, checkbook, and an accounts receivable ledger.

Skip a patient who has an outstanding bill, and who disappears, leaving no forwarding address.

Superbill a comprehensive list of examinations, procedures, and treatments, and the corresponding fee listing, which a patient receives for services rendered.

Withholding deductions made by an employer from an employee's paycheck.

If you find yourself employed by a health care facility or a clinical department which treats a large number of patients, and you discover that part of your job description also includes billing, banking, and insurance processing, you will soon realize that being involved in this aspect of health care is perhaps one of the most challenging, and in some cases, most difficult tasks which may be required of your position.

In the health care industry, we often say that the person who takes care of the billing and banking is worth his or her weight in gold! For it is this person who is most responsible for ensuring the monetary livelihood of all the members of the health care team. This includes the doctor, the clinical and administrative staff, and yes, even yourself! It is the billing and banking person whose sole task generally revolves around seeing to it that bills and statements are sent out to patients, owed monies are paid out to the appropriate people and organizations, and employees are paid for their services.

Principles of Bookkeeping in the Health Care Environment

It is impossible for any business, including the business of delivering health care, to function effectively and efficiently without well-kept financial records. And to be able to meet such a goal requires a person who is not only professional, but also one who is capable of paying attention to details, is well organized, and possesses the ability to maintain consistency throughout the completion of his or her workload.

If you are required to perform *bookkeeping* tasks in your facility, you must realize that to do so requires a well-established routine. You must also realize that there are certain guidelines, or principles, which are used in bookkeeping, and, if you follow these rules, you should be able to perform your responsibilities in an orderly and efficient manner. The key principles of bookkeeping include:

- Always record all charges and receipts into the *daily record* immediately upon receiving them.
- Always endorse all checks as soon as they are collected.
- Make sure you prepare receipts in duplicate for all currency received.
- Be sure you pay all facility bills before they are due, and remember to record the date the bill was paid and the check number on the paid bill receipt.
- Post all charges and receipts to the *general ledger* on a daily basis.
- Deposit all monies received on a daily basis.
- Check daily to make sure that the amount you have deposited in the bank, plus the money you have on hand in petty cash, equals the amount you have recorded in your daily ledger.
- Only use your petty cash fund for small expenses. Pay all other expenses by check, so that you will have an immediate record of the expenditure.
- Make all bookkeeping entries in ink, and always check your arithmetic to make sure you are keeping columns of figures straight and carrying decimals out correctly, and never rely completely on a calculator!
- Never erase an error. If you find you have made an error, draw a straight line through the incorrect figure and then rewrite the correct figure above it.

Bookkeeping Systems

There are four basic types of bookkeeping systems which are employed by most health care facilities. These include *computerized bookkeeping systems* which utilize either a batch type of service or a telephone linked service which is shared by others; a *single-entry system,* which is considered the easiest to use because it is often the basis for filing income tax returns; a *double-entry system,* which involves the concept of assets minus liabilities always equals net worth, and the *pegboard system,* considered the most popular of all the systems because of the ease with which bookkeeping procedures can be completed.

Accounts Receivable and Accounts Payable

All health care facilities must be concerned with accounts receivable and accounts payable. *Account receivables,* which are commonly referred to as *A/R,* are monies or claims which arise as a result of services rendered. *Accounts payable,* or *A/P,* deal with monies or claims which are owed to creditors for regular business operating expenses. When you are dealing with accounts receivable and accounts payable, you must also be concerned with the accounts receivable control, a summary performed on a daily basis of what remains unpaid on all the health care facility's accounts. An important point that you should remember, too, is that accounts receivable are an important and integral part of both the pegboard and the double-entry systems of bookkeeping;

however, when you are using the single-entry system, accounts receivable are always given separate consideration.

Whatever is spent by your facility must also be recorded on a daily basis. These amounts are generally itemized on a form called a *disbursement record.* This record usually has columns for the date, name of supplier or vendor, amount of the charge, amount of the check and check number, deposits, and bank balance. In most cases, there are also columns for putting in a category for every business expense, such as rent, taxes and licenses, dues and meetings, medical supplies and equipment, office expenses, utilities, travel, and employee payroll.

Petty Cash

If you work in a smaller, private health care facility, such as a doctor's office or a clinic, there's a very good possibility that the facility will have a *petty cash* fund set aside for small office expenses, such as parking, postage fees, and less frequently used office supplies. Money should never be taken out of this fund for major expenses.

If you are using a petty cash fund, you will probably use some type of petty cash voucher system, which will help you to control your expenditures. The voucher provides space to record the expenditure date, the amount paid, the purpose, and the name of the person to whom the payment has been made. All vouchers should also be numbered.

If you are required to handle petty cash, chances are that your supervisor or employer will request that you become bonded by an insurance company. This guarantees payment of a specified amount to an employer in the event of financial loss caused by an employee.

Payroll and Employee Deductions

Payroll procedures, like bookkeeping methods, can be handled in a variety of ways, depending upon the type and size of health care facility in which you are employed. Some institutions are set up for a bank to handle all payroll, while others may hire an accountant to process payroll. Larger institutions, such as hospitals and multi-specialty clinics, frequently have their payroll processed entirely by computer. This is often the method of choice for many facilities, because the computer is capable of not only issuing the payroll checks, but can also automatically calculate deductions for each individual employee.

If you are responsible for processing payroll, you will need to have a basic understanding of income tax laws and employment regulations. This means taking the time to learn about federal taxes, such as FICA, disability and unemployment insurance deductions, state tax deductions, and how to calculate an employee's gross salary into a net payroll check.

All payroll checks must include specific information regarding the employer's and employee's identification numbers, withholding allowance, FICA taxes, income tax deductions, unemployment compensation disability deductions, and unemployment taxes.

Employer's Identification Number and Employee's Withholding Allowance Certificate

An employer identification number is used for federal tax purposes. Form SS-4 from the Internal Revenue Service is filed to receive this number. The employees use their Social Security number as their individual identification number. If an employee has no Social Security number, he or she must apply for a number immediately.

Upon employment, each new person hired by your facility must complete an Employee's Withholding Allowance Certificate, also known as Form W-4. This form provides the employer with the number of exemptions claimed by the employee. Employees should be asked by December 1 of each year whether or not there has been a change in the number of exemptions since the last form filed the previous year.

FICA and Income Tax Deductions

The Federal Insurance Contributions Act, also known as Social Security, has three programs financed from one payroll tax in which employers and employees contribute at a rate as specified by the law. Old Age Survivors Insurance (OASI) provides senior citizens and their surviving dependents with retirement benefits, while *Medicare* provides them with hospitalization insurance. The Disability Insurance Program (SDI) provides all workers with insurance benefits due to disability during their working years.

Under federal law, all employers are required to *withhold* from their employees' salaries, an advance payment on income taxes. This money is remitted periodically to a regional Internal Revenue Service office.

Unemployment Compensation Disability and Unemployment Taxes

Unemployment compensation disability, a type of insurance policy that provides for temporary cash benefits to employees suffering a wage loss due to a nonwork-related injury or illness, are mandatory in some states. At the present time, these states include California, Hawaii, New Jersey, New York, Rhode Island, and Puerto Rico. About one percent of an employee's gross salary goes to unemployment compensation disability by way of a monthly deduction.

Under the Federal Unemployment Tax Act (FUTA), most employers pay a federal tax that is used for administrative costs of state employment programs. Employers may also be required to pay for a state unemployment tax program.

Preparing Tax Reports

Health care professionals who are responsible for processing employee's payroll are oftentimes involved in preparing the employer's tax reports. All health care facilities are required to prepare and file these reports, which are commonly referred to as an Employer's Federal Tax Return on a regular quarterly basis. The report must include the total number of employees, along with their names and social security numbers, the total wages paid, the amount of withholding tax paid, the amount of wages which are subject to FICA and the amount of FICA taxes which have been paid, the total periodic tax deposits, and the amount, if any, of underdeposited taxes which are due.

In addition to preparing the employer's tax report, you may also be required to prepare the employee annual reports. According to federal law, these reports, commonly referred to as Form W-2, Employee's Wage and Tax Statement, must be provided to the employee no later than January 31 for the previous tax year. The form must show the employer's identification number, the employee's social security number, the amount of total wages and other compensation, and the total income tax and social security tax paid in by the employee for the year preceding January 31.

Billing and Collection Procedures in the Health Care Environment

An important aspect of all health facilities is the proper billing and collection of fees for services rendered. Larger institutions, such as hospitals, have specially trained people and departments whose sole responsibility involves the billing and collection of patient fees. Smaller facilities, such as private physicians' offices and urgent care centers, frequently designate a member of the administrative staff to be responsible for billing and banking procedures. If you find yourself in the position of having to *bill* or collect payments from your patients, it's important that you become knowledgeable in just how such a task is completed.

The effective use of interpersonal skills and tactfulness are essential in dealing with issues involved in billing and collection. This involves being businesslike in your dealings with patients, particularly in cases in which patients may be having difficulties in paying for their health care services.

Internal and External Billing Practices

Most health care facilities use one of two ways to bill patients. The first method involves handling the billing procedures within the health care facility where the patient was seen or treated. This is called internal billing. Internal billing can be very simple, as in the case of billing in a small private doctor's office, or it can be very difficult and complex, as in the case of a large hospital which may employ a fully computerized billing system.

Some facilities may choose an external billing system, in which the institution hires an outside service to handle all patient accounts. A major advantage of the external billing system is that it cuts out much of the time-consuming tasks involved in billing.

No matter which system of billing is employed by your facility, completeness and accuracy are the keys to a successful billing and collection program. This means that all information pertaining to the patient's name, address, telephone number, health insurance coverage, and medical history must be secured at the time the patient is first seen by your facility, since all of this will be necessary at the time of billing. Most of the data obtained from the patient's registration form can provide you with the facts you will later need for collecting payments.

Collecting Fees for Services Rendered

All fees for medical services rendered by your facility must be in clear view and explained to patients. A typed itemized list of the most common and frequently employed services that the physician or department offers is often used, since it is readily available to the patient. Most states require such a list to be posted in the institution and made available to all patients.

In cases where a patient does not understand the fee schedule or is incapable of making rational decisions regarding his or her care or treatment, you must discuss the disclosure of fees with both the patient and the person responsible for paying the bill. Once it has been determined that the persons involved fully comprehend the process of billing and collection of fees, you must make a determination about collecting these fees.

Many smaller facilities require payment at the time services are provided. In this instance, the facility would be responsible for explaining the system of payment at the time the patient first calls to make an appointment. In some situations, however, this may not always be practical. If this is the case, the facility may choose to extend credit to the patient. This usually occurs when a patient faces large fees for service, such as in the case of surgery or multiple visits to the facility.

Many health care facilities have opted to use credit card billing as a method of obtaining payments for services rendered. In these cases, your employer will probably require you to carefully check the expiration date on the credit card, as well as the name of the person listed on the card. If you do accept credit cards, you should be prepared for the patient to become defensive if the card is rejected. They may become insistent that you accept the card because the "credit card company has made a mistake." Remember, you are not responsible for dealing with any problems or discrepancies between the credit card company and the patient. Your job is to be polite and not to pass judgment on the patient.

Superbill Billing

Many states throughout the country have adopted the *superbill* system, which combines a bill and an insurance claim in one statement. The statement is provided to the patient at the time he or she is seen at the facility. The superbill usually includes the patient's name, date, identification of services received, treatment codes, diagnostic information as it is classified in the *ICD-9-CM code* system, insurance requirements, *assignment of benefits,* and the physician's identification number.

A major advantage of the superbill system is that it eliminates a great deal of the paperwork needed for processing insurance claims, and encourages the patient to provide payment immediately after the services have been rendered. The patient can then submit the superbill directly to his or her insurance company, where benefits can either be assigned to the patient, or directly to the health care facility, if credit has been previously granted.

Statements, Cycle Billing, and Ledger Card Billing

Some health care facilities may choose to send their patients a monthly itemized statement as a bill for services. Sending out these statements is not always the best method of collecting payments for services rendered, since it can often increase the facility's cost for collection, as well as significantly delay the amount of time in which the payments are received.

Institutions which do use statements often use cycle billing. Cycle billing is sending out the statements according to an alphabetical breakdown. When the facility uses this system, billing goes on throughout the month and therefore can allow for continuous cash flow during the entire month.

A frequently used method of billing employed by many physician's offices and private clinics is a ledger card. Ledger cards, which generally include all charges, credits, and any adjustments that might be necessary for each patient, are copied and then mailed directly to the patient. Bills which remain unpaid are flagged by using a color strip at the top of the ledger card. When the bill is paid, the color strip can be removed.

A much more sophisticated method of billing which many larger facilities, such as hospitals and outpatient clinics, often use is a billing software application and a computer system. In this method, the computer is searched throughout the billing cycle, and printouts of patients with outstanding balances are identified. Once the system has identified patients who still owe payments to the facility, the software can provide you with a standard reminder letter to be sent to the patient regarding his or her delinquent bill.

Collecting Fees on Overdue Accounts

Unfortunately, patients are not always as prompt as they should be when it comes to paying for their medical costs. Because of this, health care facilities employ a policy regarding the collection of late payments.

There are several ways in which a facility can identify which accounts may be overdue and unpaid. One system is to use a method of aging accounts. When a patient's account is aged, it helps to identify both the accounts and the length of time the account has been delinquent. A color coding system can easily be used to identify the length of time the account has been left unpaid.

If your agency uses a computerized billing system, accounts can be aged automatically. The first notation might be a record of a superbill given at the time of the patient's visit. A statement would be sent after one month, and after two months a statement with an overdue notice might be sent. Letters would be sent after three and four months, reminding the patient of the overdue account.

If a patient's account becomes so delinquent that gentle reminders are not working, your facility may choose to send out a collection letter in an attempt to collect the overdue bill. However, before you can send out any letters, you should be aware of the Fair Debt Collections Practice Act, a federal act passed in 1978, established for the protection of people from undue harassment, and which outlaws any abusive, deceptive, and unfair collection practices by any business, including health care facilities. As long as your agency understands this legislation, after ninety days of delinquency for an account your facility may begin to write collection letters. The goal of these letters should be to encourage the patient to pay the balance due, which keeps the health care facility from having to pay a collection agency to secure the payment.

While the length of time may vary as to how long a facility is willing to wait to be paid, most facilities generally wait no longer than five or six months before they turn the patient's account over to a professional collection agency. During the seventh month, the agency will attempt to collect the payment. If the amount is worth going after, usually by the eighth month a lawsuit can be generated by the collection agency on behalf of the facility.

In some cases, you may encounter patients who have a balance due, but can no longer be reached at the address they provided on their patient record sheet. If this occurs, and no forwarding address has been left, this is called a *skip.*

When a collection letter has been sent by the facility to the patient regarding his or her overdue bill, a skip problem becomes quite evident when the letter is returned with the notation "Address Unknown." As soon as you realize that a skip has taken place, you should begin the task of locating the patient. This can be done in a number of ways. You may be able to call the patient's employer, however, if you do this, you must be very careful not to disclose the reason for your search. You may also call the person listed on the patient's registration form as his or her nearest relative. You may even attempt to locate the patient's neighbor or landlord to see if they have a forwarding address for the patient. Other ways in which you can attempt to locate a person who has skipped without paying his or her bill include checking the telephone book for last names similar to the patient's, asking the Department of Motor Vehicles if they have a change of address, calling the patient's bank if you have that information, and asking for a transfer address if one has been provided, and checking with utility companies, such as the telephone or gas and electric company to see if they have a forwarding address.

Banking Procedures in the Health Care Environment

If you are involved in billing and collection procedures for your health care facility, there's a very good possibility that you will also be in charge of banking procedures. You should understand that banking institutions are involved in many different aspects of financial transactions. They receive deposits for checking and savings accounts, loan money to businesses and individuals, and service loans for savings and loan associations. Your institution may use the bank for many of the services it provides.

The most common type of banking services health care facilities use is maintaining a *checking account,* which is a bank account against which checks can be written. A majority of the payments received by the health care facility are provided by checks.

There are many different varieties of checking accounts, including some that pay interest like a savings account. It may be your responsibility to determine which kind of checking account offered in your community will best suit your facility.

When money is not needed to pay for the facility's expenses, it is often deposited into a savings account. Savings accounts earn interest on the amount deposited. Like checking accounts, there are several kinds of savings accounts, such as a simple passbook account which draws interest at the lowest rate offered by the financial institution, and which generally does not require a minimum balance to maintain, and has no check-writing options. Another type of savings account is called a money market account, which usually requires a minimum balance, generally over $1,000, and which provides the depositor the option of writing a prearranged amount of checks per month.

As you carry out your banking responsibilities, you may encounter various types of *checks.* The most common of these include a cashier's check, which is a bank check drawn against itself and signed by a bank official; certified check, which is a customer's own check, with "certified" or "accepted" written across the face of the check; a money order, which can be sold by banks and other businesses; a bank draft, which is a written order used to pay funds drawn by a bank or its account at another bank; a traveler's check, which has been designed for travelers to use in situations in which a personal check would not be accepted; a limited check, which may be limited as to the amount as well as the time during which it can be cashed; a voucher check, which usually has a detachable form used to notate the purpose for which the check was written; and a warrant, which is a check that cannot be cashed but is evidence of a debt due. Warrants are most often used by governmental agencies and insurance companies, who use them to authorize the agency or company to pay for a specific claim.

Accepting Checks and Credit Cards for Payment of Services Rendered

If your facility takes checks from patients to pay for their fees for services rendered, there are certain things you must remember. First of all, you should never accept a check which has been erased or appears to have any visible errors. Never accept a check which has been written out to "cash," as opposed to the name of the facility. If you receive a check that has been sent back to your facility marked "account closed" or "account overdrawn," you must contact the person who wrote the check immediately, to make sure your facility is not only paid for the services provided, but also is reimbursed for any additional *service charges* incurred for the check being returned.

You must also make sure that any check you receive is properly endorsed. An *endorsement* is written on the back of a check or money order, and is an indication that all rights in the check are transferred to another party. Endorsements must always be made in ink, pen, or rubber stamp, and should be made on the left or perforated end of the check.

If your facility also accepts credit cards for payment of services rendered, you must carefully check to be sure that the name on the credit card matches the bearer's name. You should also check the expiration date of the card, and if your employer uses an automatic credit card machine, you may be required to enter the number of the credit card and amount to make sure that the card is not over the patient's credit limit. In addition, you must make sure that the information provided on the card is clear on the credit card charge slip and that you give the patient the proper receipt. There are often three parts to a charge slip, with the individual copies clearly marked as to where they should go.

Making Bank Deposits

An important part of banking procedures has to do with making accurate bank deposits of the daily checks and cash brought into your facility. All deposits should be made as soon as possible to avoid losing checks or having them stolen. Delays may cause a check to be returned for insufficient funds, or the check may eventually have a stop-payment on it. It is also a courtesy to the patient to cash checks promptly, and insurance checks often have a restricted period for their cashing.

Whenever a deposit is made, it must be accompanied by a *deposit slip*. The slip contains the name and address of your employer and the date of the deposit, as well as the checking account number. It's always a good idea to make a copy of the deposit slip for your facility.

The total amount of the deposit is immediately entered into the checkbook, and the checks are clipped together or put in bank wrappers, and all coins, currency, and checks should be put in a large bank envelope or bag.

Bank deposits can be made in several ways. Depending upon your employer, he or she may choose to make their deposits by mail, in an after-hours bank depositor, or at an automatic teller machine (*ATM*).

Processing Bank Statements

A *bank statement* is a list which provides an itemized accounting by date and amount of all deposits and withdrawals made from a specific account. Most financial institutions provide these statements at regular intervals, usually on a monthly basis. When the statement is received by your facility, it should be immediately reconciled against the checkbook stubs or check register. You may receive canceled checks, or you may have an account where checks are available upon demand.

Reconciling the bank statement should be done as soon as possible after its arrival. In some cases, the balances in the checkbook and the bank statement may be different. This is often due to some checks not yet appearing on the bank statement. The reconciliation is therefore necessary.

If after you have completed the reconciliation, the balances agree, you are finished. If they do not, you must determine the amount of the disagreement. Some of the most common mistakes leading to a disagreement on the reconciliation include forgetting to include an outstanding check, incorrect or inaccurate math, failing to record deposits or recording a deposit more than once, carrying out figures incorrectly, failing to write down a check, and transposing a figure.

Summary

In this chapter, we discussed the role of the physical medicine health care provider who finds him- or herself responsible for carrying out billing and banking procedures in the health care environment. We talked about how to perform basic bookkeeping procedures, as well as how to properly bill patients for services rendered. We also explained how to perform specific banking procedures utilized by most health care facilities, including processing payments made by check, making bank deposits, and reconciliation of bank statements.

Review Questions

1. Define the following abbreviations:
   a. A/C ____________
   b. A/R ____________
2. Briefly explain the process of *cycle billing*.
3. Briefly explain the principles of bookkeeping in the health care environment.
4. Explain the differences between the following bookkeeping systems:
   a. Single-entry
   b. Double-entry
   c. Pegboard
5. Define the following tax deductions:
   a. FICA
   b. SDI
   c. OASI
6. Briefly explain what a Superbill billing system is.
7. Why must a bank statement be reconciled as soon as possible after its arrival?

31

Insurance Coding and Indexing

Performance Objectives

Upon completion of this chapter, you will be able to:

1. Identify and briefly discuss various types of insurance programs available for health care.
2. Discuss reference manuals available for coding medical insurance claims.
3. Describe the importance of accuracy as it relates to coding an insurance claim form.
4. Explain and be able to demonstrate how to produce a rough draft copy of an insurance claim form.

Terms and Abbreviations

Alphanumeric code a code that uses both letters and numbers and sometimes other symbols, such as punctuation marks.
CHAMPUS abbreviation for Civilian Health and Medical Program for the Uniformed Services, which is a military program responsible for providing medical care for dependents of the military and retired military personnel.
CHAMPVA abbreviation for Civilian Health and Medical Program for the Veterans Administration, which is a government insurance program that covers families of veterans with 100 percent service-connected disability, or the surviving spouse and children of a veteran who died as a result of a service-connected disability.
CPT abbreviation for *Current Procedural Terminology* codes, which is a coding system published by the American Medical Association and used to communicate procedures performed by a physician.
Deductible the amount of money a patient or responsible party must pay prior to the insurance company paying the balance.
FECA/Black Lung abbreviation for Federal Employee Compensation Act, which is a program that reimburses federal employees for medical expenses related to accidents or injuries which occurred on the job.
HCFA abbreviation for Health Care Financing Administration, which is an administrative agency within the United States Department of Health and Human Services, and which is responsible for handling all issues related to Medicare and Medicaid.
ICD codes abbreviation for International Classification of Diseases codes, which is an internationally recognized coding system for all known diseases, originally designed by the World Health Organization of the United Nations.
Medicaid a state government program designed to help indigent or poor people with medical benefits.
Medicare Part A the part of Medicare that pays a portion of an inpatient's hospital care, daily skilled care received in a skilled nursing facility, home health care, and hospice care.
Medicare Part B the part of Medicare that pays a portion of a patient's physician and outpatient services.
SNF abbreviation for skilled nursing facility.
Subscriber the person who is the insurance policyholder; may also be called the insured.
Workers' compensation medical payments which are made by employers when an employee has a work-related illness or injury.

According to most health insurance providers, approximately 80 percent of the money paid to a physician's office or to a health care facility comes in the form of insurance payments from private insurance companies or government insurance programs. Since the costs of health care continue to rise on an annual basis, it is mandatory that physicians, hospitals, and clinics be paid on time. Therefore, as a member of the health care delivery team, if you find yourself responsible for processing health insurance claims for your facility, the first thing you must realize is that you have a very important task in gathering data which is necessary to accurately file claims for monies owed, as well as grouping illnesses which allow for indexing.

Careers in Insurance Coding

While this text deals more specifically with careers in physical medicine, it's important for you to realize also that with the advent of changes in health care systems, an accurate insurance coding clerk, or someone who possesses the skills and knowledge required to process health insurance claims, will be in great demand. People specializing and working with health insurance should be able to work with a high degree of accuracy and attention to details. A knowledge of medical terminology is a definite asset, and computer keyboarding skills are a major advantage. If you are really ambitious, you may choose to enroll in any one of a number of vocational schools or colleges throughout the country, and become a certified coding specialist.

Health Insurance Programs

There are two major programs which exist exclusively to pay for health care. These two systems include one which is financed by the individual and one which is financed by state and federal government funds. Approximately 2,000 different private health care programs are available, including all types of commercial plans, preferred provider organizations (PPOs), and health maintenance organizations (HMOs).

Comprehensive health care is provided by the federal government for large groups of qualified people. The groups which fall under these categories include members of the uniformed services, retired military personnel, and their dependents through *CHAMPUS* and *CHAMPVA;* coverage for the elderly through Medicare, which is administered by the Social Security Administration; coverage for the disabled and indigent through *Medicaid,* which is also administered by the Social Security System; and coverage for those with job-related injuries or illnesses, which is administered through *FECA/Black Lung* or individual *workers' compensation* insurance companies. All funds for payment through health insurance coverage are financed through general taxation or, in the case of the Social Security system, from a trust fund of contributions paid by employees, employers, and self-employed workers.

When a service or a procedure is performed by a health care provider, that person expects to be paid. In order to obtain insurance compensation, either the patient or the provider must submit a completed form which details the specific services provided. Codes are used to standardize and simplify these forms. The code numbers, which are used to identify individual physicians, diseases being treated, and procedures, services, and supplies provided to a patient are obtained from publications called manuals, which are listings referred to as coding systems.

Since payment is made according to the code that has been assigned for a diagnosis and procedure, it is imperative that if you are working as an insurance coding clerk, you be accurate in choosing the correct code. An incorrect code can result in a form being returned to the doctor's office or the health care facility, or, in some cases, a reduced amount being paid.

Understanding and Using Coding Systems

When a doctor examines a patient at his or her office or the hospital, a procedure has been performed for which the physician is expected to be paid, either by the patient or by a private insurance company or a government health care agency. In a regular sequence of events, the physician or health facility will first identify the procedures performed for the patient. For uniformity in reporting procedures and treatments, the American Medical Association has developed and published a coding system called *Current Procedural Terminology* codes, or *CPT* codes. These procedures and their codes are generally marked on a superbill, charge slip, or the medical record (Figure 31-1).

The CPT manual is used to determine the correct five-digit code. It is divided into several sections, including introduction, medicine, anesthesia, surgery (by individual body systems), radiology, nuclear

Previous Balance ______ Name ______

Date of Service ______

Diagnosis (I.C.D.A. Code) ______ ______ ______

Attending Physician's Statement

AMA Current Procedural Terminology, 3rd Edition

Patient: ______

1. OFFICE VISIT	New	Established	Fee
Brief	90000	90040	___
Limited	90010	90050	___
Intermediate	90015	90060	___
2. INJECTIONS			
Special Immunization		( )	___
		( )	___
Injection (Medicine)		90750	___
Injection (Antibiotic)		90780	___
Immun. Therapy - 1 Inj.		90785	___
3. HOSPITAL SERVICE		Name	
· Visit	Initial	Subsequent	Fee
Brief	90200	90240	___
Limited		90250	___
Intermediate	90215	90260	___
___	thru ___		
4. EMERGENCY ROOM SERVICE			
Limited	90510	90550	___
Intermediate	90515	90560	___
Extended		90570	___

5. Surgery & Lab Procedures			Other Services
Routine Newborn	90285	___	______
Vaginal Delivery	59410	___	______
Cesarean Section	59520	___	______
ECG Interpretation	93000	___	
Cardiac catherization	93525	___	
Chest X-ray	71020	___	
Flat film abdomen	74000	___	
Intravenous pylogram	74400	___	
Upper Gastro. Intest.	74240	___	
Small Intestine Series	74250	___	
Barium enema	74270	___	
Air contrast enema	74280	___	
Gall bladder series	74290	___	
Urinalysis	81000	___	
CBC	85010	___	
Sedimentation rate	85650	___	
T & A (under 12)	42820	___	
T & A (over 12)	42821	___	

RETURN ___ Days ___ Weeks ___ Month Next Appt. ______ AM / PM
Day Month Date Time

Figure 31-1
Example of patient charge slip.

medicine, diagnostic ultrasound, pathology and laboratory, and the appendix. When your responsibilities include insurance coding, it is extremely important that you code the procedure accurately because insurance companies and government agencies will only pay according to the correct coding.

Identifying CPT Codes

If you are working with insurance codes, there are three steps you must follow to obtain a correct procedure.

1. Refer to the alphabetical index at the end of the CPT manual to locate the procedure.
2. Note the five-digit code which has been provided for the procedure.
3. Locate the correct numerical code in the manual for the exact description of the procedure.

In order for you to gain an understanding of how procedures are assigned a specific code number, let's look at the two examples provided below. In Figure 31-2a, the codes represented are those which would be found under medicine, while the codes shown in Figure 31-2b are codes found under surgery, procedures for the integumentary system.

Coding Under the International Classification of Diseases

Several years ago, the World Health Organization (WHO) of the United Nations devised a list of all known diseases. Once this list was developed, WHO assigned code numbers to the various diseases. Ultimately, the *International Classification of Diseases,* or *ICD* codes were developed and are now used internationally.

90000 office and other outpatient medical service, NEW PATIENT; *brief service*
90010 *limited* service
90015 *intermediate* service
90017 *extended* service
90020 *comprehensive* service
(a)

10000 incision and drainage of infection or noninfected sebaceous cyst; *one* lesion
10001 *second* lesion
10002 *more than two* lesions
10003 incision and drainage of infected or noninfected epithelial inclusion cyst (sebaceous cyst) with complete removal of sac and treatment of cavity
(b)

Figure 31-2
(a) Codes found under medicine; (b) codes found under surgery, procedures for the integumentary system.

ICD codes are identified in three bound volumes known as ICD books. Volume I is a tabular list of diseases with a three-digit number and, at times, a two-digit extension, such as 003.22 Salmonella pneumonia. Volume II of the ICD code book is an alphabetic index of diseases. An insurance clerk would look first in Volume II at the alphabetic name, and then use the number given to refer to Volume I. It's important to remember that you should never code from Volume II alone. It should be used only as a reference. Coding from Volume I will provide you with much more extensive information.

Volume III of the ICD code books is both a tabular and an alphabetic index of procedures used for the purpose of billing hospital patients, and it coordinates with the HCPCS coding used for all government claims.

Coding Under the Health Care Procedural Coding System (HCPCS)

In 1983, HCPCS, which is pronounced "hicpics," was created by Medicare to standardize procedural coding for all Medicare and Medicaid claims. It is an *alphanumeric code* system developed by the federal *Health Care Financing Administration (HCFA),* to be used as a supplement to the CPT codes for filing insurance claims for Medicare, CHAMPUS, and Medicaid. These codes relay information about nonphysician procedures, services, and specific supplies.

There are three levels of coding found in the HCPCS system. Level I uses the CPT codes from the *Current Procedural Terminology* manual to code the services and procedures provided by physicians. The five-digit code represents Level I, such as 90040, brief office visit. Level II codes are published and updated on an annual basis by the Health Care Financing Administration and are used to code nonphysician procedures, services, and supplies. Level II codes are represented by one alphabetic character followed by four numbers, such as A0040, ambulance service, air, helicopter service. Level III codes may be assigned by the Medicare office responsible for a specific geographic region. Local codes will have an alphabetic letter *S* through *Z* and four digits, and are provided by the regional Medicare office as they are updated. Local codes have the highest priority and should always be used first.

Processing Coding Changes and Charges

As a member of the administrative medical services staff, you have a responsibility to stay current with the different coding procedures, government rules and regulations, and newly assigned coding numbers. Updates are printed every year for each of the coding manuals, and if you are assigned to process insurance claims, you must make sure that you are using the very latest edition of your coding manuals. If an update, addendum, or appendix is printed, it should be placed immediately in the appropriate manual so that you are using the current codes.

Each year, Medicare changes the amounts for deductible charges and pricing for procedures that can be charged by the physician who is a Medicare provider. Medicaid also changes its rules and regulations very often. Medical office workers who are responsible for handling Medicare and Medicaid are also responsible for noting any changes and charging the patients for their deductible part accordingly. In addition, you must also bill the government for the Medicare/Medicaid approved amount.

Processing Insurance Claim Forms

In order for the physician's office or the health care facility to receive payment from an insurance company or government insurance system, an insurance claim form must be properly filled out. The form most widely used by private insurance companies and government insurance agencies is FORM HCFA-1500 (Figure 31-3 on p. 370). It is commonly referred to as the "universal insurance claim form" because it can easily be adopted for almost every private and government insurance agency. If you are responsible for filling out this form, you must remember that there are two types of information that are required. The first includes all routine information regarding the patient, his or her *subscriber,* and the insurance company. The second type of information involves all of the medical information and health-related issues which are provided by the patient's physician.

The most accurate way to obtain information regarding health insurance is to ask the patient or the person insured for his or her insurance identification card and then make a copy of both the front and the back of the card. This card contains essential information that is required for processing the claim, and usually includes the person's Social Security number and group number. In addition, the insurance company's name, address, telephone, and service representative are usually printed on the back of the identification card.

If you are responsible for processing Medicare claims, you should also make a copy of the patient's or subscriber's identification card, so that verification can be made concerning coverage under Parts A and B. Part B is currently optional for all patient's receiving Medicare benefits.

Filling Out the Insurance Claim Form

If you plan on receiving payment for your physician or the health care facility, especially in a timely manner, it's extremely important that the claim form be accurately filled out, since any errors can result in either not receiving the payment, or in waiting an undue amount of time to be paid. Therefore, when processing the HCFA-1500 insurance claim form, there is a specific way you must respond to each and every section of the form.

At the top of the form in Block 1, you must first check the applicable program block. If the patient has private or employer's group insurance, check "Other" and write the name of the insurance company in the top right-hand corner. Then complete the form using the following information.

- Block 2: Type the patient's name; last name first.
- Block 3: Type the patient's date of birth, such as 02/17/55, and indicate sex.
- Block 4: Type the name of the insured, that is, the name of the person who purchased the insurance policy.
- Block 5: Type the patient's address, city, state, zip code, and telephone number.
- Block 6: Check the appropriate box for the relationship of patient to insured.
- Block 7: Type the insured's address and telephone number.
- Block 8: Check the appropriate boxes for the patient's marital and employment status.
- Block 9: If the patient or the insured has another insurance policy in force that may also pay, type in the information here.
- Block 10: Check whether the condition was related to the patient's employment or an accident. This box is very important because a determination will be made regarding the type of insurance that will be filed.
- Block 11: Type the insured's group number, indicate date of birth, and name of employer's health benefit plan.
- Block 12: Have the patient sign the insurance form in order to release medical information from your facility to the insurance company; if your office or institution has a "Release of Information" form with the patient's signature already on file, type "Signature on File" in the blank.
- Block 13: Have the insured person sign for authorization to pay medical benefits to the physician or provider for service; if the patient has already signed the "Release of Information," you may once again type "Signature on File" in the blank.
- Block 14: Type in the date of illness, accident, or pregnancy.
- Block 15: Type in the date your office or institution was first consulted for this condition.
- Block 16: Type in dates that patient was unable to work.
- Block 17: Fill in name of referring physician.
- Block 17a: Fill in I.D. number of referring physician.
- Block 18: Fill in hospitalization dates.
- Block 19: N/A
- Block 20: Indicate if an outside lab was used, and their charges.
- Block 21: Fill in diagnosis or nature of illness or injury.
- Block 22: Indicate Medicaid resubmission code.
- Block 23: Fill in prior authorization number.
- Block 24a: Type in digit form; use six digits, such as 01 08 97 for January 8, 1997.

PLEASE
DO NOT
STAPLE
IN THIS
AREA

CARRIER

PICA

HEALTH INSURANCE CLAIM FORM

PICA

1. MEDICARE (Medicare #) MEDICAID (Medicaid #) CHAMPUS (Sponsor's SSN) CHAMPVA (VA File #) GROUP HEALTH PLAN (SSN or ID) FECA BLK LUNG (SSN) OTHER (ID)

1a. INSURED'S I.D. NUMBER (FOR PROGRAM IN ITEM 1)

2. PATIENT'S NAME (Last Name, First Name, Middle Initial)

3. PATIENT'S BIRTH DATE MM | DD | YY SEX M F

4. INSURED'S NAME (Last Name, First Name, Middle Initial)

5. PATIENT'S ADDRESS (No., Street)

6. PATIENT RELATIONSHIP TO INSURED Self Spouse Child Other

7. INSURED'S ADDRESS (No., Street)

CITY STATE

8. PATIENT STATUS Single Married Other

CITY STATE

ZIP CODE TELEPHONE (Include Area Code) ( )

Employed Full-Time Student Part-Time Student

ZIP CODE TELEPHONE (INCLUDE AREA CODE) ( )

9. OTHER INSURED'S NAME (Last Name, First Name, Middle Initial)

10. IS PATIENT'S CONDITION RELATED TO:

11. INSURED'S POLICY GROUP OR FECA NUMBER

a. OTHER INSURED'S POLICY OR GROUP NUMBER

a. EMPLOYMENT? (CURRENT OR PREVIOUS) YES NO

a. INSURED'S DATE OF BIRTH MM | DD | YY SEX M F

b. OTHER INSURED'S DATE OF BIRTH MM | DD | YY SEX M F

b. AUTO ACCIDENT? PLACE (State) YES NO

b. EMPLOYER'S NAME OR SCHOOL NAME

c. EMPLOYER'S NAME OR SCHOOL NAME

c. OTHER ACCIDENT? YES NO

c. INSURANCE PLAN NAME OR PROGRAM NAME

d. INSURANCE PLAN NAME OR PROGRAM NAME

10d. RESERVED FOR LOCAL USE

d. IS THERE ANOTHER HEALTH BENEFIT PLAN? YES NO *If yes*, return to and complete item 9 a-d.

READ BACK OF FORM BEFORE COMPLETING & SIGNING THIS FORM.

12. PATIENT'S OR AUTHORIZED PERSON'S SIGNATURE I authorize the release of any medical or other information necessary to process this claim. I also request payment of government benefits either to myself or to the party who accepts assignment below.

SIGNED ______ DATE ______

13. INSURED'S OR AUTHORIZED PERSON'S SIGNATURE I authorize payment of medical benefits to the undersigned physician or supplier for services described below.

SIGNED ______

PATIENT AND INSURED INFORMATION

14. DATE OF CURRENT: MM | DD | YY ILLNESS (First symptom) OR INJURY (Accident) OR PREGNANCY(LMP)

15. IF PATIENT HAS HAD SAME OR SIMILAR ILLNESS. GIVE FIRST DATE MM | DD | YY

16. DATES PATIENT UNABLE TO WORK IN CURRENT OCCUPATION FROM MM | DD | YY TO MM | DD | YY

17. NAME OF REFERRING PHYSICIAN OR OTHER SOURCE

17a. I.D. NUMBER OF REFERRING PHYSICIAN

18. HOSPITALIZATION DATES RELATED TO CURRENT SERVICES FROM MM | DD | YY TO MM | DD | YY

19. RESERVED FOR LOCAL USE

20. OUTSIDE LAB? YES NO $ CHARGES

21. DIAGNOSIS OR NATURE OF ILLNESS OR INJURY. (RELATE ITEMS 1,2,3 OR 4 TO ITEM 24E BY LINE)

1. ___ . ___

2. ___ . ___

3. ___ . ___

4. ___ . ___

22. MEDICAID RESUBMISSION CODE ORIGINAL REF. NO.

23. PRIOR AUTHORIZATION NUMBER

24. A DATE(S) OF SERVICE From MM DD YY To MM DD YY	B Place of Service	C Type of Service	D PROCEDURES, SERVICES, OR SUPPLIES (Explain Unusual Circumstances) CPT/HCPCS | MODIFIER	E DIAGNOSIS CODE	F $ CHARGES	G DAYS OR UNITS	H EPSDT Family Plan	I EMG	J COB	K RESERVED FOR LOCAL USE
1										
2										
3										
4										
5										
6										

25. FEDERAL TAX I.D. NUMBER SSN EIN

26. PATIENT'S ACCOUNT NO.

27. ACCEPT ASSIGNMENT? (For govt. claims, see back) YES NO

28. TOTAL CHARGE $

29. AMOUNT PAID $

30. BALANCE DUE $

31. SIGNATURE OF PHYSICIAN OR SUPPLIER INCLUDING DEGREES OR CREDENTIALS (I certify that the statements on the reverse apply to this bill and are made a part thereof.)

SIGNED DATE

32. NAME AND ADDRESS OF FACILITY WHERE SERVICES WERE RENDERED (If other than home or office)

33. PHYSICIAN'S, SUPPLIER'S BILLING NAME, ADDRESS, ZIP CODE & PHONE #

PIN# GRP#

PHYSICIAN OR SUPPLIER INFORMATION

FOLD HERE / USE ENVELOPE NO. 1500E

(APPROVED BY AMA COUNCIL ON MEDICAL SERVICE 8/88) ***PLEASE PRINT OR TYPE*** APPROVED OMB-0938-0008 FORM HCFA-1500 (12-90), FORM RRB-1500, APPROVED OMB-1215-0055 FORM OWCP-1500, APPROVED OMB-0720-0001 (CHAMPUS)

Figure 31-3
HCFA-1500 Insurance Claim Form. (Reprinted with permission from Weiss, R.C. *Your Career in Administrative Medical Services.* Philadelphia: W. B. Saunders, 1996, p. 212.)

- Block 24b: Type in the location where the services were performed. Use the place of service codes as found on the back of the insurance claim form HCFA-1500.
- Block 24c: Leave blank.
- Block 24d: Type in the 5-digit procedure code found in the CPT or HCPC manuals. In the modifier code box, type in the 2-digit modifier from the CPT manual.
- Block 24e: Type in the diagnosis code. The code is in conjunction with diagnosis 1, 2, 3, or 4 in field 21.
- Block 24f: Type in the amount of the charges.
- Block 24g: Type in the number of times identical procedures were performed during the time the patient was treated (according to field 24a). Usually the number is 1; however, if a patient is treated more than once on a specific day, the number would be changed.
- Block 24h: Leave this blank.
- Block 24i: If service was performed in a hospital emergency room, this code should match the service code listed in item 24b.
- Block 24j: This is the coordination of benefits. Using a Y for yes or an N for no, indicate whether or not any other insurance plans or policies may be responsible for payment on this claim.
- Block 24k: Leave this blank.
- Block 25: Type in physician's Federal Tax I.D. number.
- Block 26: Type in patient's account number.
- Block 27: Type in yes or no as to whether the provider accepts assignment of payment for services.
- Block 28: Type in total charge.
- Block 29: Type in amount paid.
- Block 30: Indicate balance due.
- Block 31: Obtain physician's signature.
- Block 32: Type in name and address where services were rendered.
- Block 33: Type in name, address, and telephone number of physician or supplier providing services.

Upon completion of the insurance claim form, make sure you double-check it for accuracy and completeness. Check for any omissions of information and for any math errors. Once you have made copies for your billing records, send the completed form to the appropriate insurance company.

Summary

In this chapter, we discussed the process and skills involved in coding procedures and treatments performed by the physician or health care provider. We talked about how to use the *Current Procedural Terminology* manual for coding descriptions of procedures, the *International Classification of Diseases* for coding a diagnosis or disease, and the *Health Care Procedural Coding System* (HCPCS) when coding nonphysician procedures, services, and supplies for Medicare and Medicaid. Finally, we discussed the purpose of health insurance claim forms, including how to properly code and fill out the HCFA-1500, which is a universal health insurance claim form used by most private and government insurance agencies.

Review Questions

1. Briefly explain the following types of insurance programs:
   a. CHAMPUS ____________
   b. CHAMPVA ____________
   c. Workers' Compensation ____________
   d. Medicare ____________
   e. Medicaid ____________
2. Define the following abbreviations:
   a. HMO ____________
   b. ICD codes ____________
   c. CPT ____________
   d. HCFA ____________
   e. FECA/Black Lung ____________
3. What does the term *subscriber* mean?
4. Briefly explain what an *alphanumeric code* is.

Index

Page numbers followed by t indicate a table. Italic page numbers indicate figures.